THE NETTER COLLECTION OF MEDICAL ILLUSTRATIONS

3rd Edition

Musculoskeletal System

Part II—Spine and Lower Limb

VOLUME 6

A compilation of paintings prepared by **FRANK H. NETTER, MD**

Edited by

Joseph P. Iannotti, MD, PhD
Lang Family Distinguished Chair in Orthopedics
Chief of Staff
Chief Academic and Innovations Officer
Cleveland Clinic Weston Hospital
Weston, Florida

Richard D. Parker, MD
Professor of Surgery at the Cleveland Clinic Lerner College of Medicine
President, Hillcrest Hospital and East Region
Past Chairman, Department of Orthopaedic Surgery
Cleveland Clinic
Cleveland, Ohio

Thomas E. Mroz, MD
Chairman, Orthopaedic and Rheumatologic Institute
Director, Spine Research
Cleveland Clinic
Cleveland, Ohio

Brendan M. Patterson, MD, MBA
Chair, Department of Orthopaedic Surgery
Cleveland Clinic Health Care System
Professor, Orthopaedic Surgery
Case Western Reserve University School of Medicine
Cleveland, Ohio

Additional Illustrations by

Carlos A.G. Machado, MD

CONTRIBUTING ILLUSTRATORS

John A. Craig, MD
Tiffany S. DaVanzo, MA, CMI
DragonFly Media
Paul Kim, MS
Kristen W. Marzejon, CMI
James A. Perkins, MS, MFA

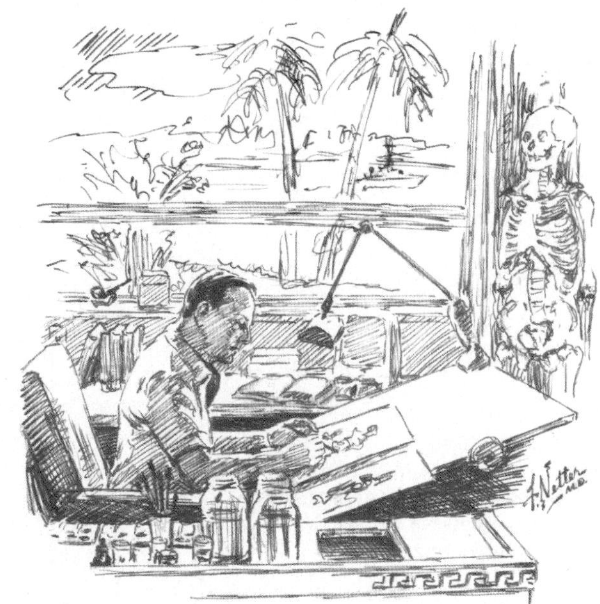

Self portrait by Dr. Netter

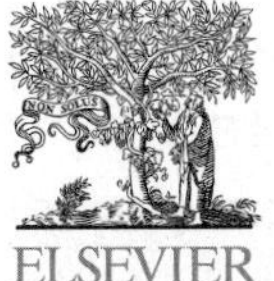

ELSEVIER

ELSEVIER
1600 John F. Kennedy Blvd.
Suite 1600
Philadelphia, Pennsylvania

THE NETTER COLLECTION OF MEDICAL ILLUSTRATIONS:
MUSCULOSKELETAL SYSTEM, PART II: SPINE AND LOWER LIMB,
VOLUME 6, THIRD EDITION ISBN: 978-0-323-88128-9

Notices

Knowledge and best practice in this field are constantly changing. As new research and experience broaden our understanding, changes in research methods, professional practices, or medical treatment may become necessary.

Practitioners and researchers must always rely on their own experience and knowledge in evaluating and using any information, methods, compounds, or experiments described herein. In using such information or methods they should be mindful of their own safety and the safety of others, including parties for whom they have a professional responsibility.

With respect to any drug or pharmaceutical products identified, readers are advised to check the most current information provided (i) on procedures featured or (ii) by the manufacturer of each product to be administered, to verify the recommended dose or formula, the method and duration of administration, and contraindications. It is the responsibility of practitioners, relying on their own experience and knowledge of their patients, to make diagnoses, to determine dosages and the best treatment for each individual patient, and to take all appropriate safety precautions.

To the fullest extent of the law, neither the Publisher nor the authors, contributors, or editors, assume any liability for any injury and/or damage to persons or property as a matter of products liability, negligence or otherwise, or from any use or operation of any methods, products, instructions, or ideas contained in the material herein.

Publisher: Elyse O'Grady
Senior Content Strategist: Marybeth Thiel
Publishing Services Manager: Catherine Jackson
Project Manager: Rosanne Toroian
Book Design: Patrick Ferguson

Printed in India

Last digit is the print number: 9 8 7 6 5 4 3 2 1

"Clarification is the goal. No matter how beautifully it is painted, a medical illustration has little value if it does not make clear a medical point."

—Frank H. Netter, MD

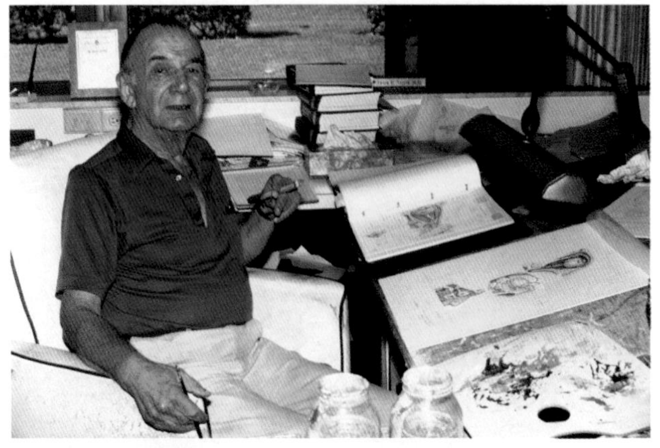

Dr. Frank Netter at work.

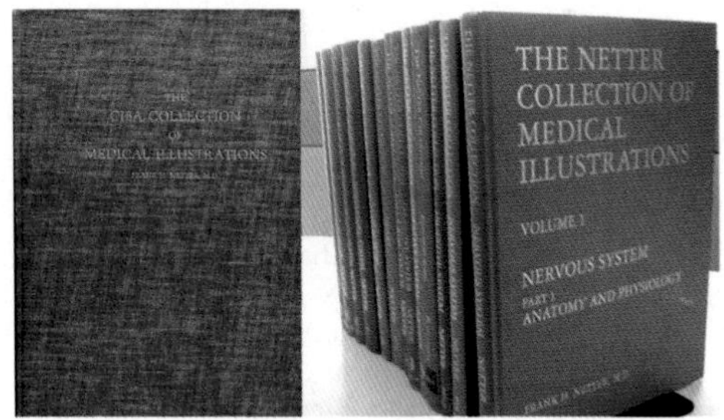

The single-volume "Blue Book" that preceded the multivolume *Netter Collection of Medical Illustrations* series, affectionately known as the "Green Books."

The
Netter Collection
OF MEDICAL ILLUSTRATIONS
3rd Edition

Volume 1 **Reproductive System**
Volume 2 **Endocrine System**
Volume 3 **Respiratory System**
Volume 4 **Integumentary System**
Volume 5 **Urinary System**
Volume 6 **Musculoskeletal System**
Volume 7 **Nervous System**
Volume 8 **Cardiovascular System**
Volume 9 **Digestive System**

Dr. Frank Netter created an illustrated legacy unifying his perspectives as physician, artist, and teacher. Both his greatest challenge and greatest success was charting a middle course between artistic clarity and instructional complexity. That success is captured in *The Netter Collection,* beginning in 1948 when the first comprehensive book of Netter's work was published by CIBA Pharmaceuticals. It met with such success that over the following 40 years the collection was expanded into an 8-volume series—with each title devoted to a single body system. Between 2011 and 2016, these books were updated and rereleased. Now, after another decade of innovation in medical imaging, renewed focus on patient-centered care, conscious efforts to improve inequities in healthcare and medical education, and a growing understanding of many clinical conditions, including multisystem effects of COVID-19, we are happy to make available a third edition of Netter's timeless work enhanced and informed by modern medical knowledge and context.

Inside the classic green covers, students and practitioners will find hundreds of original works of art. This is a collection of the human body in pictures—Dr. Netter called them *pictures,* never paintings. The latest expert medical knowledge is anchored by the sublime style of Frank Netter that has guided physicians' hands and nurtured their imaginations for more than half a century.

Noted artist-physician Carlos Machado, MD, the primary successor responsible for continuing the Netter tradition, has particular appreciation for the Green Book series. *The Reproductive System* is of special significance for those who, like me, deeply admire Dr. Netter's work. In this volume, he masters the representation of textures of different surfaces, which I like to call 'the rhythm of the brush,' since it is the dimension, the direction of the strokes, and the interval separating them that create the illusion of given textures: organs have their external surfaces, the surfaces of their cavities, and texture of their parenchymas realistically represented. It set the style for the subsequent volumes of *The Netter Collection*—each an amazing combination of painting masterpieces and precise scientific information.

This third edition could not exist without the dedication of all those who edited, authored, or in other ways contributed to the second edition or the original books, nor, of course, without the excellence of Dr. Netter. For this third edition, we also owe our gratitude to the authors, editors, and artists whose relentless efforts were instrumental in adapting these classic works into reliable references for today's clinicians in training and in practice. From all of us with the Netter Publishing Team at Elsevier, thank you.

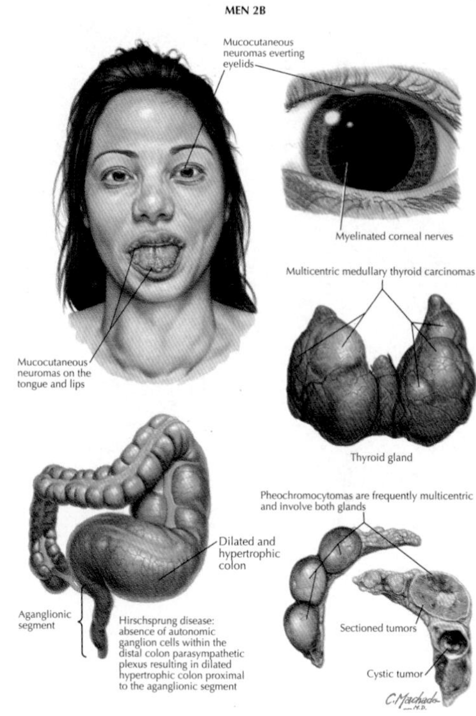

An illustrated plate painted by Carlos Machado, MD.

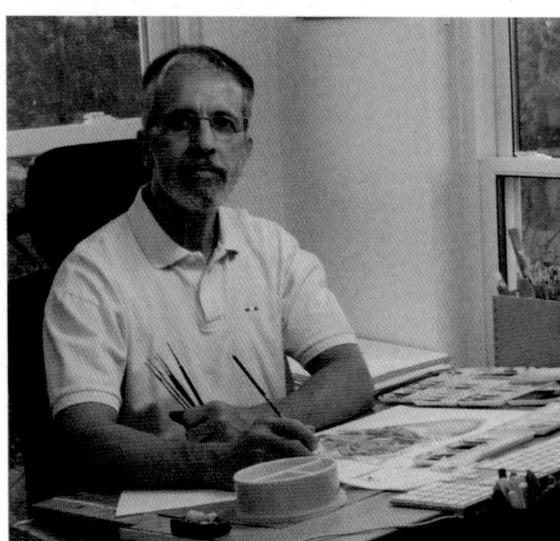

Dr. Carlos Machado at work.

ABOUT THE EDITORS

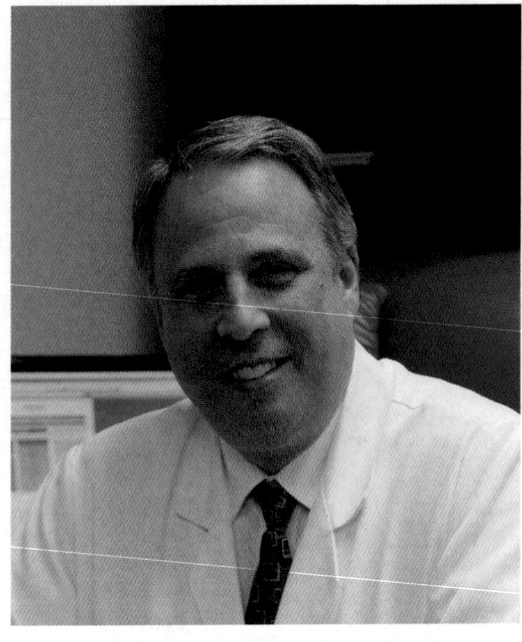

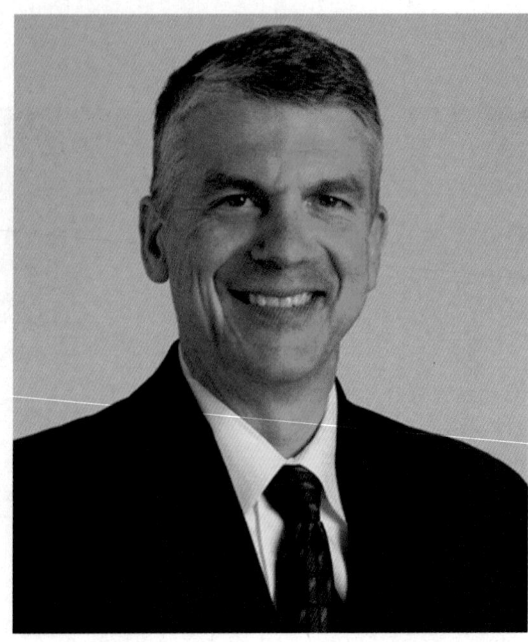

EDITORS-IN-CHIEF

Joseph P. Iannotti, MD, PhD, is Lang Family Distinguished Chair of Orthopaedics and Chief of Staff and Chief Academic and Innovation Officer for Cleveland Clinic Florida. He has a joint appointment in the Department of Bioengineering at the Lerner Research Institute.

Dr. Iannotti joined the Cleveland Clinic in 2000 as Chair of Orthopaedic Surgery (2000–2009) and Chair of the Orthopaedic and Rheumatology Institute (2008–2019). He came to the Cleveland Clinic from the University of Pennsylvania, leaving there as a tenured professor of orthopaedic surgery and Head of the Shoulder and Elbow Service. Dr. Iannotti received his medical degree from Northwestern University in 1979, completed his orthopedic residency training at the University of Pennsylvania in 1984, and earned his doctorate in cell biology from the University of Pennsylvania in 1987.

Dr. Iannotti's clinical and basic science research program focuses on innovative treatments for tendon repair and tendon tissue engineering, prosthetic design, software planning, and patient-specific instrumentation. Dr. Iannotti has had continuous extramural funding for his research since 1981. He has been the principal or co-principal investigator of dozens of research grants. He has been an invited lecturer and visiting professor at nearly 100 national and international academic institutions and societies, delivering more than 800 lectures both nationally and internationally.

Dr. Iannotti has published two textbooks on the shoulder, one in its second edition and the other in its third edition. He has authored over 350 original peer-reviewed articles, review articles, and book chapters. Dr. Iannotti has more than 100 US and international patents related to shoulder prosthetics, surgical instruments, and tissue-engineered implants. He is member of the National Academy of Innovators.

He has received awards for his academic work from the American Orthopaedic Association, including the North American and American-British-Canadian traveling fellowships and the Neer Research Award in 1996, 2001, and 2015 from the American Shoulder and Elbow Surgeons. He won the orthopedic resident teaching award in 2006 for his role in research education. He was awarded the Mason Sones Innovator of the Year award in 2012 and the Lifetime Achievement Award for Innovation in 2019 from the Cleveland Clinic.

He has served in many leadership roles at the national level, including as past Chair of the Academic Affairs Council and the Board of Directors of the American Academy of Orthopaedic Surgery. In addition, he has served and chaired several committees of the American Shoulder and Elbow Surgeons and was President of the International Society of Shoulder and Elbow Surgeons from 2005 to 2006 and Chairman of the Board of Trustees of the *Journal of Shoulder and Elbow Surgery.* He currently serves on several not-for-profit boards.

Richard D. Parker, MD, is President of Hillcrest Hospital and East Region President of Cleveland Clinic Ohio. He is Professor of Surgery at the Cleveland Clinic Lerner College of Medicine and Past Chairman of the Department of Orthopaedic Surgery at the Cleveland Clinic. Dr. Parker is an expert on the knee, ranging from nonoperative treatment to all aspects of surgical procedures, including articular cartilage, meniscus, ligament, and joint replacement. He has published more than 200 peer-reviewed manuscripts and numerous book chapters and has presented his work throughout the world. Dr. Parker received his undergraduate degree at Walsh College in Canton, Ohio, and his medical education at The Ohio State University College of Medicine, and he completed his orthopedic residency at The Mount Sinai Medical Center in Cleveland, Ohio. He received his fellowship training with subspecialization in sports medicine through a clinical research fellowship in sports medicine, arthroscopy, knee and shoulder surgery in Salt Lake City, Utah. He obtained his Certificate of Subspecialization in orthopedic sports medicine in 2008, which was the first year it was available.

Before joining the Cleveland Clinic in 1993, Dr. Parker acted as head of the section of sports medicine at The Mount Sinai Medical Center. His current research focuses on clinical outcomes focusing on articular cartilage, meniscal transplantation, posterior cruciate ligament, and the Multicenter Orthopaedic Outcomes Network (MOON) ACL registry. In addition to his clinical and administrative duties, he also serves as the assistant team physician for the Cleveland Cavaliers and serves as a knee consultant to the Cleveland Guardians. He lives in the Chagrin Falls area with his wife, Jana, and enjoys biking, golfing, and walking in his free time.

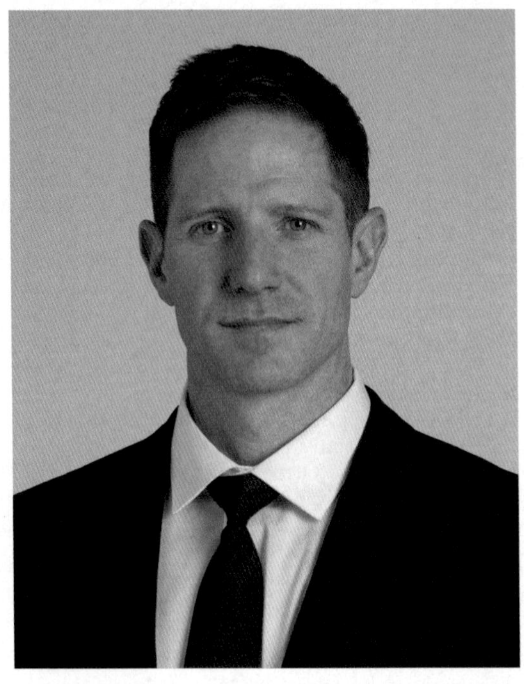

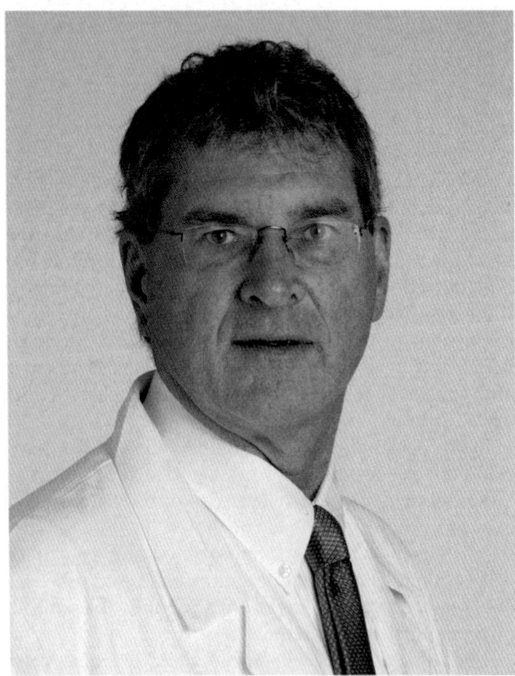

Associate Editors

Thomas E. Mroz, MD, is the Chairman of the Orthopaedic and Rheumatologic Institute and Director of Spine Research at Cleveland Clinic. He is a board-certified orthopedic surgeon who graduated from Case Western Reserve University and Case Western Reserve University School of Medicine, Cleveland, Ohio. Thereafter, he completed his residency in orthopaedic surgery at the George Washington University Medical Center, Washington, DC. He then completed two spinal surgery fellowships, one at the University of California Los Angeles, and the other in the Department of Neurosurgery at the University of Tennessee in Memphis. The focus of his second fellowship was minimally invasive spine surgery.

Dr. Mroz specializes in all aspects of spinal surgery and has a dedicated interest in minimally invasive surgery and cervical spine surgery.

He is very active in research and has lectured nationally and internationally on minimally invasive surgery and cervical spine surgery. He has authored more than 400 abstracts, research articles, and textbook chapters, and he is the Deputy Editor for the *Global Spine Journal*. He is a member in good standing in the North American Spine Society and the American Academy of Orthopaedic Surgeons, a Diplomate of the American Board of Orthopaedic Surgery, and a Board Member of the Cervical Spine Research Society.

Brendan M. Patterson, MD, MBA, joined the staff at the Cleveland Clinic in 2017 after more than 25 years of service at MetroHealth, a public hospital health system. He joined the faculty of MetroHealth in 1992 after an orthopedic residency at the Hospital for Special Surgery in New York City and an orthopedic trauma fellowship at Harborview Medical Center, University of Washington in Seattle. He served as Chairman of Orthopaedic Surgery at MetroHealth System for over 10 years and was promoted to Professor, Orthopaedic Surgery at Case Western Reserve University School of Medicine in 2012. Currently, he serves as Chair of Orthopaedic Surgery at the Cleveland Clinic. His areas of expertise include complex fractures and adult reconstruction.

Dr. Patterson graduated magna cum laude from Amherst College in 1981, majoring in economics and chemistry. He graduated from Case Western Reserve University School of Medicine as a member of the Alpha Omega Alpha Honor Society and was elected as the society's President in his fourth year. He received his MBA from the Weatherhead School of Management at Case Western Reserve University in 2000.

He is a Fellow of the American Academy of Orthopaedic Surgery and an active member of the Orthopaedic Trauma Association (OTA). Dr. Patterson was a member of the Board of Directors of the OTA for 10 years and served as its Chief Financial Officer for 4 years. Dr. Patterson led the development of the OTA knowledge portal that moved all of its educational materials to a digital format. In 2009 he established the Center for Orthopaedic Trauma Advancement, a 501(c)(3) organization whose primary mission is to develop funding for the education of orthopedic trauma fellows. He began his term as President of the OTA in the fall of 2022.

PREFACE

Frank Netter produced nearly 20,000 medical illustrations spanning the entire field of medicine over a five-decade career. There is no physician who has not used his work as part of their education. Many educators use his illustrations to teach others. One of the editors of this series had the privilege and honor to be an author of portions of the original "Green Book" of musculoskeletal medical illustrations as a junior faculty member and considers it a special honor to be part of this updated series.

Many of Frank Netter's original illustrations have stood the test of time. His work depicting basic musculoskeletal anatomy and relevant surgical anatomy and exposures have remained unaltered in the current series. His illustrations demonstrated the principles of treatment or the manifestation of musculoskeletal diseases and were rendered in a manner that only a physician-artist could render.

This edition of musculoskeletal illustrations has been updated with modern text and our current understanding of the pathogenesis, diagnosis, and treatment of a wide array of diseases and conditions. We have added new illustrations and radiographic and advanced imaging to supplement the original art. We expect that this series will prove to be useful to a wide spectrum of both students and teachers at every level.

Part I covers specific disorders of the upper limb, including anatomy, trauma, and degenerative and acquired disorders. Part II covers these same areas in the lower limb and spine. Part III covers the basic science of the musculoskeletal system, metabolic bone disease, rheumatologic diseases, musculoskeletal tumors, the sequelae of trauma, and congenital deformities.

The series is jointly produced by the clinical and research staff of the Orthopaedic and Rheumatologic Institute of the Cleveland Clinic and Elsevier. The editors thank each of the many talented contributors to this three-volume series. Their expertise in each of their fields of expertise has made this publication possible. We are both very proud to work with these colleagues. We are thankful to Elsevier for the opportunity to work on this series and for their support and expertise throughout the long development and editorial process.

Joseph P. Iannotti, MD, PhD
Richard D. Parker, MD

INTRODUCTIONS TO THE FIRST EDITION

INTRODUCTION TO PART I—ANATOMY, PHYSIOLOGY, AND METABOLIC DISORDERS

I had long looked forward to undertaking this volume on the musculoskeletal system. It deals with the most humanistic, the most soul-touching, of all the subjects I have portrayed in The CIBA Collection of Medical Illustrations. People break bones, develop painful or swollen joints, are handicapped by congenital, developmental, or acquired deformities, metabolic abnormalities, or paralytic disorders. Some are beset by tumors of bone or soft tissue; some undergo amputations, either surgical or traumatic; some occasionally have reimplantation; and many have joint replacement. The list goes on and on. These are people we see about us quite commonly and are often our friends, relatives, or acquaintances. Significantly, such ailments lend themselves to graphic representation and are stimulating subject matter for an artist.

When I undertook this project, however, I grossly underestimated its scope. This was true also in regard to the previous volumes of the CIBA Collection, but in the case of this book, it was far more marked. When we consider that this project involves every bone, joint, and muscle of the body, as well as all the nerves and blood vessels that supply them and all the multitude of disorders that may affect each of them, the magnitude of the project becomes enormous. In my naiveté, I originally thought I could cover the subject in a single book, but it soon became apparent that this was impossible. Even two books soon proved inadequate for such an extensive undertaking and, accordingly, three books are now planned. This book, Part I, Volume 8 of the CIBA Collection, covers basic gross anatomy, embryology, physiology, and histology of the musculoskeletal system, as well as its metabolic disorders. Part II, now in press, covers rheumatic and other arthritic disorders, as well as their conservative and surgical management (including joint replacement), congenital and developmental disorders, and both benign and malignant neoplasms of bones and soft tissues. Part III, on which I am still at work, will include fractures and dislocations and their emergency and definitive care, amputations (both surgical and traumatic) and prostheses, sports injuries, infections, peripheral nerve and plexus injuries, burns, compartment syndromes, skin grafting, arthroscopy, and care and rehabilitation of handicapped patients.

But classification and organization of this voluminous material turned out to be no simple matter, since many disorders fit equally well into several of the above groups. For example, osteogenesis imperfecta might have been classified as metabolic, congenital, or developmental. Baker's cyst, ganglion, bursitis, and villonodular synovitis might have been considered with rheumatic, developmental, or in some instances even with traumatic disorders. Pathologic fractures might be covered with fractures in general or with the specific underlying disease that caused them. In a number of instances, therefore, empiric decisions had to be made in this connection, and some subjects were covered under several headings. I hope that the reader will be considerate of these problems. In addition, there is much overlap between the fields of orthopedics, neurology, and neurosurgery, so that the reader may find it advantageous to refer at times to my atlases on the nervous system.

I must express herewith my thanks and appreciation for the tremendous help which my very knowledgeable collaborators gave to me so graciously. In this Part I, there was first of all Dr. Russell Woodburne, a truly great anatomist and professor emeritus at the University of Michigan. It is interesting that during our long collaboration I never actually met with Dr. Woodburne, and all our communications were by mail or phone. This, in itself, tells of what a fine understanding and meeting of the minds there was between us. I hope and expect that in the near future I will have the pleasure of meeting him in person.

Dr. Edmund S. Crelin, professor at Yale University, is a long-standing friend (note that I do not say "old" friend because he is so young in spirit) with whom I have collaborated a number of times on other phases of embryology. He is a profound student and original investigator of the subject, with the gift of imparting his knowledge simply and clearly, and is in fact a talented artist himself.

Dr. Frederick Kaplan (now Freddie to me), assistant professor of orthopaedics at the University of Pennsylvania, was invaluable in guiding me through the difficult subjects of musculoskeletal physiology and metabolic bone disease. I enjoyed our companionship and friendship as much as I appreciated his knowledge and insight into the subject.

I was delighted to have the cooperation of Dr. Henry Mankin, the distinguished chief of orthopaedics at Massachusetts General Hospital and professor at Harvard University, for the complex subject of rickets in its varied forms—nutritional, renal, and metabolic. He is a great but charming and unassuming man.

There were many others, too numerous to mention here individually, who gave to me of their knowledge and time. They are all credited elsewhere in this book but I thank them all very much herewith. I will write about the great people who helped me with other parts of Volume 8 when those parts are published.

Finally, I give great credit and thanks to the personnel of the CIBA-GEIGY Company and to the company itself for having done so much to ease my burden in producing this book. Specifically, I would like to mention Mr. Philip Flagler, Dr. Milton Donin, Dr. Roy Ellis, and especially Mrs. Regina Dingle, all of whom did so much more in that connection than I can tell about here.

Frank H. Netter, 1987

INTRODUCTION TO PART II—DEVELOPMENTAL DISORDERS, TUMORS, RHEUMATIC DISEASES, AND JOINT REPLACEMENT

In my introduction to Part I of this atlas, I wrote of how awesome albeit fascinating I had found the task of pictorializing the fundamentals of the musculoskeletal system, both its normal structure as well as its multitudinous disorders and diseases. As compactly, simply, and succinctly as I tried to present the subject matter, it still required three full books (Parts I, II, and III of Volume 8 of The CIBA Collection of Medical Illustrations). Part I of this trilogy covered the normal anatomy, embryology, and physiology of the musculoskeletal system as well as its diverse metabolic diseases, including the various types of rickets. This book, Part II, portrays its congenital and developmental disorders, neoplasms—both benign and malignant—of bone and soft tissue, and rheumatic and other arthritic diseases, as well as joint replacement. Part III, on which I am still at work, will cover trauma, including fractures and dislocations of all the bones and joints, soft-tissue injuries, sports injuries, burns, infections including osteomyelitis and hand infections, compartment syndromes, amputations, both traumatic and surgical, replantation of limbs and digits, prostheses, and rehabilitation, as well as a number of related subjects.

As I stated in my above-mentioned previous introduction, some disorders, however, do not fit exactly into a precise classification and are therefore covered piece-meal herein under several headings. Furthermore, a considerable number of orthopedic ailments involve also the fields of neurology and neurosurgery, so readers may find it helpful to refer in those instances to my atlases on the anatomy and pathology of the nervous system (Volume 1, Parts I and II of The CIBA Collection of Medical Illustrations).

Most meaningfully, however, I herewith express my sincere appreciation of the many great physicians, surgeons, orthopedists, and scientists who so graciously shared with me their knowledge and supplied me with so much material on which to base my illustrations. Without their help I could not have created this atlas. Most of these wonderful people are credited elsewhere in this book under the heading of "Acknowledgments" but I must nevertheless specifically mention a few who were not only collaborators and consultants in this undertaking but who have become my dear and esteemed friends. These are Dr. Bob Hensinger, my consulting editor, who guided me through many puzzling aspects of the organization and subject matter of this atlas; Drs. Alfred and Genevieve Swanson, pioneers in the correction of rheumatically deformed hands with Silastic implants, as well as in the classification and study of congenital limb deficits; Dr. William Enneking, who has made such great advances in the diagnosis and management of bone tumors; Dr. Ernest ("Chappy") Conrad III; the late Dr. Charley Frantz, who first set me on course for this project, and Dr. Richard Freyberg, who became the consultant on the rheumatic diseases plates; Dr. George Hammond; Dr. Hugo Keim; Dr. Mack Clayton; Dr. Philip Wilson; Dr. Stuart Kozinn; and Dr. Russell Windsor.

Finally, I also sincerely thank Mr. Philip Flagler, Ms. Regina Dingle, and others of the CIBA-GEIGY organization who helped in more ways than I can describe in producing this atlas.

Frank H. Netter, MD, 1990

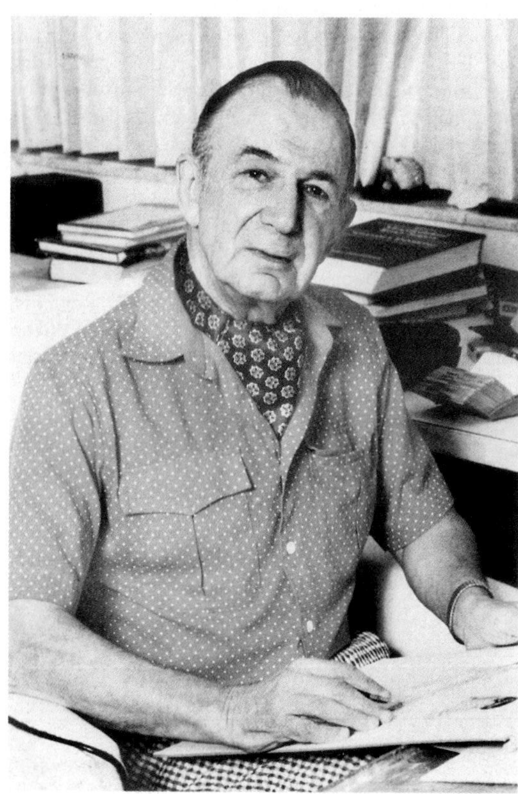

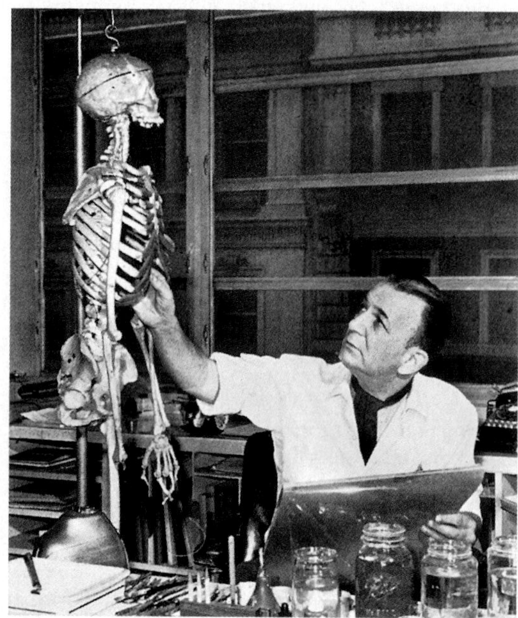

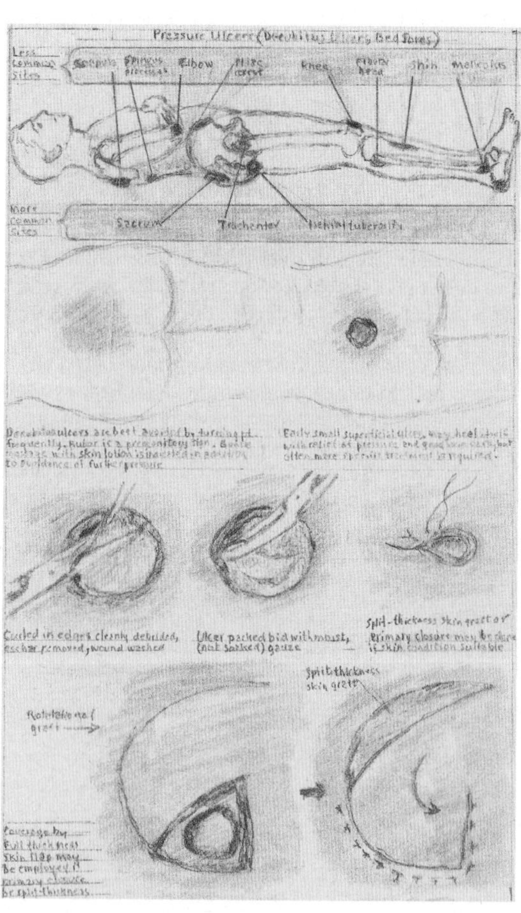

Sketch appearing in front matter of Part III of the first edition.

CONTRIBUTORS

EDITORS-IN-CHIEF

Joseph P. Iannotti, MD, PhD
Lang Family Distinguished Chair in Orthopedics
Chief of Staff
Chief Academic and Innovations Officer
Cleveland Clinic Weston Hospital
Weston, Florida

Richard D. Parker, MD
Professor of Surgery, Cleveland Clinic Lerner College of Medicine
President, Hillcrest Hospital and East Region
Past Chairman, Department of Orthopaedic Surgery
Cleveland Clinic
Cleveland, Ohio

ASSOCIATE EDITORS

Abby G. Abelson, MD, FACR
Clinical Assistant Professor of Medicine
Chair, Department of Rheumatic and Immunologic Diseases
Cleveland Clinic Lerner College of Medicine at Case Western Reserve University
Cleveland, Ohio
EDITOR: PART III: SECTIONS 3, 5
AUTHOR: PART III: PLATES 3.26–3.29, 3.34–3.37, 3.45–3.47, 5.45, 5.52–5.54

Thomas E. Mroz, MD
Chair, Enterprise Orthopaedic Surgery and Rehabilitation
Cervical Spine Surgery
Director, Spine Research
Cleveland Clinic
Cleveland, Ohio
EDITOR: PART II: SECTION 1

Brendan M. Patterson, MD, MBA
Chair, Department of Orthopaedic Surgery
Cleveland Clinic Health Care System
Professor, Orthopaedic Surgery
Case Western Reserve University School of Medicine
Cleveland, Ohio
EDITOR: PART II: SECTIONS 2, 3, 4, 5; PART III: SECTIONS 1, 2, 4, 6, 7, 8, 9
AUTHOR: PART II: PLATES 2.63–2.77, 3.1–3.26, 3.42–3.43, 4.1–4.13; PART III: PLATES 1.1–1.21, 2.1–2.15, 2.27–2.41, 7.1–7.11, 9.2, 9.3, 9.9, 9.10

CONTRIBUTORS

Robert Tracy Ballock, MD
Professor Emeritus of Surgery
Cleveland Clinic Lerner College of Medicine at Case Western Reserve University
Cleveland, Ohio
PLATES 2.22–2.24, 5.34–5.43

Mark J. Berkowitz, MD
Staff Surgeon, Foot and Ankle Center
Orthopaedic and Rheumatologic Institute
Cleveland Clinic
Cleveland, Ohio
PLATES 5.19–5.30, 5.44–5.49

Bilal B. Butt, MD
Spine Fellow, Center for Spine Health
Cleveland Clinic
Cleveland, Ohio
PLATES 1.1–1.16

William A. Cantrell, MD
Resident, Department of Orthopaedic Surgery
Cleveland Clinic
Cleveland, Ohio
PLATES 3.1–3.26, 4.1–4.13

Ryan C. Goodwin, MD, MBA
Director, Center for Pediatric Orthopaedic Surgery
Cleveland Clinic
Cleveland, Ohio
PLATES 2.25–2.41, 3.30, 4.16–4.17

Kathryn E. Huff, DO
Pediatric Orthopedic Surgeon
Essentia Health St. Mary's Medical Center
Duluth, Minnesota
PLATES 2.25–2.41, 3.30, 4.16–4.17

Thomas E. Kuivila, MD
Vice Chair for Education, Department of Orthopaedic Surgery
Cleveland Clinic
Cleveland, Ohio
PLATES 1.31–1.46

Sara Lyn Miniaci-Coxhead, MD, MEd
Orthopaedic Surgeon, Orthopaedic and Rheumatologic Institute
Cleveland Clinic
Cleveland, Ohio
PLATES 5.1–5.18, 5.31–5.33

Robert M. Molloy, MD
Staff Surgeon, Adult Reconstruction Center
Department of Orthopaedic Surgery
Orthopaedic and Rheumatologic Institute
Cleveland Clinic
Cleveland, Ohio
PLATES 2.42–2.59, 3.27–3.28, 3.31–3.41

Anokha Padubidri, MD
Orthopaedic Surgeon, Orthopaedic and Rheumatologic Institute
Cleveland Clinic
Cleveland, Ohio
PLATES 3.29, 4.14–4.15

Arpan Ajit Patel, MD
Resident, Neurosurgery
Cleveland Clinic
Cleveland, Ohio
PLATES 1.17–1.30

Dominic W. Pelle, MD
Assistant Professor Spine Surgery, Center for Spine Health
Cleveland Clinic
Cleveland, Ohio
PLATES 1.1–1.16

James T. Rosneck, MD
Orthopaedic Surgeon, Sports Health Center
Cleveland Clinic
Cleveland, Ohio
PLATES 2.1–2.21, 2.60–2.62

Jason W. Savage, MD
Staff Spine Surgeon, Center for Spine Health
Cleveland Clinic
Cleveland, Ohio
PLATES 1.1–1.16, 1.31–1.46

Michael Steinmetz, MD
Professor and Chairman, Department of Neurosurgery
Cleveland Clinic Lerner College of Medicine
Cleveland, Ohio
PLATES 1.17–1.30

Benjamin Bernard Whiting, MD
Resident, Neurosurgery
Cleveland Clinic Foundation
Cleveland, Ohio
PLATES 1.17–1.30

Ernest Young, MS, MD
Orthopaedic Surgeon, Department of Orthopaedic Surgery
Cleveland Clinic
Cleveland, Ohio
PLATES 4.18–4.22

CONTRIBUTORS TO SECOND EDITION

We acknowledge the work of the contributors to the previous edition.

Kalil G. Abdullah

Robert Tracy Ballock, MD

Gordon R. Bell, MD

Mark J. Berkowitz, MD

Ryan C. Goodwin, MD

David P. Gurd, MD

Thomas Kuivila, MD

Sean Matuszak, MD

Adam F. Meisel, MD

Nathan W. Mesko, MD

Robert M. Molloy, MD

Thomas E. Mroz, MD

James T. Rosneck, MD

David L. Schub, MD

Stephen Tolhurst, MD

CONTENTS OF COMPLETE VOLUME 6—MUSCULOSKELETAL SYSTEM: THREE-PART SET

PART I **Upper Limb**

SECTION 1 Shoulder

SECTION 2 Upper Arm and Elbow

SECTION 3 Forearm and Wrist

SECTION 4 Hand and Finger

ISBN: 978-0-3238-8088-6

PART II **Spine and Lower Limb**

SECTION 1 Spine

SECTION 2 Pelvis, Hip, and Thigh

SECTION 3 Knee

SECTION 4 Lower Leg

SECTION 5 Ankle and Foot

ISBN: 978-0-3238-8128-9

PART III **Biology and Systemic Diseases**

SECTION 1 Embryology

SECTION 2 Physiology

SECTION 3 Metabolic Disorders

SECTION 4 Congenital and Development Disorders

SECTION 5 Rheumatic Diseases

SECTION 6 Tumors of Musculoskeletal System

SECTION 7 Injury to Musculoskeletal System

SECTION 8 Soft Tissue Infections

SECTION 9 Fracture Complications

ISBN: 978-0-3238-8087-9

CONTENTS

SECTION 1

SPINE

Vertebral Column

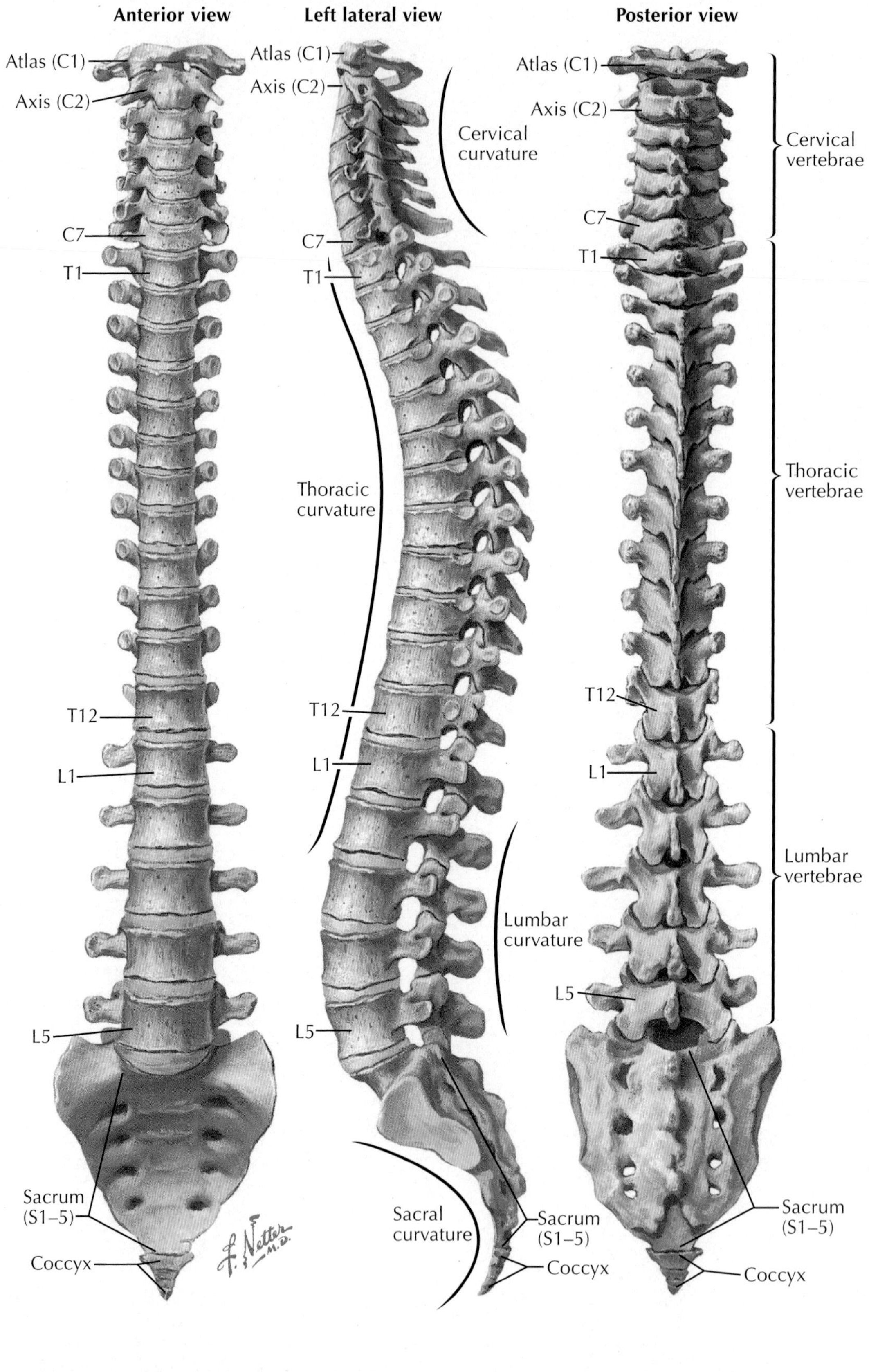

The vertebral column is built from individual units of alternating bony vertebrae and fibrocartilaginous discs. These units are intimately connected by strong ligaments and supported by paraspinal muscles with tendinous attachments to the spine. The individual bony elements and ligaments are described in Plates 1.9 to 1.18.

There are 33 vertebrae (7 cervical, 12 thoracic, 5 lumbar, 5 sacral, and 4 coccygeal), although the sacral and coccygeal vertebrae are usually fused to form the sacrum and coccyx. All vertebrae conform to a basic plan, but morphologic variations occur in the different regions. A typical vertebra is made up of an anterior, more or less cylindrical *body* and a posterior *arch* composed of two *pedicles* and two *laminae,* the latter united posteriorly in the midline to form a *spinous process.* These processes vary in shape, size, and direction in the various regions of the spine. On each side, the arch also supports a *transverse process* and *superior and inferior articular processes;* the latter form synovial joints that are the posterior sites of contact (left and right) for adjacent vertebral segments. The disc is the anterior site of attachment. The spinous and transverse processes provide levers for the many muscles attached to them. The increasing size of the vertebral bodies from above downward is related to the increasing weights and stresses borne by successive segments, and the sacral vertebrae are fused to form a solid wedge-shaped base—the keystone in a bridge whose arches curve down toward the hip joints. The *intervertebral discs* act as elastic buffers to absorb the many mechanical shocks sustained by the vertebral column.

Only limited movements are possible between adjacent vertebrae, but the sum of these movements confers a considerable range of mobility on the vertebral column. Flexion, extension, lateral bending, rotation, and translation are all possible, and these actions are freer in the cervical and lumbar regions than in the thoracic region. Such differences exist because the discs are thicker in the cervical and lumbar areas, and they lack the splinting effect produced by the thoracic rib cage and sternum. Additionally, the cervical and lumbar spinous processes are shorter and less closely apposed, and the articular processes are shaped and arranged differently.

At birth, the vertebral column presents a general dorsal convexity; later, the cervical and lumbar regions become curved in the opposite directions—when the infant reaches the stages of holding up the head (3–4 months) and sitting upright (6–9 months). The dorsal convexities are *primary curves* associated with the fetal uterine position, whereas the cervical and lumbar ventral *secondary curves* are compensatory to permit the assumption of the upright position. There may be additional slight lateral deviations resulting from unequal muscular traction in right-handed and left-handed persons.

The evolution of the human from a quadrupedal to a bipedal posture has been mainly attributed to the tilting of the sacrum between the hip bones, by an increase in lumbosacral angulation, and by minor adjustments of the anterior and posterior depths of various vertebrae and discs. An erect posture greatly increases the load on the lower spinal joints; however, as good as these ancestral adaptations were, some static and dynamic imperfections remain and predispose to the effects of gradual strain.

The length of the vertebral column averages 72 cm in the adult male and 7 to 10 cm less in the female. The *vertebral canal* extends through the entire length of the column and provides excellent protection for the spinal cord, the exiting nerve roots, and the cauda equina. Vessels and nerve roots pass through *intervertebral foramina* between the superior and inferior borders of the pedicles of adjacent vertebrae, bound anteriorly by the corresponding vertebral body and intervertebral discs and posteriorly by the joints between the articular processes of adjoining vertebrae.

ANATOMY OF CRANIOCERVICAL JUNCTION

BONY ANATOMY

The craniocervical junction consists of the occiput and the first two cervical vertebrae (C1 and C2). It is the complex bony and ligamentous articulations of this region that facilitate its unique biomechanic properties, accounting for 25% of flexion and extension and 50% of rotation of the neck. The occiput is the skull's most inferior bone, and it retains a cupped shape posteriorly that gives way to the triangular foramen magnum inferiorly. This foramen harbors the cervical spine cord as it ascends and transitions into the medulla and upper brainstem. At the anterolateral border of the foramen magnum are the occipital condyles, which are articulation points for the atlas (C1). These articulations are relatively flat to limit axial rotation of the atlantooccipital joint.

The atlas has two superior protuberances, known as its lateral masses, that articulate with the occipital condyles. The atlas is the only vertebral body to lack a spinous process, and in rare cases it may entirely lack a posterior arch. The atlas is a ring-shaped structure that lacks a vertebral body and does not make contact with an intervertebral disc. Embryologically, the body of the atlas becomes the dens (odontoid process) of the axis (C2). The dens articulates with the atlas anteriorly as it projects upward from the axis. The other points of articulation between the atlas and axis are the synovial joints of the articulating processes. The C1–C2 joints are biconcave, as opposed to the flatter articulation of the occiput and C1. Whereas the occiput–C1 joint is designed mainly to flex and extend, the C1–C2 joint is designed to provide axial rotation.

ATLAS AND AXIS

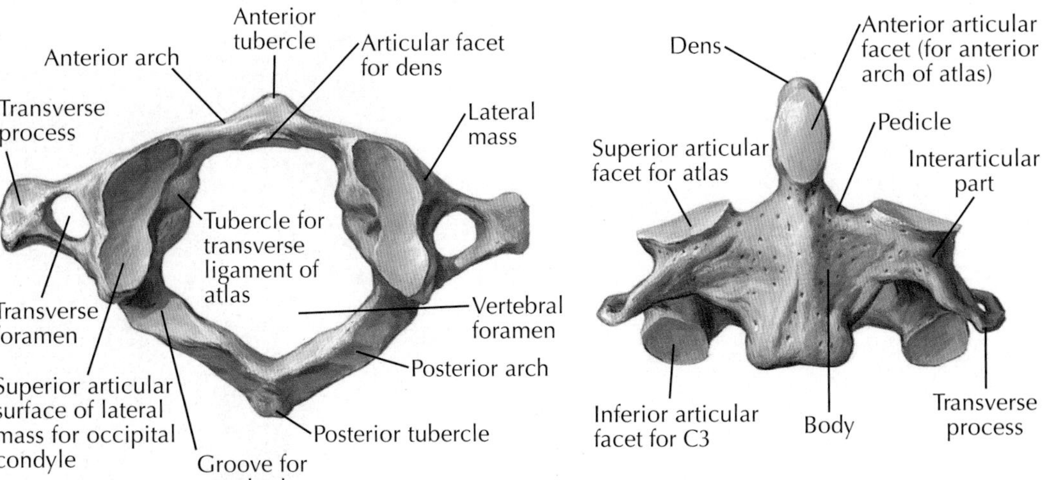

Atlas (C1): superior view

Axis (C2): anterior view

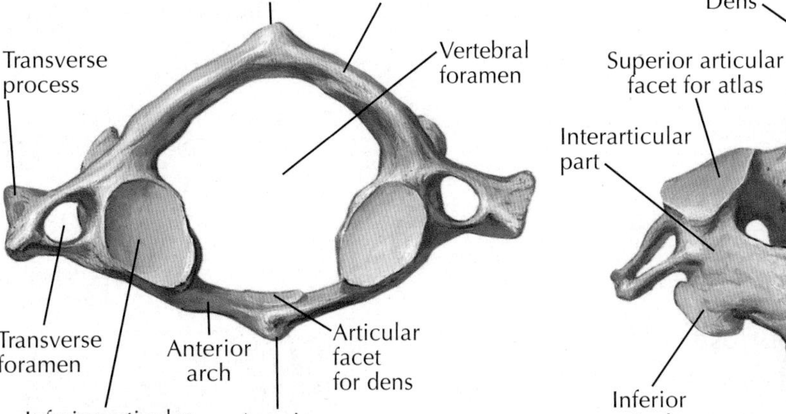

Atlas (C1): inferior view

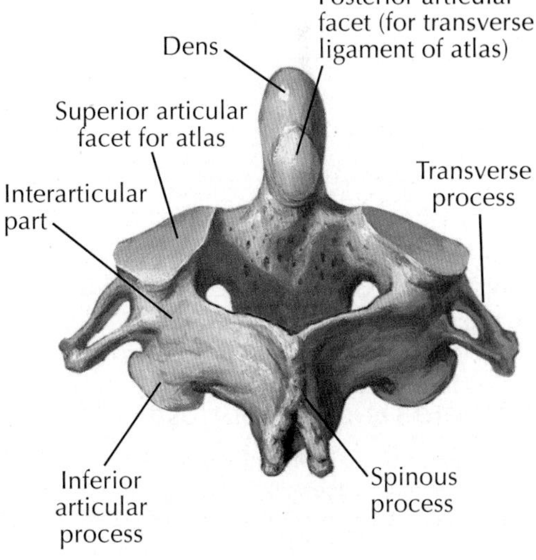

Axis (C2): posterosuperior view

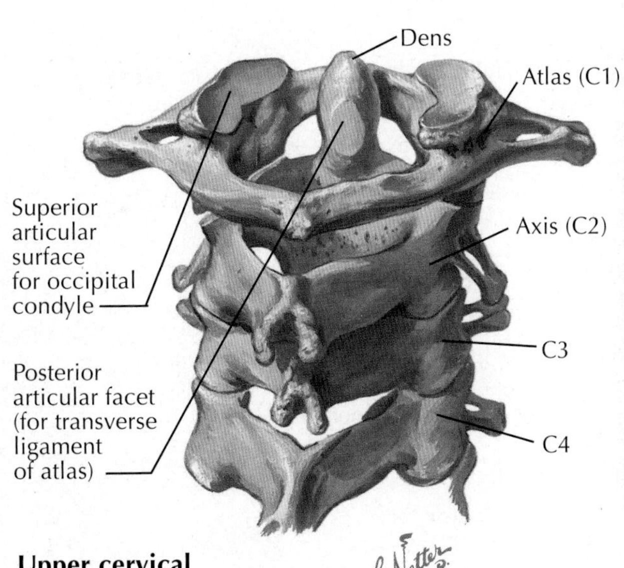

Upper cervical vertebrae, assembled: posterosuperior view

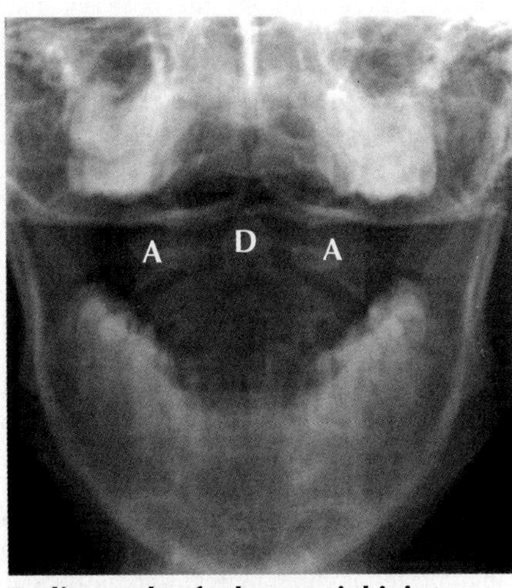

Radiograph of atlantoaxial joint (open mouth odontoid view). *A,* Lateral masses of atlas (C1 vertebra). *D,* Dens of axis (C2 vertebra).

EXTERNAL CRANIOCERVICAL LIGAMENTS

Anterior view

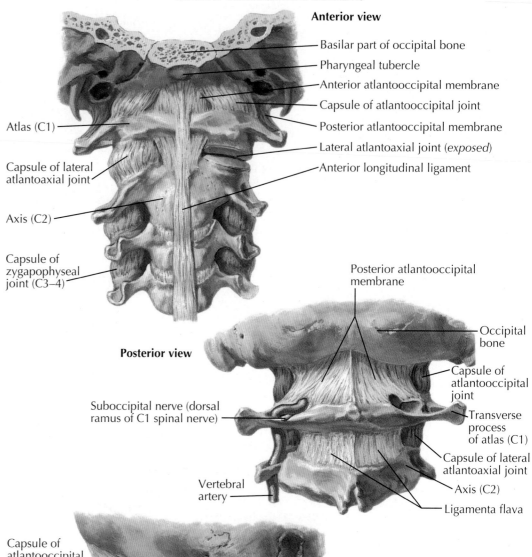

Basilar part of occipital bone
Pharyngeal tubercle
Anterior atlantooccipital membrane
Capsule of atlantooccipital joint
Posterior atlantooccipital membrane
Lateral atlantoaxial joint (*exposed*)
Anterior longitudinal ligament
Atlas (C1)
Capsule of lateral atlantoaxial joint
Axis (C2)
Capsule of zygapophyseal joint (C3–4)

Posterior view

Posterior atlantooccipital membrane
Occipital bone
Capsule of atlantooccipital joint
Transverse process of atlas (C1)
Capsule of lateral atlantoaxial joint
Axis (C2)
Ligamenta flava
Suboccipital nerve (dorsal ramus of C1 spinal nerve)
Vertebral artery

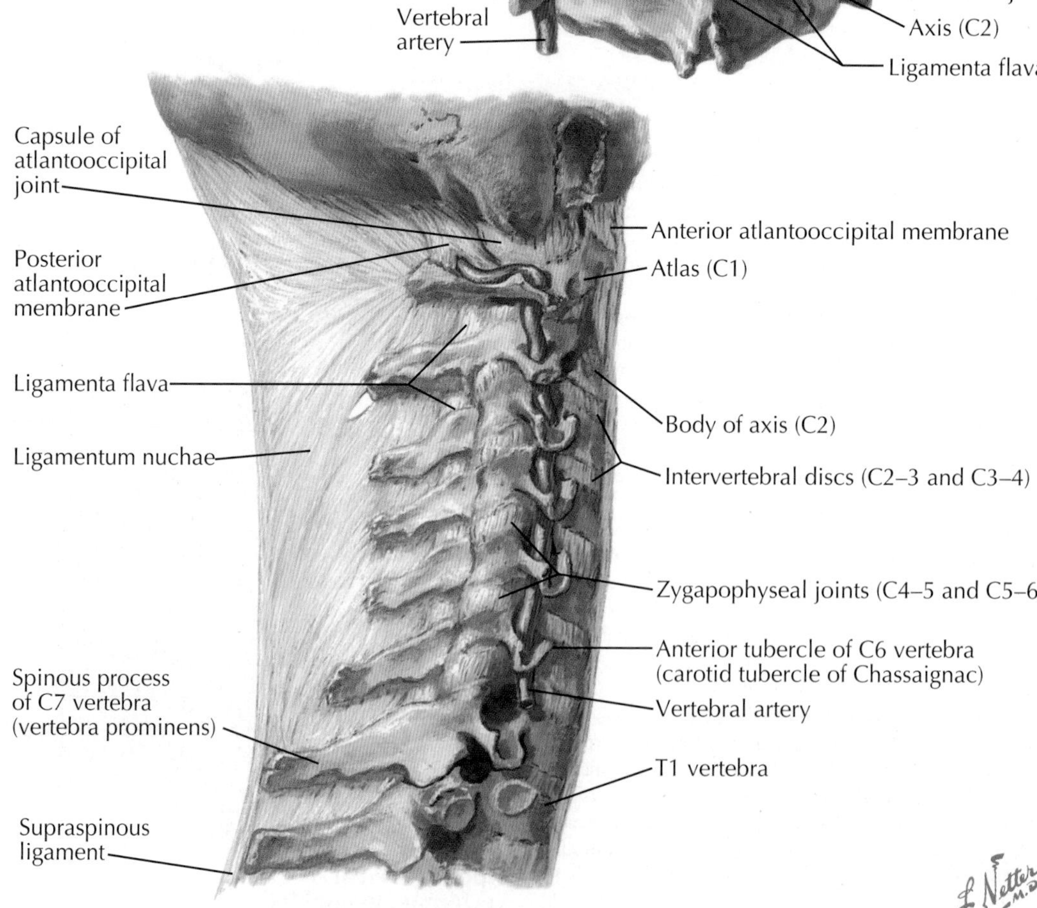

Right lateral view

ANATOMY OF CRANIOCERVICAL JUNCTION (Continued)

LIGAMENTS AND MUSCULATURE

The ligamentous complex of the craniovertebral junction is a sophisticated network that plays a crucial role in maintaining the physical stability of the vertebra that protects the body's most critical neurologic structures. Of the eight ligaments that support the craniovertebral junction, several have notable clinical relevance. The tectorial membrane is contiguous with the cranial dura mater and inserts onto the clivus. It originates as a superior continuation of the posterior longitudinal ligament and is thought to prevent anterior spinal cord compression by the clivus and possibly by the dens. The left and right alar ligaments function to limit axial rotation and connect the anterior and superior aspects of the dens to the occiput. The cruciate ligament is composed of vertical and horizontal components. The horizontal component is known as the *transverse ligament,* and it connects the two medial walls of the atlas, snugly securing the dens as it articulates with the anterior ring of the atlas. It acts to effectively limit the movement of C1 on C2 in the anteroposterior plane. The vertical components of the cruciate ligament consist of inferior and superior bands, but their function is not as well understood.

The *suboccipital muscles* extend the head and rotate it and the atlas ipsilaterally. At the suboccipital region there exist the rectus capitis posterior major and rectus capitis posterior minor muscles and the obliquus capitis inferior and obliquus capitis superior muscles of the head (see Plate 1.5). These muscles are directly deep to the semispinalis capitis muscle, and three of them bound the suboccipital triangle.

INTERNAL CRANIOCERVICAL LIGAMENTS

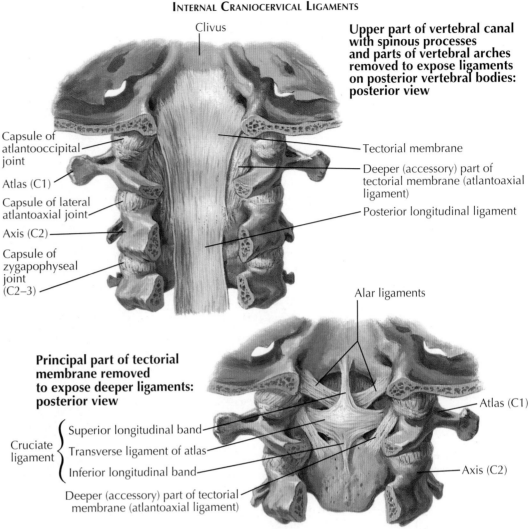

Clivus

Upper part of vertebral canal with spinous processes and parts of vertebral arches removed to expose ligaments on posterior vertebral bodies: posterior view

Capsule of atlantooccipital joint
Atlas (C1)
Capsule of lateral atlantoaxial joint
Axis (C2)
Capsule of zygapophyseal joint (C2–3)
Tectorial membrane
Deeper (accessory) part of tectorial membrane (atlantoaxial ligament)
Posterior longitudinal ligament

Alar ligaments

Principal part of tectorial membrane removed to expose deeper ligaments: posterior view

Cruciate ligament: Superior longitudinal band; Transverse ligament of atlas; Inferior longitudinal band
Deeper (accessory) part of tectorial membrane (atlantoaxial ligament)
Atlas (C1)
Axis (C2)

ANATOMY OF CRANIOCERVICAL JUNCTION (Continued)

The *rectus capitis posterior major muscle* arises from the spinous process of the axis. Broadening as it ascends, it inserts into the middle of the inferior nuchal line of the occipital bone and into the bone below this line. The *obliquus capitis inferior muscle* arises from the spinous process of the axis and, passing horizontally, ends in the transverse process of the atlas. The *obliquus capitis superior muscle* arises from the transverse process of the atlas. Passing upward and medially, this muscle inserts into the occipital bone above the inferior nuchal line, where it overlaps the insertion of the rectus capitis posterior major. The *rectus capitis posterior minor muscle* lies medial to the rectus capitis posterior major muscle. It originates from the posterior tubercle of the atlas and, widening as it ascends, inserts into the medial part of the inferior nuchal line and into the occipital bone.

It is the area between the two oblique muscles and the rectus capitis major muscle that is defined as the *suboccipital triangle* (see Plate 1.5). Its floor is the posterior atlantooccipital membrane, which is attached to the posterior margin of the posterior arch of the atlas. Deep to this membrane, the vertebral artery occupies the groove on the upper surface of the posterior arch of the atlas as it passes medially toward the foramen magnum.

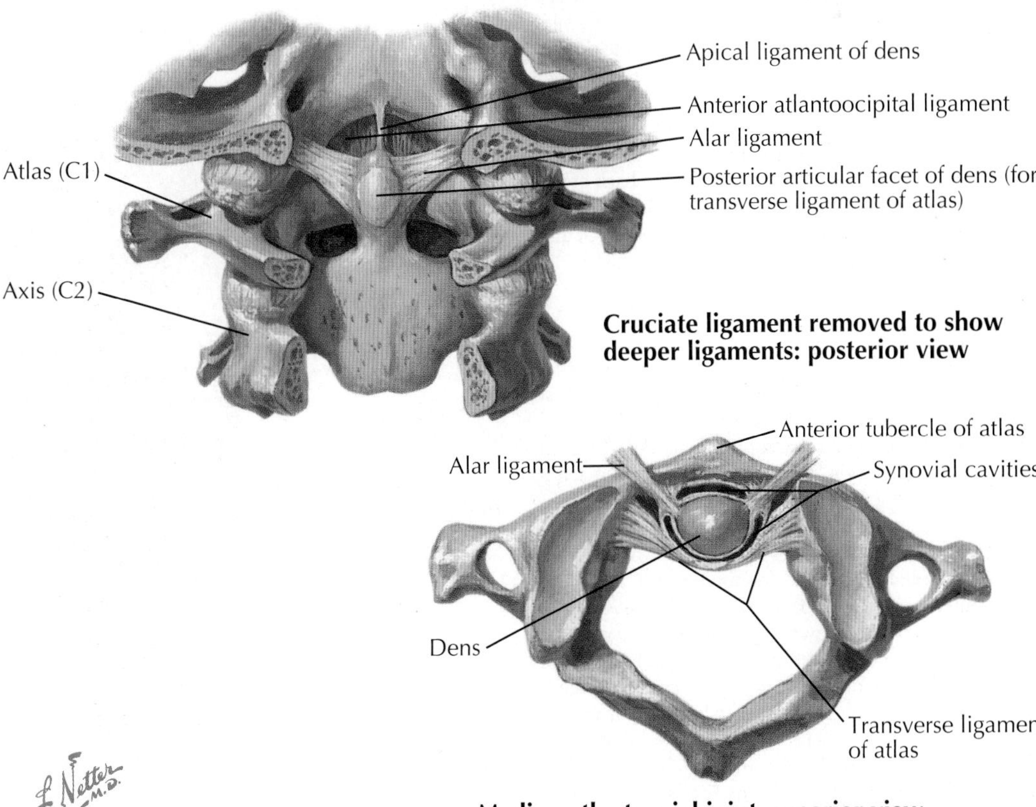

ANATOMY OF CRANIOCERVICAL JUNCTION (Continued)

NERVES

The suboccipital nerve emerges from between the vertebral artery and the posterior arch of the atlas. It divides in the dense tissue of the suboccipital triangle and branches into the suboccipital muscles. The *suboccipital nerve* (dorsal ramus of C1) has no cutaneous distribution. The medial branch of the dorsal ramus of C2 is known as the *greater occipital nerve* (dorsal ramus of C2), which has a distribution as high as the vertex of the scalp. It emerges below the obliquus capitis inferior muscle and turns upward to cross the suboccipital triangle and reach the scalp by piercing the semispinalis capitis and trapezius muscles. The *lesser occipital nerve* of the cervical plexus (ventral ramus of C2) supplies the skin of the scalp behind the ear as well as the skin of the back of the ear itself. The *third occipital nerve,* the medial branch of the dorsal ramus of C3, distributes in the upper neck and to the scalp, to just beyond the superior nuchal line.

VASCULATURE

By far the most important of the vascular structures that traverse the craniovertebral junction are the vertebral arteries. In 90% of individuals the vertebral arteries typically enter the transverse foramina at C6. The path of the vertebral artery is relatively linear until it reaches C2, where the foramina are oriented obliquely compared with the more horizontal orientation of the more caudal foramina. It continues through the more horizontally oriented transverse foramen of C1 and then arches anteromedially until it lies in the groove of the posterior arch of C1 known as the sulcus arteriosus. It then continues medially and pierces the atlantooccipital membrane. The venous drainage of the craniovertebral junction is via the jugular venous feeders and ultimately the subclavian vein. There is often a well-developed venous plexus at the C1–C2 junction just lateral to the dura and around the C2 roots that surgeons must contend with when exposing the C1–C2 region.

SUBOCCIPITAL TRIANGLE

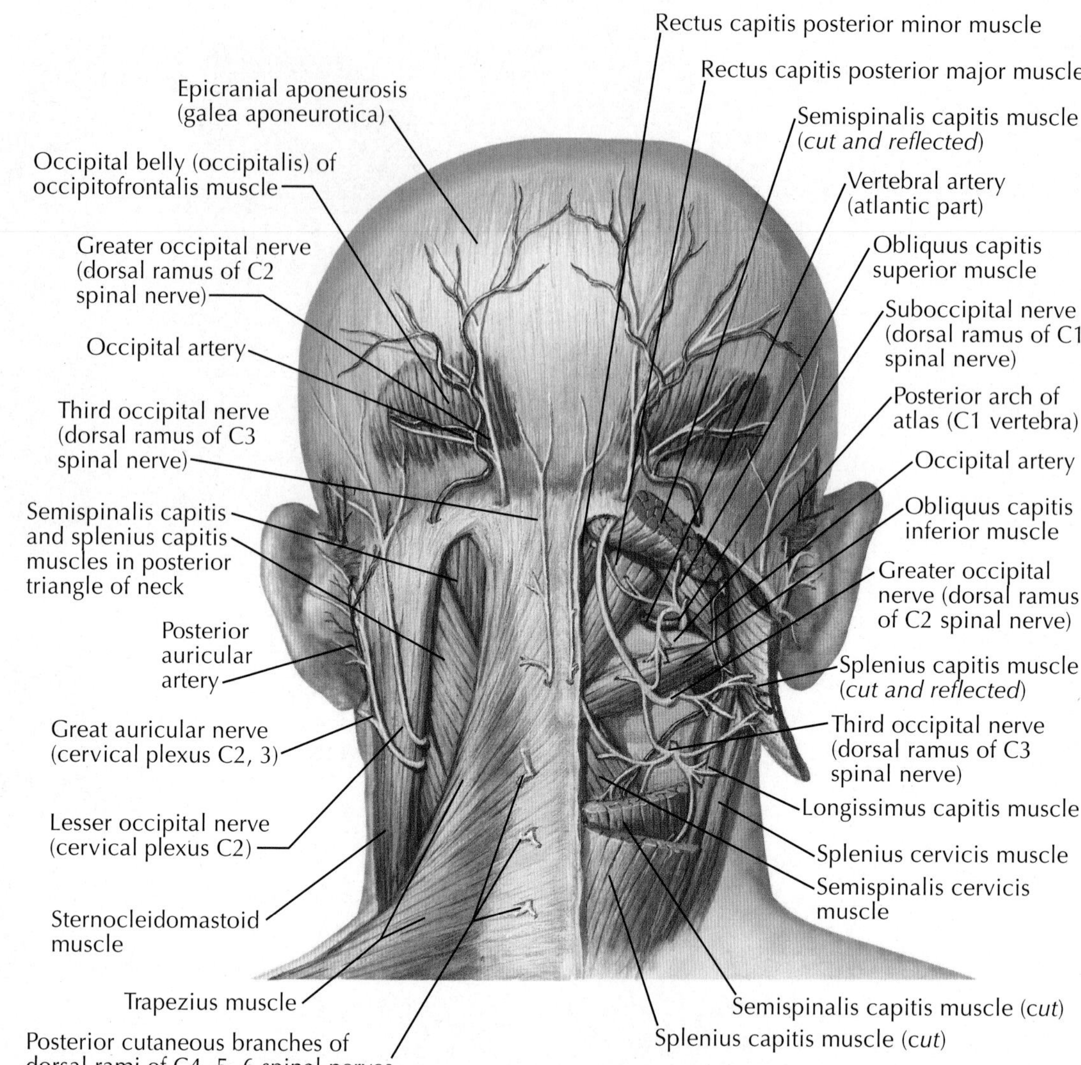

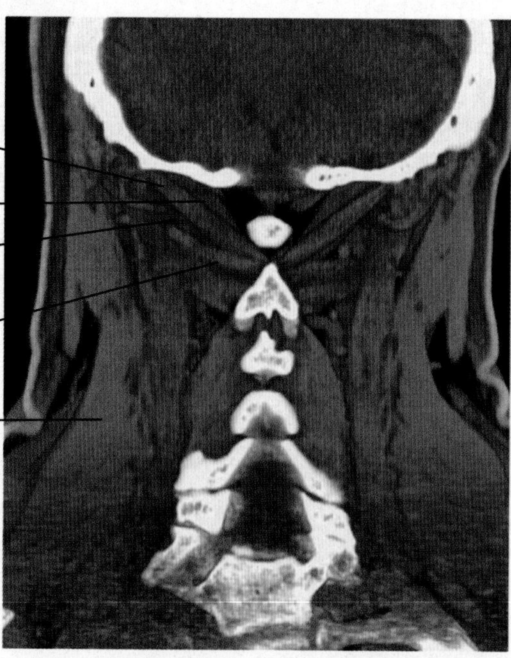

Volume-rendered display. Cervical spine CT scan.
From Weber EC, Vilensky JA, Carmichael SW. Netter's Concise Radiologic Anatomy. Elsevier; 2008.

Clinical Problems and Correlations of Craniovertebral Junction

DENS FRACTURES

Among pathologic entities at the craniocervical junction, one of the most common is the dens fracture, which may constitute nearly 20% of all fractures of the cervical spine. It is the most common cervical fracture in elderly patients. The mean age at onset of odontoid fractures is 47 years, with a bimodal distribution. Younger patients tend to present with dens fractures as a component of a constellation of severe injuries that result from a high-speed, high-energy injury. Elderly patients comprise the second, larger peak group of those affected. These fractures are typically the result of a low-speed trauma, such as a fall from the standing position. A high proportion of the dens volume is cancellous bone, and osteopenia and osteoporosis predispose older people to these types of fractures. The latter deserve special consideration in the elderly, in whom mortality rates have been reported as high as 40%.

Dens fractures are generally classified as types I, II, and III. Type I fractures involve just the tip of the dens and are the least common. Type II fractures involve the base of the odontoid process and do not extend into the C2 vertebral body. They are considered the most common and the least stable. Type III fractures extend into the body of C2. Differentiating the type of dens fracture is of significant clinical importance. Dens fractures in younger patients tend to be discovered during imaging after high-energy trauma such as motor vehicle accidents or falls and are most clearly evident on sagittal and coronal reconstructions of axial computed tomography (CT). In these patients it is important to rule out atlantooccipital dislocation, which is associated with type I dens fractures. A more common clinical scenario is an elderly patient presenting after a fall with upper cervical neck pain and reduced range of motion. On arrival, these patients often undergo CT of the head and neck, and the practitioner should scrutinize both coronal and sagittal reconstructions to evaluate for a dens fracture. If CT is unavailable or the patient presents in an ambulatory setting, three plain radiographs with anteroposterior, open-mouth odontoid, and cross-table lateral views should be obtained.

Isolated type I fractures that have occurred from low-energy injuries can generally be treated with application of a hard cervical collar and are associated with a high healing rate without surgical intervention. Type I fractures in younger patients or after high-impact injury should be evaluated with magnetic resonance imaging (MRI) to rule out atlantooccipital dislocation because these fractures involve the alar ligament.

Type II fractures are considered unstable fractures and have a low healing rate, which is due to disruption of cancellous bone blood supply. The vascular supply to C2 runs from caudal to cranial, making the dens a watershed area, and this underscores the reason for the high nonunion rate observed in this fracture pattern. Historically, intervention of some sort has been advocated, whether it be surgical stabilization or nonsurgical immobilization (e.g., use of a halo vest orthosis). The treatment of type II fractures has become an area of

Dens Fracture

Type I. Fracture of tip

Type II. Fracture of base or neck

Type III. Fracture extends into body of axis

Superior articular facet

Inferior articular facet

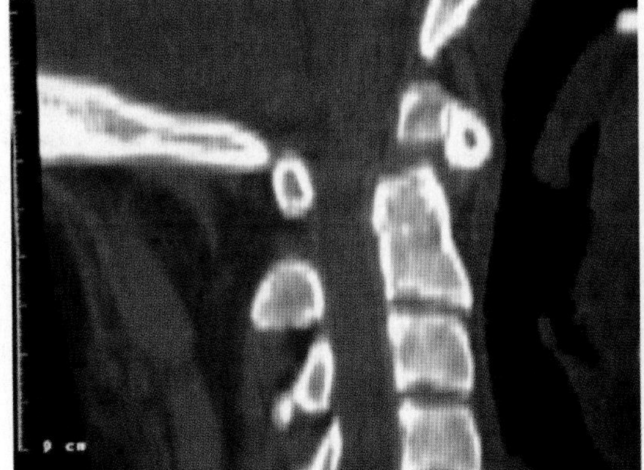

Reformatted sagittal CT scan of type II dens fracture

Plain radiograph of post C1–2 transarticular fixation and fusion

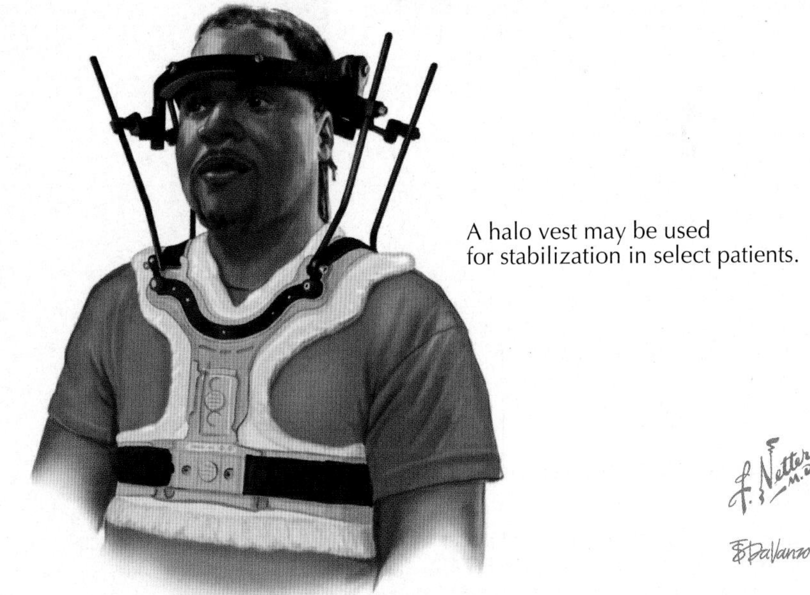

A halo vest may be used for stabilization in select patients.

From Jones HR, Srinivasan J, Allam GJ, Baker RA. Netter's Neurology. 2nd ed. Elsevier; 2011.

considerable clinical controversy. The benefit of surgical fixation is that it may greatly decrease the risk of nonunion, avoid cord compression that may occur as a sequela of nonunion, and possibly obviate the need for immobilization with an orthosis. However, surgical intervention must be weighed against the patient's comorbidities and the risks of surgical intervention. The alternative to surgery is a halo vest orthosis, which immobilizes the cervical spine to promote fracture healing. A well-described danger of halo vest immobilization is a high mortality rate observed with its use in elderly patients. These patients are at high risk for falls, and use of this device confers an even more morbid scenario should they fall and reinjure themselves. This has caused many surgeons to avoid the use of these devices in elderly patients. An alternative treatment regimen is a period of rigid collar immobilization followed by flexion and extension radiographs. A pain-free, radiographically stable fibrous union is an acceptable outcome in an elderly patient with substantial comorbidities. In patients deemed to be acceptable surgical candidates, type II dens fractures can be treated

Clinical Problems and Correlations of Craniovertebral Junction (Continued)

anteriorly with an odontoid screw or posteriorly with wiring techniques, transarticular screws, or segmental screw fixation across C1–C2. The type of surgical treatment is dependent on both fracture morphology and surgeon expertise.

Type III fractures extend into the cancellous, well-vascularized portion of the C2 body and portend a good prognosis. They tend to heal well with a cervical collar owing to the large contact area between the fracture surfaces.

JEFFERSON FRACTURE

A specific burst fracture pattern of the atlas is the eponymously named Jefferson fracture. A complete Jefferson fracture requires that the atlas be fractured at both the anterior and posterior arches bilaterally, disrupting the atlantooccipital and atlantoaxial articulations. The classic definition of a Jefferson fracture results in four distinct bone fragments, but variations with any number of fragments are common. This fracture type is a result of severe axial loading, which transmits stress from the skull to the lateral masses of the atlas. The lateral masses undergo some element of lateral distraction, and the axial forces are transmitted to the thin anterior and posterior arches of the atlas.

This fracture type is often seen in patients presenting after a dive into a shallow pool or who have been launched upward in a motor vehicle accident, striking their head on the car's roof. Patients are usually neurologically intact but may complain of neck pain. All patients should receive a CT scan on arrival in the emergency department after this type of trauma. Stable fractures generally have minimal displacement and can be treated in a brace. Unstable fractures are associated with greater displacement, and a halo vest orthosis or surgical intervention may be required.

HANGMAN'S FRACTURE AND FRACTURES OF THE AXIS

Classic hangman's fracture consists of bilateral fractures through the pars interarticularis of C2. Its namesake is a reference to the type of fractures once thought to contribute to the cause of death during judicial hangings. This type of fracture is now most commonly seen in motor vehicle accidents, where the head lurches forward past a restrained torso and then snaps abruptly backward when motion ceases. This hyperextension is likely the cause of the observed fracture pattern. Patients with this injury may complain of pain but most often are neurologically intact because this fracture effectively expands the spinal canal. Most of these patients can be treated with halo immobilization, although highly displaced or angulated fractures may require operative treatment. The fracture is generally associated with good, long-term outcome and recovery.

Jefferson and Hangman's Fractures

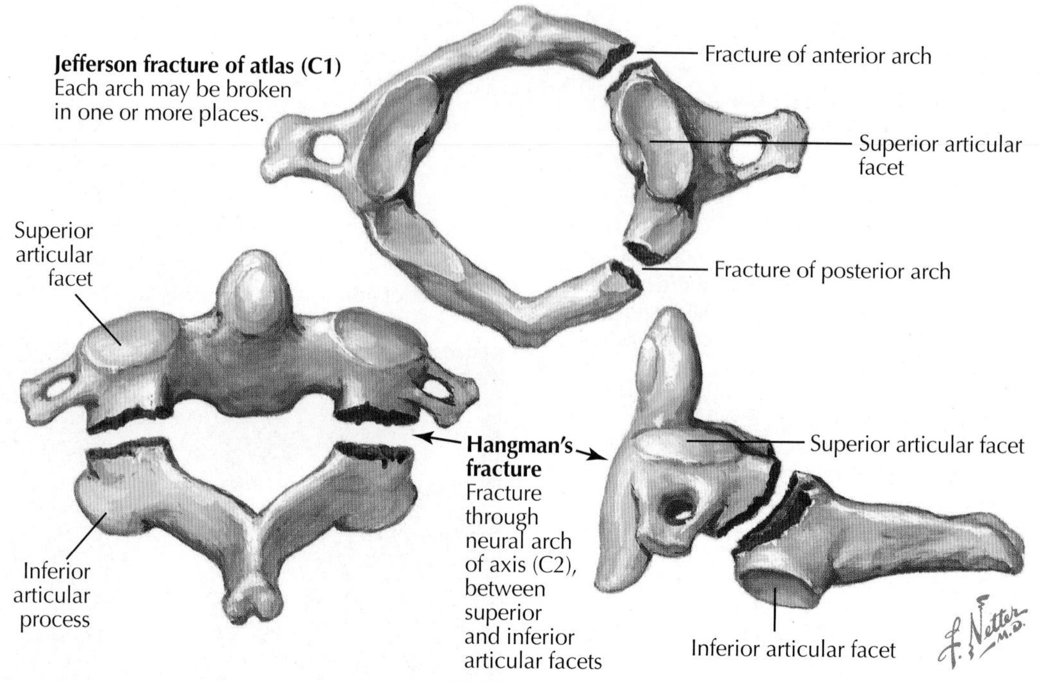

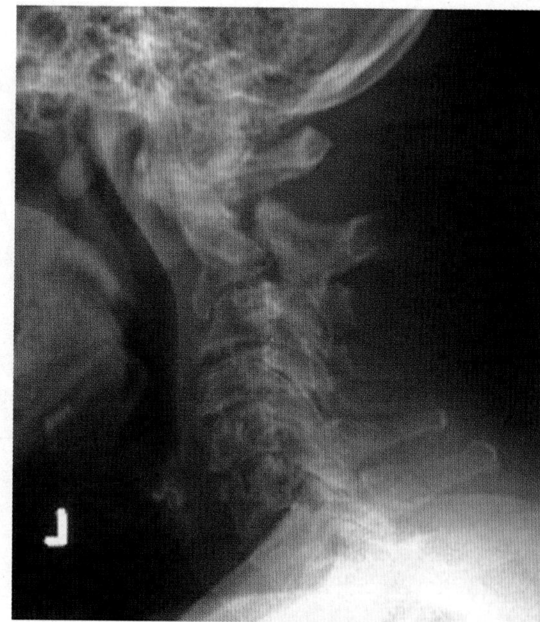

Hangman's fracture. *From Jones HR, Srinivasan J, Allam GJ, Baker RA. Netter's Neurology. 2nd ed. Elsevier; 2011.*

ATLANTOOCCIPITAL DISLOCATION

Sometimes morbidly referred to as "internal decapitation," atlantooccipital dislocation is a rare clinical entity remarkable for its change in reporting over the past several years. It does not have a strict, universally accepted definition, but it generally indicates that there is instability at the craniocervical junction that allows for an inappropriate amount of displacement or mobility of the occiput relative to the atlas. Atlantooccipital dislocation is a result of extremely high-energy trauma. These patients frequently present with serious trauma to other organ systems, including the chest and abdomen, and are often clinically unstable. Owing to the severity of the associated injuries, atlantooccipital dislocation was once thought to be fatal and usually found only at autopsy. With the advent of on-site intubation and maturation of support systems outside the hospital, atlantooccipital dislocation has become a much more recognized and treatable pathologic process. This is a highly unstable injury and requires prompt surgical treatment with instrumented occipital-cervical fusion.

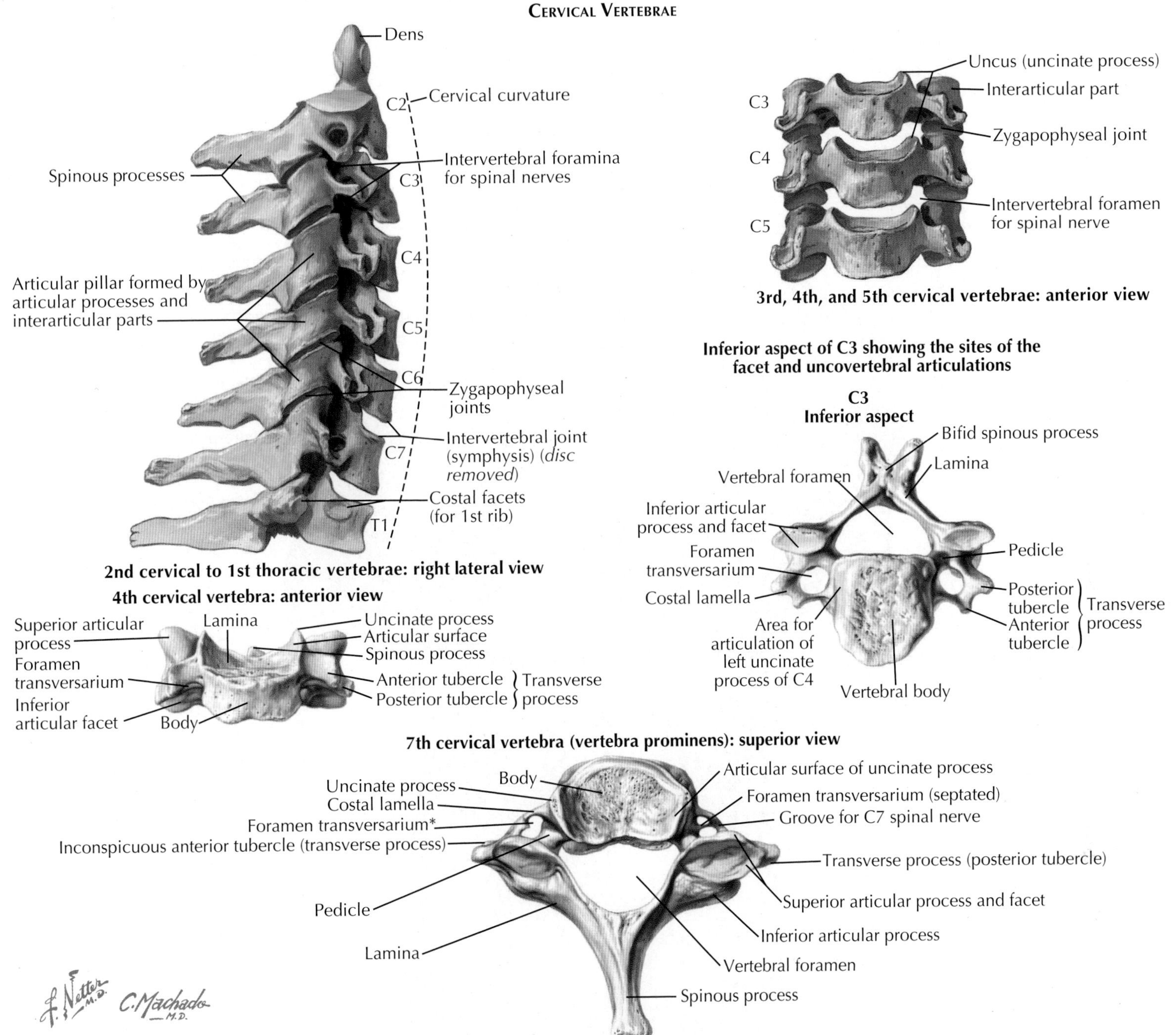

**The foramina transversaria of C7 transmit vertebral veins, but usually not the vertebral artery, and are asymmetric in this specimen.*

Anatomy of Subaxial Cervical Spine

BONY ANATOMY

The subaxial cervical spine consists of five cervical vertebrae. These vertebrae begin with C3 and end at C7. The overall balance of the cervical spine is slightly lordotic, which contributes to normal global sagittal alignment with the head appropriately aligned over the pelvis. This transition begins at the cervicothoracic junction, where the normal kyphosis of the thoracic spine gives way to the lordotic cervical spine. The cervical vertebrae have a common fundamental design but are unique from all other vertebral types owing to the presence of their transverse foramen and uncovertebral joints.

The subaxial cervical *vertebral bodies* are morphologically unique and smaller than those of the other movable vertebrae and increase in size caudally. The superior surfaces of the vertebral bodies are concave from side to side and slightly convex from front to back. The inferior surfaces are slightly curved. The lateral edges of the superior body are slightly raised, and the lower surfaces are beveled with small clefts. These clefts, which seem to articulate with the slightly raised lateral edges of the inferior vertebral body, are known as *uncovertebral joints,* although their actual function is unclear and they do not seem to be true joints. Surgically, they provide a marker for the lateral extent of decompression of the spinal cord and nerve roots during ventral surgery.

The *spinal canal* in the subaxial region is comparatively large to accommodate the cervical enlargement of the spinal cord; it is bound by the bodies, pedicles, and laminae of the vertebrae. The *pedicles* project posterolaterally from the bodies and are grooved by superior and inferior vertebral notches, almost equal in depth, which form the intervertebral foramina by connecting with similar notches on adjacent vertebrae. The medially directed *laminae* are thin and relatively long and fuse posteriorly to form short, bifid *spinous processes* (C3–C6). Projecting laterally from the junction of the pedicles and laminae are articular pillars supporting *superior* and *inferior articular facets.*

Each *transverse process* is pierced by a *foramen,* through which the vertebral artery passes. Foramina are bound by narrow bony bars ending in anterior and posterior tubercles; these are interconnected lateral to the foramen by the so-called *costotransverse bar.* Only the medial part of the posterior bar represents the true

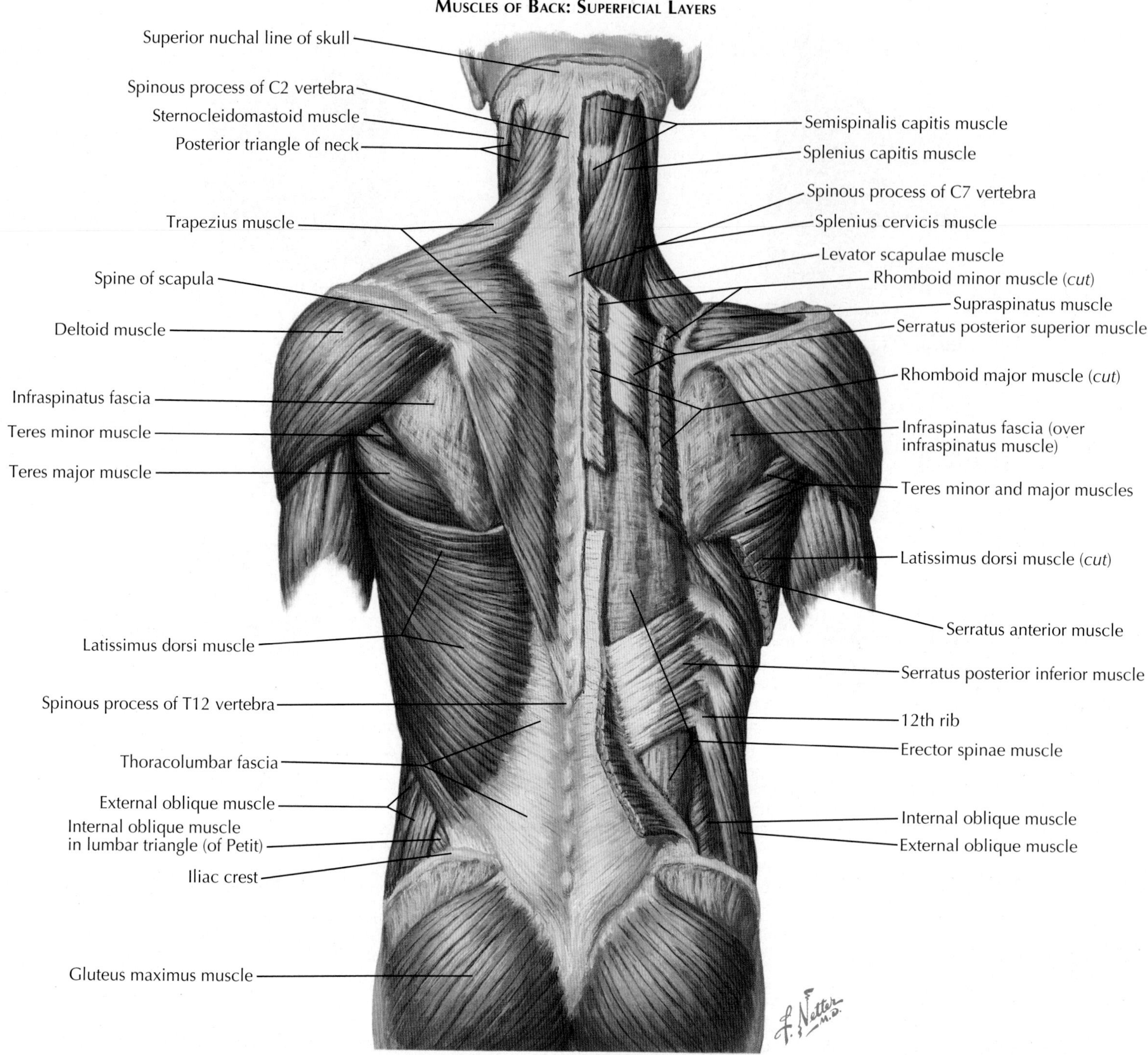

Anatomy of Subaxial Cervical Spine (Continued)

transverse process; the anterior and costotransverse bars and the lateral portion of the posterior bar constitute the costal element. If these elements overgrow in the lower subaxial spine, this can lead to the formation of cervical ribs. This occurs most commonly in the C6 and C7 levels. The upper surfaces of the costotransverse bars are grooved and lodge the anterior primary rami of the spinal nerves. The anterior tubercles of C6 are large and are termed *carotid tubercles* because the common carotid arteries lie just anteriorly and can be compressed against them. The dorsal facet joints formed from the inferior and superior articulating processes of adjacent vertebrae form the dorsum, or roof, of the neural foramina through which the spinal nerves exit the spinal column. Clinically, the foramen is very important because it is a common site of nerve root compression as people age. The surgically relevant borders of the foramen are the disc ventrally, the lateral dura medially, the inferior articular process dorsally, and the pedicle inferiorly.

The seventh cervical vertebra (C7) is called the *vertebra prominens,* because its spinous process is long and "proud" and ends in a tubercle that is easily palpable at the base of the neck.

Ligaments and Musculature

The splenius muscle serves as a strap, covering and holding in the deeper muscles of the back of the neck. It originates from the ligamentum nuchae and the spinous processes of C7 to T6. The muscle may be divided into two parts—the *splenius capitis muscle,* which inserts on the mastoid process and the lateral third of the superior nuchal line of the skull, and the *splenius cervicis muscle,* which terminates in the posterior tubercles of the first two or three cervical vertebrae. The cervicis portion is the outer and lower portion of the splenius muscle, and its inserting bundles curve deeply along its lateral margin.

The splenius muscle draws the head and neck backward and rotates the face toward the side of the muscle that is acting. Both sides contracting together act to extend the head and neck. The muscle is innervated by the lateral branches of the dorsal rami of the second to fifth or sixth cervical nerves. It lies directly under the trapezius and is covered by the nuchal fascia; its mastoid insertion is deep to that of the sternocleidomastoid, and it overlies the erector spinae and the

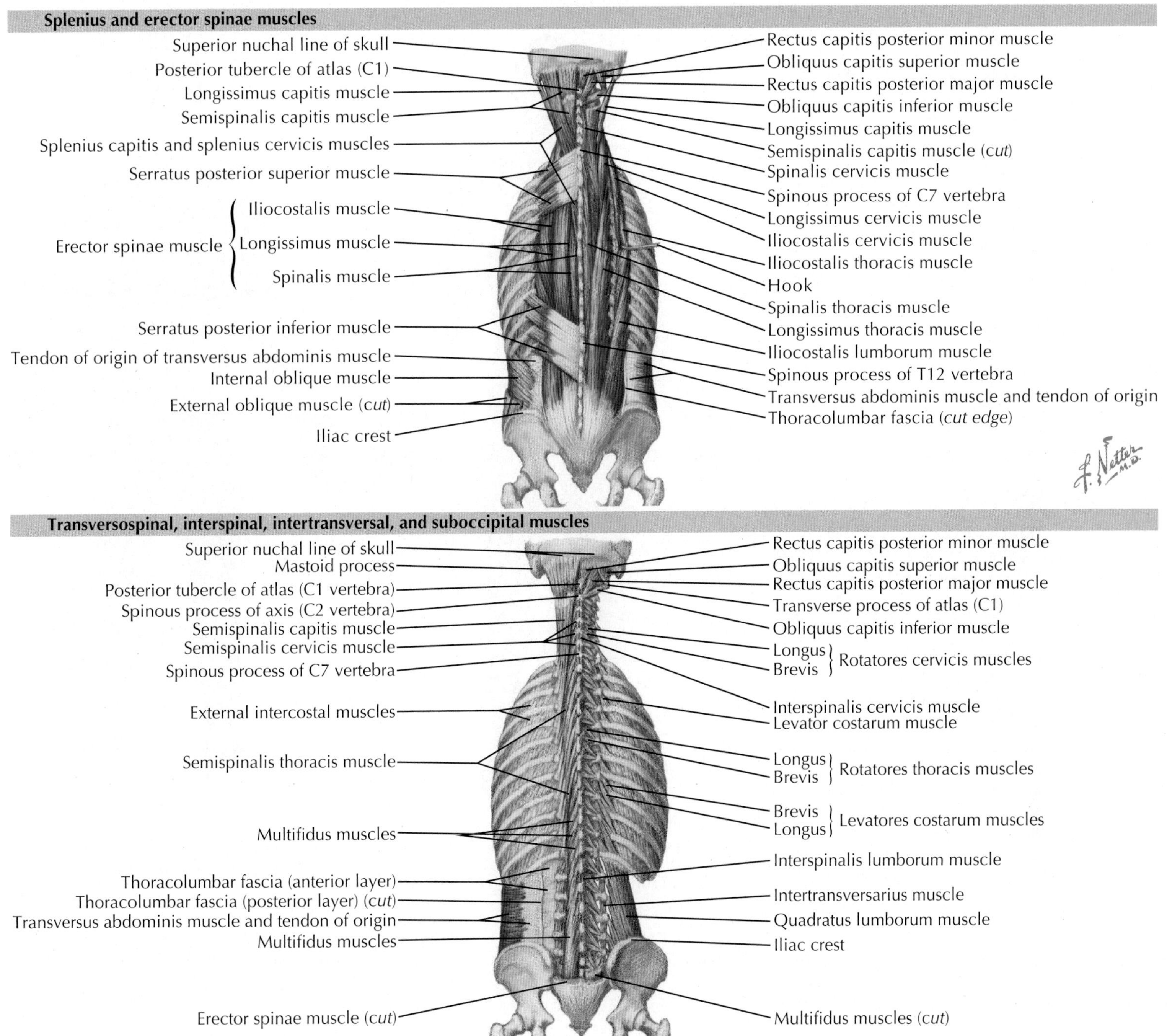

ANATOMY OF SUBAXIAL CERVICAL SPINE (Continued)

semispinalis. The longissimus cervicis muscle arises medial to the upper end of the longissimus thoracis, from the transverse processes of about the upper four to six thoracic vertebrae. Its slips of insertion end in the transverse processes of C2 to C6. The longissimus capitis muscle connects the articular processes of the lower four cervical vertebrae with the posterior margin of the mastoid process.

The spinalis cervicis muscle is frequently absent or poorly developed. When completely represented, it arises from the ligamentum nuchae and from the spinous processes of C7 and, perhaps, the upper thoracic vertebrae. Its insertion may reach the spinous processes of the axis and sometimes extends to the C3 and C4 vertebrae. The spinalis capitis muscle is not a separate muscle but is blended laterally with the semispinalis capitis.

The *ligamentum nuchae* is a fibroelastic membrane stretching from the external occipital protuberance and crest to the posterior tubercle of the atlas and the spinous processes of all the other cervical vertebrae. It provides areas for muscular attachments and forms a midline septum between the posterior cervical muscles. Previously thought to be of minimal biomechanical significance, the ligamentum nuchae now seems to play a role in the preservation of range of motion in humans. The *ligamentum flavum* is also known as the yellow ligament because of its high elastin content. This ligament acts to connect the laminae of adjacent vertebrae. As in the remainder of the spine, the *anterior longitudinal ligament* and *posterior longitudinal ligament* border the anterior and posterior components of the spinal canal, respectively.

NERVES

The cervical spinal nerves are similar in form and function to the nerves found in the other areas of the spine. The dorsal and ventral ramus combine to form the distal nerve, which then branches to provide sensory and motor function to its appropriate dermatome and myotome. What differs importantly is the numbering of spinal nerves. There are eight cervical nerves with only seven cervical vertebrae. This occurs because the first through seventh cervical nerves exist above the level of the corresponding vertebral body. As a result, the eighth cervical nerve exits below the C7 vertebra.

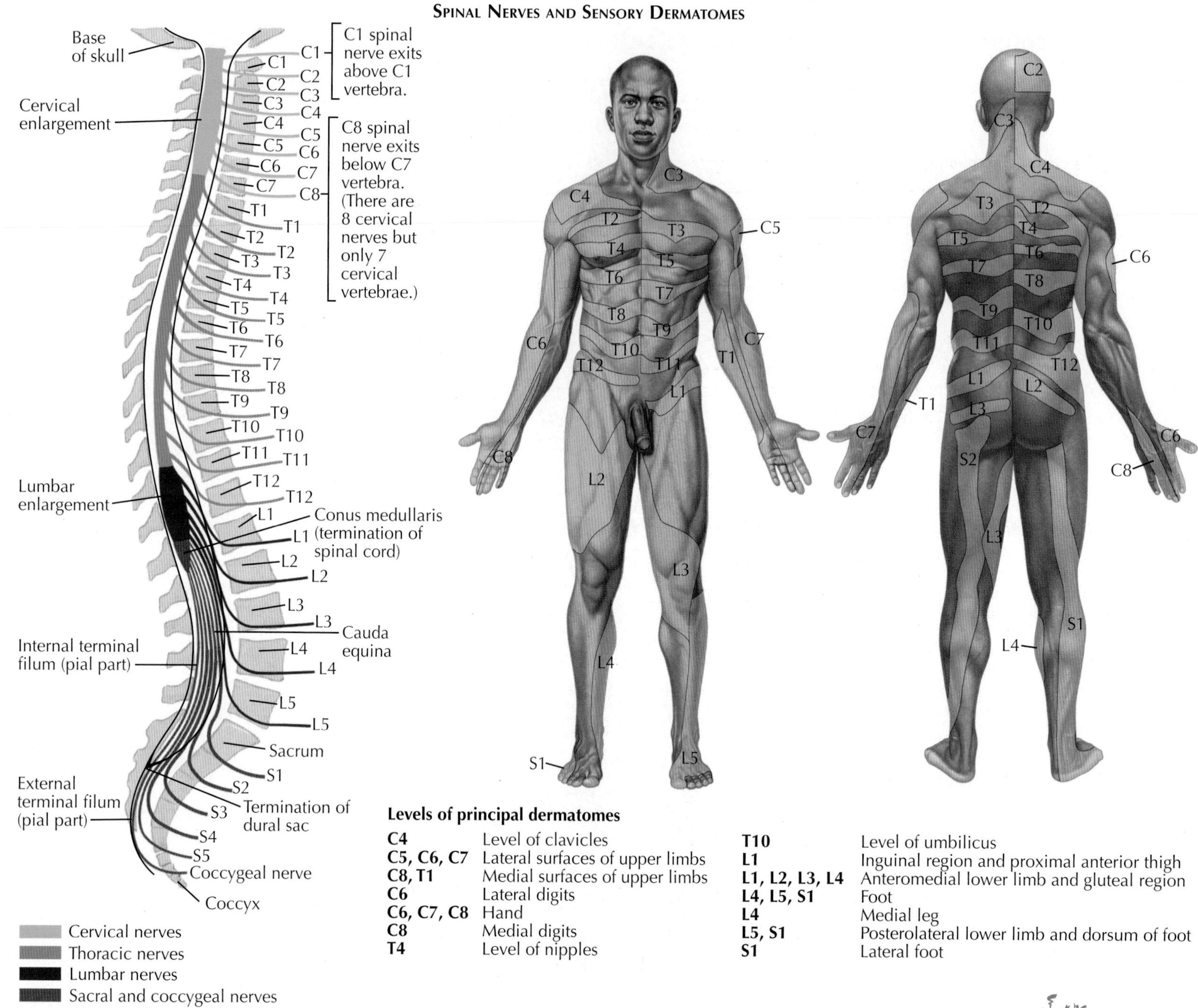

ANATOMY OF SUBAXIAL CERVICAL SPINE (Continued)

VASCULATURE

The vertebral artery enters the spine through the transverse foramen of C6 in approximately 90% of people. On the right it originates from the subclavian artery, and on the left it comes from the aortic arch; the arteries course upward into the craniovertebral junction. It is divided into four segments (V1–V4). The first (extraosseous) segment originates from its respective parent artery and ends at the transverse foramen of C6. The V2 (foraminal) segment consists of the vertebral artery as it lies within the transverse foramina from C6 to the atlas. The V3 (extraspinal) segment originates at the foramen of C1 and terminates as the vertebral artery pierces the dura at the level of the foramen magnum. The V4 (intradural) segment makes up the remainder of the vertebral artery until the two arteries unite in the midline of the brainstem at the junction of the pons and midbrain and create the basilar artery. In humans, one vertebral artery is almost always dominant, with 75% of individuals possessing a dominant left vertebral artery. The blood supply to the musculature and bones of the cervical spine is supplied through a series of innominate small vessels that originate from the subclavian artery, including the anterior spinal artery and posterior spinal artery.

It is critical that surgeons understand the potential for anomalous positions of the vertebral artery. The artery will enter the foramen transversarium at levels other than C6 in approximately 10% of people. This has implications for anterior surgical approaches to the cervical spine. The vertebral artery may also course through the lateral aspect of the vertebral body. This occurs in approximately 2.7% of people. It is critical that surgeons evaluate for these anomalies with a thorough preoperative review of advanced imaging (i.e., MRI or CT).

CLINICAL PROBLEMS AND CORRELATIONS OF SUBAXIAL CERVICAL SPINE

CERVICAL SPONDYLOSIS

Of all the pathologic processes found in the cervical spine, cervical spondylosis (degeneration) is the most common (see Plate 1.13). It can be found to some extent in all humans as we age. Spondylosis begins with the nucleus pulposus region of the intervertebral disc progressively losing the ability to maintain its water content (desiccation). Disc dehydration and other molecular changes to the disc composition result in a decrease in disc height. This increases stress forces on the annulus fibrosis. This diseased disc changes the normal biomechanics of the cervical spine leading to a variety of downstream effects. This cascade of events is termed the degenerative cascade. With biomechanic changes, there is an increased frequency of disc herniations into the spinal canal or cervical foramen. With altered bearing surfaces, secondary cervical spine deformities may result, often leading to flattening of the cervical spine and sometimes into an overt kyphotic position. As spondylosis progresses, osteophytes form ventrally and dorsally and the uncovertebral and facet joints hypertrophy. The longer this process continues, the larger the facets hypertrophy, eventually resulting in neural compression and symptoms to the patient. It is important to remember, however, that most people remain clinically asymptomatic during this process until a certain patient specific threshold is reached.

If the central canal is compressed, myelopathic symptoms will prevail. If the nerve root is primarily compressed, then radiculopathic symptoms will be evident. These entities can exist in isolation or in conjunction with each other in a syndrome termed *myeloradiculopathy*. The pathology of these entities is discussed next.

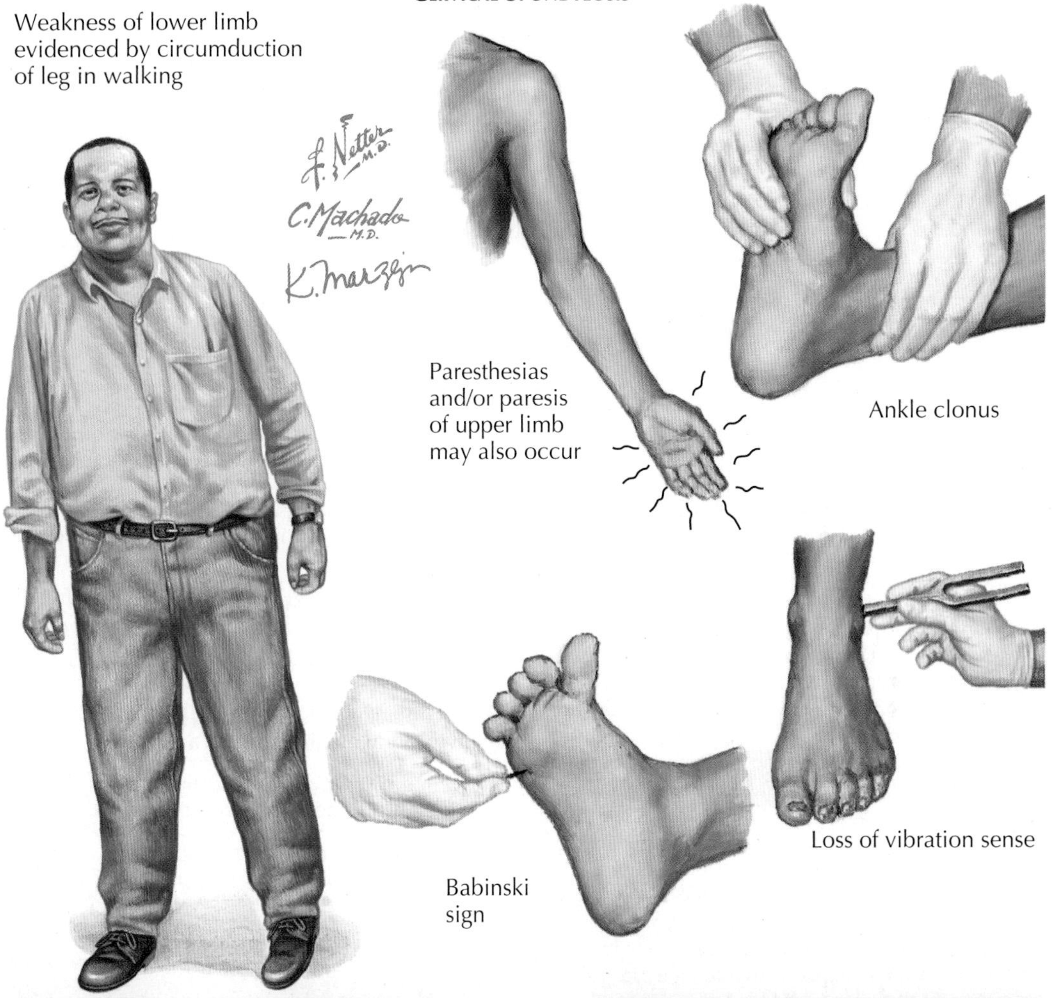

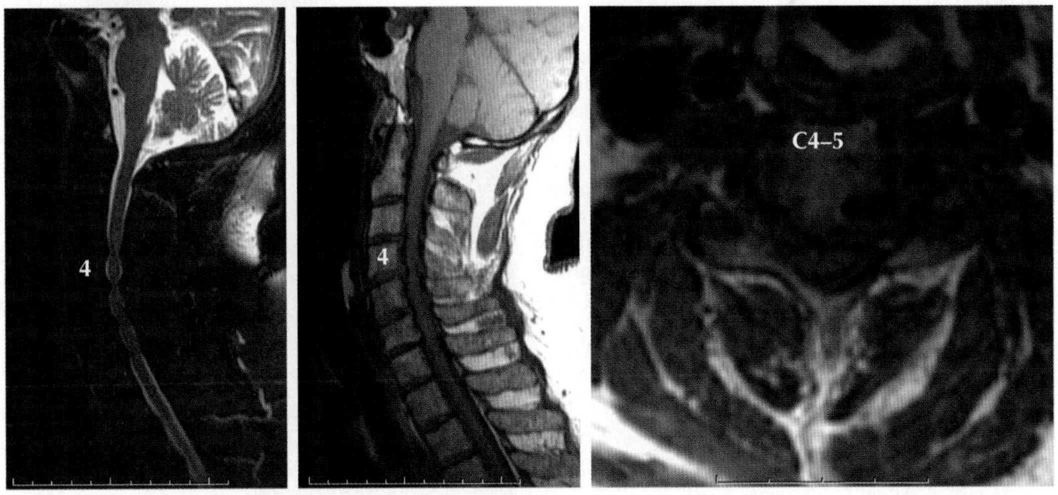

Left to right, T2-weighted sagittal, T1-weighted sagittal, and T1-weighted axial MR images showing degenerative disease with spinal cord compression. Idiopathic spinal stenosis with disc protrusion anteriorly and hypertrophy of ligamentum flavum posteriorly, most extreme at C4–5.

CERVICAL MYELOPATHY

Cervical myelopathy is a result of encroachment on the spinal cord (see Plate 1.13). As just described, the process of cervical spondylosis results in a loss of spinal canal space by several processes. The first is the propensity for cervical disc herniation, which is caused by disc degeneration but can be aggravated by thickening, or hypertrophy, of the posterior longitudinal ligament. The other cause is encroachment by osteophytic processes that result from the communication of vertebral bodies or uncinate joints that lack cervical disc buffering. Osteophyte formation is postulated to be a protective mechanism of the spine to increase the surface area of each vertebral body to better distribute the normal forces of daily activity. Cervical myelopathy may result from one or both of these processes. It is a relatively common clinical entity and has significant effects on a patient's quality of life. Additionally, preexisting myelopathy can significantly predispose a patient to serious spinal cord injury after only minor trauma.

Cervical myelopathy is a constellation of signs and symptoms resulting from spinal cord dysfunction. Patients with cervical myelopathy present a classic picture of upper motor neuron signs. They have difficulty with gait, balance, and fine motor coordination in the upper extremities, particularly in movements such as buttoning a shirt or tying one's shoes. Weakness and stiffness of the legs are common, and urinary symptoms of urgency or retention are also possible in later stages.

CERVICAL SPONDYLOSIS AND MYELOPATHY

Degenerative changes in the cervical spine (ankylosing spondylitis)

Atlas (C1)
Axis (C2)
C3 vertebral body (*sectioned in coronal plane*)
Complete transverse cleft in intervertebral disc
Uncovertebral joint with cleft formation
Spread of cleft formation into central portion of intervertebral disc with age leading to progressive degenerative changes in the disc
Deformed vertebral bodies and lipping of vertebral margins
Spondylophytes (osteophytes) on uncinate processes
Narrowing of intervertebral foramen
C7 vertebra
C. Machado — M.D.

Advanced ankylosing spondylitis with uncovertebral arthrosis in C4 and C5

Advanced spondylophyte (osteophyte) formation on uncinate processes
Uncovertebral joint fused due to extensive spondylophyte formation and ossification
Vertebral body
C4
C5
Potential for compression of vertebral artery within foramen transversarium
Superior articular process
Facet joint ossified due to advanced osteoarthritic change
Markedly narrowed intervertebral foramen may lead to compression of spinal nerve
Inferior articular process with facet
Groove for spinal nerve on transverse process
Spinous process

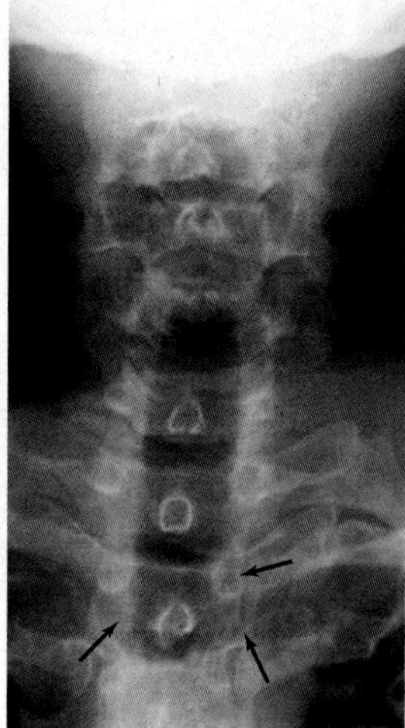

Radiograph showing stenosis secondary to cervical spondylosis and bridging of vertebral bodies by osteophytes

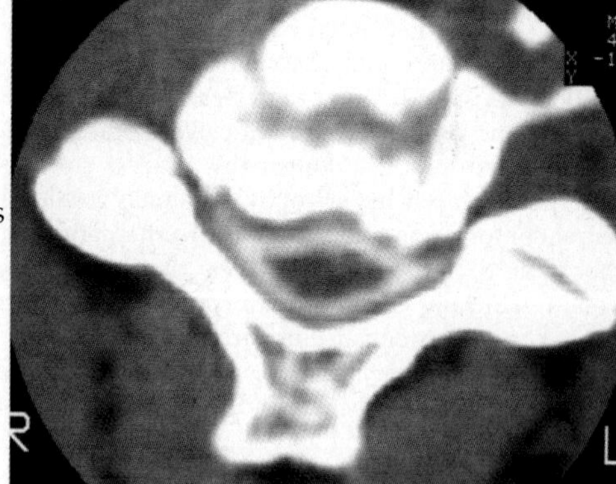

Metrizamide myelogram with CT scan showing spinal cord compression secondary to severe cervical spondylosis

CLINICAL PROBLEMS AND CORRELATIONS OF SUBAXIAL CERVICAL SPINE (Continued)

On examination, patients frequently have hyperactive reflexes below the level of the spinal cord compression (generally exacerbated in the lower extremities) and may demonstrate pathologic signs of the corticospinal tracts. Two common exam signs in patients presenting with cervical myelopathy are the Hoffman and Babinski reflexes. In brief, the Hoffman reflex is a pathologic flexion and adduction of the thumb and index finger when the middle finger is flicked down. Similarly, the Babinski reflex is a pathologic extension of the great toe after the lateral plantar aspect of the foot has been stroked forcefully enough to stimulate the nociceptive fibers of the foot. Motor testing may demonstrate weakness in any of the upper extremity muscle groups, depending on the severity and level of spinal cord compression. In advanced disease, the intrinsic muscles of the hand demonstrate impressive wasting ("myelopathy hand"). Lower extremity strength is variable, with proximal muscle weakness being more common than distal muscle weakness. Examination of gait is a valuable clinical tool because patients with myelopathy often exhibit a stiff, spastic, or wide-based gait. The clinical phenomenon of *central cord syndrome* generally occurs when a patient with preexisting myelopathy sustains a hyperextension injury. These patients present acutely with upper greater than lower extremity weakness and sensory changes below the level of their injury. Urinary or fecal incontinence may also be present. The prognosis for central cord syndrome is favorable, especially in younger patients.

Observation of these signs and symptoms warrants MRI of the cervical spine and referral to a spine surgeon. A thorough imaging evaluation with radiographs and MRI provides adequate assessment of spinal alignment and the location(s), pattern, and degree of neural compression. Cervical myelopathy is a surgical disease in the majority of patients because it is usually progressive and, as such, neurologic deterioration may be permanent. The natural history of cervical myelopathy is periods of disease stability with intermittent, stepwise decreases in function. The goal of surgery is to halt disease progression, although some degree of functional recovery is often observed postoperatively.

CERVICAL RADICULOPATHY

When a cervical nerve root is inflamed or impinged at the level of the cervical foramen, cervical radiculopathy may occur. It most commonly occurs as a result of disc herniation in the younger patient or from nerve root compression due to cervical spondylotic changes. Compression of the nerve root can result in pain, weakness, or sensory deficits that correspond to the dermatomal and myotomal distribution of the nerve itself.

Patients may present with acute or chronic cervical radiculopathy due to isolated nerve root compression. Patients with existing cervical myelopathy may also have a radicular pain component, termed *cervical myeloradiculopathy.* More than 90% of patients with cervical radiculopathy improve with nonoperative care. Examination of a patient with cervical radiculopathy includes a typical motor and sensory examination but also maneuvers intended to compress the nerve root or to relieve tension on the root and exacerbate or alleviate symptoms. This may include the shoulder abduction sign, in which the examiner holds the patient's hand

CERVICAL DISC HERNIATION: CLINICAL MANIFESTATIONS

Herniated disc compressing nerve root

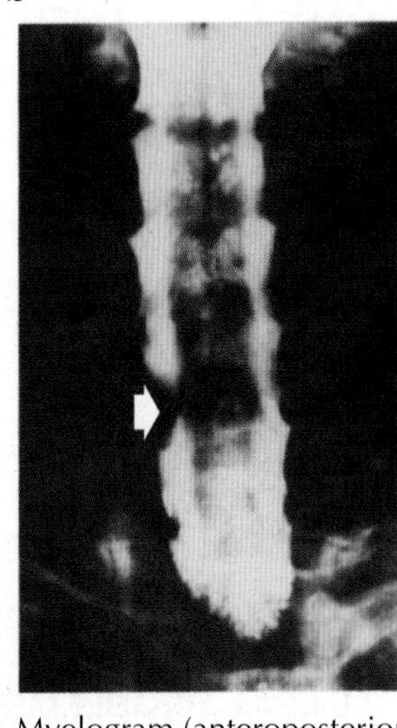

Myelogram (anteroposterior view) showing prominent extradural defect (open arrow) at C6–7

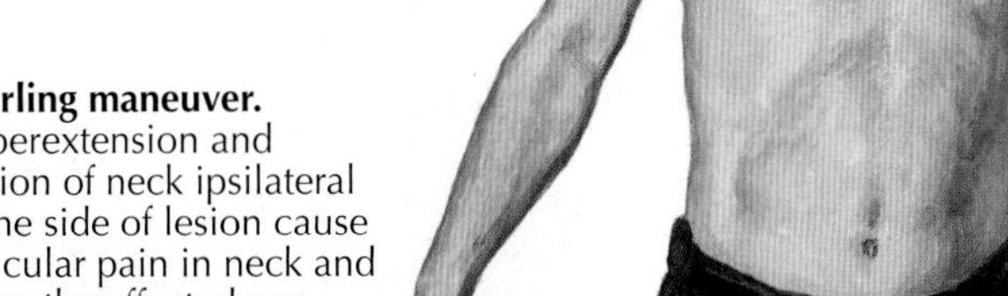

Spurling maneuver. Hyperextension and flexion of neck ipsilateral to the side of lesion cause radicular pain in neck and down the affected arm.

Level	Motor signs (weakness)	Reflex signs	Sensory loss
C5	Deltoid	0	
C6	Biceps brachii	Biceps brachii Weak or absent reflex	
C7	Triceps brachii	Triceps brachii Weak or absent reflex	
C8	Interossei	0	

CLINICAL PROBLEMS AND CORRELATIONS OF SUBAXIAL CERVICAL SPINE (Continued)

over the head to alleviate symptoms. The Spurling maneuver is a provocative test in which the head of the patient is turned to the side of the symptoms and axial pressure is then applied by the examiner. This is thought to narrow the intervertebral foramen and exacerbate the patient's symptoms. A "positive" Spurling sign is exacerbation of arm pain. It has been found to be very sensitive but not specific for radiculopathy. Observation of the patient in late stages of the disease may demonstrate wasting of the intrinsic hand muscles if one of the lower cervical nerves is involved, but, unlike in cervical spondylotic myelopathy, the findings are unilateral.

Diagnosis of cervical radiculopathy is aided by a thorough review of plain radiographs (including oblique views), MR images, or a CT myelogram of the cervical spine. It allows appropriate visualization of the cervical discs and nerve roots and aids the clinician in preoperative decision-making.

SURGICAL APPROACHES FOR THE TREATMENT OF MYELOPATHY AND RADICULOPATHY

The decision to employ surgery for cervical myelopathy or radiculopathy requires a high degree of consideration of its risks, benefits, and preference of the patient. Surgical treatment of cervical myelopathy is less controversial given its positive effect on a patient's quality of life and the well-known benefits of spinal cord decompression. The treatment of cervical radiculopathy depends on the etiology (disc herniation or foraminal narrowing) and on the number of affected nerve roots. Complicating the surgical approach is that these conditions often occur together, so surgery may be aimed at alleviating both myelopathy and radiculopathy in a single operation. An important distinction to remember between radiculopathy and myelopathy is the former is typically a nonoperative disease, whereas the latter is a surgical one. That is, radiculopathy usually responds very favorably to nonoperative care.

Anterior Approach to the Cervical Spine

One of the most common spine surgeries performed is the anterior cervical discectomy and fusion. Patients who have degenerative changes of the spine involving mainly the ventral aspect of the spinal cord or nerve root(s) are likely to benefit from this procedure. The surgery involves an incision just lateral to the midline of the neck, and a dissection lateral to the trachea and medial to the carotid sheath of the neck to approach the anterior cervical spine. From there, the prevertebral fascia is incised, and the intervertebral disc is exposed and removed, as is the posterior longitudinal ligament. This exposes the ventral dura and exiting roots. This may be performed at one or multiple levels in the spine. An intervertebral graft (tricortical iliac crest autograft, cadaveric allograft, or synthetic cage) is used to replace the intervertebral disc to facilitate fusion of the adjacent vertebrae. The addition of an anterior cervical plate improves fusion rates and prevents graft dislodgment. Another option for ventral treatment of both radiculopathy and myelopathy is cervical disc replacement,

Clinical Problems and Correlations of Subaxial Cervical Spine (Continued)

which uses the same approach to the spinal column but acts to preserve motion rather than fuse the regions of the spine. Cervical corpectomy (removal of the central vertebral body) is indicated for spinal cord compression occurring behind the vertebral body or in cases of osteomyelitis or tumor.

Posterior Approaches to the Cervical Spine

For select patients with myelopathy or myeloradiculopathy, decompressive posterior surgery may be appropriate. Two common procedures are laminectomy with instrumented fusion and laminoplasty of the cervical spine. In both procedures, a midline incision is made in the neck and the overlying muscles are dissected from bone to expose the spinous processes and laminae. The laminae and spinous processes are either removed (laminectomy) or are altered to expand the cervical spinal canal (laminoplasty). There are multiple laminoplasty techniques, and their discussion is beyond the scope of this chapter.

Radiculopathy can often be treated posteriorly via a decompression of the foramen and lamina (laminoforaminotomy). These procedures are typically attempted at one or two levels, are performed unilaterally, and may offer significant symptomatic improvement to the appropriately selected patient.

VERTEBRAL ARTERY DISSECTION

Like all arteries, the vertebral artery consists of an intima, media, and adventitia. Whereas the term *dissection* is often applied to any vertebral artery injury, there exists a gradient of damage that is observed. A small intimal tear, for example, may have minimal, if any, clinical consequences. A true dissection of the vertebral artery refers to the creation of a tear through the intima, allowing blood to enter the arterial wall. The arterial pulsations result in a growing amount of blood in the arterial wall and lead to thrombosis. If blood ruptures through the wall entirely, a hematoma is created. This is known as a pseudoaneurysm, which may also be catastrophic if the lumen becomes occluded. The furthest end of the spectrum is vertebral artery transection, which is frequently fatal regardless of which vertebral artery is affected.

The vertebral artery is well protected by the transverse foramina between C6 and C1. This bony protection comes at a cost: whereas the bony ring of the transverse foramen prevents injury of the artery during low-energy trauma, fracture of the transverse foramen from a high-energy mechanism places the vertebral artery at risk of injury from bony impingement. The majority of patients found to have a vertebral artery dissection after blunt trauma have associated cervical spine trauma. Nontraumatic dissections are often spontaneous.

Much attention is paid to rare, but nonetheless important, causes of vertebral artery injury. These include chiropractic manipulation, contact sports, and yoga. There are several anatomic considerations that make these events more likely to occur. First, the vertebral artery is relatively susceptible to different forces at two points during its course. The first is between the atlas and the axis, where high rotary potential allows for the possibility that a forced, high-energy, high-velocity

Surgical Approaches for the Treatment of Myelopathy and Radiculopathy

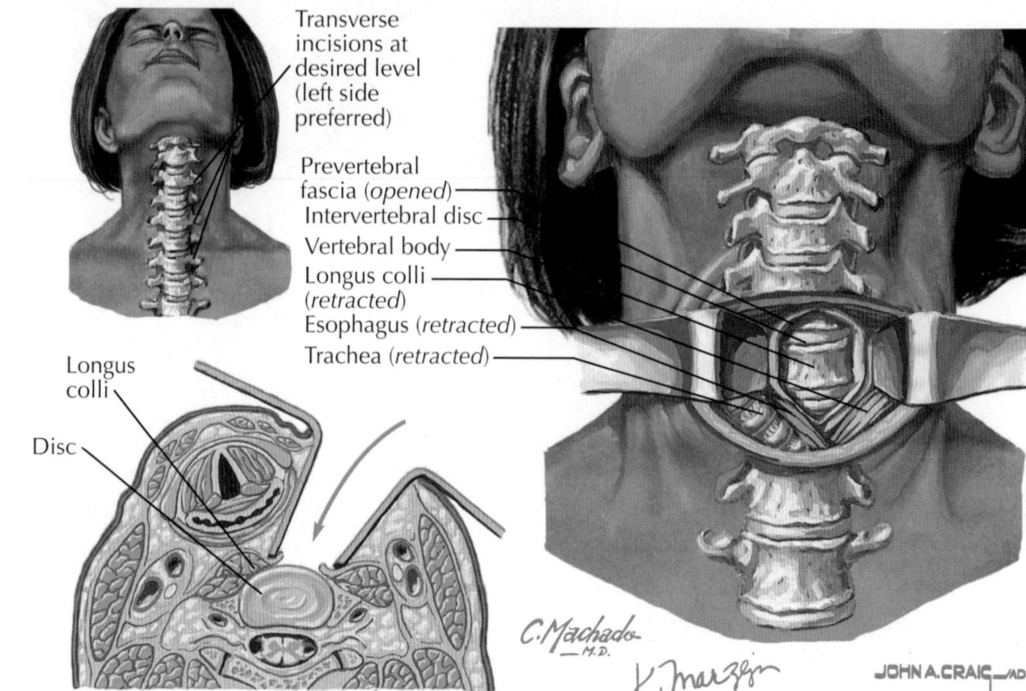

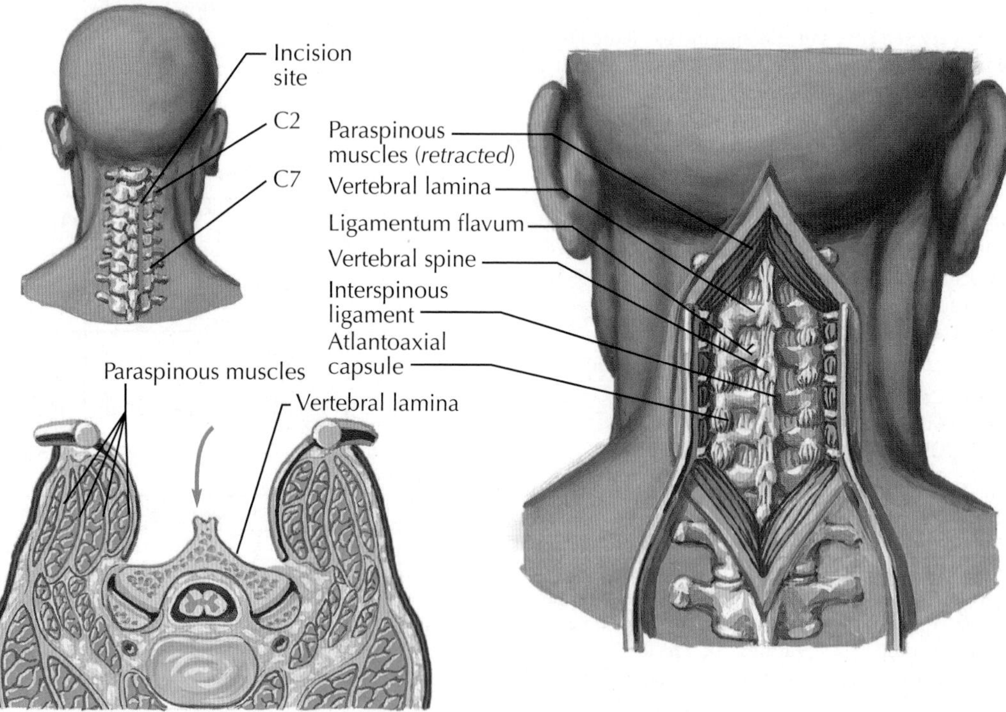

Extravascular Compression of Vertebral Arteries

When head is turned sharply to right, rotation of atlas causes sharp angulation of left vertebral artery resulting in obstruction of lumen.

When head is returned to neutral position, sharp angulation of artery disappears; vessel fills normally.

Osteophytes at the C5–6 level displace and compress right vertebral artery. Such spondylotic compression of vertebral arteries is not likely to produce symptoms unless the collateral flow is inadequate and/or the compression is aggravated by turning the head.

Clinical Problems and Correlations of Subaxial Cervical Spine (Continued)

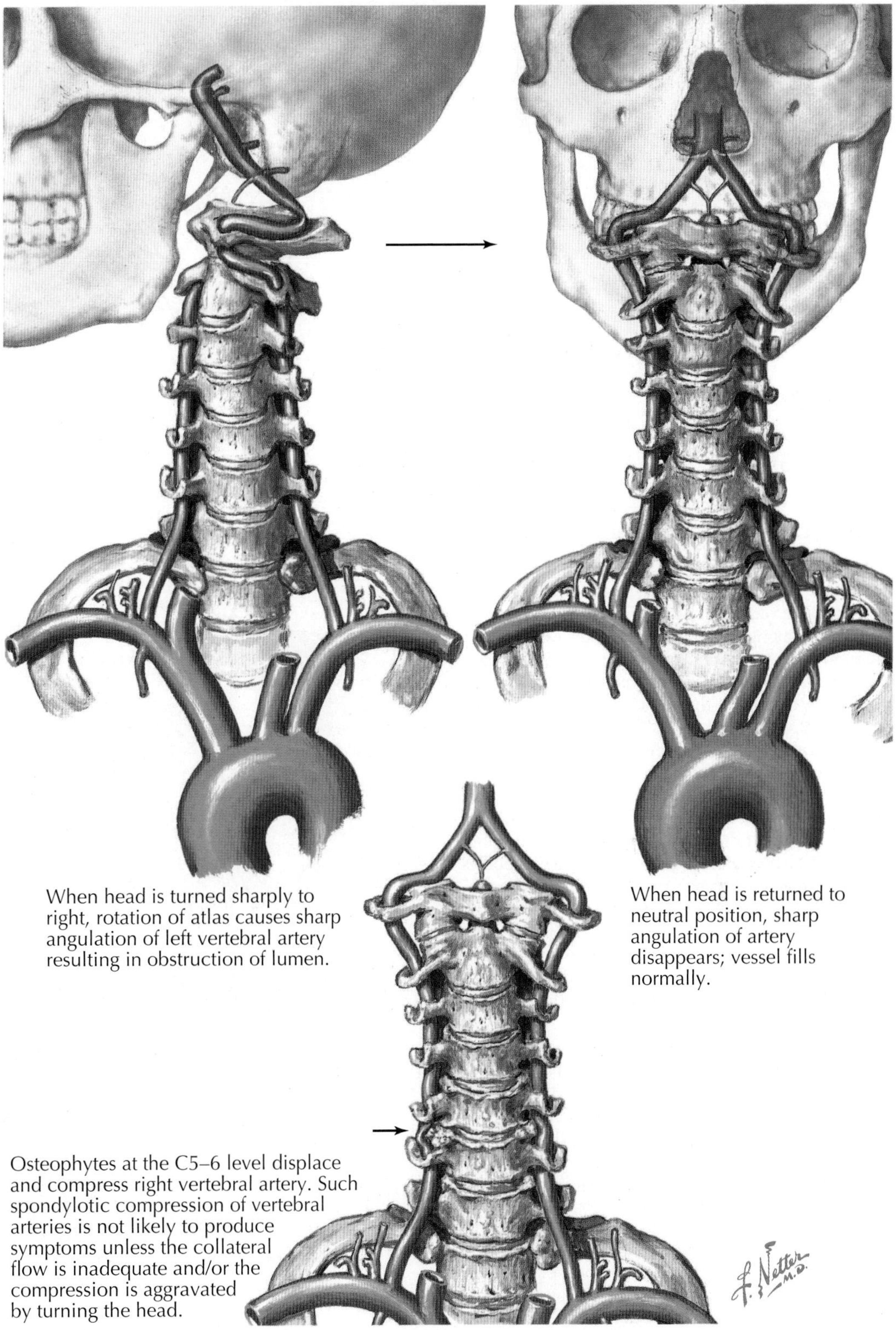

rotation may cause damage. This is what may occur during certain chiropractic manipulations. The other site is at the extraosseous (V3) segment where the vertebral artery lies in the sulcus arteriosus before piercing the dura on its course to the brain. At this level, the vertebral artery is truly unprotected by major bony landmarks, and activities causing prolonged hyperextension may result in vertebral artery damage.

The effects of vertebral artery dissection are related to the neurologic structures that it sustains, and damage can occur via several mechanisms. Dissection or embolism can cause occlusion or diminished flow to the posterior circulation, creating vertebrobasilar insufficiency. Clinically, dizziness, ataxia, altered level of consciousness, and visual changes may be observed. Rarely, blood supply to the anterior spinal cord may be compromised if the anterior spinal artery (which arises from the vertebral artery) is affected. If the damaged vertebral artery is anomalous and feeds the posterior inferior cerebellar artery without joining to form the basilar artery, then lateral medullary syndrome (Wallenberg syndrome) can result. A constellation of symptoms results, including an ipsilateral Horner syndrome, facial numbness, and cerebellar deficits, as well as contralateral numbness below the neck.

If a vertebral artery dissection is suspected, the gold standard diagnostic tool is the angiogram. If angiography is unavailable or not clinically advisable, a CT angiogram may be obtained. The treatment of a dissection ranges from medical treatment alone with anticoagulation and blood pressure support to endovascular stenting or surgical intervention depending on the type and severity of the pathologic process.

LOCKED FACETS

Locked facets (also known as "jumped facets") are the result of spinal trauma and can occur unilaterally or bilaterally. This occurs when the inferior articulating process of the cranial vertebrae becomes locked ventral to the superior articular process of the caudal vertebrae. The consequences of this distinction are significant because the resultant differences in treatment and outcomes diverge greatly. Bilateral locked facets are the result of traumatic hyperflexion injuries, and a majority of those patients presenting with bilateral locked facets are quadriplegic. Those with incomplete spinal cord injury have some potential for recovery, but the overall prognosis remains poor. There exists debate as to whether reduction should be undertaken closed (with traction) or open (using pins to distract the spine intraoperatively before surgical fixation). Unilateral locked facets are also the result of hyperflexion, but a component of rotational subluxation occurs. Clinically these patients tend to present with their heads deviated away from the side of injury. Because these are unilateral injuries, patients often are noted to have less severe neurologic injuries. Depending on the concurrent fractures present in the spine, these patients may undergo closed reduction and stabilization with a high rate of success.

Thoracic Vertebrae and Ligaments

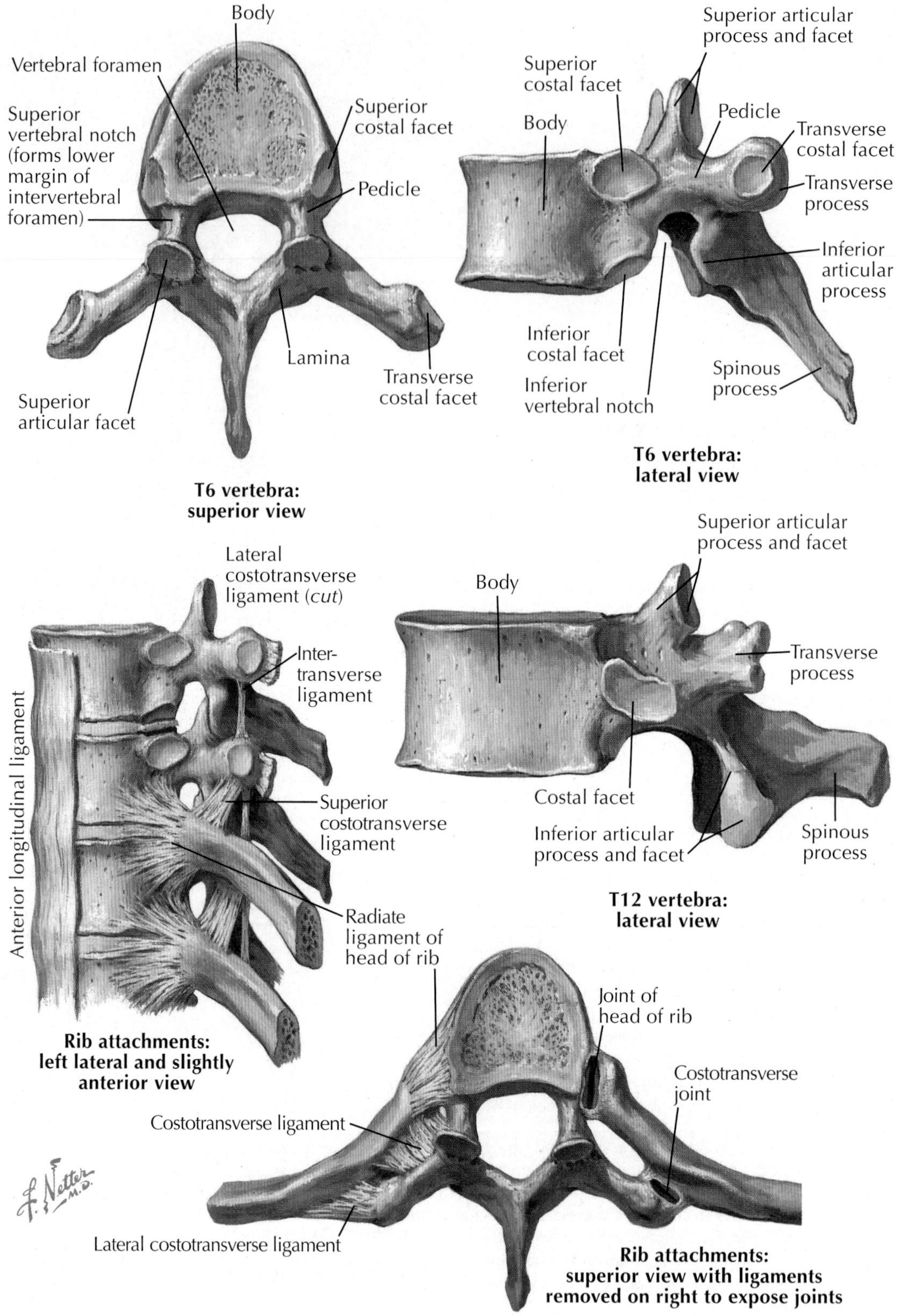

T6 vertebra: superior view

T6 vertebra: lateral view

Rib attachments: left lateral and slightly anterior view

T12 vertebra: lateral view

Rib attachments: superior view with ligaments removed on right to expose joints

Anatomy of the Thoracolumbar and Sacral Spine

THORACIC VERTEBRAE AND LIGAMENTS

The 12 thoracic vertebrae (T1–T12) are intermediate in size between the smaller cervical and the larger lumbar vertebrae. The vertebral bodies are slightly taller posteriorly than anteriorly, producing a slight wedge shape and producing a natural kyphotic curve in the thoracic spine. Vertebrae are easily recognized by their costal facets on both sides of the bodies and on all the transverse processes except those of T11 and T12. The costal facets articulate with the facets on the heads and tubercles of the corresponding ribs. The spinal canal is narrower and more rounded than in the cervical spine and corresponds to the more circular shape of the spinal cord in the thoracic region. The spinal canal is formed by the posterior surfaces of the vertebral bodies anteriorly, the medial aspect of the pedicles laterally, and the anterior aspect of the lamina posteriorly. The stout pedicles are directed posterolaterally from the vertebral bodies; they have shallow superior and much deeper inferior vertebral notches. The laminae are short and relatively thick, and they partially overlap, creating a shingled appearance.

The typical thoracic superior articular processes project upward from the junction of the pedicles and the laminae, facing posteriorly and slightly upward and outward. The inferior articular processes project downward from the anterior parts of the laminae, and their facets face forward and slightly downward and inward, mirroring the superior articular process.

Thoracic spinous processes are typically long and project inferiorly and posteriorly, with the exception of the upper and lower thoracic spinous processes, which take on a horizontal course. The transverse processes, which form at the junction of the pedicle and laminae, are also relatively long and extend posterolaterally. Except for the lowest two (or occasionally three) thoracic vertebrae, the transverse processes have small oval facets on the anterolateral aspect that articulate with similar facets on their corresponding rib tubercles, creating the costotransverse joint.

Each adjacent vertebral component is connected by an associated soft tissue structure as follows: vertebral bodies via intervertebral discs and anterior and posterior longitudinal ligaments, transverse processes via intertransverse ligaments, laminae via ligamentum flavum, and spinous processes via supraspinous and interspinous ligaments. Finally, the facet joints are formed by adjacent vertebrae's superior and inferior articular processes (i.e., such that the inferior articular process of T1 forms a facet joint with the superior articular process of T2). These facets are synovial joints that are covered by a fibrous articular capsule.

Costovertebral Joints

The ribs are connected to the vertebral bodies and the transverse processes by various ligaments. The costovertebral joints, between the vertebral bodies and the rib heads, have articular capsules. The second to tenth costal heads, each of which articulates with two vertebrae, are also connected to the corresponding vertebral discs by interarticular ligaments. Radiate (stellate) ligaments unite the anterior aspects of the rib heads with the sides of the vertebral bodies above and below the discs. The rib head articulates with both the superior border of its corresponding vertebra and the inferior border of the vertebra above (i.e., the ninth rib articulates with the vertebral bodies of both T8 and T9). The

Lumbar Vertebrae and Intervertebral Discs

Intervertebral disc

L2 vertebra: superior view

Lumbar vertebrae, assembled: left lateral view

L3 and L4 vertebrae: posterior view

ANATOMY OF THE THORACOLUMBAR AND SACRAL SPINE (Continued)

costotransverse joints between the facets on the transverse processes and on the tubercles of the ribs are also surrounded by articular capsules. They are reinforced by several ligaments, including a (middle) costotransverse ligament between the rib neck and transverse process of the vertebra above and a lateral costotransverse ligament interconnecting the end of a transverse process with the nonarticular part of the related costal tubercle.

LUMBAR VERTEBRAE AND INTERVERTEBRAL DISCS

The five lumbar vertebrae (L1–L5) are the largest separate vertebrae and are distinguished by the absence of costal facets. The vertebral bodies are wider in the medial to lateral aspect than from anterior to posterior, with superior and inferior surfaces that are concave and almost parallel, except in the case of the fifth vertebral body, which is slightly wedge shaped. The vertebral foramina are pear shaped and are formed by the superior and inferior pedicle. The pedicles are short and strong, arising from the upper and posterolateral aspects of the vertebral bodies. The pedicles of the inferior lumbar spine (L4–L5) are more medially oriented than the pedicles of the upper lumber spine. The laminae are short, broad plates that meet in the middle to form nearly horizontal spinous processes that are perpendicular to the lamina. The craniocaudal (or superior to inferior) intervals between adjacent laminae and spinous processes, referred to as the interlaminar spaces, are larger than in the cervical and thoracic spine.

As in the cervical and thoracic spines, the facet joints are formed from the superior and inferior articular processes of adjacent vertebrae. These processes respectively project superiorly and inferiorly from the area between the pedicles and laminae. The facet joints are in a relatively sagittal orientation, which allows for flexion and extension motion but little rotation. The portion of bone that connects the superior and inferior articular processes of a single vertebra is known as the pars interarticularis. The transverse processes of L1 to L3 are long and slender, whereas those of L4 and L5 are more pyramidal. Near the base of each transverse process are small accessory processes; small, rounded mammillary processes protrude from the posterior margins of the superior articular processes.

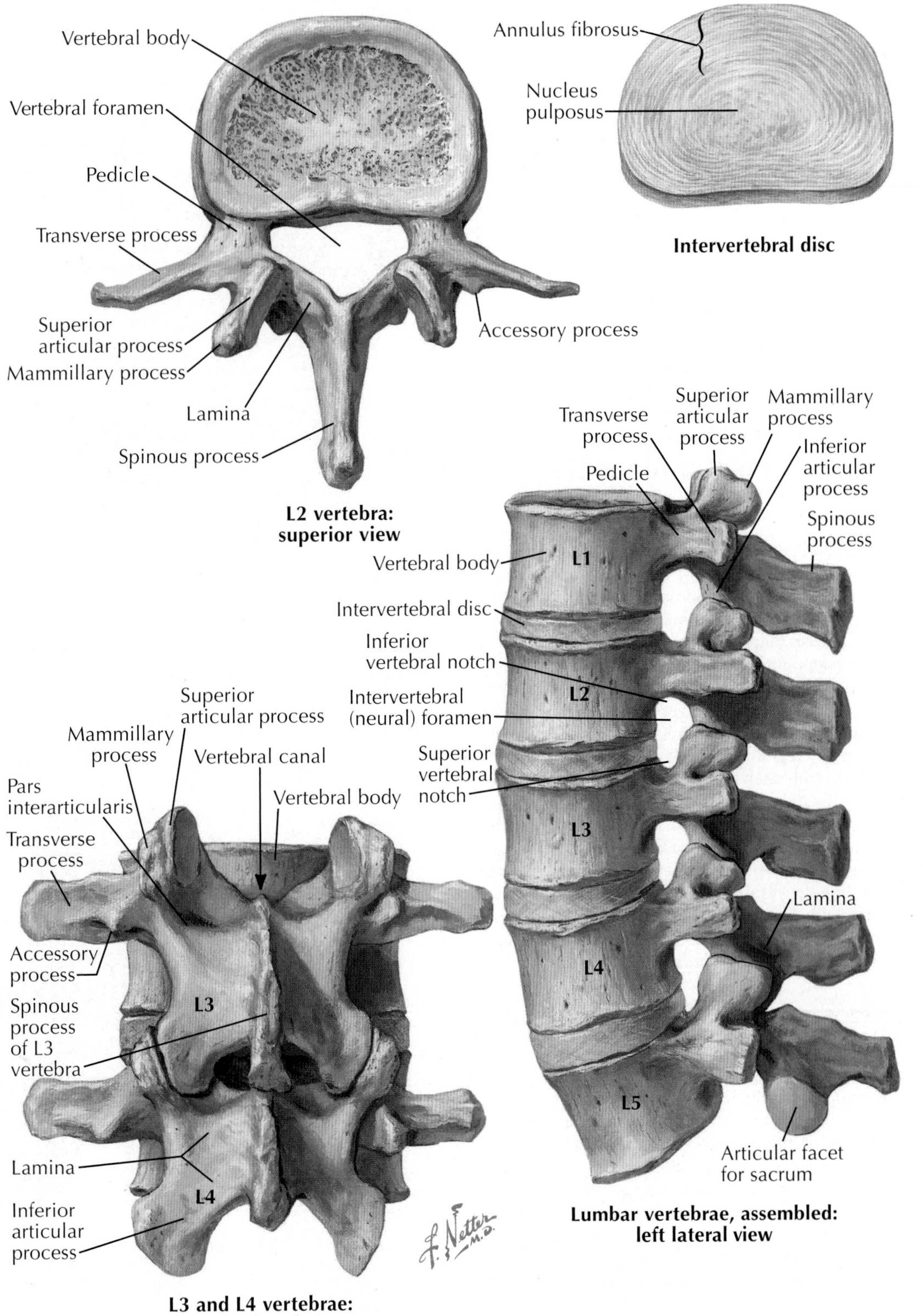

The fifth lumbar vertebra is atypical. It is the largest vertebra in the lumbar spine, with the anterior aspect of the vertebral body having greater height than the posterior aspect. This creates a wedge-shaped vertebral body that contributes to the significant lordotic curve formed in the lumbosacral spine. The L5 inferior articular processes face almost forward and are set more widely apart, and the roots of their thick transverse processes are continuous with the entire lateral surfaces of the pedicles.

Intervertebral Discs

Interposed between the adjacent vertebral bodies are intervertebral discs. These are immensely strong fibrocartilaginous structures that provide powerful bonds between vertebrae and act to buffer axial loads. The discs consist of outer concentric layers of fibrous tissue, the annulus fibrosus. The fibers in adjacent layers of the annulus are arranged obliquely but in opposite directions to resist torsion. The annulus fibrosus contains a central elastic and pulpy zone called the nucleus pulposus. The

ANATOMY OF THE THORACOLUMBAR AND SACRAL SPINE (Continued)

SACRAL SPINE AND PELVIS

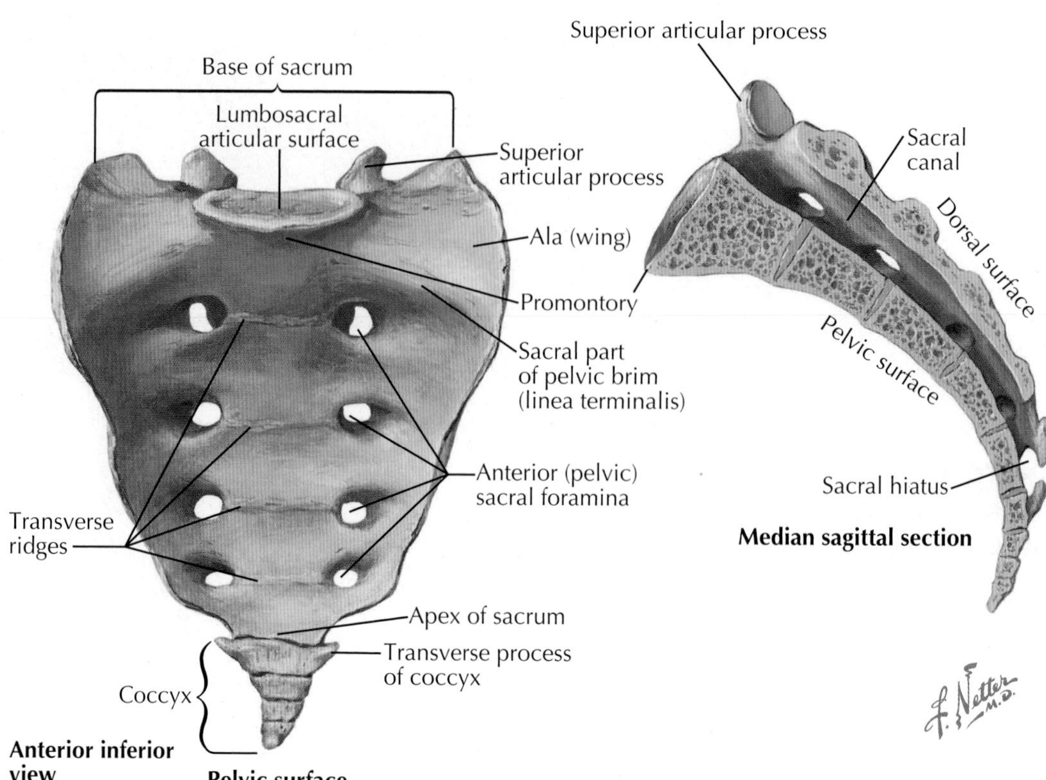

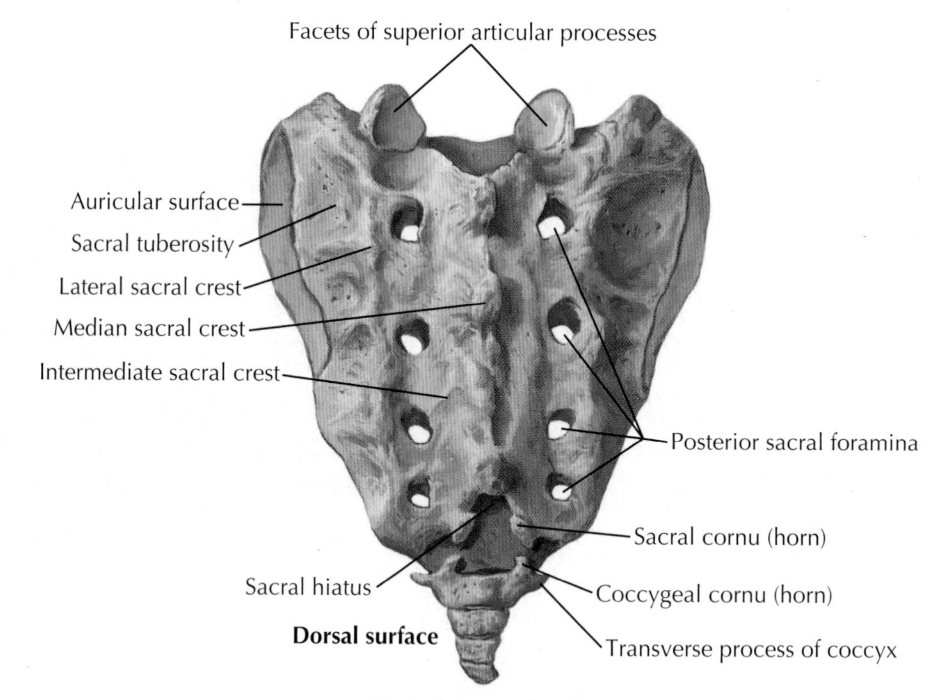

vascular and nerve supply to the discs is minimal. If the fibers of the annulus fail as a result of injury or disease, the enclosed nucleus pulposus may extrude posteriorly through the defect in the annulus. Disc bulges or herniation of nucleus pulposus outside the annulus fibrosus can lead to symptomatic compression of neural structures.

In the normal spine, the discs account for almost 25% of the height of the vertebral column; they are thinnest in the upper thoracic region and thickest in the lumbar region. In the sagittal plane, the lumbar discs are moderately wedge shaped, with greater height anteriorly. The normal lordosis of the lumbar spine (20–45 degrees) is due more to the shape of the discs than to the shape of the vertebral bodies. With aging, the nucleus pulposus undergoes various changes, including dehydration and replacement of mucoid matrix with fibrocartilage. This degenerative process can contribute to loss of normal curvature in the spine and abnormal load displacement.

LUMBOSACRAL TRANSITIONAL VERTEBRAE

Lumbosacral transitional vertebrae are common variants that are present in approximately 25% of people. It is important to identify on radiographic imaging, as failure to recognize this variant can lead to surgical procedures performed at the incorrect level. Lumbarization of the S1 vertebra is present in approximately 2% of the population. In this scenario, there are six rib-free vertebrae between the last rib-bearing vertebra (T12) and the sacrum. The S1/S2 vertebra may additionally have a facet joint present and an intervertebral disc. Sacralization of the L5 vertebra is a more common variant, occurring in approximately 17% of patients. The L5 vertebra is either partially or completely fused to the sacrum. The L5/S1 segment will typically have absent intervertebral discs and absent or hypoplastic facets. Additionally, the L5 transverse processes may be enlarged with either fusion or pseudoarticulation with the sacrum. This transitional vertebra is typically classified using the Castellvi classification system. Pseudoarticulation between the transverse process and the sacrum with associated low back pain is eponymously named Bertolotti syndrome. This pathology is typically managed with conservative treatment; however, refractory symptoms can require surgical resection of the pseudoarticulation or instrumented fusion of the L5 or L6 and S1 segments.

SACRAL SPINE AND PELVIS

The principal function of the pelvis is to transmit body weight to the limbs and absorb the muscular stresses of an upright posture. The center of gravity of the body passes just anterior to the sacral promontory.

The sacrum, composed of five fused vertebrae, broadens laterally into the sacral ala. The sacral nerve roots emerge through the anterior and posterior sacral foramina just medial to the sacral ala. The anterior surface of the sacrum is smooth. Dorsally, the surface is highly irregular to facilitate ligamentous attachments. The lateral articular surfaces of the sacrum articulate with the pelvis, forming the sacroiliac joints. The joint surfaces contain complementary elevations and depressions to diminish motion. Additionally, the anterior and posterior sacroiliac joint capsules have overlying sacroiliac ligaments, which are among the strongest in the body.

ANATOMY OF THE THORACOLUMBAR AND SACRAL SPINE (Continued)

LUMBOSACRAL LIGAMENTS

The anterior longitudinal ligament is a strap-like band that increases in width as it descends the spine. It extends from the anterior tubercle of the atlas (C1) to the sacrum. It is firmly attached to the anterior margins of the vertebral bodies and discs. The posterior longitudinal ligament is broader in the upper spine and becomes narrower as it traverses caudally. It lies within the vertebral canal immediately behind the vertebral bodies. Its upper end is continuous with the tectorial membrane, and it extends from the axis (C2) to the sacrum. The edges of the ligament are serrated, particularly in the lower thoracic and lumbar regions, with digitations extending out at the level of the disc. At these intervertebral points, the ligament blends with the annular fiber of the disc. The ligament is separated from the posterior vertebral body surfaces by basivertebral veins that join the anterior internal venous plexus. The posterior longitudinal ligament is stronger in the midline and weaker laterally, which helps to explain the propensity for lumbar disc herniations to occur posterolaterally.

The ligamentum flavum is largely composed of yellow, elastic tissue and connects adjacent laminae. It extends from the anteroinferior surface of the lamina above to the posterosuperior aspect of the lamina below, and from the midline to the facet joint capsules laterally. There is a midline raphe separating the right and left ligaments. The ligaments increase in thickness from the cervical to the lumbar spine. With aging and degenerative changes, the ligamentum flavum can become thickened and contribute to spinal canal stenosis and narrowing.

The supraspinous ligaments connect the tips of adjacent spinous processes from the seventh cervical vertebra to the sacrum. They are continuous with the nuchal ligament in the cervical spine and the interspinous ligaments immediately anterior, and they increase in thickness caudally. The interspinous ligaments are thin, membranous structures between the roots and apices of the spinous processes and are best developed in the lumbar region. These posterior ligamentous structures provide strong resistance to abnormal or excessive flexion motion.

The interosseous sacroiliac ligaments are formed by short, thick bundles of fibers connecting the sacral and iliac tuberosities. The dorsal sacroiliac ligaments fill the deep depression between the sacrum and the iliac bones dorsally. The sacrotuberous ligament is long, flat, and triangular. It arises from the posterior superior and posterior inferior iliac spines and from the posterior and lateral aspects of the sacrum. The fibers converge on the ischial tuberosity. The sacrospinous ligament arises from the lateral aspect of the lower sacrum and coccyx and attaches to the ischial spine. This ligament converts the greater sciatic notch into the greater sciatic foramen and with the sacrotuberous ligament forms the lesser sciatic foramen. The lumbosacral joint unites L5 and the sacrum. These vertebrae are united by the same ligamentous structures found throughout the lumbar spine with the addition of the strong iliolumbar ligament traversing laterally from the transverse process of L5 to the posterior part of the iliac crest. The iliolumbar ligament resists the tendency of the lumbar vertebra to slip down the slope of the sacral promontory.

LUMBOSACRAL LIGAMENTS

Anterior longitudinal ligament
Body of L1 vertebra
Intervertebral discs
Ventral ramus of L2 spinal nerve
L4 spinal nerve
Body of L5 vertebra
Dorsal ramus of L5 spinal nerve
Auricular surface of sacrum (for articulation with ilium)
Sacrum
Coccyx
Superior articular process
Transverse process
Lamina
Inferior articular process
Pedicle
Intervertebral foramen
Spinous process
Interspinous ligament
Supraspinous ligament

Left lateral view

Pedicle (*cut*)
Posterior longitudinal ligament
Superior articular processes; facet tropism (difference in facet axis) on right side
Spinous process
Lamina
Transverse process
Inferior articular process
Ligamentum flavum
Iliolumbar ligament
Iliac crest
Posterior superior iliac spine
Posterior inferior iliac spine
Posterior sacroiliac ligaments
Greater sciatic foramen
Spine of ischium
Sacrospinous ligament
Lesser sciatic foramen
Sacrotuberous ligament
Ischial tuberosity
Lateral, Posterior sacrococcygeal ligaments

Posterior view

F. Netter M.D.

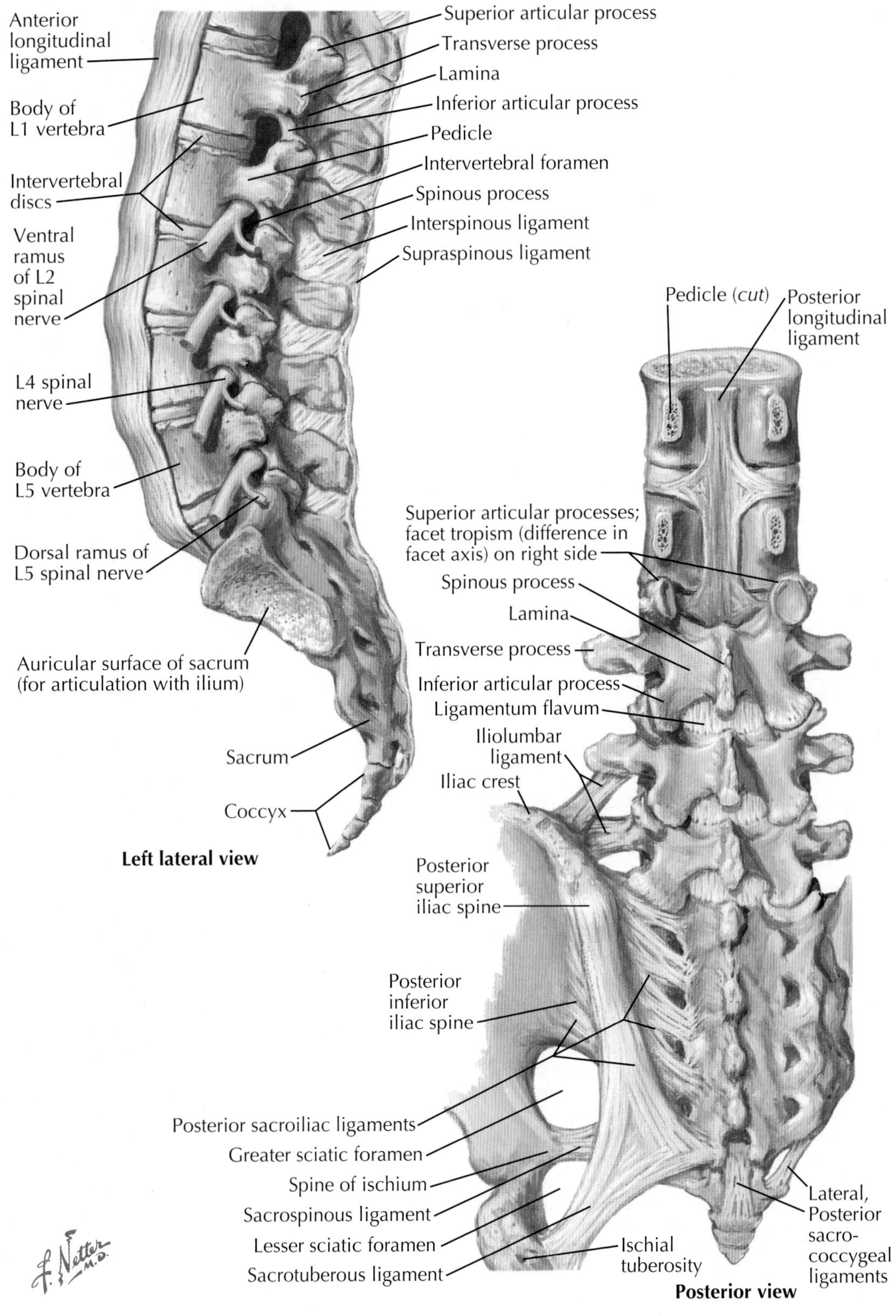

Clinical Problems and Correlations of the Thoracolumbar Spine

DEGENERATIVE DISC DISEASE

Low back pain, with or without leg pain, is very common in the population, particularly in middle-aged and older adults, with close to 80% of all people experiencing some form of back pain in their lifetime. Degeneration of the intervertebral discs and some degree of low back pain and stiffness are nearly universal features of aging. Disc degeneration, beginning as early as the second decade of life, is considered an irreversible process. Degenerated discs have decreased height, increased posterior and lateral bulging, and reduced ability to dissipate compression forces. As a result, associated changes occur, including abnormal loading of the facet joints with development of facet arthritis and overgrowth, osteophyte formation, greater stress on adjacent ligaments and muscles, and thickening of the ligamentum flavum. In some patients these degenerative changes can contribute to pathologic back pain. Loss of disc height can additionally lead to compression of neuroforamen, particularly in the lumbar spine. In combination with facet and ligamentum flavum hypertrophy, the lumbar thecal sac or exiting nerve roots can become compressed leading to symptoms of back and/or leg pain. However, despite these anatomic changes associated with aging and degenerative disc disease, it can be clinically difficult to isolate the primary source of low back pain.

In some cases, back pain may become chronic. Chronic low back pain, defined as persistent symptoms for longer than 6 to 8 weeks, is common among people older than 40 to 50 years and those working in occupations requiring frequent bending, lifting, or exposure to repetitive vibration (e.g., truck drivers). Although obesity, smoking, and poor physical fitness are all known environmental risk factors for disc degeneration, genetic factors are considered to contribute up to 74% of the etiology of disc degeneration.

Degenerative Disc Disease

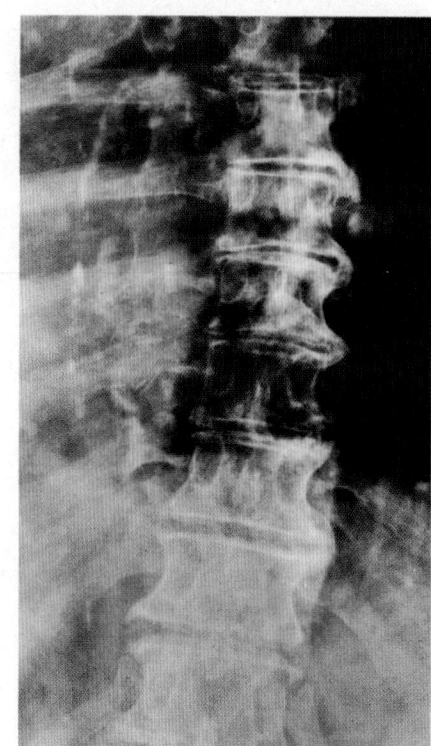

Radiograph of thoracic spine shows narrowing of intervertebral spaces and spur formation.

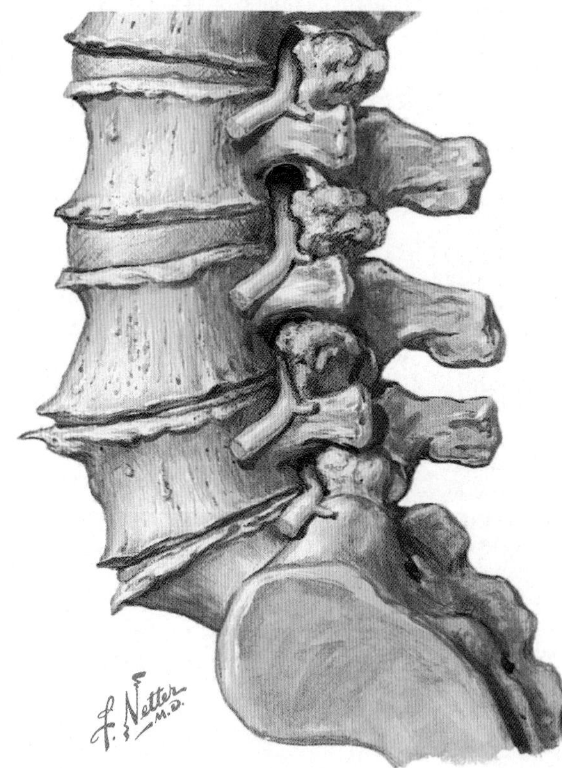

Degeneration of lumbar intervertebral discs and hypertrophic changes at vertebral margins with spur formation. Osteophytic encroachment on intervertebral foramina compresses spinal nerves.

A typical feature of back pain is its frequent radiation to one or both buttocks. The pain can additionally radiate to the posterior thigh. It is frequently exacerbated by lifting and bending activities and relieved with rest. Examination typically shows mild tenderness in the lower back or sacroiliac region. Flexion and extension of the spine may be limited and painful. Patients with associated psychological issues may display nonorganic findings, such as exaggerated pain behaviors and nonanatomic localization of symptoms.

Radiographs and MR images of the spine reveal changes that are difficult to differentiate from normal age-related changes. These include decreased disc height, anterior vertebral body osteophytes, and facet hypertrophy. Screening radiographs to rule out tumor, infection, or an inflammatory arthritic process are appropriate for patients with pain lasting longer than 6 weeks. MRI is typically reserved for patients with symptoms suggestive of infection, neoplasm, or neural compression. When evaluating for neural compression,

LUMBAR DISC HERNIATION

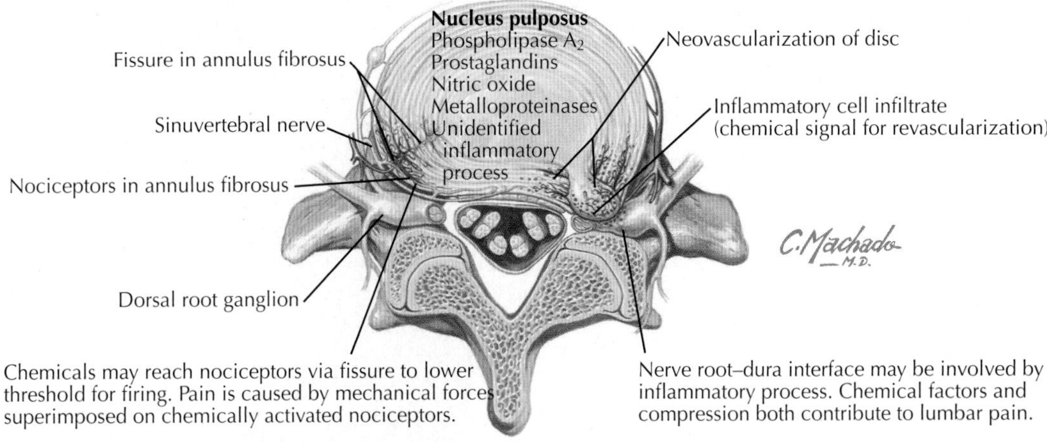

Chemicals may reach nociceptors via fissure to lower threshold for firing. Pain is caused by mechanical forces superimposed on chemically activated nociceptors.

Nerve root–dura interface may be involved by inflammatory process. Chemical factors and compression both contribute to lumbar pain.

Disc Rupture and Nuclear Herniation

Rim lesion

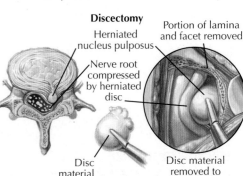

Tears in internal annular lamellae

Herniated nucleus pulposus

Peripheral tear of annulus fibrosus and cartilage end plate (rim lesion) initiates sequence of events that weaken and tear internal annular lamellae, allowing extrusion and herniation of nucleus pulposus.

Discectomy

Herniated nucleus pulposus

Portion of lamina and facet removed

Nerve root compressed by herniated disc

Disc material removed

Disc material removed to decompress nerve root

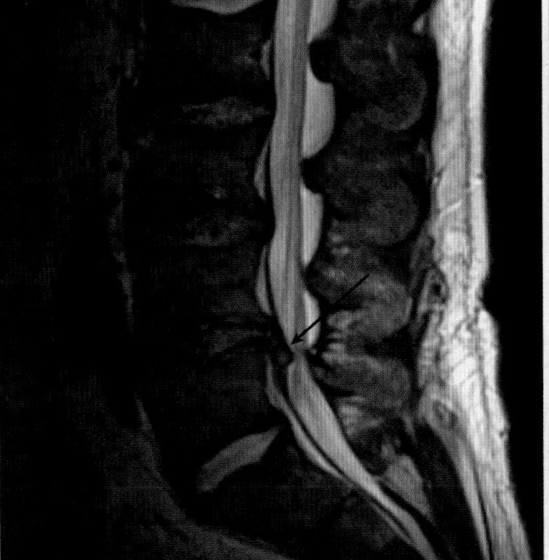

T2-weighted sagittal MR image showing herniation at L4–5 (*arrow*) with small portion lying below level of the disc space

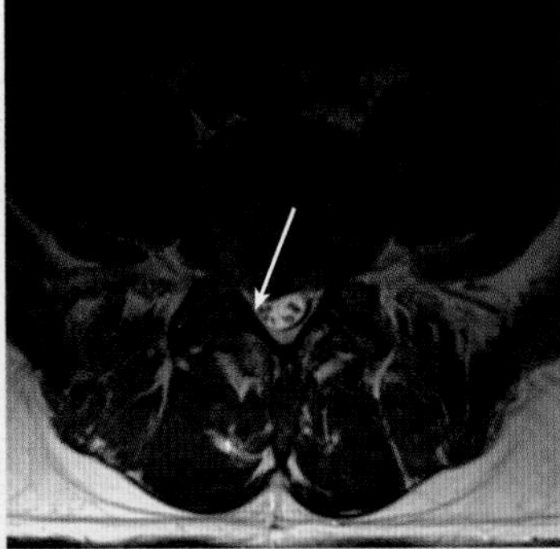

T2-weighted axial MR image showing disc herniation (*arrow*) at the level of disc space and contiguous with disc

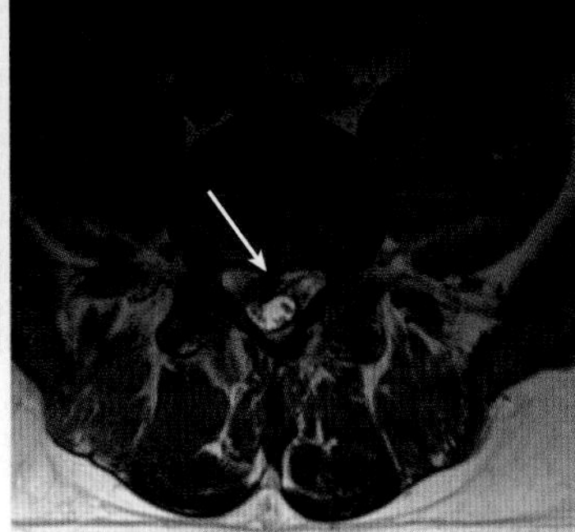

T2-weighted axial MR image showing disc fragment (*arrow*) lying slightly below level of disc space and not attached to disc

CLINICAL PROBLEMS AND CORRELATIONS OF THE THORACOLUMBAR SPINE (Continued)

CT myelography can be used in patients unable to obtain MRI.

Recurrent episodes of back pain are typical, and most can be managed nonoperatively with nonsteroidal anti-inflammatory drugs (NSAIDs), general conditioning exercises, active physical therapy, weight reduction, and smoking cessation. Unremitting pain necessitates further evaluation. Operative treatment is rarely indicated for back pain, and the role of fusion or arthroplasty for patients with isolated discogenic low back pain is controversial.

LUMBAR DISC HERNIATION

The nucleus pulposus may herniate posteriorly or posterolaterally and compress a nerve root, resulting in lumbar radiculopathy (leg pain in a dermatomal distribution). The herniation may be *protruded* (with the annulus intact), *extruded* (through the annulus but contained by the posterior longitudinal ligament), or *sequestered* (free within the spinal canal). Pain results from nerve root compression and from an inflammatory response initiated by various cytokines released from the nucleus pulposus.

Patients with lumbar disc herniation typically are young and middle-aged adults with a history of previous low back pain. Lumbar disc herniations are rare in the elderly population, as the mucoid nucleus pulposus is typically replaced by fibrocartilage with aging. The pain may be exacerbated or initiated by a bending, twisting, or lifting event but may also develop insidiously. The central portion of the posterior longitudinal ligament is the strongest portion of the ligament and resists midline posterior extrusions. More than 90% of lumbar disc herniations occur posterolaterally at L4–L5 and L5–S1. Posterolateral disc herniations may cause neural compression and radicular pain involving the traversing spinal nerve. For example, an L4–L5 posterolateral disc herniation will typically affect the L5 nerve root. This is due to the L4 nerve root exiting the neural foramen just cranially to the level of the L4–L5 disc and thus is lateral to the disc herniation. Occasionally, a disc herniation will be located far lateral and can affect the more proximal exiting nerve root within the foramen. This can cause radicular pain corresponding to the vertebral level cephalad to the disc (e.g., an L4–L5 far lateral disc herniation will affect the proximally exiting L4 nerve root).

Increasing pressure or stretch on the compressed nerve root exacerbates pain. Pain can also increase with any activity that increases intraabdominal pressure, such as sitting, sneezing, and lifting. It is typically decreased by lying down with a pillow under the legs or by lying on the side with the hips and knees flexed (fetal position). Symptoms can be variable, but pain

Lumbar Spinal Stenosis

Patient assumes characteristic bent-over posture, with neck, spine, hips, and knees flexed; back is flat or convex, with absence of normal lordotic curvature. Pressure on cauda equina and resultant pain are thus relieved.

Inferior articular process of superior vertebra

Superior articular process of inferior vertebra

Lateral recess

Central spinal canal narrowed by enlargement of inferior articular process of superior vertebra. Lateral recesses narrowed by subluxation and osteophytic enlargement of superior articular processes of inferior vertebra.

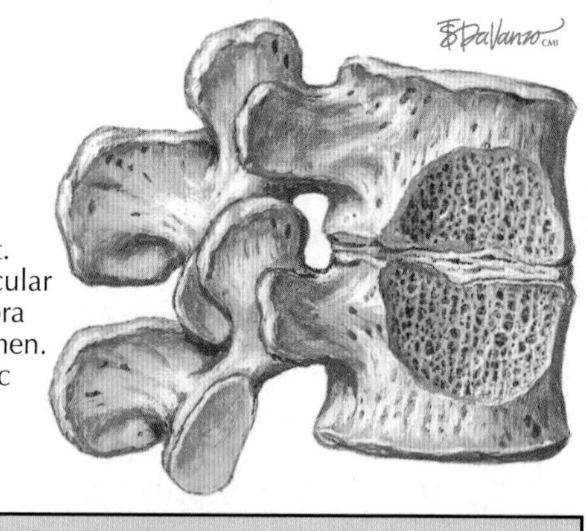

Vertebrae approximated due to loss of disc height. Subluxated superior articular process of inferior vertebra has encroached on foramen. Internal disruption of disc shown in cut section.

Vascular vs. Neurogenic Claudication

Evaluation	Vascular	Neurogenic
Walking distance	Fixed	Variable
Palliative factors	Standing	Sitting/bending
Provocative factors	Walking	Walking/standing
Walking uphill	Painful	Painless
Bicycle test	Positive (painful)	Negative (painless)
Pulses	Absent	Present
Skin	Loss of hair/shiny	Normal
Weakness	Rarely	Occasionally
Back pain	Occasionally	Commonly
Back motion	Normal	Limited
Pain character	Cramping/distal to proximal	Numbness/aching/proximal to distal
Atrophy	Uncommon	Occasionally

Clinical Problems and Correlations of the Thoracolumbar Spine (Continued)

and sensory disturbances typically follow the dermatome of the nerve root(s) affected.

On examination, the patient may lean away from the affected side to relieve compression on the affected root. The straight-leg raise test (lifting the leg with the knee straight) is a classic sciatic nerve tension sign that indicates L5 or S1 root inflammation and should be performed on both legs. A positive test typically reproduces the patient's radicular symptoms below the knee. The specificity of the test is heightened when raising the contralateral leg provokes symptoms on the affected side (the cross-leg sign). The comparable test for a more proximal lesion affecting the L4 root or higher is the femoral nerve stretch test, which is performed by having the patient lie on the nonaffected side and by having the examiner extend the affected hip with the knee flexed. A positive test reproduces the patient's proximal leg pain.

Radiographs of the lumbar spine may be normal but are useful in ruling out other conditions such as fracture. MRI is the study of choice to delineate the location and type of disc herniation. Most patients respond to symptomatic treatment such as NSAIDs, muscle relaxants, oral narcotics, a short course of oral corticosteroids, or epidural corticosteroid injection and will note improvement of symptoms by 6 weeks. Often in these cases the herniated disc fragment resorbs over this time while the symptoms are managed.

Indications for surgery include cauda equina syndrome, urinary retention or incontinence, progressive neurologic deficit, severe single nerve root paralysis, and radicular pain lasting longer than 6 to 12 weeks. The goal of surgery is to relieve pressure on the affected nerve root or cauda equina. The procedure usually involves a small laminotomy (drilling a window in the lamina) and excision of the herniated disc fragment (see Plate 1.22). The procedure can be performed in an "open" fashion with a midline skin incision, through a tubular retractor with a paramedian incision, or endoscopically. Removal of the herniated disc fragment is typically a delicate procedure requiring the use of an operative microscope. Lumbar microdiscectomy typically provides dramatic relief of symptoms in 85% to 90% of patients. Recurrent disc herniations may occur in 5% to 10% of patients. Possible complications of surgery include injury to the neural elements, postoperative infection, durotomy, and persistent pain.

Cauda Equina Syndrome

Multiple nerve roots of the cauda equina may be severely compressed by a large central disc herniation or other pathologic process such as epidural abscess, epidural hematoma, or fracture resulting in a rapid onset of neurologic deficit. Midline sacral nerve roots

LUMBAR SPINAL STENOSIS (CONTINUED)

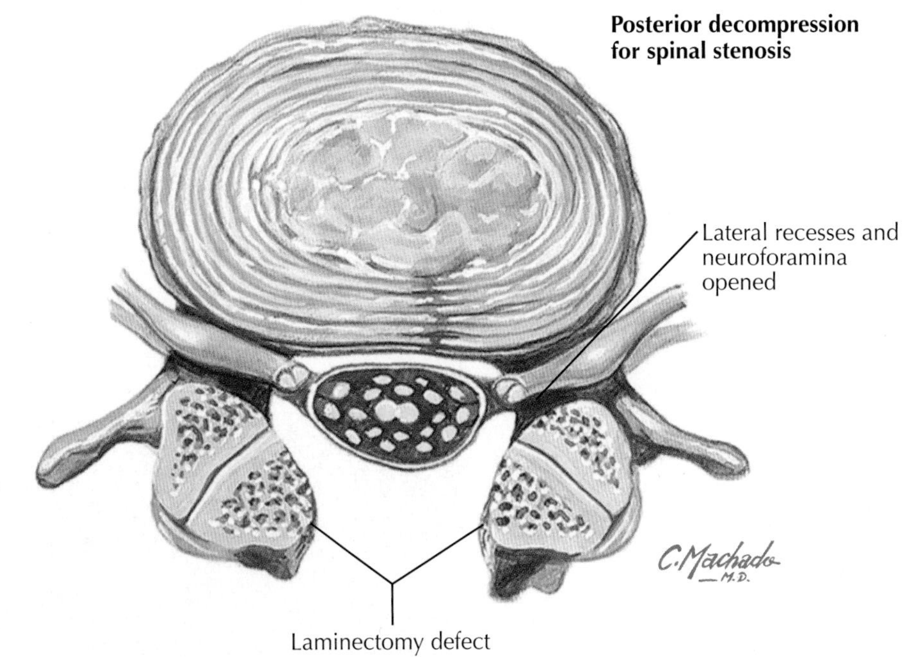

CLINICAL PROBLEMS AND CORRELATIONS OF THE THORACOLUMBAR SPINE (Continued)

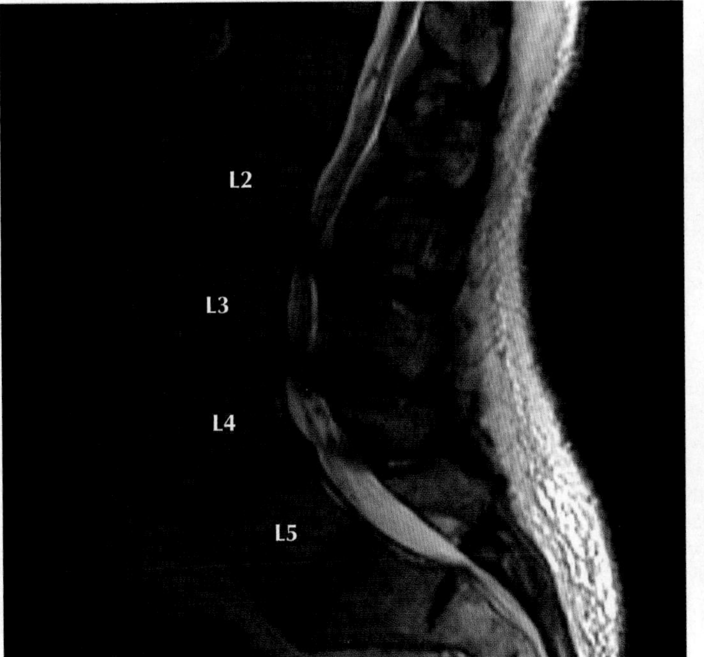

T2-weighted sagittal MRI showing multilevel stenosis, most severe at L2–3 and L3–4, less severe at L4–5

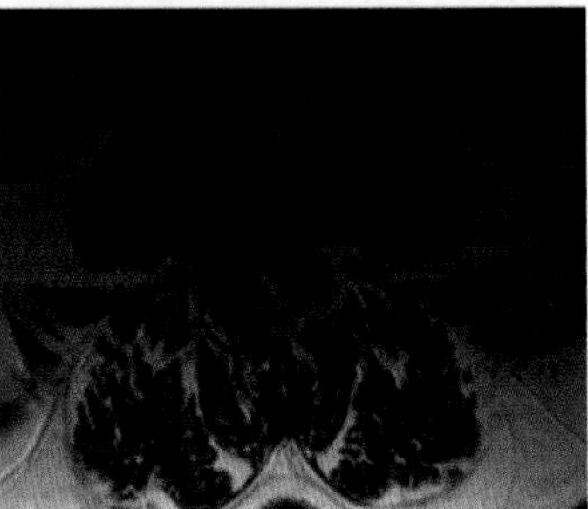

T2-weighted axial MRI showing severe canal stenosis at L3–4

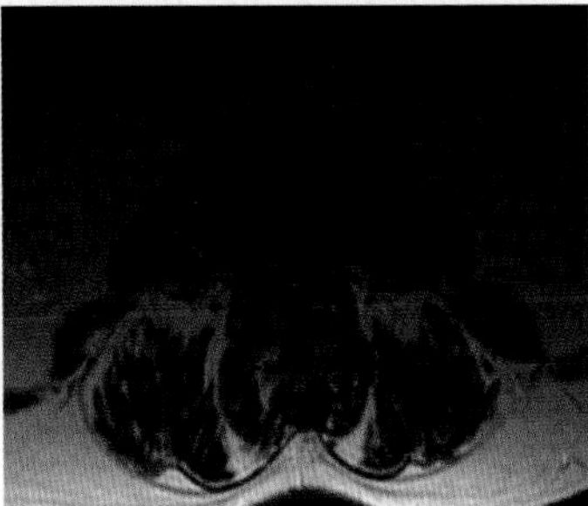

T2-weighted axial MRI showing severe canal stenosis at L2–3

that control bowel and bladder function are particularly vulnerable to such compression. Typical symptoms include bilateral lower extremity radicular pain and motor/sensory dysfunction, anesthesia in the perineum in a "saddle" distribution, urinary retention with or without overflow incontinence, and bowel incontinence. Patients with cauda equina syndrome require emergent surgical decompression. Even with prompt treatment, however, the return of neurologic function may be incomplete.

LUMBAR SPINAL STENOSIS

Lumbar spinal stenosis may result from any condition that causes narrowing of the spinal canal or neural foramina with subsequent compression of the nerve roots at one or more levels. The most common cause is degenerative changes in the disc and facet joints. These degenerative changes can be associated with spondylolisthesis, which is an anterior slipping (anterolisthesis) of one vertebra on the subjacent level. Patients with achondroplasia or other conditions that alter growth of the posterior vertebral arch may also develop stenosis with progressive symptoms in the second or third decade of life. Lumbar stenosis may also be congenital or may be caused by traumatic or postoperative changes.

Narrowing of the spinal canal is common in persons older than 60 years, but most have minimal symptoms. The spine is a three-joint complex comprising the intervertebral disc anteriorly and the two facet joints posteriorly. It is thought that the pathology of spinal stenosis begins anteriorly in the disc and involves the facet joints secondarily. Skeletal changes associated with stenosis in the older population include facet hypertrophy, osteophyte formation, and occasionally spondylolisthesis leading to central and/or neural foraminal stenosis. Soft tissue changes associated with stenosis include buckling or thickening of the ligamentum flavum and posterior longitudinal ligament, as well as bulging or frank herniation of the disc.

Symptomatic lumbar spinal stenosis afflicts both sexes and typically does not develop until after 40 years of age unless there is a congenital component. Typical symptoms include a diffuse pain in the buttocks and posterior thighs or pain in a dermatomal/radicular pattern. Back pain may or may not be present. Symptoms are frequently bilateral, but one extremity may be more severely affected than the other. Patients note pain and often numbness or weakness when walking, usually beginning in the buttocks or thighs, and often progressing to the calves and feet. This condition is also termed *neurogenic claudication*. Symptoms are typically relieved by sitting, bending forward, or leaning on an object. Forward-flexion of the lumbar spine reduces

Degenerative Lumbar Spondylolisthesis

Types of Spondylolisthesis	
Type	**Description**
I. Isthmic	Stress defect, attenuation, or acute fracture of pars interarticularis
II. Degenerative	Segmental instability, facet joint degeneration
III. Dysplastic	Congenital incompetency of facets
IV. Traumatic	Acute fracture of the pedicles
V. Pathologic	Metastatic or metabolic disease causing instability of the neural arch
VI. Postsurgical	Result of surgical decompression that removes too much of facets or pars interarticularis

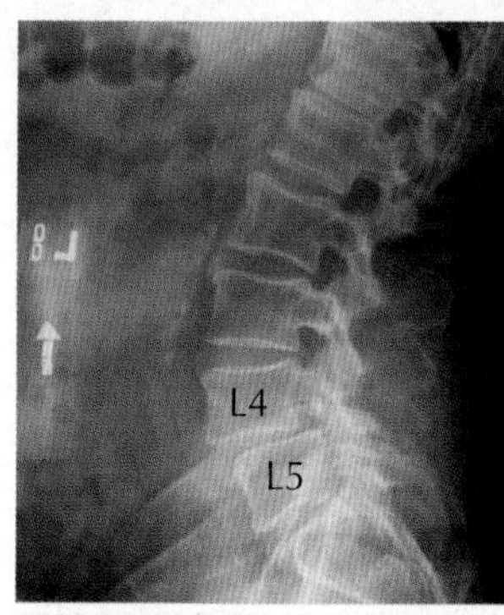

Standing lateral radiograph showing L4–5 spondylolisthesis

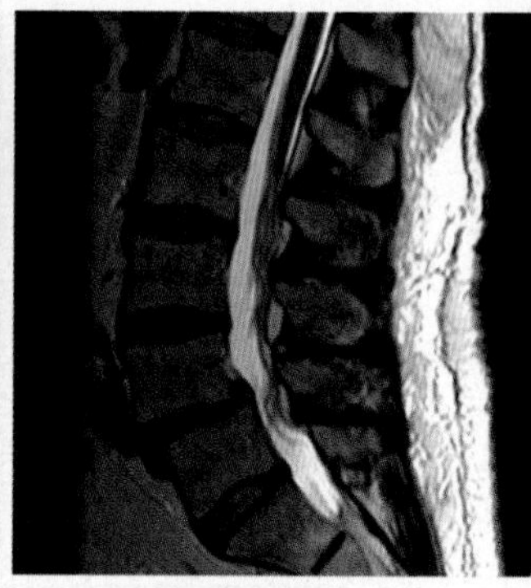
T2 sagittal MRI showing canal narrowing at level of the L4–5 spondylolisthesis

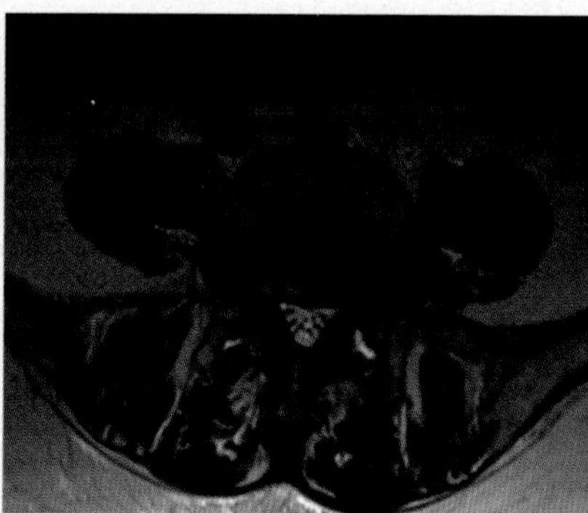
T2 axial MRI showing canal narrowing at L4–5

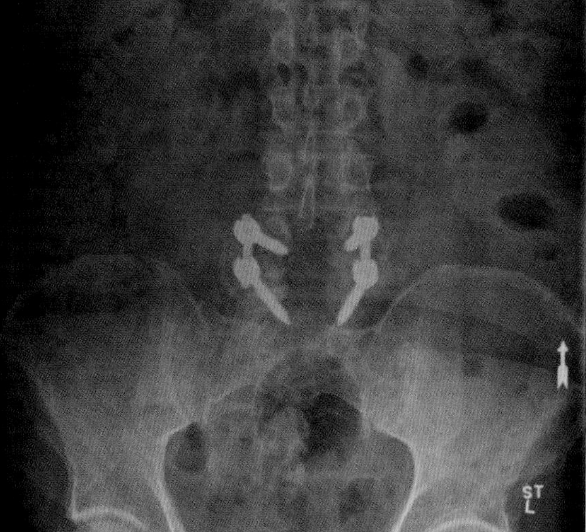
Standing postoperative anteroposterior radiograph showing L4–5 instrumented fusion

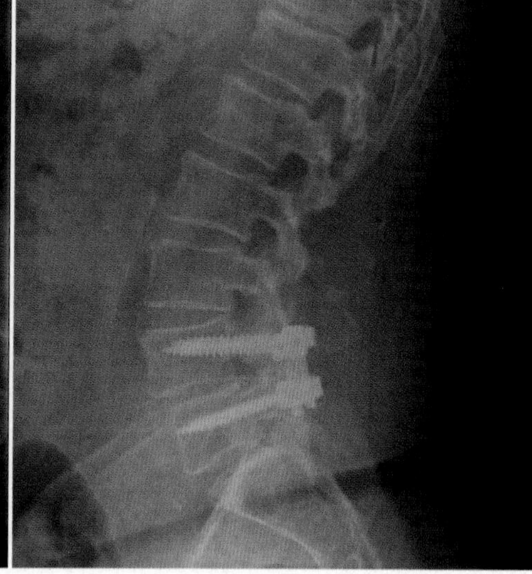
Standing postoperative lateral radiograph showing instrumented L4–5 fusion with reduction of the slip at L4–5

Clinical Problems and Correlations of the Thoracolumbar Spine (Continued)

discomfort and improves exercise tolerance by expanding the spinal canal, thereby relieving neural compression. As a result, patients with symptomatic spinal stenosis sometimes walk with their hips and knees flexed to allow for lumbar flexion (see Plate 1.23). Patients typically report improved symptoms when leaning on a shopping cart (the "shopping cart sign"), walking up hills, or exercising on a recumbent bike, all of which permit a slight degree of lumbar flexion, thereby relieving neural compression.

Vascular claudication may mimic neurogenic claudication and should be ruled out as the primary cause of symptoms as they may coexist. Similar to neurogenic claudication, patients with vascular claudication may have increased leg pain with exercise that is relieved by rest. However, patients with vascular claudication do not have pain relief with lumbar flexion or walking uphill, have a fixed claudication distance, rarely have back pain, often have loss of calf hair, and typically have diminished or absent peripheral pulses (see Plate 1.23). The progression or primary location of the pain in vascular claudication tends to be distal to proximal as opposed to the proximal to distal progression in neurogenic claudication.

Findings on examination are often limited in patients with lumbar spinal stenosis. Lumbar range of motion may be either normal or diminished. Muscle weakness, if present, is often subtle and may only be observed after having the patient walk. Weight-bearing radiographs should be obtained and usually demonstrate typical age-related changes of facet joint arthrosis, diminished disc height, or a degenerative spondylolisthesis, most common at L4–L5 and L3–L4. The differential diagnosis includes vascular claudication, peripheral neuropathy associated with diabetes mellitus or vitamin B_{12} or folic acid deficiency, abdominal aortic aneurysm, infection, and tumor.

Nonoperative management is initially symptom directed and includes physical therapy, NSAIDs, epidural corticosteroid injections, weight reduction, and smoking cessation. Membrane-stabilizing agents such as gabapentin or pregabalin have also been useful in reducing symptoms. When symptoms persist and surgery is an option, diagnostic imaging with either MRI or CT myelography should be performed. Weight-bearing lumbar radiographs are important to obtain to rule out an associated degenerative spondylolisthesis. If spondylolisthesis is present, decompression is usually accompanied by spinal fusion of the affected levels. If no degenerative spondylolisthesis is present, surgical therapy usually involves neural decompression alone.

Surgery is most effective to relieve leg symptoms of neurogenic claudication. It is less successful in patients in whom back pain is the predominant symptom and in patients with significant comorbidities such as smoking, obesity, or diabetes. This is most commonly achieved by removal of midline spinous process followed by

Degenerative Spondylolisthesis: Cascading Spine

Pedicle screws inserted through pedicles into vertebral body

C. Machado M.D.

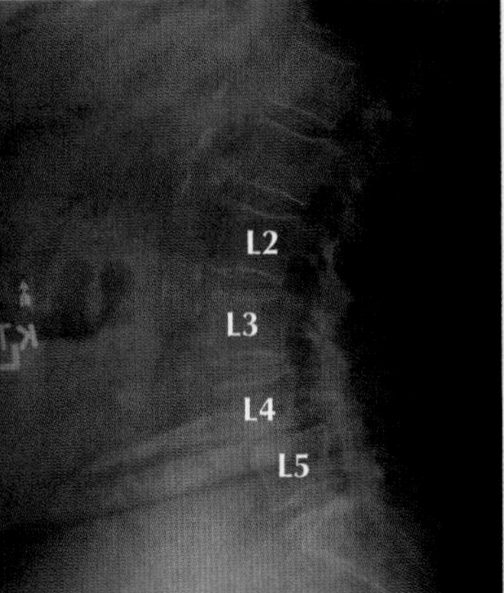

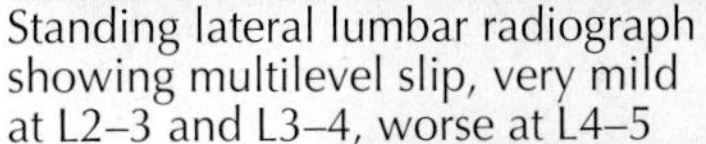
Standing lateral lumbar radiograph showing multilevel slip, very mild at L2–3 and L3–4, worse at L4–5

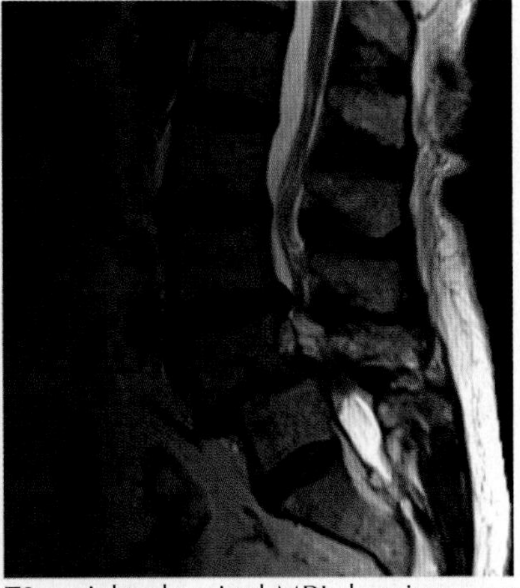
T2-weighted sagittal MRI showing severe stenosis at L4–5 and L3–4 and slightly less at L2–3

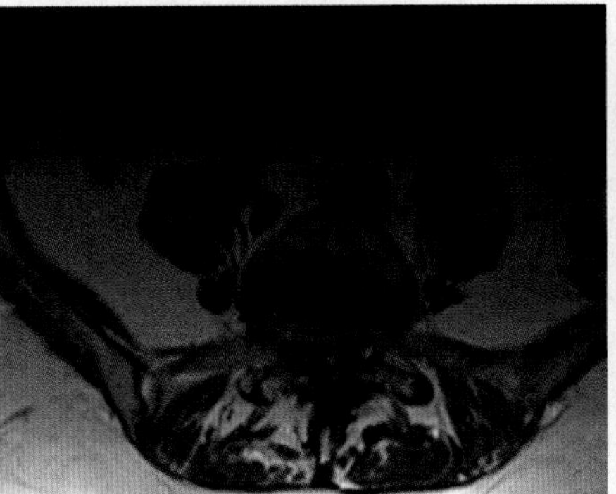
T2-weighted sagittal MRI showing severe stenosis at L4–5 level with near-complete obliteration of the spinal canal

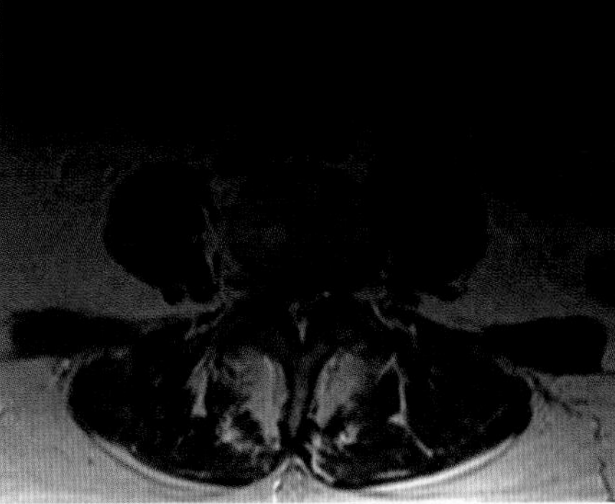
T2-weighted sagittal MRI showing moderately severe stenosis at L3–4 level

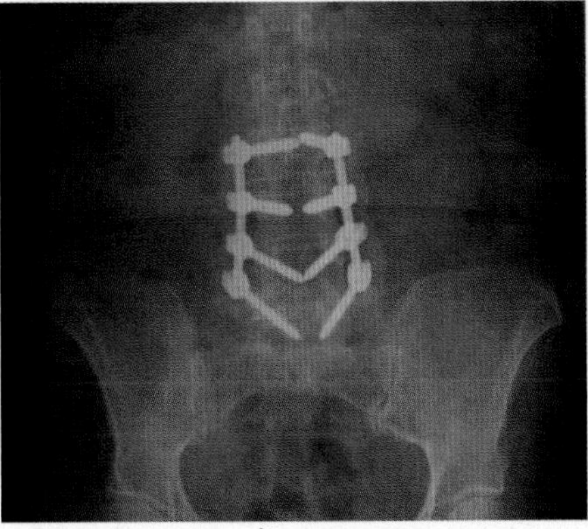
Postoperative standing anteroposterior radiograph showing instrumented spinal fusion

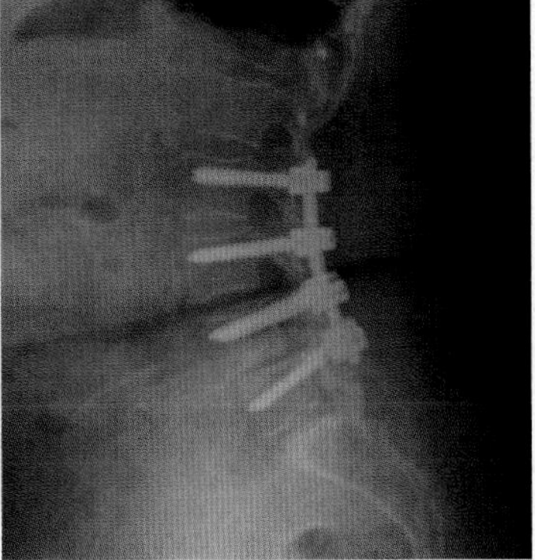
Postoperative standing lateral lumbar radiograph showing instrumented fusion with improvement of the slip at all levels

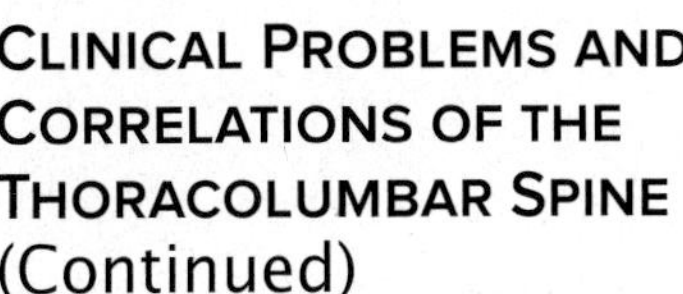

Clinical Problems and Correlations of the Thoracolumbar Spine (Continued)

laminectomy and unilateral or bilateral foraminotomy as needed (see Plate 1.24). Iatrogenic instability can occur after complete removal of a unilateral facet joint, by more than 50% facet resection bilaterally, or by removal of more than one-third of the pars interarticularis bilaterally. Thus care must be taken to avoid exceeding these limits in surgery unless necessary to perform satisfactory neural decompression. In such cases, spinal fusion should be considered. Recurrence of stenosis after decompression may occur, particularly at adjacent levels to a concomitant spinal fusion, often due to altered spine biomechanics and load distribution.

DEGENERATIVE LUMBAR SPONDYLOLISTHESIS

Spondylolisthesis is translation (slippage) of one vertebra in relation to an adjacent segment. The superior vertebra typically slips in an anterior direction in relation to the inferior vertebra (anterolisthesis). Retrolisthesis, in which the superior vertebra slips posteriorly, can also occur. This is occasionally observed in degenerative spondylolisthesis involving the upper lumbar levels. The causes of spondylolisthesis vary, but most patients have either an isthmic or degenerative spondylolisthesis (see Plate 1.25). Isthmic spondylolisthesis typically occurs at L5–S1, begins during adolescence, and is discussed elsewhere.

In degenerative spondylolisthesis (spondylolisthesis with an intact neural arch), erosion and narrowing of the disc and facet joints lead to segmental instability. Because the posterior arch is intact, the slippage causes stenosis, which can be aggravated with flexion. This condition typically occurs in adults over age 40 years, is more common in women, and is most common at the L4–L5 level. It is less likely to occur at L5/S1 due to the more anterior to posterior orientation of the facet joint. Spondylolisthesis can occur at multiple levels, however, and can result in the appearance of a "cascading spine."

Symptoms include back pain, radicular pain, and neurogenic claudication. Indications for surgical management include severe, progressive back pain, persistent claudicatory leg pain, neurologic weakness, and, rarely, cauda equina syndrome. Because the affected segments are unstable, decompression is usually combined with arthrodesis. Achieving arthrodesis in the setting of lumbar degenerative disease can be a challenge, and multiple techniques are typically used to help achieve a successful fusion. These include fixation devices, osseous autograft or allograft, and/or substitutes including demineralized bone matrix and bone morphogenetic proteins. Spinal fixation is accomplished by placement of segmental instrumentation that may include pedicle screws, cortical screws, interspinous fixation devices, or interbody cages. The bony surface of the posterior elements is typically decorticated to provide a suitable surface for bone growth.

Sagittal Plane Deformity

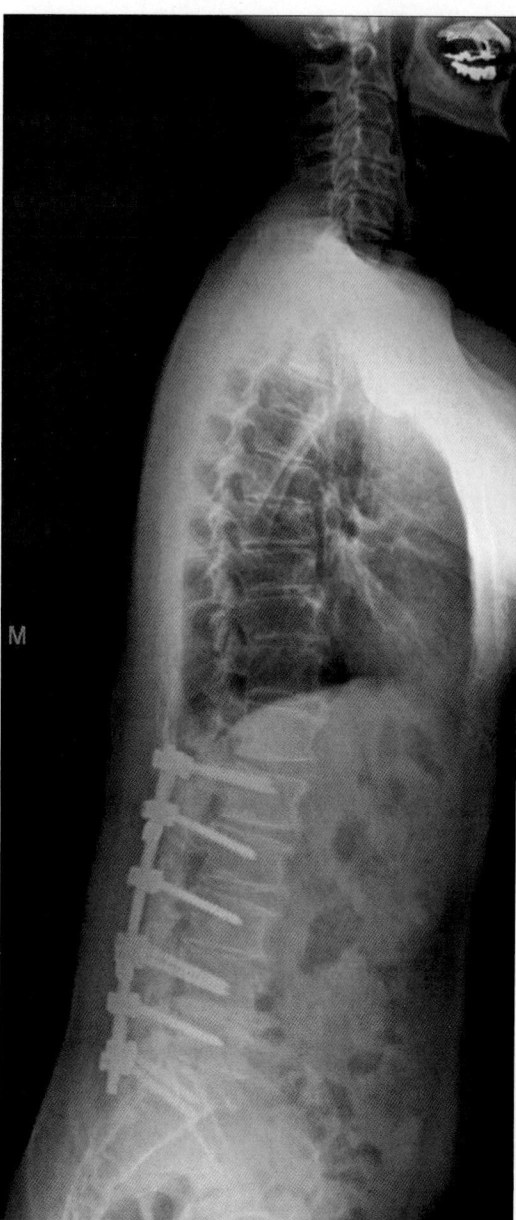

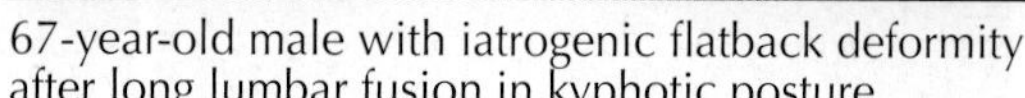

67-year-old male with iatrogenic flatback deformity after long lumbar fusion in kyphotic posture

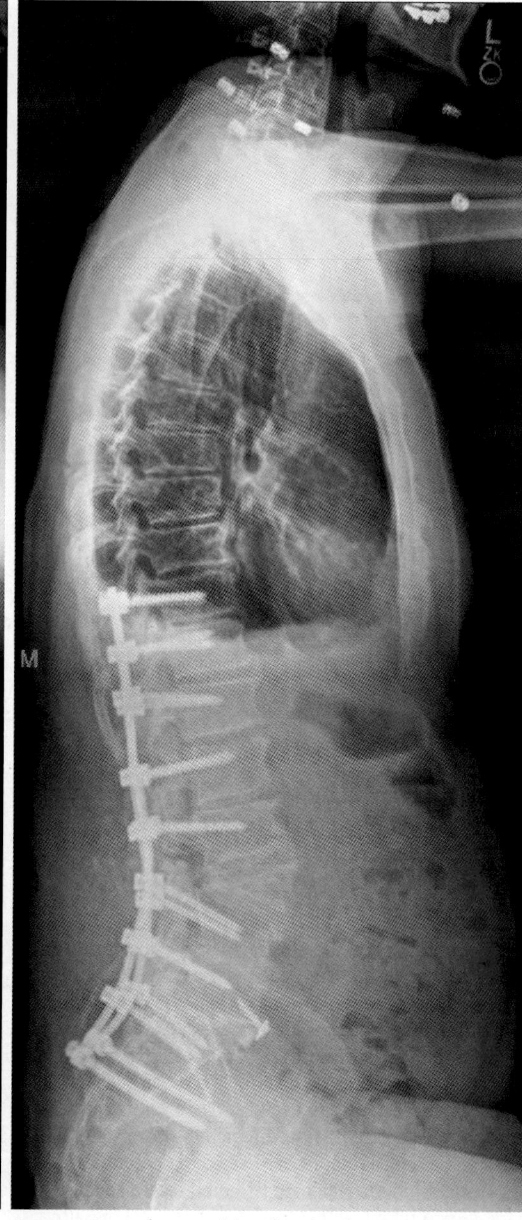

Restoration of normal lumbar lordosis and sagittal balance by L3 pedicle subtraction osteotomy and instrumented fusion

ADULT DEFORMITY

SCOLIOSIS IN ADULTS

Scoliosis is a coronal curvature of the spine of more than 10 degrees. In adults, scoliosis either presents as the sequela of adolescent idiopathic scoliosis or develops de novo secondary to degenerative changes in the disc, osteoporosis, or both (see Plates 1.36 to 1.39 for congenital scoliosis). Other less common causes include neuromuscular conditions such as posttraumatic paralysis, muscular dystrophy, or cerebral palsy.

Curve progression may occur in adults with preexisting adolescent idiopathic scoliosis. Progression is less likely when the curve is less than 30 degrees but occurs more frequently with 50- to 75-degree thoracic curves and unbalanced thoracolumbar or lumbar curves of greater than 30 degrees. Older adults with adolescent idiopathic scoliosis who develop degenerative changes are more likely to have curve progression. Osteoporosis may accelerate curve progression in patients with degenerative scoliosis.

Many patients with milder degrees of adult scoliosis are completely asymptomatic. Those with symptoms most commonly report pain localized to the area of curvature. The overall incidence of back pain in adults with scoliosis may not differ from those without scoliosis, but the incidence of severe pain is greater. As with back pain, the source of the pain can be difficult to localize and is often multifactorial. Causes include trunk imbalance with subsequent muscle fatigue; overload of facets, discs, and ligaments; and spinal stenosis. Radicular symptoms are more common in patients with degenerative scoliosis because the curve may narrow the neural foramen, particularly in the concavity of the curve. Significant pulmonary compromise from the curve is unlikely unless the patient has a significant thoracic curve (>70–80 degrees).

Nonoperative management of painful adult scoliosis is similar to management of other chronic spine conditions. Indications for surgical management include structurally significant curves with documented progression, progressive neurologic symptoms, or intractable pain.

Operative management includes decompression for stenotic symptoms and spinal fusion with instrumentation, as this facilitates curve correction and allows for early ambulation. The most important goal of fusion surgery is to restore coronal and sagittal balance (i.e., the head should be positioned over the pelvis in both planes) and to arrest curve progression. In rigid, nonflexible curves, vertebral osteotomies of varying degrees may be required to achieve curve correction; posterior osteotomies can be combined with anterior release with discectomy or complete vertebral column resection (VCR) to assist in curve correction. The Schwab classification system is one method of categorizing osteotomy types/grades. The incidence of major complications for deformity surgery is much higher in adults than adolescents. Possible adverse outcomes include pseudarthrosis, subsequent surgery, persistent pain, neurologic injury, thromboembolism, infection, and, rarely, death.

SAGITTAL PLANE DEFORMITY

Alterations in the normal sagittal alignment of the spine can be a debilitating problem in adults. As with scoliosis, significant sagittal plane malalignment can cause back pain, most likely as a result of disc, ligament, and muscle overload and the need for accessory muscles to combat the deformity and to maintain an erect position. Lumbar kyphosis is among the most common causes of sagittal plane deformity. Aging of the spine is normally kyphogenic, with loss of the normal lumbar lordosis. Further sagittal deformity can occur from multiple causes, such as genetic disease like ankylosing spondylitis, metabolic bone disease, and osteoporosis. It can also be caused, or accentuated, by iatrogenic factors, such as fusion using distraction instrumentation (e.g., Harrington rods) or spinal fusion without contouring lordosis into the fusion construct. Kyphosis commonly presents as pain, fatigue, and change in posture. Loss of lumbar lordosis with a kyphotic posture can predispose patients to tripping and easy fatigue while walking and may necessitate the use of a walker or other assistive device that will support a flexed posture. Without such support, hip and knee flexion is frequently required to allow for forward gaze. Stance and gait in this position are extremely fatiguing. The constellation of pain and deformity in patients with lumbar kyphosis has been called "flat back."

Nonoperative management is similar to that of adult scoliosis. For symptomatic patients with sagittal imbalance, surgery is the mainstay of treatment. This frequently involves an osteotomy in the lumbar spine to re-create lordosis with instrumentation and fusion to maintain the correction. Osteotomy in the lumbar spine can vary greatly based on the need for correction. Surgeons may employ a small osteotomy with resection of unilateral facet to slightly more invasive with resection of bilateral facet, pedicle, and partial vertebral body (pedicle subtraction osteotomy) to complete VCR of multiple vertebral segments. Potential complications of this type of surgery are significant and are similar to those for surgical treatment of adult scoliosis.

THREE-COLUMN CONCEPT OF SPINAL STABILITY AND COMPRESSION FRACTURES

Three-Column Concept of Spinal Stability

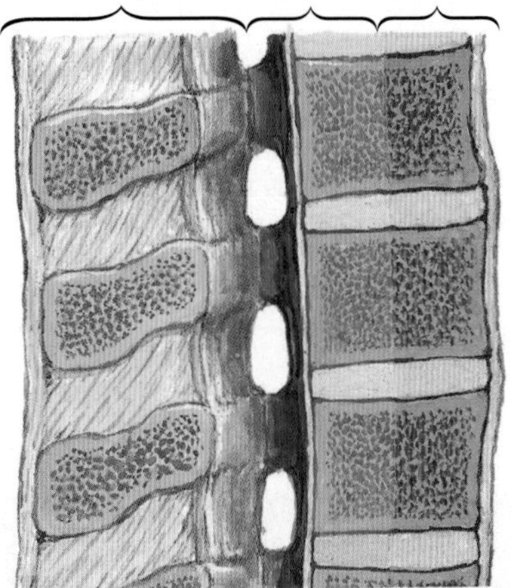

Three-column concept. If more than one column is involved in fracture, then instability of spine usually results.

Posterior column Middle column Anterior column

Lateral view. Note that lateral facet (zygapophyseal) joints are in posterior column, with intervertebral foramina in middle column.

Compression Fractures

Axial

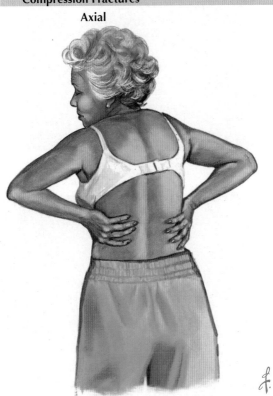

Vertebral compression fractures cause continuous (acute) or intermittent (chronic) back pain from midthoracic to midlumbar region, and occasionally to lower lumbar region.

Progressive thoracic kyphosis, or dowager's hump, with loss of height and abdominal protrusion

THORACOLUMBAR SPINE TRAUMA

Most thoracic and lumbar fractures result from vertical compression or flexion-distraction injuries. These injuries frequently occur around the thoracolumbar junction (T11–L2) because it represents a transition from the stiffer thoracic to the more flexible lumbar spine. The upper thoracic region (T1–T10) is more injury resistant because it is stabilized by the ribs, and the lower lumbar region (L3–L5) has larger, stronger, and more injury-resistant vertebrae.

Multiple classification systems exist for thoracolumbar trauma, but the three-column theory of Denis is among the simplest to conceptualize. This concept divides the vertebral body into three columns: the anterior column extending from the anterior longitudinal ligament through the anterior two-thirds of the vertebral body; the middle column containing the posterior third of the vertebral body and the posterior longitudinal ligament; and the posterior column, which includes the posterior spinal elements (lamina, pedicles, spinous processes) and posterior ligamentous complex (supraspinous and interspinous ligaments, facet capsules, and ligamentum flavum). Injuries involving one column can frequently be treated nonoperatively, two-column injuries may require surgical management, and three-column injuries generally mandate surgical fixation with or without decompression.

COMPRESSION FRACTURES

Compression fractures result from failure of the anterior vertebral column when a flexion or axial loading force is applied. This most commonly occurs at the thoracolumbar junction in elderly patients with osteoporosis. It is generally a stable fracture, and treatment is usually symptomatic with pain medication and a thoracolumbar orthosis for comfort. The fracture typically becomes stable once the bone heals. Surgical treatment can include cement augmentation of the vertebral body to provide immediate stability and to minimize the risk of progressive kyphosis. Multiple compression fractures in patients with severe osteoporosis can cause a kyphotic posture (see Plate 1.29). In such cases, cement augmentation or spinal instrumentation should be considered. Although less common than osteoporosis, compression fractures can also be attributable to metastatic disease to the spine. Medical professionals should have a high index of suspicion in patients with oncologic history and without identifiable trauma.

BURST FRACTURES

Burst fractures involve failure of the anterior and middle columns of the spine from an axial load and are generally associated with higher energy trauma than simple compression fractures. Because the posterior vertebral

Compression Fractures (Continued)

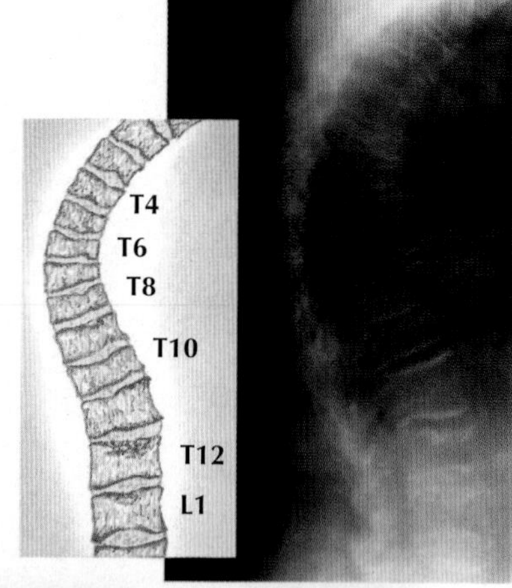

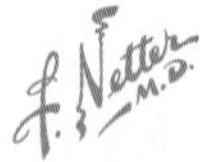

Multiple compression fractures of lower thoracic and upper lumbar vertebrae in patient with severe osteoporosis (radiograph of same patient)

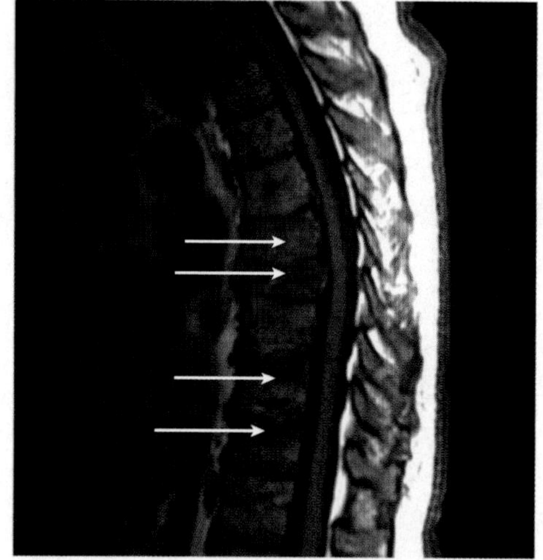

T1-weighted sagittal MRI showing multiple vertebral compression fractures (*arrows*) from multiple myeloma

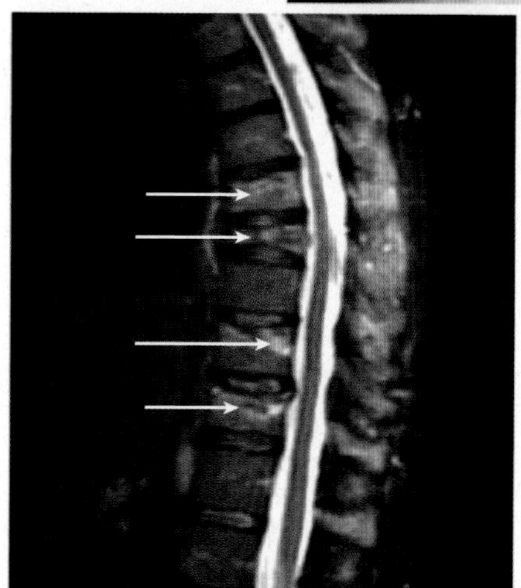

T2-weighted sagittal MRI showing multiple compression fractures (*arrows*) from multiple myeloma. Note that middle vertebra has not fractured.

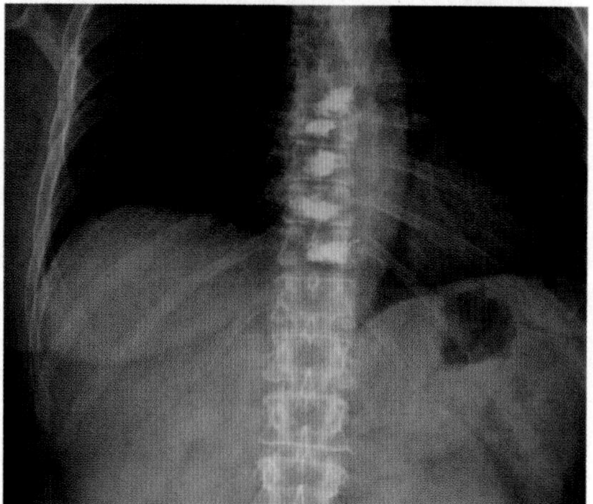

Anteroposterior chest radiograph showing the four compression fractures and the intervening normal level after cement augmentation

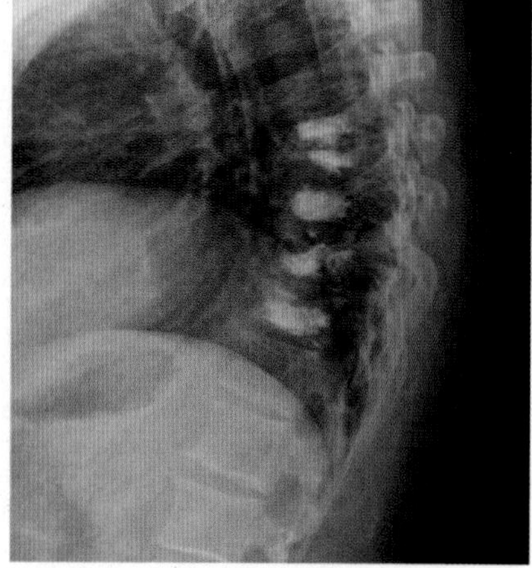

Lateral chest radiograph showing the four compression fractures and the intervening normal level after cement augmentation

Thoracolumbar Spine Trauma (Continued)

body (middle column) is fractured, bony fragments can migrate posteriorly and retropulse into the spinal canal, causing spinal cord or nerve root injury (see Plate 1.30). Suspected burst fractures should be evaluated by CT or MRI to assess the degree of spinal canal compromise and the integrity of the bony and ligamentous structures of the posterior column. Posterior column injury denotes a more severe fracture pattern (a three-column injury) that frequently requires surgery.

Treatment of burst fractures varies and has been the subject of some controversy. Stable burst fractures without neurologic injury can be treated with pain medication, activity restriction, and a thoracolumbar orthosis to relieve pain and promote bony healing. Relative indications for surgery include greater than 25 degrees of kyphosis, greater than 50% height loss of the vertebral body, or greater than 50% spinal canal compromise. A complete or incomplete neurologic injury and an injury to the posterior column (a three-column injury) constitute absolute indications for surgery. Surgery typically involves instrumented spinal fusion two levels above and two levels below the fractured vertebra. If there is a neurologic injury or concern for severe canal stenosis, then decompression is also performed. Posterior-only procedures can be performed when decompression is not indicated or adequate decompression of the spinal canal can be achieved through a posterior approach. It can also be performed in patients requiring decompression with an acute fracture (<5 days after injury) because such fracture fragments are mobile and can usually be reduced by a combination of distraction and lordosis. Anterior procedures are appropriate for subacute injuries requiring decompression, in patients with a severe neurologic deficit and significant canal intrusion by fracture fragments, and in patients with severely comminuted vertebral body fractures with no anterior column support (see Plate 1.30).

Chance Fractures

A Chance fracture is a bony injury through the vertebra in the thoracolumbar spine. It is best visualized on the lateral radiograph or CT scan. The Chance fracture is also known as a "seat belt" fracture because it frequently results from motor vehicle accidents in which the patient wears a lap belt without a shoulder belt. With sudden deceleration, the patient simultaneously experiences flexion anteriorly, with the lap belt acting as the pivot point, and distraction (tension) of the posterior column of the spine. As the distraction continues, a fracture propagates from posterior to

Thoracolumbar Spine Trauma (Continued)

anterior through the spine, involving all three columns. Although the fracture often reduces spontaneously, it is inherently unstable. Fractures must be treated surgically or immobilized in a thoracolumbar orthosis (with spinal stability verified with a standing radiograph in the brace). Occasionally, this flexion-distraction injury affects only the discoligamentous structures in the spine, resulting in a "soft tissue Chance" injury. In this variant of the injury, the transverse cleavage plane propagates through the posterior ligamentous complex (supraspinous and interspinous ligaments, ligamentum flavum, and facet capsules) and anteriorly through the intervertebral disc. Signs of this injury on the lateral radiograph include gapping at the facet joint and widening of the distance between spinous processes. This injury must be treated by surgical fixation, as these discoligamentous structures will not spontaneously heal after being disrupted.

Unstable Injuries of the Thoracolumbar Spine

The thoracolumbar junction is vulnerable to several different mechanisms of injury: flexion, rotation, axial loading, or any combination of those forces. Fracture-dislocations are relatively common in this region, where the less mobile thoracic spine meets the highly mobile segments of the lumbar spine. A fracture-dislocation of the thoracolumbar spine is severe and involves disruption of all three columns of the spine. These fractures are inherently unstable and are associated with a high rate of neurologic injury. Treatment of these injuries typically involves instrumented spinal fusion and is directed at restoring stability to this area.

Sacral Fractures

Traumatic sacral fractures can present as a solitary injury but often are observed in association with a pelvic ring or lumbosacral facet injuries in a patient with multiple injuries. The closer the fracture is to the midline (either involving the sacral neural foramina or central canal), the higher is the rate of neurologic injury. Most sacral fractures are stable and do not require surgery. In patients with neurologic injury and objective evidence of neurologic compression, however, surgical decompression and stabilization may be indicated.

Burst, Chance, and Unstable Fractures

Burst fractures

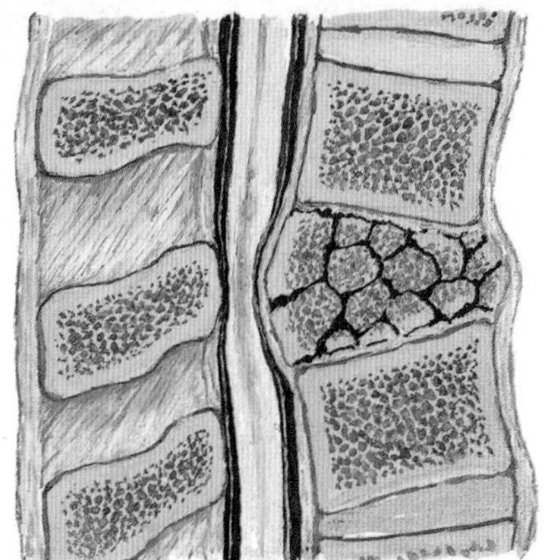

Burst fracture of vertebral body involving both anterior and middle columns resulted in instability and spinal cord compression.

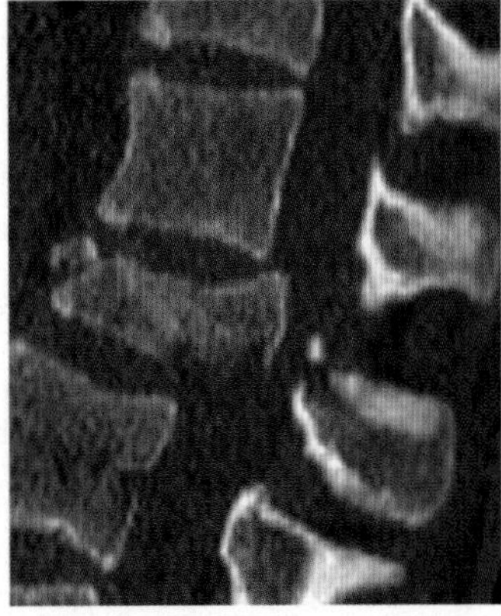

Midsagittal CT reconstruction showing markedly compressed and disrupted L1

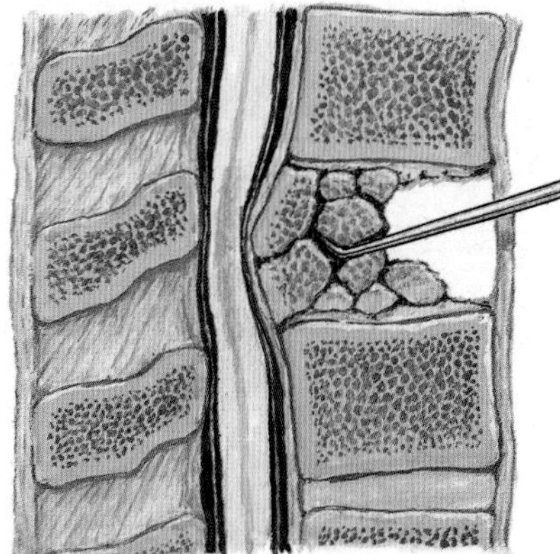

Anterior decompression of burst fracture (corpectomy) with hooked curet

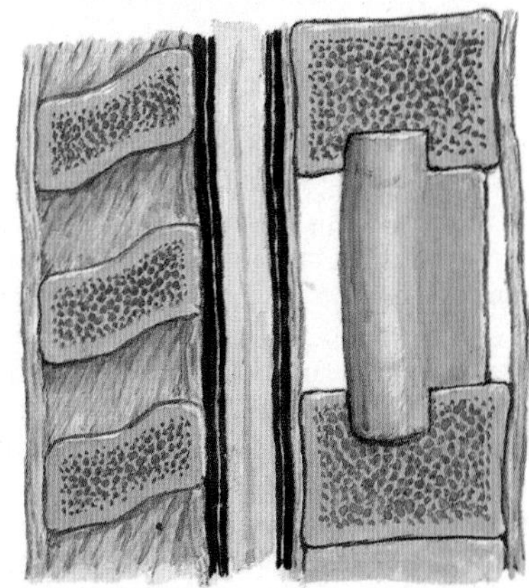

Bone graft from iliac crest restores vertebral height and stability after bone compressing spinal cord had been removed with corpectomy.

Chance fracture

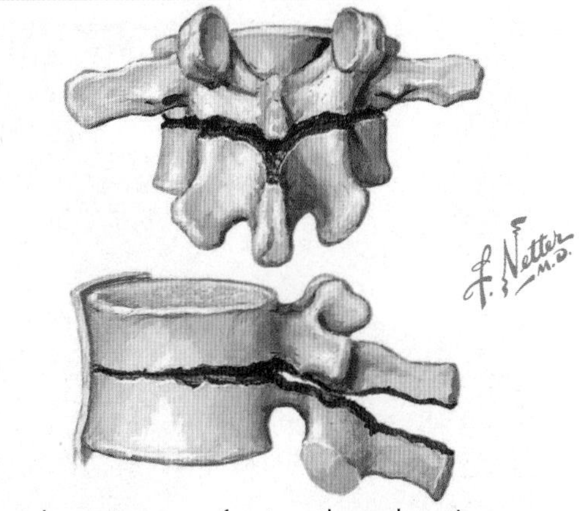

Complete transverse fracture through entire vertebra. Note hinge effect of anterior longitudinal ligament.

Fracture-dislocation

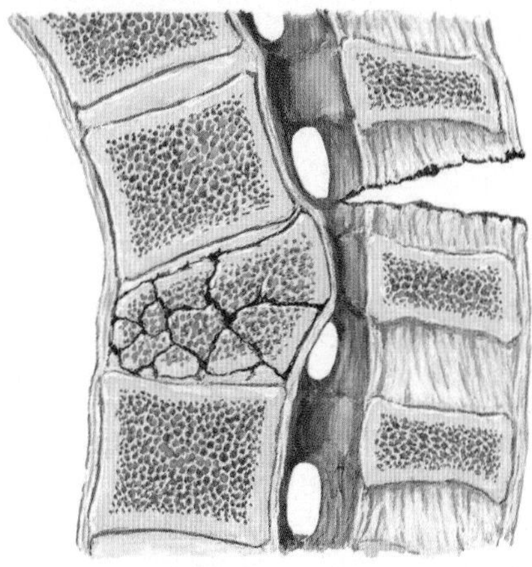

All three columns moved.

Congenital Anomalies of Occipitocervical Junction

The articulation of the atlas (C1) and axis (C2) is the most mobile part of the vertebral column and consequently the least stable. The dens (odontoid process) of the axis acts as a bony buttress to prevent hyperextension of the neck, but the rest of the normal range of motion—and the protection of the spinal cord in the area—is maintained by the integrity of the surrounding ligaments and capsular structures. Atlantoaxial instability may result from occipitalization of the atlas, basilar impression, odontoid malformations, and laxity of the dens-retaining ligaments. It is often associated with Down syndrome (trisomy 21) and some of the skeletal dysplasias that cause dwarfism. The most significant risk is compression of the spinal cord.

OCCIPITALIZATION OF ATLAS

This condition is characterized by partial or complete fusion of the bony ring of the atlas to the base of the occiput. The clinical signs—torticollis, short neck, a low posterior hairline, and restricted neck motions—are similar to those of Klippel-Feil syndrome (see Plate 1.33). One-fifth of patients have associated congenital abnormalities, including jaw malformations, incomplete cleft of the nasal cartilage, cleft palate, external ear deformities, cervical ribs, hypospadias, and urinary tract anomalies.

Fusion of the atlantooccipital joint increases the strain on the C1–C2 articulation and leads to instability in greater than 50% of patients, particularly when a C2–C3 fusion is also present. The dens may gradually encroach anteriorly into the spinal cord or medulla, or the posterior ring of C1 may be pulled forward into the spinal cord.

"Relative" basilar impression is seen in about 50% of patients. It is caused by diminished vertical height of the ring of the atlas, which brings the tip of the dens of the axis closer to the foramen magnum and the medulla oblongata. Neurologic symptoms develop if the dens projects into the opening of the foramen magnum.

CONGENITAL ODONTOID ANOMALIES

Odontoid anomalies include agenesis, hypoplasia, and os odontoideum, in which the body of the dens is a free ossicle separated from the axis by a wide gap, suggesting a nonunion (see Plate 1.32). In normal children younger than 2 years, the bony dens is "separated" from the body of the axis by a broad cartilaginous band that corresponds to a rudimentary intervertebral disc. Complete fusion of this vestigial structure typically occurs after age 5 years. Abnormalities of the dens are more commonly associated with bone dysplasias and Down and Klippel-Feil syndromes.

Minor trauma is commonly associated with the onset of symptoms, which may range from local irritation of the atlantoaxial articulation to neurologic impairment resulting from C1–C2 instability, decreased space available for the spinal cord, and spinal cord compression. The abnormality is often marked by the insidious onset of slowly progressive neurologic impairment of both posterior and anterior spinal cord structures. In children, presenting symptoms may be subtle and nonspecific, such as generalized weakness, frequent falling, or requests to be carried.

Congenital anomalies of occipitocervical junction

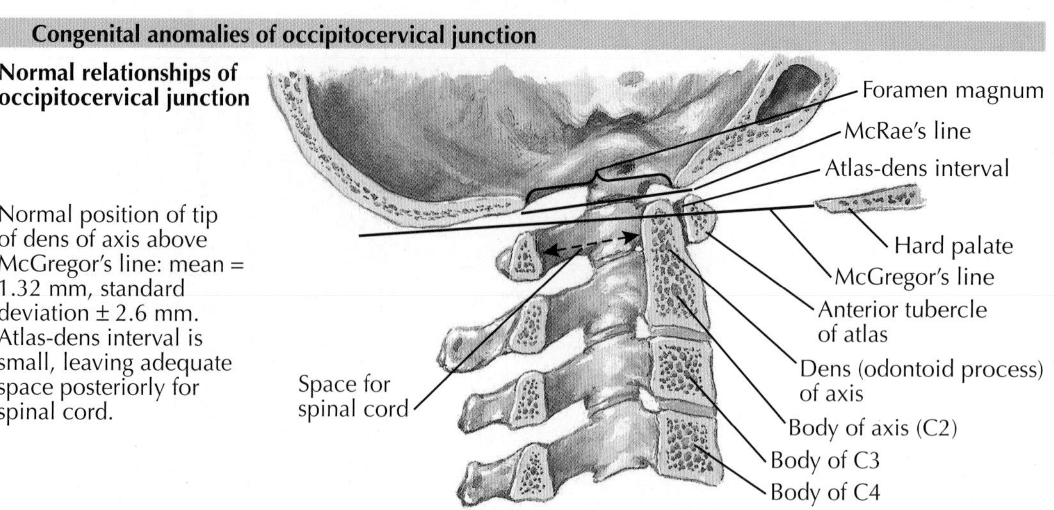

Occipitalization of atlas with instability of C1–2 (atlantooccipital fusion)

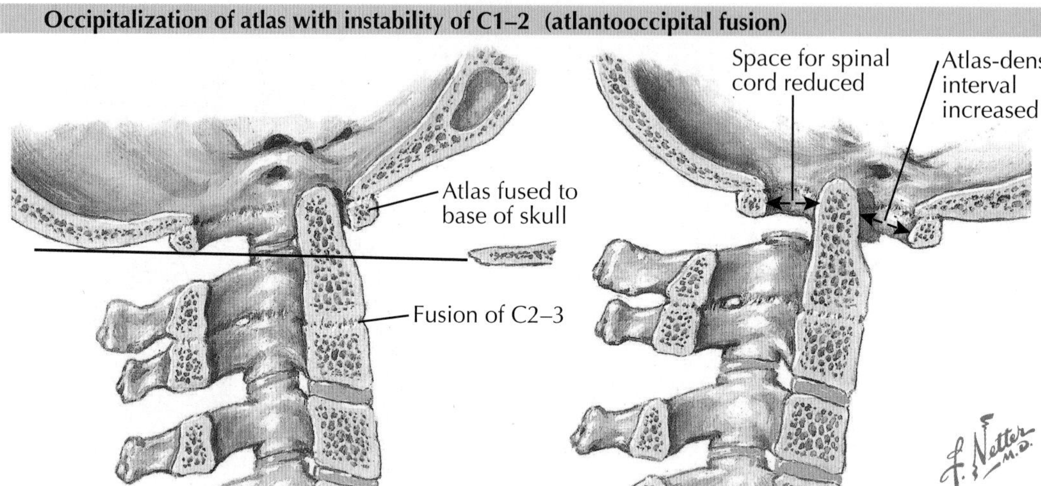

Atlas fused to base of skull. Dens projects into foramen magnum well above McGregor's line; 70% of patients with occipitalization of atlas and fusion of C2–3 develop C1–2 instability.

When neck is flexed, space available for spinal cord may be considerably reduced as atlas-dens interval increases. Fusion of C2–3 accentuates instability.

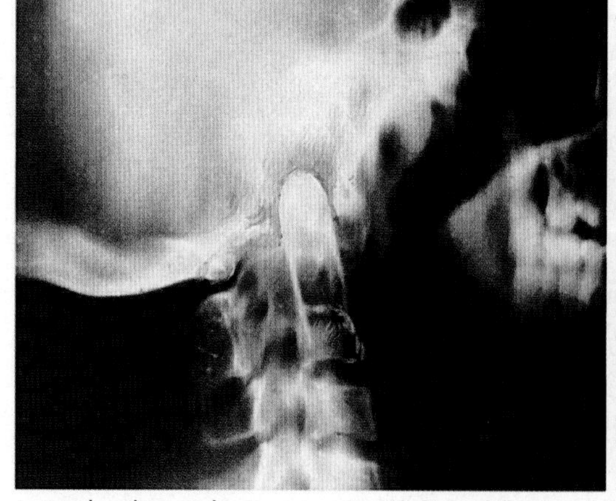

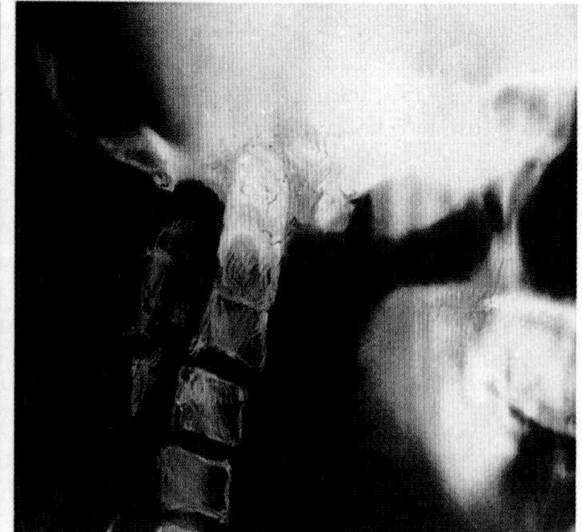

Lateral radiographs in extension (*left*) and flexion (*right*) of patient with occipitalization of atlas and hypermobile dens extending well into foramen magnum (basilar impression)

LAXITY OF TRANSVERSE LIGAMENT OF ATLAS

Laxity of the transverse ligament (see Plate 1.32) may be due to acute or repetitive trauma, or the attachment may be weakened by inflammation from infection or rheumatologic conditions. In Down syndrome, the laxity may be due to rupture or attenuation of the transverse ligament and may lead to severe C1–C2 instability. Lateral flexion-extension radiographs are required in children with Down syndrome who have neurologic problems or plan to participate in sports (most typically, Special Olympics) that may cause stress or trauma to the head and neck.

PSEUDOSUBLUXATION OF C2 ON C3

Cervical spine flexibility is greater in children than in adults. A common and normal finding in children is the anterior displacement of C2 on C3 when the neck is

CONGENITAL ANOMALIES OF OCCIPITOCERVICAL JUNCTION (Continued)

flexed. This pseudosubluxation is due to the normal laxity of the intervertebral ligaments, and nearly 50% of children younger than 8 years have anteroposterior movement of 3 mm or more. The straight-line relationship of the posterior elements in flexion (the posterior cervical line eponymically known as Swischuk's line) is helpful in differentiating physiologic from pathologic anterior displacement of C2 on C3. The posterior cervical line drawn from the anterior aspect of the spinous process of C1 to the anterior aspect of the spinous process of C3 should pass no more than 2 mm anteriorly to the same point of C2. Also common in typical children is subtle overriding of the atlas on the dens with the neck in extension.

Clinical Manifestations. The clinical signs and symptoms of instability of the C1–C2 junction are inconsistent. Only a few patients report a trauma or pain of the head or neck or exhibit torticollis, quadriparesis, or signs of high spinal cord compression.

The clinical signs of basilar impression or occipitalization of the atlas suggest that major neurologic damage is occurring as the dens encroaches on the spinal cord (see Plate 1.31). Muscle weakness and wasting, ataxia, spasticity, hyperreflexia, and pathologic reflexes—the signs of pyramidal tract irritation—are common. Posterior impingement from the rim of the foramen magnum or the posterior ring of the atlas is typical of odontoid anomalies; symptoms include alterations of sensation for deep pressure, vibration, and proprioception. Nystagmus, ataxia, and incoordination may be due to an associated cerebellar herniation, and signs and symptoms of vertebral artery compression—dizziness, seizures, mental deterioration, and syncope—may occur alone or in combination with symptoms of spinal cord compression.

Radiographic Findings. The atlas-dens interval (see Plate 1.2) is the space between the anterior aspect of the dens of the axis and the posterior aspect of the anterior ring of the atlas. In children, the atlas-dens interval should be no greater than 4.5 mm, particularly on neck flexion. (In adults, the upper limit of normal is 3 mm.) A subtle increase in the atlas-dens interval with the neck in neutral position may indicate disruption of the transverse ligament of the atlas. This is a valuable sign in evaluation of acute injury when standard flexion-extension views are potentially hazardous.

The atlas-dens interval is of limited value in evaluating chronic atlantoaxial instability resulting from congenital anomalies of the occipitocervical junction, rheumatoid arthritis, and Down syndrome. In patients with these conditions, the dens is frequently hypermobile, resulting in an increased atlas-dens interval, and measurement of the amount of space available for the spinal cord is more valuable. This is accomplished by measuring the distance from the posterior aspect of the dens to the nearest posterior structure (foramen magnum or posterior ring of the atlas). This measurement is particularly helpful in evaluating a nonunion of the dens or os odontoideum, because in both conditions the atlas-dens interval may be normal but on neck flexion or extension the space available for the spinal cord may be considerably reduced. A reduction of the lumen of the vertebral canal to 13 mm or less may be associated with neurologic problems.

Laxity or tear of dens-retaining ligaments

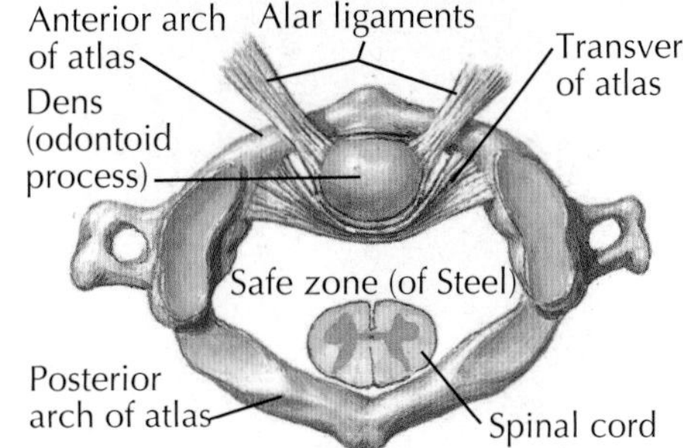

Dens normally held in place by transverse ligament of atlas and by alar ligaments attached to anterior margin of foramen magnum. Dens occupies anterior third of area enclosed by arches of atlas. Spinal cord occupies posterior third. Middle third is safe zone (of Steel).

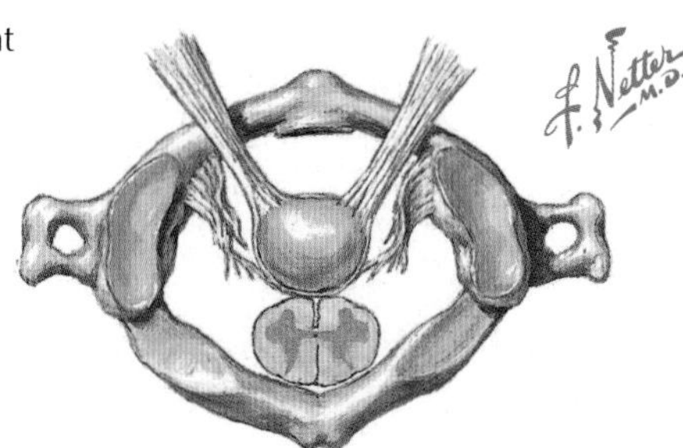

If transverse ligament is attenuated or torn, dens may drop back into safe zone on neck flexion but alar ligaments act as checkreins and may prevent spinal cord injury. If alar ligaments also give way, spinal cord damage may result. Laxity or tear of retaining ligaments is also a factor in odontoid hypermobility in occipitalization of atlas.

Os odontoideum

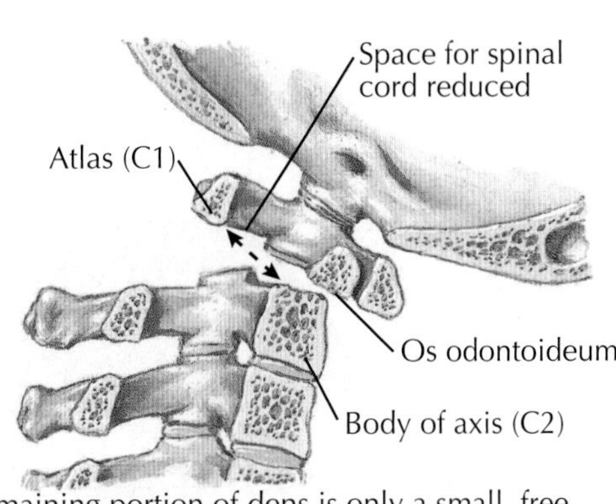

Remaining portion of dens is only a small, free ossicle that cannot stabilize atlantoaxial joint. On neck flexion, atlas slides forward with skull, carrying ossicle with it and reducing space for spinal cord.

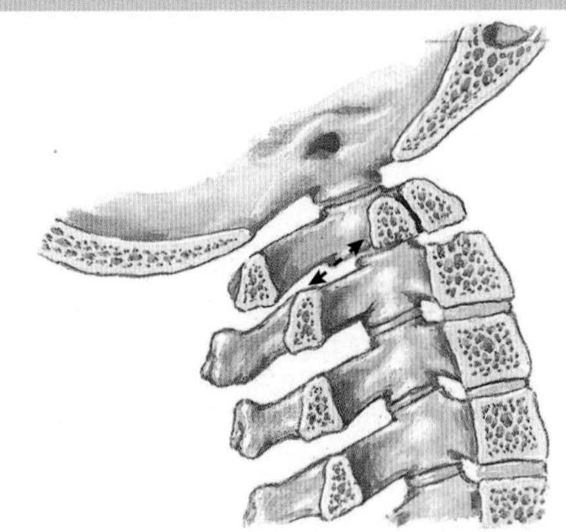

On neck extension, reverse occurs but space for spinal cord may also be compromised. Os odontoideum is functionally equivalent to odontoid fracture. Odontoid aplasia or hypoplasia has similar effects.

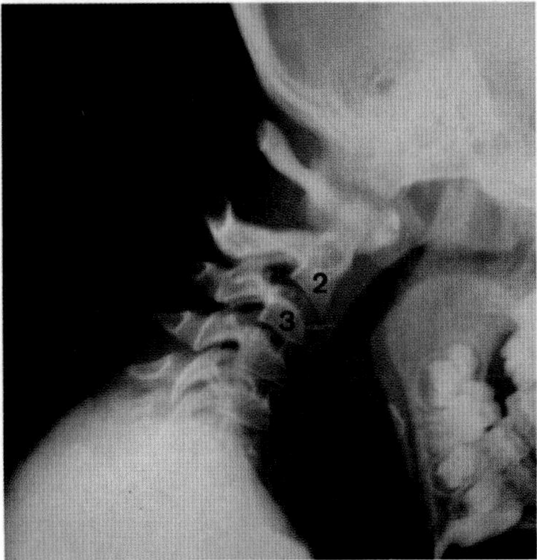

Pseudosubluxation of C2 on C3. In young children, normal laxity of ligaments may allow anterior displacement of C2 on C3. This usually improves with maturation.

Obtaining a satisfactory radiograph is often hampered by the patient's limited ability to cooperate, by fixed bony deformity, and by overlapping shadows from the mandible, occiput, and foramen magnum. Directing the x-ray beam 90 degrees to the lateral of the skull usually produces a satisfactory view. Visualization may be enhanced with flexion-extension radiographs or CT, and motion studies are frequently necessary.

Treatment. Effective treatment of atlantoaxial instability can be provided only if the exact cause of the symptoms is determined. Before surgical intervention, reduction of the atlantoaxial articulation should be achieved either by positioning or by traction with the patient awake. Surgical reduction should be avoided because it has been associated with increased morbidity and mortality.

SYNOSTOSIS OF CERVICAL SPINE (KLIPPEL-FEIL SYNDROME)

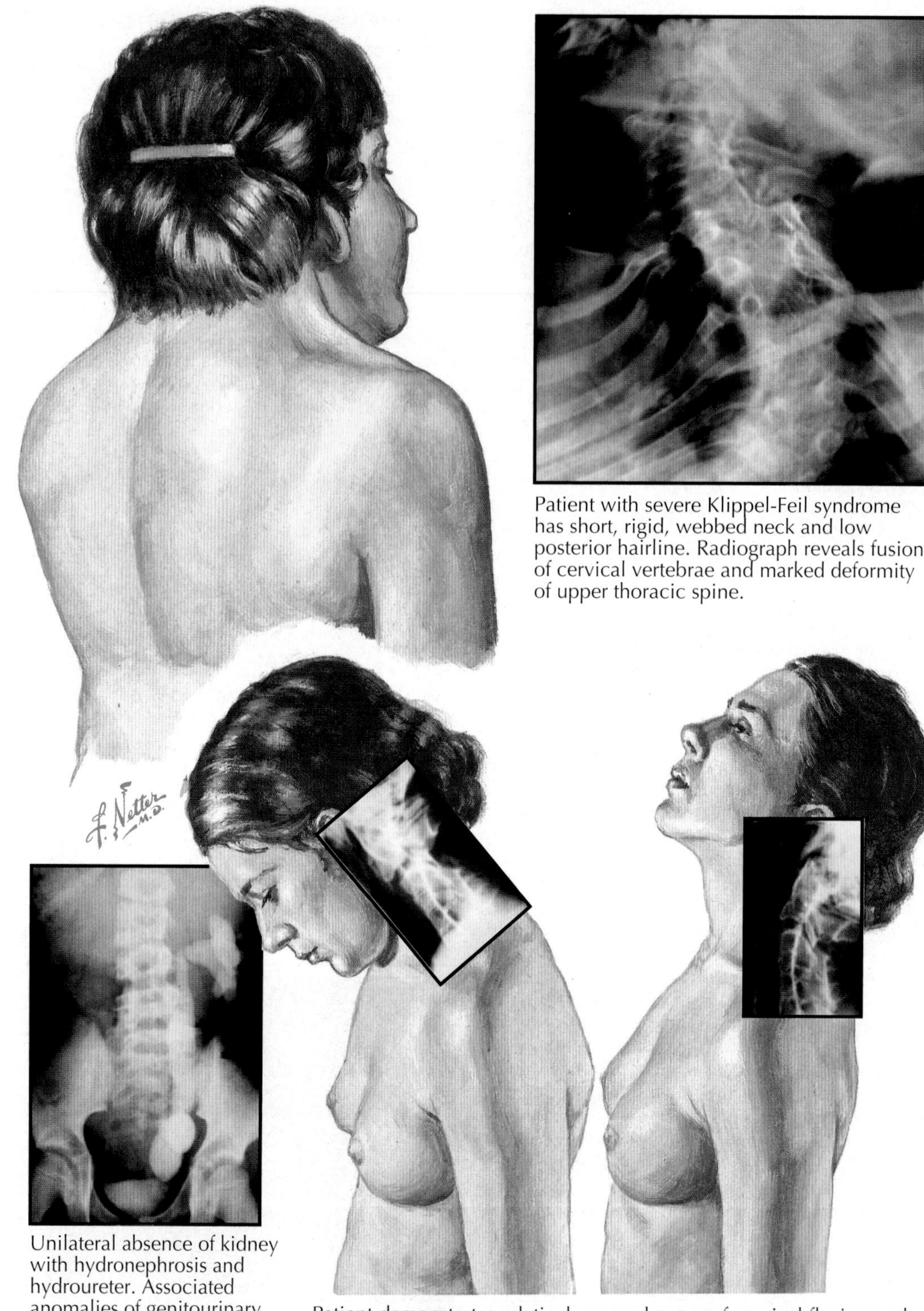

Patient with severe Klippel-Feil syndrome has short, rigid, webbed neck and low posterior hairline. Radiograph reveals fusion of cervical vertebrae and marked deformity of upper thoracic spine.

Unilateral absence of kidney with hydronephrosis and hydroureter. Associated anomalies of genitourinary tract or other systems may be less apparent yet more serious than cervical spine fusions.

Patient demonstrates relatively normal range of cervical flexion and extension despite fusion of most cervical vertebrae; motion occurs chiefly at one open disc space. No cervical webbing or abnormality of posterior hairline is evident.

Klippel-Feil syndrome refers to the congenital fusion of two or more cervical vertebrae. In some patients, the entire cervical spine is involved. The fusion is a result of failure of segmentation of the cervical somites during the third to eighth weeks of embryonic development. Although the etiology is not yet determined, the developmental defect is not limited to the cervical spine. Unilateral or bilateral elevation of the scapula occurs in 25% to 30% of these patients. Other, less apparent defects in the genitourinary, nervous, and cardiopulmonary systems and hearing loss often occur in patients with Klippel-Feil syndrome.

Clinical Manifestations. The classic clinical signs of the syndrome—low posterior hairline, short neck, and limitation of neck motion—are not consistent findings; fewer than one-half of patients exhibit all three signs. Although the most common finding is limitation of neck motion, many patients with marked cervical involvement maintain a deceptively good range of motion.

Whereas anomalies of the atlantoaxial joint (C1–C2) may be symptomatic, fusion of lower cervical vertebrae causes no symptoms. Rather, the problems commonly associated with Klippel-Feil syndrome originate at the open segments adjacent to the area of synostosis, which may become compensatorily hypermobile. As a result of trauma or increased demands placed on these joints, hypermobility can lead to frank instability or degenerative osteoarthritis. Symptoms may be due to mechanic irritation at open articulations, nerve root irritation, or spinal cord compression. The development of symptoms is most likely with fusion of more than four vertebrae; occipitalization of the atlas plus a C2–C3 fusion, leading to excessive demands on the atlantoaxial articulation; and an open articulation between two zones of vertebral fusion.

Potentially serious conditions that are associated with Klippel-Feil syndrome include scoliosis or kyphosis (60% of patients), urinary tract abnormalities (33%), congenital heart disease (14%), and deafness (30%). Because the urinary tract problems are often asymptomatic in children but if present require treatment or monitoring, ultrasonography or evaluation by MRI should be performed routinely.

Radiographic Findings. Radiographic examination can be problematic because fixed bony deformities frequently prevent proper positioning of the patient for standard views, and overlapping shadows from the mandible, occiput, and foramen magnum may obscure the upper vertebrae. Standard radiographic views of the neck on flexion and extension are therefore helpful, and CT with reconstruction views are helpful in delineating the bony anatomy. MRI is a powerful tool in assessing spinal cord morphology and nerve root impingement.

Ossification of the vertebral body is not complete until adolescence, and in children the unossified physes may give the false impression of a normal disc space. Therefore a suspected fusion in a child should be confirmed with lateral flexion-extension radiographs.

The bony cervical defects may extend to the upper thoracic area, particularly in patients with severe involvement. However, narrowing of the vertebral canal, which is due to degenerative changes or developmental hypermobility, does not usually occur until adulthood.

Treatment. Children with minimal involvement usually lead a normal, active life with minor or no restrictions or symptoms. Symptoms referable to the cervical spine may occur in adulthood as a result of osteoarthritis or instability of the hypermobile articulations. Although conservative treatment is sufficient in most patients, a few require judicious surgical stabilization. Scoliosis must be monitored carefully and treated if necessary. However, the relatively good prognosis of the cervical condition is overshadowed by the hidden or unrecognized associated anomalies. Early recognition and treatment of these problems may spare the patient further deformity or serious illness.

CONGENITAL MUSCULAR TORTICOLLIS (WRYNECK)

Congenital muscular torticollis (congenital wryneck) is a common condition, usually discovered in the first 6 to 8 weeks of life. Contracture of the sternocleidomastoid muscle tilts the head toward the involved side, rotating the chin to the contralateral shoulder. The cause is believed to be ischemia of the sternocleidomastoid muscle, particularly the sternal head, due to intrauterine positioning, prolonged labor, or increased pressure during passage through the birth canal. The contracture usually occurs on the right side, and 20% of children with congenital muscular torticollis also have congenital dysplasia of the hip. These observations support the hypothesis that both problems are related to intrauterine malpositioning or presentation.

Clinical Manifestations. In the first month after delivery, a soft, nontender enlargement, or "tumor," is noted beneath the skin and attached to the body of the sternocleidomastoid muscle. The tumor usually resolves in 6 to 12 weeks, after which contracture, or tightness, of the sternocleidomastoid muscle and the torticollis become apparent. With time, fibrosis of the sternal head of the muscle may entrap and compromise the branch of the accessory nerve to the clavicular head, further increasing the deformity.

If the contracture does not improve, deformities of the face and skull (plagiocephaly) can develop in the first year. The face becomes flattened on the side of the contracted sternocleidomastoid muscle. The deformity is related to the sleeping position. Children who sleep prone are more comfortable with the affected side down; consequently, that side of the face becomes distorted. Children who sleep supine develop flattening of the back of the head.

Treatment. In the first year of life, conservative measures comprising stretching and range-of-motion exercises and positioning produce good results in 85% to 90% of patients. If conservative measures fail, surgical intervention is required. Surgery should be considered in patients with a persistent sternocleidomastoid contracture at age 11 months. Allowing the deformity to persist results in permanent facial asymmetry, vision difficulties, and a poor cosmetic result.

Surgery usually consists of resection of a portion of the distal sternocleidomastoid muscle. The incision should be placed transversely in the neck to coincide with the normal skin folds. It should not be placed near the clavicle, because scars in this area tend to spread. Postoperative treatment includes passive stretching exercises and, occasionally, a brace or cast to maintain the corrected position.

CLINICAL APPEARANCE OF CONGENITAL MUSCULAR TORTICOLLIS (WRYNECK)

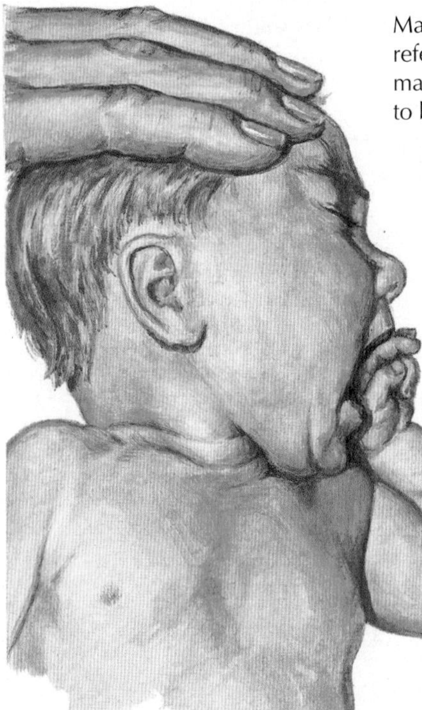

Mass in neck within sternocleidomastoid muscle often referred to as sternocleidomastoid tumor. This earliest manifestation of congenital muscular torticollis regresses, to be followed by contracture of muscle.

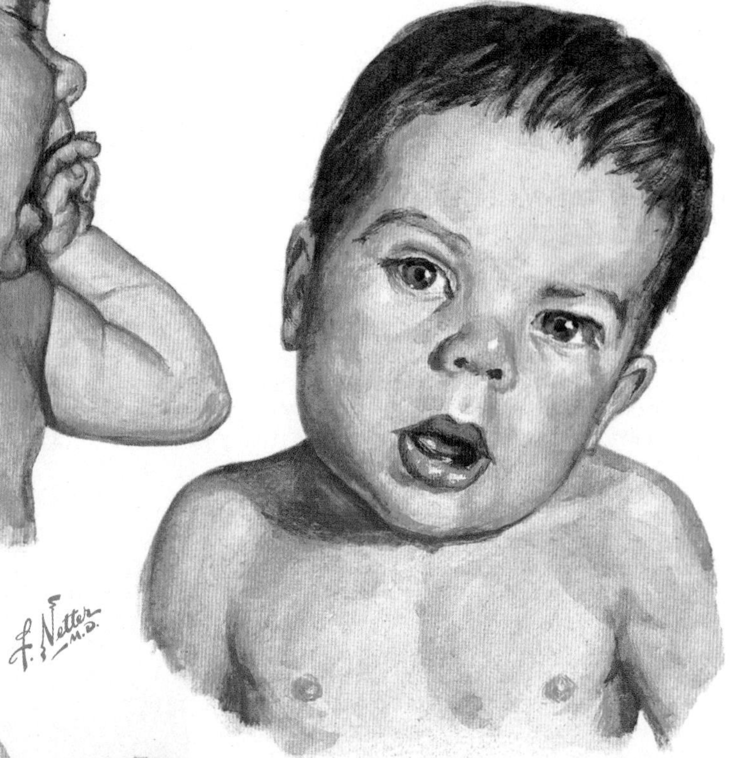

Child with muscular torticollis. Head tilted to left with chin turned slightly to right because of contracture of left sternocleidomastoid muscle. Note facial symmetry (flattening of left side of face).

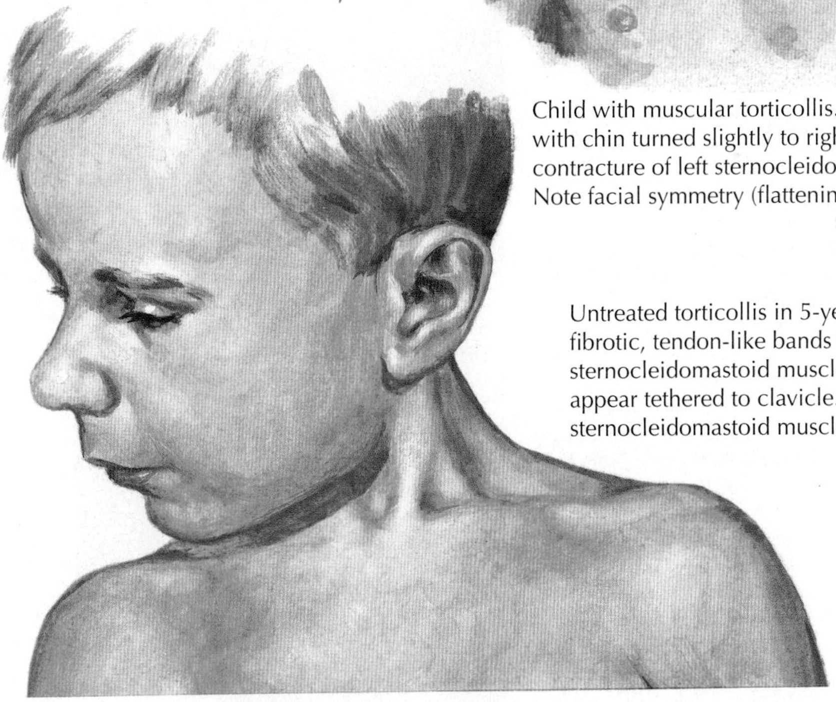

Untreated torticollis in 5-year-old boy. Thick, fibrotic, tendon-like bands have replaced sternocleidomastoid muscle, making head appear tethered to clavicle. Two heads of left sternocleidomastoid muscle are prominent.

NONMUSCULAR CAUSES OF TORTICOLLIS

Torticollis is a common childhood complaint that can be caused by a wide variety of problems, but identifying the cause can be difficult (see Plate 1.35). If the characteristic posture of the head and neck is noted shortly after birth, congenital anomalies of the cervical spine should be considered, particularly those of the occipitocervical junction. Torticollis may be a sign of Klippel-Feil syndrome, basilar impression, or occipitalization of the atlas. In these conditions, however, the sternocleidomastoid muscle on the short side is not contracted.

Wryneck that appears several weeks after birth is usually congenital muscular torticollis. Less commonly, soft tissue problems such as abnormal skin webs or folds (pterygium colli) maintain the neck in a twisted position.

Congenital Muscular Torticollis (Wryneck) (Continued)

Tumors in the region of the sternocleidomastoid muscle, such as cystic hygroma, branchial cleft cysts, and thyroid teratomas, are rare but must be considered.

Intermittent torticollis can occur in the young child. A seizure-like condition called benign paroxysmal torticollis of infancy can be the result of a variety of neurologic causes, including drug intoxication. Similarly, sudden posturing of the trunk and torticollis associated with gastroesophageal reflux are often reported.

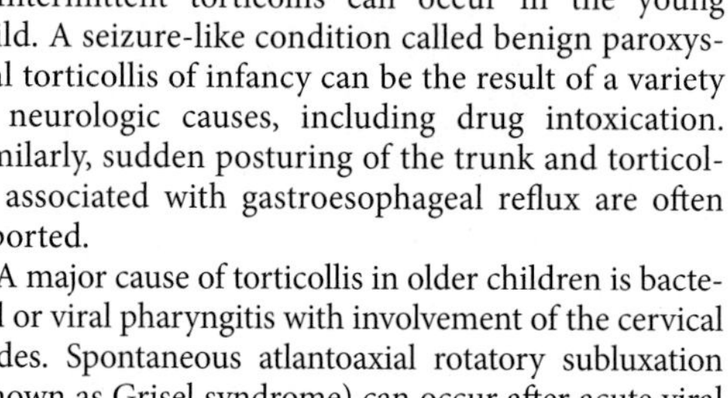

A major cause of torticollis in older children is bacterial or viral pharyngitis with involvement of the cervical nodes. Spontaneous atlantoaxial rotatory subluxation (known as Grisel syndrome) can occur after acute viral or bacterial pharyngitis and in association with flares of autoimmune disorders.

Surgery in the upper pharynx, such as a tonsillectomy, may also precipitate rotatory subluxation. Inflammation and local edema in the retropharyngeal region can lead to transient laxity of the ligamentous restraints, allowing greater motion of C1–C2. Standard radiographic techniques are inadequate for diagnosis, and special views, including tomography and fine cut CT limited to the upper cervical spine, are often required. Bed rest, NSAIDs, and use of a soft collar may be sufficient if the diagnosis is made early. A head halter or halo brace may be necessary for long-standing problems or if the simple measures fail. If the torticollis persists beyond 3 weeks, recurs, or becomes subacute, postreduction immobilization in a Minerva cast brace or halo brace is indicated. Surgical stabilization is required for the rare recalcitrant cases.

Traumatic causes should be considered and carefully excluded in the diagnosis of torticollis. Unrecognized and untreated injuries may have serious neurologic consequences. Torticollis commonly follows an injury to the C1–C2 articulation. It may also be due to fractures and dislocations of the dens, which may not be apparent on initial radiographs. Skeletal dysplasia, Morquio syndrome, spondyloepiphyseal dysplasia, and Down syndrome are commonly associated with C1–C2 instability and accompanying torticollis.

Torticollis is also a sign of certain neurologic problems, particularly space-occupying lesions of the central nervous system, such as tumors of the posterior cranial fossa or the spinal cord, chordoma, and syringomyelia. Uncommon neurologic causes include dystonia musculorum deformans and hearing and vision problems, which can lead to head tilt. Although hysterical and psychogenic causes have been described, they are very uncommon and should be considered only a diagnosis of exclusion.

Calcification of the vertebral disc, an uncommon problem of childhood, most often involves the cervical vertebrae. The C6–C7 disc space is the most frequent site, but any disc space can be involved. In 30% of children, trauma is the apparent cause; 15% of children report an upper respiratory tract infection. The onset of symptoms is abrupt, with torticollis, neck pain, and limitation of neck motion the usual presenting complaints. Only 25% of patients are febrile on presentation. Rarely, the disc herniates posteriorly, causing spinal cord compression, or anteriorly, causing dysphasia. Typically, the clinical manifestations resolve rapidly and the radiographic signs more gradually. Two-thirds of children are symptom free within 3 weeks and 95% within 6 months. Resolution of associated neurologic symptoms occurs in 90% of patients.

Nonmuscular Causes of Torticollis

Atlantoaxial rotatory subluxation and fixation (after Fielding and Hawkins)

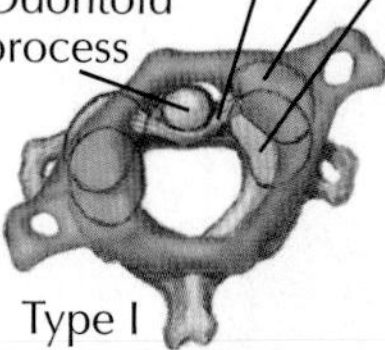

Type I
Rotatory subluxation of atlas about dens but transverse ligament intact. No anterior displacement.

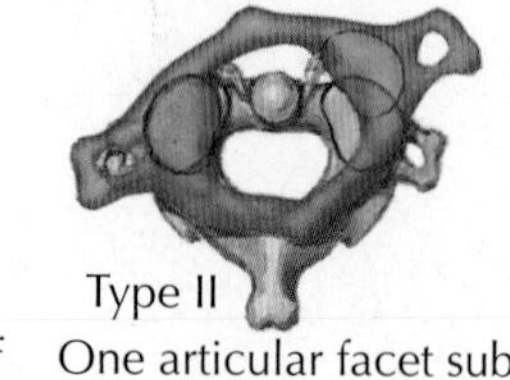

Type II
One articular facet subluxated, other acts as pivot; transverse ligament defective. Anterior displacement of 3–5 mm.

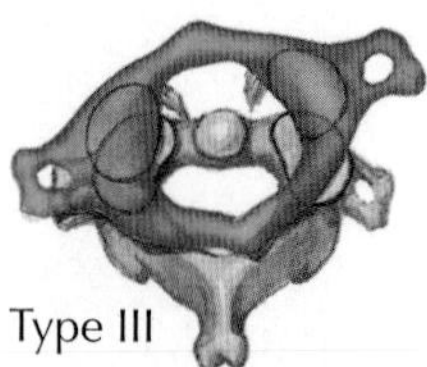

Type III
Both articular facets subluxated, transverse ligament defective. Anterior displacement of >5 mm.

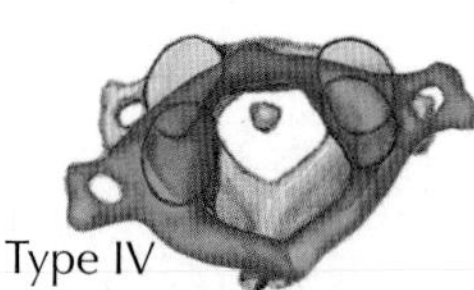

Type IV
Posterior rotatory subluxation (rare). Os odontoideum or absent or defective dens.

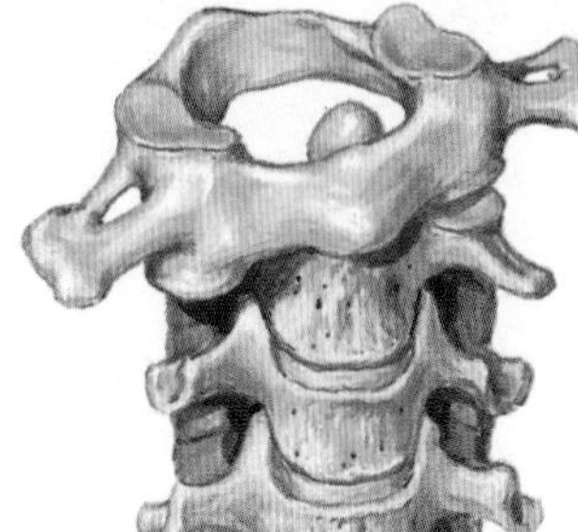

Type I rotatory subluxation

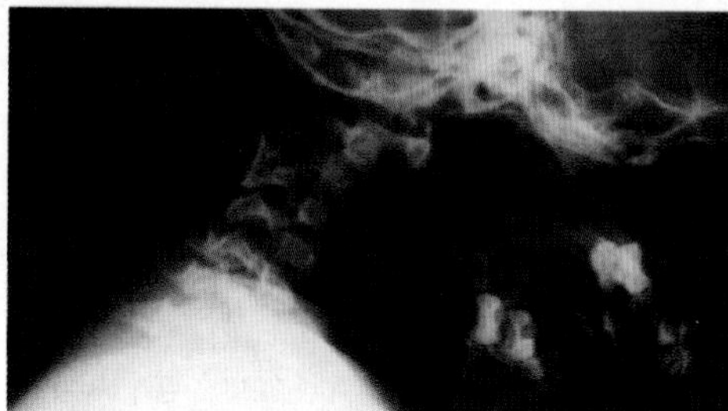

Radiograph shows lateral mass of atlas rotated anteriorly. CT scans helpful in confirming diagnosis.

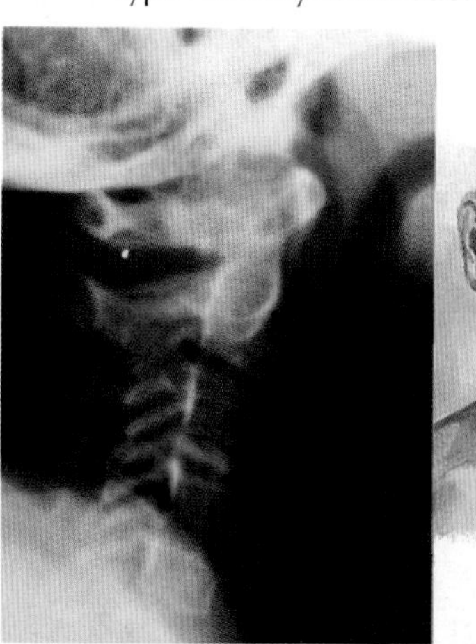

Acute intervertebral disc calcification
Seven-year-old girl with spontaneous onset of torticollis. Radiograph reveals calcification of C3–4 disc.

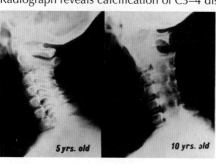

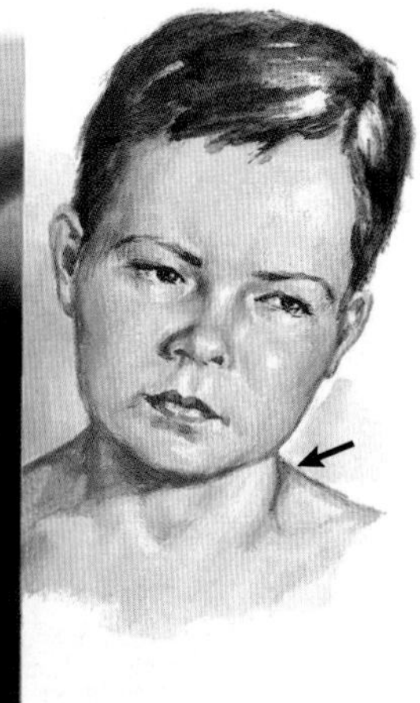

Cervical adenitis

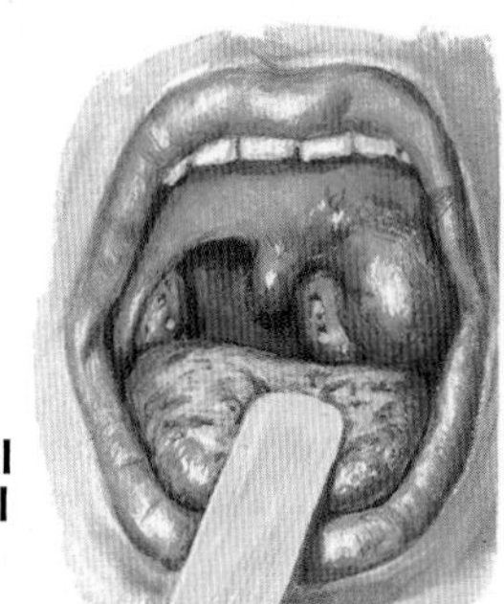

Retropharyngeal abscess or tonsil infection

Juvenile arthritis of cervical spine
Radiographs show progression.

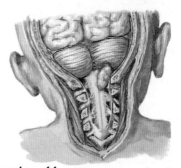

Tumor in region of foramen magnum (rare)

Scoliosis

Scoliosis is a rotational deformity of the spine and ribs. Although in most cases the cause of scoliosis is unknown (idiopathic scoliosis), more than 50 genetic markers have been identified as having a major role in adolescent idiopathic curves. Scoliosis may also result from a variety of congenital, neuromuscular, mesenchymal, and traumatic conditions, and it is commonly associated with neurofibromatosis.

PATHOLOGY

A complicated three-dimensional deformity, scoliosis is characterized by both lateral curvature and vertebral rotation. Although degree of vertebral rotation and lateral curvature do not necessarily proceed in concert, typically, as the curve progresses, the vertebrae and spinous processes in the area of the major curve rotate toward the concavity of the curve (see Plate 1.37). Because the ribs are attached to the vertebral body, the ribs subsequently rotate dorsally on the convexity and volarly on the concave side. The entire thoracic cage can become ovoid, and anterior prominence can become as noticeable as posterior prominence. Most idiopathic curves are noteworthy for relative hypokyphosis of the thoracic spine. Kyphotic curves are more common in congenital and certain neuromuscular conditions. Lordosis (swayback) of the lumbar spine may accompany the scoliotic deformity.

In addition to rotation, scoliosis also causes other pathologic changes in the vertebrae and related structures in the area of the curve. The disc spaces become narrower on the concave side of the curve and wider on the convex side. The vertebrae also may become wedged (i.e., thicker on the convex side). On the concave side of the curve, the pedicles and laminae are frequently shorter and thinner, and the vertebral canal is narrower.

The structural changes described are most common in idiopathic forms of scoliosis; the pathologic process may vary somewhat in paralytic and congenital forms. In general, in the paralytic curve, which is caused by severe muscle imbalance, the ribs assume an almost vertical position on the convex side.

IDIOPATHIC SCOLIOSIS

About 85% of patients with scoliosis exhibit an idiopathic (genetic) form. The disease is not primarily a problem of bone and joints but likely a manifestation of genetically mediated neuromuscular imbalance. Significant scoliosis (i.e., curves severe enough to require treatment) occurs up to seven times more often in girls than boys, whereas mild scoliosis affects boys and girls in equal numbers.

About 90% of all idiopathic curves are probably genetic, and thus the two terms are used synonymously. The scoliotic trait may not pass on to every generation (incomplete penetrance) and may cause a severe curve in a parent and a mild curve in a child, or vice versa (variable expressivity). If a person with idiopathic scoliosis has children, about one-third of all offspring will have scoliosis; if both parents have genes for scoliosis, even if one parent does not exhibit the disease, the odds that offspring will be afflicted are even greater.

Curve Patterns

For years, the curve pattern classification system used to evaluate adolescent scoliosis was as described by Moe, Winter, and King—the so-called King classification. In recognition of subtleties with newer surgical management of advanced curves not well addressed by this older classification, the Lenke classification system of adolescent idiopathic scoliosis was developed to provide a comprehensive and interobserver reliable means to categorize curves. Upright posteroanterior and lateral radiographs along with the supine side-bending radiographs are required. The classification system consists of a triad that uses a curve type (1–6) (see Plate 1.37), a lumbar spine modifier (A, B, C), and a sagittal thoracic modifier (−, N, +). All three regions of the radiographic coronal and sagittal planes—the proximal thoracic, main thoracic, and thoracolumbar/lumbar—are designated as either the major curve (largest Cobb measurement) or minor curves, with the minor curves separated into structural (rigid, with correction limited on supine bending films) and nonstructural types

Pathologic Anatomy of Scoliosis

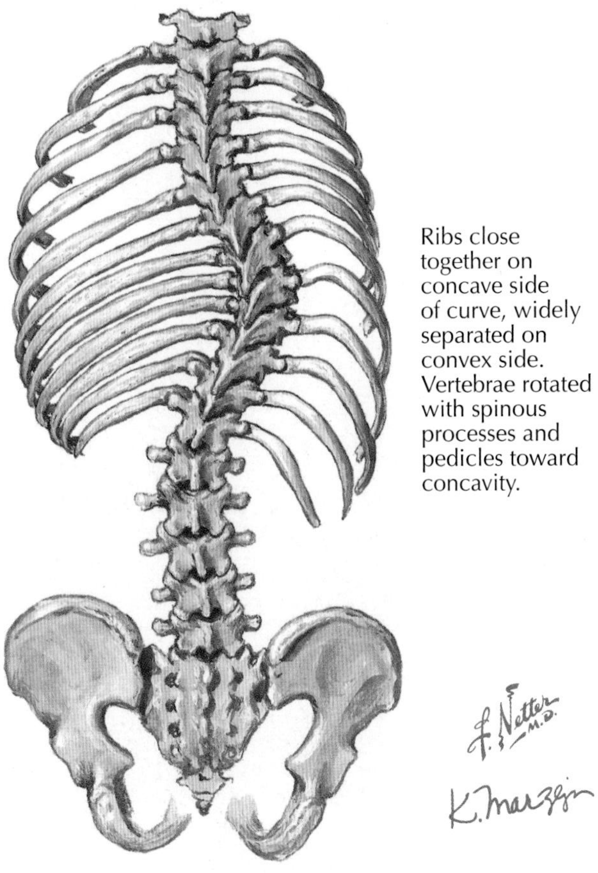

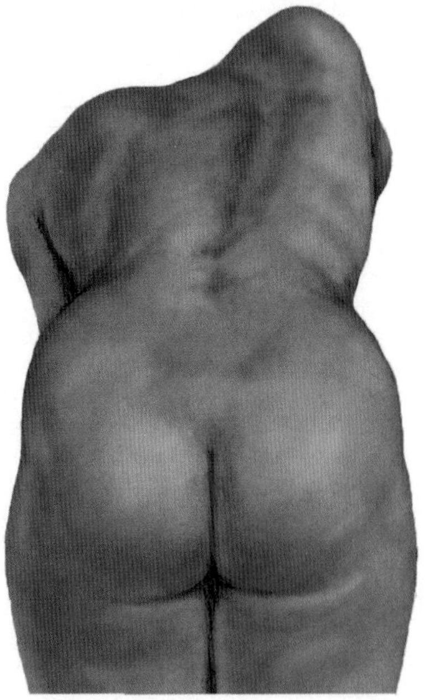

Ribs close together on concave side of curve, widely separated on convex side. Vertebrae rotated with spinous processes and pedicles toward concavity.
F. Netter M.D.
K. Marzen

Posterior bulge of ribs on convex side forms characteristic rib hump in thoracic scoliosis

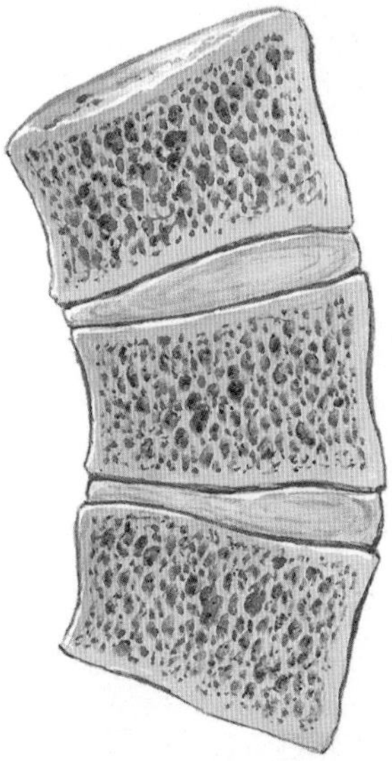

Section through scoliotic vertebrae. Decreased vertebral height and disc thickness on concave side.

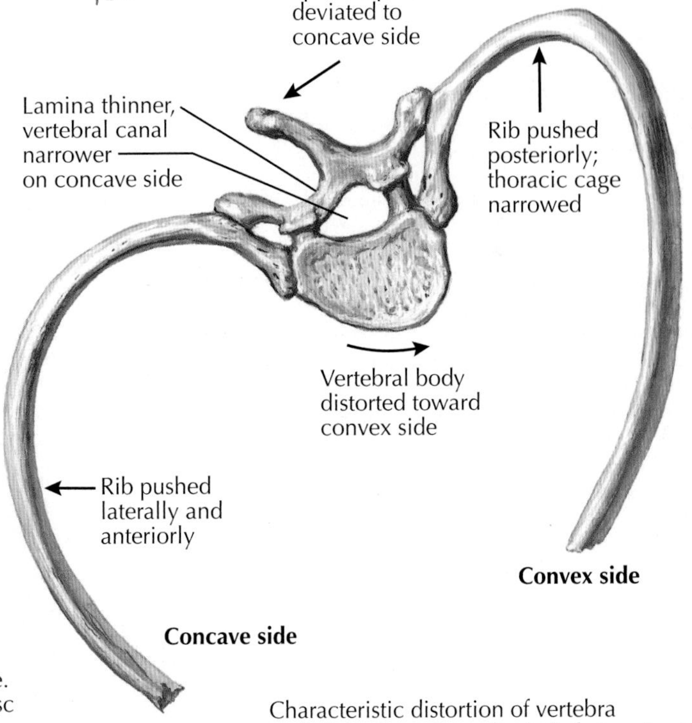

Characteristic distortion of vertebra and rib in thoracic scoliosis (inferior view)

Scoliosis (Continued)

(flexible, with correction on bending film to <25 degrees). The current recommendations are that the major and structural minor curves be included in the instrumentation and fusion and the nonstructural minor curves be excluded. Overall, this classification system is treatment directed; however, there are other aspects of the deformity that may suggest deviation from the recommendations of the classification system. The goal of this system is to allow organization of curve patterns to provide comparisons of treatment methods to provide the best treatment for each scoliosis patient.

In general, *right thoracic curves* are the most common. The curve usually extends to and includes T4, T5, or T6 at its upper end and T11, T12, or L1 at its lower limit. Typically, these curves do not correct on side bending. Because of severe vertebral rotation, the ribs on the convex side become badly deformed, resulting in a severe cosmetic defect and serious impairment of cardiopulmonary function when the curve exceeds 60 degrees. Right thoracic curves can develop rapidly and therefore must be treated early.

The right thoracic curve is always a *major* curve (i.e., the curve is structural and of great significance). There are usually smaller curves in the opposite direction above and below the right thoracic curve. These *secondary* curves are usually referred to as *minor* curves. A minor curve usually forms as a compensatory mechanism to help keep the head aligned over the pelvis and may be structural or nonstructural.

The *thoracolumbar curve* is also a common idiopathic curve pattern. It is longer than the right thoracic curve and may be to either right or left. The upper end of the curve extends to and includes T4, T5, or T6 and the lower end includes L2, L3, or L4, usually with minor upper thoracic and lower lumbar curves. The thoracolumbar curve is usually less cosmetically deforming than the thoracic curve; however, it can cause severe rib and flank distortion due to vertebral rotation.

The *double major curve* consists of two structural curves of almost equal prominence. Double major curves can be any of the following combinations: right thoracic/left lumbar (most common); right thoracic/left thoracolumbar; left thoracolumbar/right lower lumbar; and right thoracic/left thoracic (double thoracic).

The *lumbar major curve* is quite common and usually runs from T11 or T12 to L5. In 65% of cases, the curve is to the left. The thoracic spine above the curve usually does not develop a structural compensatory curve and remains flexible. Lumbar major curves are not very deforming but can become quite rigid, leading to severe arthritis pain in later life and during pregnancy.

The extent of deformity varies with the underlying curve pattern, tending to be most severe with the right thoracic and thoracolumbar curves and less severe with balanced double major curves. Severe right thoracic and thoracolumbar curves often produce a marked overhang of the thorax toward the convexity of the curve and a rib hump, and the torso tilts to the convex side. In contrast, with a balanced double major curve, the shoulders are level over the pelvis, and the rib and lumbar prominences are not too severe. The major deformity with this type of curve is trunk shortening.

Typical Scoliosis Curve Patterns

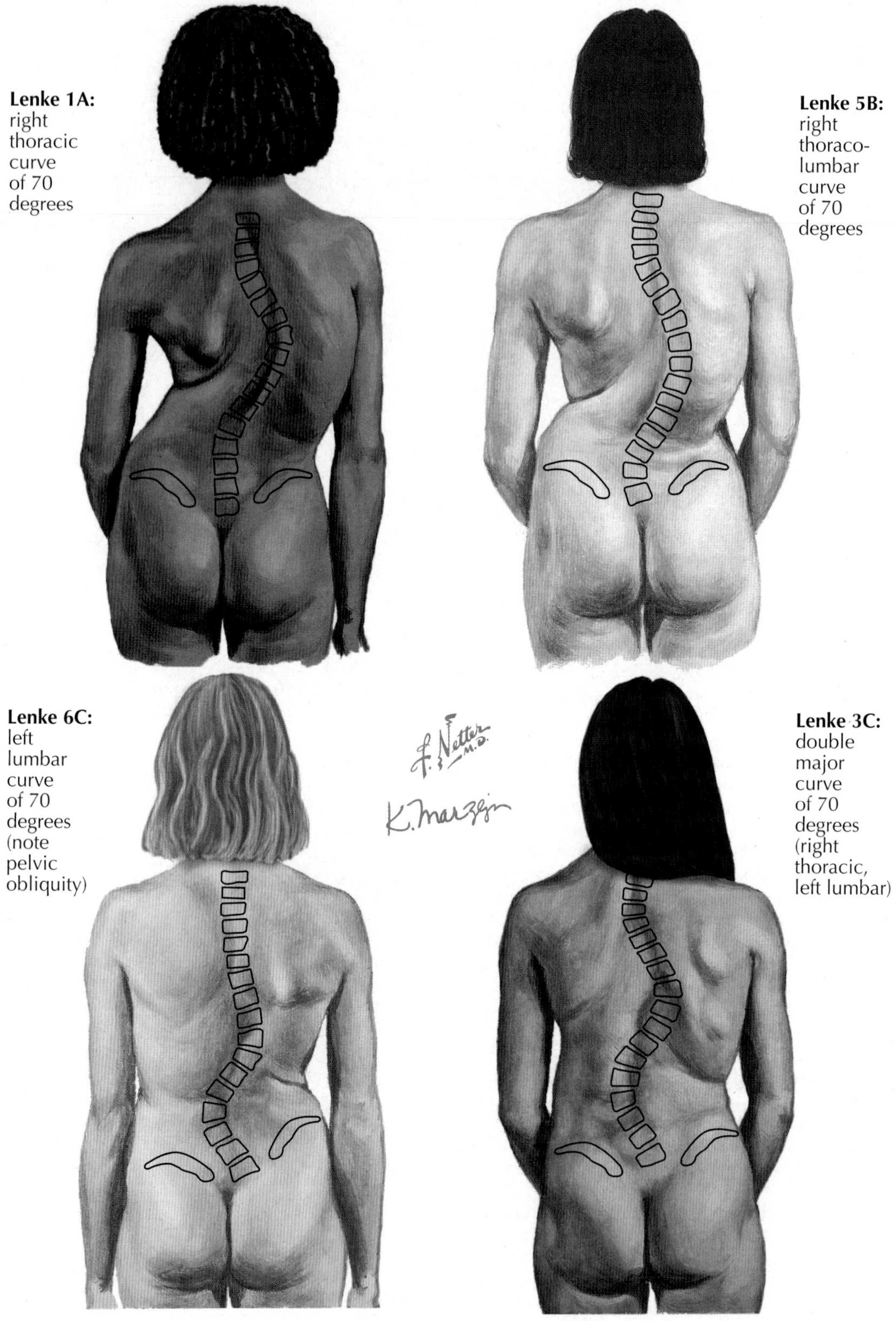

Lenke 1A: right thoracic curve of 70 degrees

Lenke 5B: right thoraco-lumbar curve of 70 degrees

Lenke 6C: left lumbar curve of 70 degrees (note pelvic obliquity)

Lenke 3C: double major curve of 70 degrees (right thoracic, left lumbar)

Age at Onset

Idiopathic scoliosis is classified into infantile, juvenile, and adolescent types according to peak periods of onset.

Infantile idiopathic scoliosis, which occurs between birth and 3 years of age, is usually noticed in the first year of life. Curiously, it is far more common in England, usually occurs in boys, and generally results in a left thoracic curve. The majority of these curves, thought to be a result of molding in the uterus, resolve spontaneously, even if untreated. Some, however, progress to severely rigid structural curves unless treated early and aggressively with serial casting as advocated by Mehta or with bracing.

Juvenile idiopathic scoliosis occurs between the ages of 4 and 10 years and is most often detected at or after age 6. Both sexes are affected equally. Most curves in this group are right thoracic curves. Unless early standing and side-bending radiographs are available, it is almost impossible to distinguish cases of late infantile onset from those of early juvenile onset.

Scoliosis (Continued)

Adolescent idiopathic scoliosis is diagnosed when the curve is noticed between 10 years of age and skeletal maturity. Many curves first noticed at this age are probably present before age 10 but are not recognized until the adolescent growth spurt. Although adolescent scoliosis occurs in both boys and girls equally, 70% of cases that progress and need treatment occur in girls. The double major and right thoracic patterns predominate.

Progression

Idiopathic curves may or may not progress during growth. The risk of progression may be linked to various factors such as sex, age at onset, delayed maturation, and vertebral anatomy. Usually, the younger the child is when the structural curve develops, the less favorable the prognosis will be. In general, structural curves have a strong tendency to progress rapidly during the adolescent growth spurt, whereas small, nonstructural curves may remain flexible for long periods, never becoming severe. Nevertheless, the worst advice a physician can give a patient with scoliosis is "as soon as you finish growing, your curve will stop." In a significant number of adults, scoliosis remains progressive, eventually causing pain and disability.

The curve is most likely to progress 1 to 2 degrees a year during adult life; if the curve is greater than 60 degrees at maturity, the curve pattern throws the trunk out of balance, or the patient has extremely poor muscle tone. Generally, a curve that is less than 30 degrees at age 25 years is unlikely to progress.

CONGENITAL SCOLIOSIS

Congenital scoliosis is probably the result of some form of trauma to the zygote or embryo in the early embryonic period that causes a vertebral or extravertebral defect. Because many organ systems develop at the same time, children with congenital scoliosis almost always have some urinary tract or cardiac anomaly as well. Children with congenital scoliosis should also be examined for cervical spine anomalies such as Klippel-Feil syndrome (see Plate 1.33) and scapular deformities such as Sprengel deformity.

Congenital curves must be observed carefully. Although most do not progress significantly, some become severe and irreversible. Posterior vertebral defects can be open or closed. The open (dysraphic) defect caused by myelomeningocele can be very severe and is usually associated with partial or complete neurologic deficit with paraplegia and urinary tract problems.

Closed vertebral defects are classified into four types: (1) partial unilateral failure of vertebral formation (wedge vertebra), (2) complete unilateral failure of vertebral formation (hemivertebra), (3) unilateral failure of segmentation (congenital bar), and (4) bilateral failure of segmentation (block vertebra). Other congenital combinations, some of which are extravertebral (e.g., rib fusions), are so mixed and bizarre they defy classification.

In hemivertebral conditions, as the anomalous vertebrae grow, they cause the spine to lengthen on the convex side, leading to severe curves. Unilateral bars can also cause severe curvature. The worst possible congenital curve results from hemivertebrae on one side of the spine and several unilateral bars on the opposite side.

The best treatment for a progressive congenital curve is a short, in situ spinal fusion performed as soon as progression is noted.

CONGENITAL SCOLIOSIS: CLOSED VERTEBRAL TYPES (MACEWEN CLASSIFICATION)

A. Partial unilateral failure of formation (wedge vertebrae)

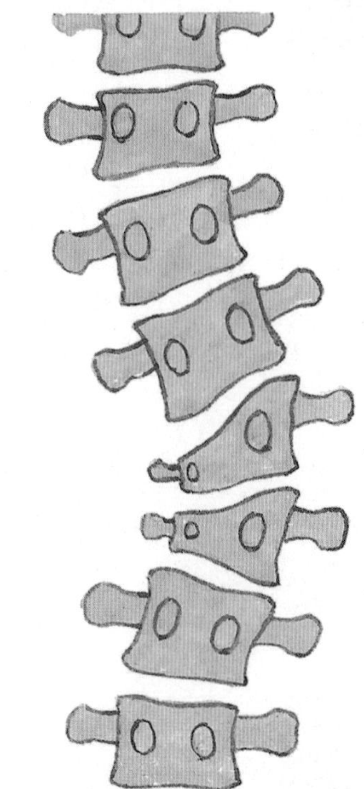

B. Complete unilateral failure of formation (hemivertebra)

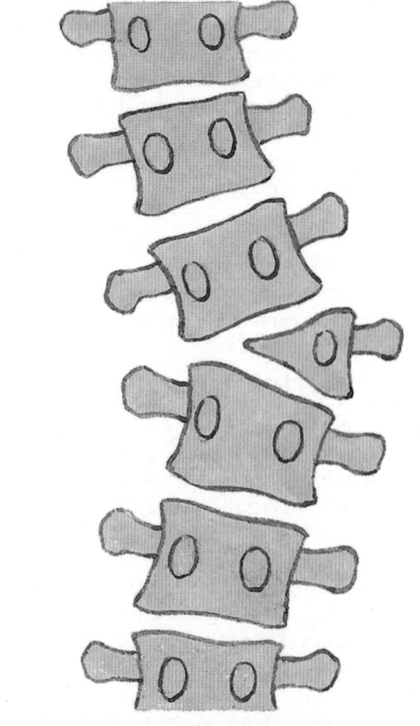

C. Unilateral failure of segmentation (congenital bar)

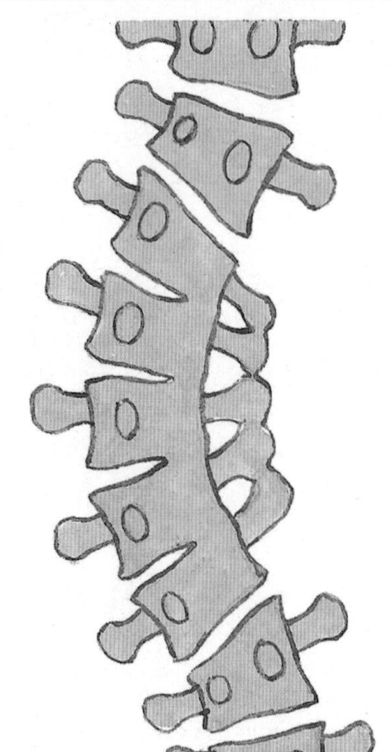

D. Bilateral failure of segmentation (block vertebra)

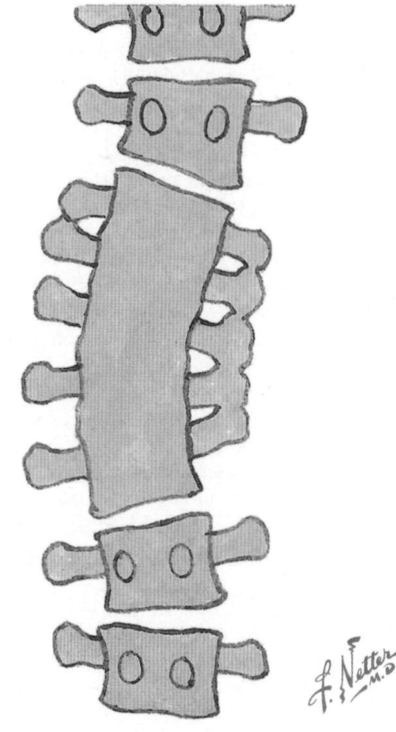

NEUROMUSCULAR SCOLIOSIS

Neuropathic forms of neuromuscular scoliosis are caused by a variety of disorders. Muscle imbalance due to poliomyelitis, a lower motor neuron disease, and cerebral palsy, an upper motor neuron disease, may lead to severe, long C-shaped curves that may extend from the lower cervical region to the sacrum. Curves caused by syringomyelia also tend to become quite severe, often necessitating surgery. Because many patients with syringomyelia live well beyond their teenage years, treatment is indicated when progression of the curve is noticed. Occasionally, neurosurgical drainage of the syrinx can help control the curve.

Myopathic forms of neuromuscular scoliosis are caused by both progressive and static disorders. The

Scoliosis (Continued)

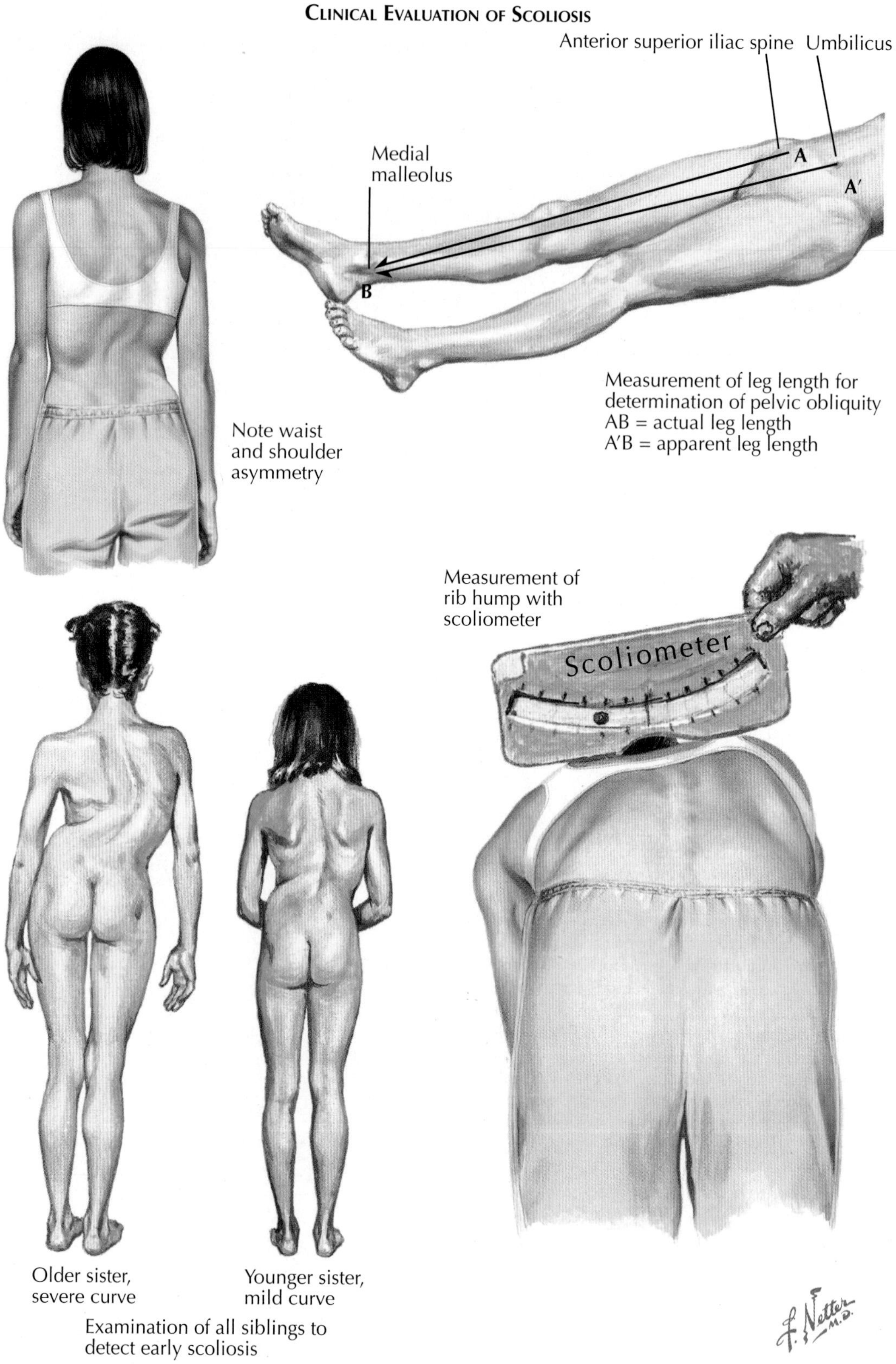

progressive disorders are exemplified by muscular dystrophies. These disorders cause muscle imbalance, generally producing long C-shaped curves. Some children with scoliosis due to muscular dystrophy are so weak that their spines appear to collapse when they assume the erect posture. Judicious bracing or surgery may be helpful in some patients, but the prognosis is always guarded.

Other neuromuscular forms may be caused by mixed disorders, such as Friedreich ataxia, in which a muscle imbalance causes muscle weakness plus overpull by the stronger trunk and paraspinal muscles.

MESENCHYMAL AND TRAUMATIC DISORDERS

Congenital mesenchymal disorders leading to scoliosis can occur with various types of dwarfism and in Marfan syndrome. Because patients with Marfan syndrome are usually very tall, their curves can become quite severe.

In osteogenesis imperfecta, the extreme brittleness of the bones results in hundreds of microfractures of the spine, eventually producing a scoliotic deformity. Scheuermann disease, if not properly treated, may also lead to a progressive kyphotic deformity in adolescents (see Plate 1.42).

Direct vertebral trauma such as a fracture with wedging or nerve root irritation can cause scoliosis. In some instances, the scoliosis may be secondary to irradiation for cancer treatment that, though saving the child's life, destroys the growth plates of the vertebral body, resulting in unequal growth and causing spinal deformity.

Physical Examination. As part of the thorough physical examination, the development of secondary sexual characteristics should be noted. Their presence or absence, in addition to a height comparison with siblings and parents, can be significant in predicting future growth patterns. The skin is examined for café-au-lait markings indicative of neurofibromatosis, and the lumbar spine is searched for pigmented areas or patches of hair that can indicate an underlying congenital condition, such as spina bifida or diastematomyelia.

After the general examination, a more specific examination of the deformity is done, beginning with evaluation of trunk alignment, which is used to gauge balance or displacement of the torso. A tape measure dropped as a plumb line from the occiput can show if the head and trunk are aligned. In patients with a very severe double major curve, however, alignment may remain perfect.

The shoulder girdle should be examined for symmetry, and scapular prominence should be noted. The neck-shoulder angle may be distorted by asymmetry of the trapezius muscle caused by cervical or high thoracic curves.

The type of curve is recorded, and its flexibility is evaluated on side bending and distraction. Lifting the patient gently by the head distracts the curve, allowing the degree of rigidity and flexibility of the spine to be assessed.

Deformities of the thoracic cage are carefully recorded. With the patient bending forward, a scoliometer is used to measure the rib hump. Anterior rib and breast asymmetry should also be noted.

Pelvic obliquity must be carefully assessed. It can be nonstructural, occurring because of a habit, or structural, resulting from a lower limb-length discrepancy.

Clinical Evaluation of Scoliosis

Anterior superior iliac spine

Umbilicus

Medial malleolus

A

A′

B

Measurement of leg length for determination of pelvic obliquity
AB = actual leg length
A′B = apparent leg length

Note waist and shoulder asymmetry

Measurement of rib hump with scoliometer

Scoliometer

Older sister, severe curve

Younger sister, mild curve

Examination of all siblings to detect early scoliosis

Structural pelvic obliquity can also be caused by contractures of muscle groups either above or below the iliac crests.

A brief but thorough neuromuscular examination including evaluation of all reflexes, response to stimuli, and motor capabilities is an important part of the scoliosis work-up. In children with congenital conditions, sensory or motor loss can indicate an internal spinal condition, such as diastematomyelia. Decreased vibratory sensation in the limbs is a consistent sign in idiopathic scoliosis, which is due to a brainstem dysfunction; a more extensive neurologic examination is usually not warranted. The findings of the neuromuscular examination should be carefully correlated with the physical examination of the back. Painful scoliosis is uncommon in children, and its presence suggests the possibility of osteoid osteoma,

Scoliosis (Continued)

spinal cord tumors, spondylolysis or spondylolisthesis, or infection.

Imaging. A single erect anteroposterior radiograph from the occiput to the iliac crest is sufficient for the initial examination of a new scoliosis patient. A spot lateral view of the lumbosacral spine is indicated if spondylolisthesis or spondylolysis (see Plate 1.44) is suspected. The thyroid, breasts, and gonads should be shielded, and radiation exposure should be kept to a minimum.

Side-bending radiographs are taken to distinguish structural from nonstructural curves. Right side bending allows a right thoracic curve to uncoil, and the radiograph provides evidence of the suppleness of the ligaments and other soft tissue structures. Left side bending uncoils a left lumbar curve. Bending radiographs are typically reserved for preoperative evaluation.

The curve is measured on the initial radiograph using the Cobb method, which is preferred by the Scoliosis Research Society. The accuracy of the Cobb method relies on determining the upper and lower end-vertebrae of the curve. The end-vertebrae at both the upper and lower limits are those that tilt most severely *toward* the concavity of the curve. In other words, the superior end-vertebra is the last vertebra whose superior border inclines toward the concavity of the curve to be measured and the inferior end-vertebra is the last one whose inferior border inclines toward the concavity of the curve. Horizontal lines are drawn at the superior border of the superior end-vertebra and the inferior border of the inferior end-vertebra. Perpendicular lines are then drawn from each of the horizontal lines and the intersecting angles measured. (The broken arrows do not converge toward the concavity being measured, indicating that these vertebrae are not end-vertebrae but are in another curve above or below the curve being measured.)

Vertebral rotation is measured most accurately by estimating the amount that the pedicles of the vertebrae have rotated, as seen in the anteroposterior radiograph.

Skeletal maturation must also be determined accurately because scoliosis progression may slow (although it does not always stop) when a patient is fully mature. Girls generally cease growing and mature at about 14.5 years of age; this occurs in boys at age 16 to 17 years.

Several methods are used to estimate skeletal age. Radiographs of the left hand and wrist are compared with the *Radiographic Atlas of Skeletal Development of the Hand and Wrist* by Greulich and Pyle. Presence of an open triradiate physis in the acetabulum is an indication of significant skeletal immaturity. Pelvic radiographs can be used to determine the degree of iliac crest secondary ossification center excursion known as the Risser sign. When the iliac crest meets the sacroiliac joint and the physis closes, maturation is nearly complete. Another technique involves examining the superior and inferior growth plates of the thoracic and lumbar vertebrae on high-quality radiographs. If the growth plates are mottled in appearance, the skeletal growth is not complete. Solid union of the growth plates with the vertebral bodies indicates that maturation is complete.

Treatment. A variety of treatment modalities are available.

School Screening. The best treatment for scoliosis is early detection and prompt referral to a center equipped to provide complete scoliosis care. Most curves can be treated without surgery if detected before they become too severe. Scoliosis screening is still being done in schools across the United States and in other countries. A physician, midlevel provider, or school nurse can typically screen scores of children in less than 1 hour. The screening procedure is simple: the child bends from the waist with the arms hanging freely (see Plate 1.39). This position accentuates even a slight asymmetry in the ribs or lumbar area. School screening should begin in the fifth grade, and both boys and girls should be examined every 6 to 9 months. If scoliosis or kyphosis is detected in a child, all siblings should be screened.

Exercises. Exercises are mentioned under treatment only to be strongly condemned as a cure for scoliosis. Unfortunately, physicians under the mistaken impression that exercises help improve or eliminate a curve continue to prescribe an exercise program to many patients, who

Determination of Skeletal Maturation, Measurement of Curvature, and Measurement of Rotation

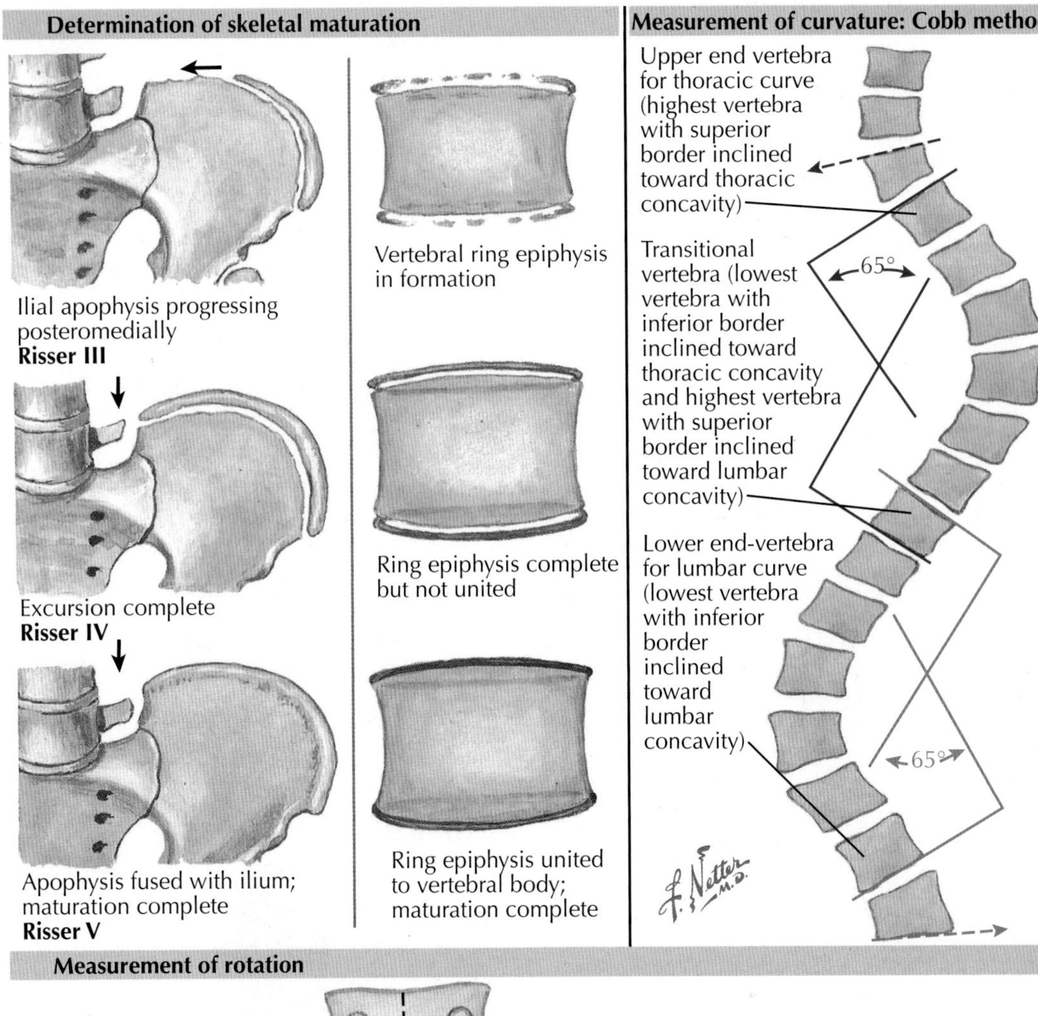

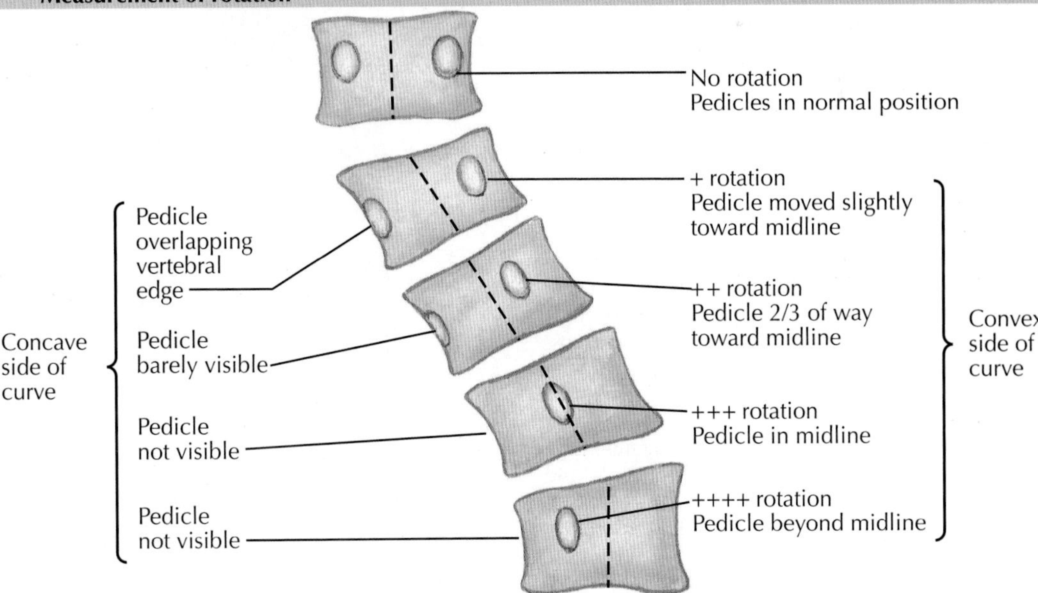

SCOLIOSIS (Continued)

are then lost to follow-up until their curve becomes more severe. Basically, only two treatments effectively correct scoliosis: spinal bracing and surgery.

Braces. With close supervision, a properly constructed, well-fitted brace, such as the Boston, Charleston, or Providence brace, can successfully halt progression of a curve in approximately 70% of patients, if the patient and family are cooperative. Some curves, however, progress to greater deformity no matter what is done. Unfortunately, there is currently no way to predict if a curve will respond successfully to bracing.

Low-profile braces have gained broad acceptance among patients and physicians alike. The now "historical" Milwaukee brace, the first brace demonstrated to alter the natural history of a curve, is rarely used in the contemporary management of scoliosis. Patient acceptance is much greater with these braces because they are barely visible under clothing or worn only at night. The inner pad is adjustable to add further pressure on the apex of the curve as the curve improves. The braces can be modified depending on the curve pattern and the presence or absence of kyphosis.

The Boston brace is generally worn over a long undershirt for 16 hours a day. Children can run and play in it relatively freely. Exercises are done daily both in and out of the brace to maintain muscle strength. The Charleston and Providence braces are "bending braces" that exert corrective force on the curve by virtue of a side-bending moment.

Patients using braces are seen every 6 months for brace adjustment. At 4- to 6-month intervals, new radiographs are taken with the patient erect and not wearing the brace. When radiographs show that skeletal maturation is nearly complete, the bracing is discontinued. Some physicians will stop bracing abruptly, whereas others wean from the brace. Neither regimen has demonstrated superiority.

Electrical Stimulation. In years past, electrical stimulation of muscle gained popularity in the treatment of scoliosis. It has been abandoned because it was not proven to alter the natural history of curve progression. In one study, patients who were treated with electrical stimulation fared worse than controls.

Surgery. The main indication for scoliosis surgery is relentless curve progression—typically progression of thoracic curves to values more than 45 degrees and progression of thoracolumbar curves to values more than 40 degrees. Pain, spinal balance, and general cosmesis are other factors that need to be considered with respect to surgical decision-making. Because the first spinal fusion was performed in 1911, many different surgical techniques and types of instrumentation have been developed, each with its own advantages and risks, including neurologic impairment. Regardless of the method and hardware, the goal of surgery is to produce a solid arthrodesis of a balanced spine in the frontal and sagittal planes over a level pelvis.

Posterior fusion techniques began using Harrington rod instrumentation. In some patients, a compression rod was added, and the rods were further attached to the vertebrae with wires passed through holes drilled in the spinous processes. Harrington rods are now primarily of historical interest. The relative lack of restoration of sagittal balance was a major long-term problem.

In the Luque technique, still employed in certain neuromuscular curve types, the spine is straightened with two rods attached to sublaminar wires or cables. The Cotrel-Dubousset method was the first segmental instrumentation that allowed for rotation correction of individual spinal elements and employed two rods coupled together with transverse traction rods and hooks, which effectively derotated the spine.

Current state-of-the-art instrumentation uses primarily pedicle screws that in comparison to hooks or sublaminar wires allow for far greater restoration of sagittal and coronal balance, as well as a more rigid construct that typically obviates the need for postoperative bracing.

With the broad acceptance of pedicle screw technology, as well as the recognition of its derotational strength, anterior surgery is less common and is typically reserved for exceptionally rigid curves requiring disc space release or curves with absent posterior bony elements.

The technique and approach used should be based primarily on the surgeon's preference and expertise.

BRACES FOR SCOLIOSIS

Providence brace

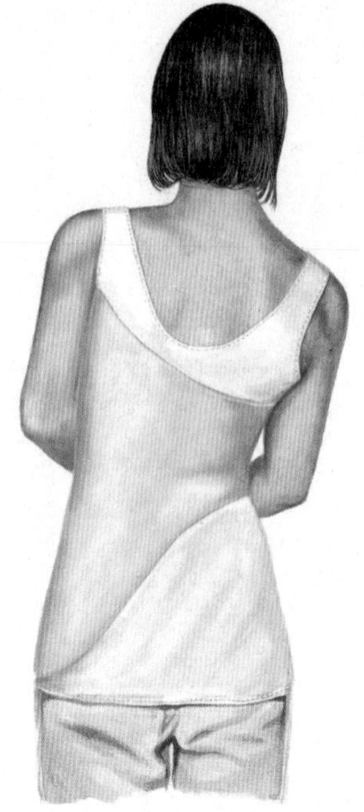

The Providence brace is seen exerting a significant yet comfortable bending moment on the curve.

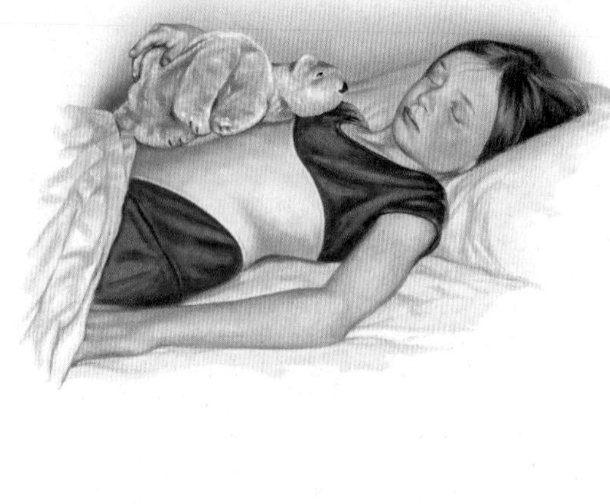

The nighttime bending brace is well tolerated, is efficacious, and has good patient compliance.

Boston brace

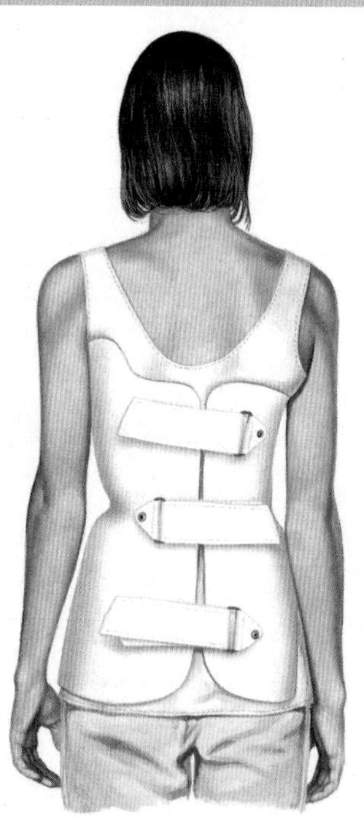

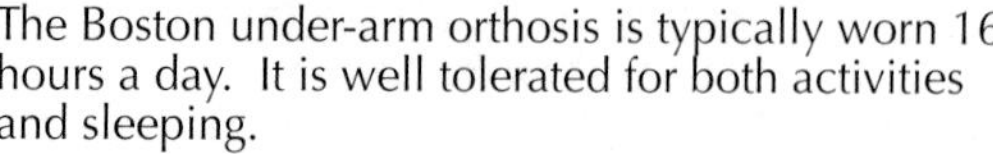

The Boston under-arm orthosis is typically worn 16 hours a day. It is well tolerated for both activities and sleeping.

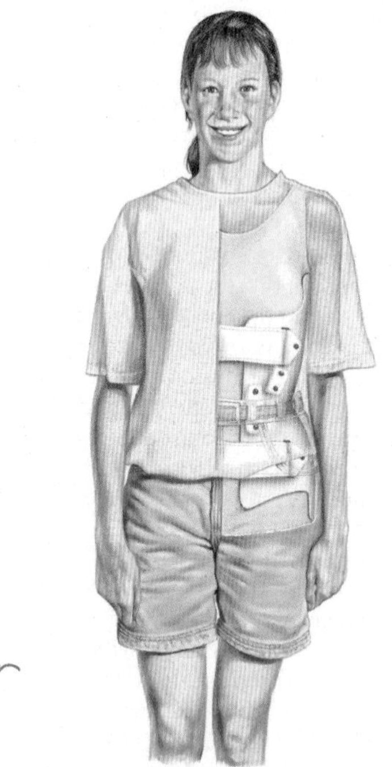

Clothing easily covers the Boston brace and therefore is better accepted than older alternatives such as the Milwaukee brace.

SCHEUERMANN DISEASE

Although an exaggerated thoracic kyphosis has been documented for centuries, it was only with the advent of medical radiography that Scheuermann was able to identify the disease. This progressive disorder occurs in patients near puberty, manifested by an increase in the normal kyphosis in the thoracic spine with an abnormal degree of wedging of the vertebrae at the apex of the kyphotic curve. The diagnosis of Scheuermann disease is limited to patients with a kyphotic curve greater than 60 degrees. (Measurements are done in a manner similar to the coronal plane Cobb method; see Plate 1.40.) Typically the curve is measured from T4 to T12 on the lateral view. Normal kyphosis is 20 to 45 degrees in which at least three adjacent vertebrae are wedged 5 degrees or more and where disc space narrowing and end plate irregularity are noted. Although Schmorl nodules are common radiographic findings, they are not part of the diagnostic criteria of Scheuermann disease.

The etiology of Scheuermann disease is not yet understood, but there appears to be a genetic factor. Scheuermann speculated that the disease was caused by avascular necrosis of the anterior portion of the cartilage ring apophysis of the vertebral body, similar to the pathogenesis of Legg-Calvé-Perthes disease. Mechanical factors (particularly heavy labor), contractures of the hamstring and pectoral muscles, and herniation of the intervertebral disc through the anterior portion of the epiphyseal plate have also been suggested as contributing factors. Specimens obtained from patients undergoing anterior spinal fusion for Scheuermann kyphosis have revealed wedge-shaped vertebral bodies and a contracted, thickened anterior longitudinal ligament that acts as a tether across the kyphosis, maintaining a relatively inflexible deformity. Subsequent histologic studies, although confirming a disruption of the epiphyseal plates and extravasation of disc material into the bony spongiosa of the vertebral body, have revealed no evidence of avascular necrosis or inflammatory changes in bone, disc, or cartilage.

Clinical Manifestations. Characteristic signs of Scheuermann disease are the exaggerated, rounded appearance of the back, round shoulders, and poor posture; pain and deformity are uncommon. In adolescents, so-called poor posture may be an important clue to significant structural alterations of the vertebral column that can only be identified with radiography. Despite urging by their parents, children with a true structural problem like Scheuermann disease cannot stand straight. As a result of the exaggerated thoracic kyphosis and lumbar lordosis, affected children typically stand slumped, with the arms folded across a prominent abdomen. The kyphosis is relatively inflexible, is not fully corrected when the patient attempts thoracic hyperextension in the prone position, and is accentuated by forward bending. Mild scoliosis is an associated finding in 20% to 30% of patients, and contracture of the hamstring and pectoral muscles, which leads to forward protrusion of the shoulder girdle, is common. Neurologic examination, usually normal, may reveal a more serious condition such as kyphosis secondary to congenital vertebral deformity or trauma.

Scheuermann disease is often misdiagnosed as postural round-back deformity, which also occurs in preadolescent children. However, this type of kyphosis is supple (i.e., it is corrected with prone hyperextension) and is not accompanied by muscle contractures, wedging of the vertebral bodies, or irregularities of the epiphyseal plates. Differential diagnosis includes infectious spondylitis, hypoparathyroidism and hyperparathyroidism, rickets, osteogenesis imperfecta, idiopathic juvenile osteoporosis, neurofibromatosis, tumors, Morquio and Hurler syndromes, and traumatic injuries.

Treatment. In growing children, treatment is instituted to arrest progression of the deformity, improve the cosmetic appearance of the back, and alleviate any pain. The deformity has been shown in some cases to be correctable if there is potential for further vertebral growth and the kyphotic deformity is flexible. The spine is held in a corrected position with a cast (not well tolerated) or a high thoracic brace. The kyphosis can correct to a normal curvature in the first year as evidenced by reconstruction of the wedged vertebral bodies and anterior portion of the vertebral apophysis. If untreated, the deformity may progress to a large degree and require surgical correction. Many kyphotic deformities are recognized when the patient is older and less flexible. Although individuals vary, the indications for surgery usually begin with curves more than 60 degrees.

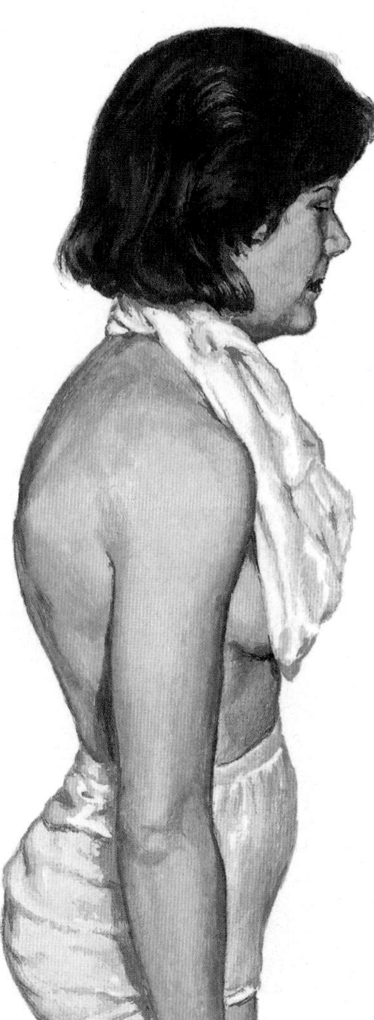

In adolescent, exaggerated thoracic kyphosis and compensatory lumbar lordosis due to Scheuermann disease may be mistaken for postural defect.

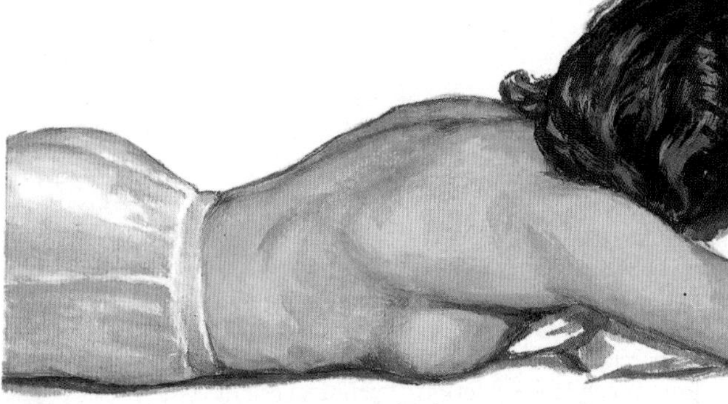

Unlike postural defect, kyphosis of Scheuermann disease persists when patient is prone and thoracic spine extended or hyperextended (*above*) and accentuated when patient bends forward (*below*).

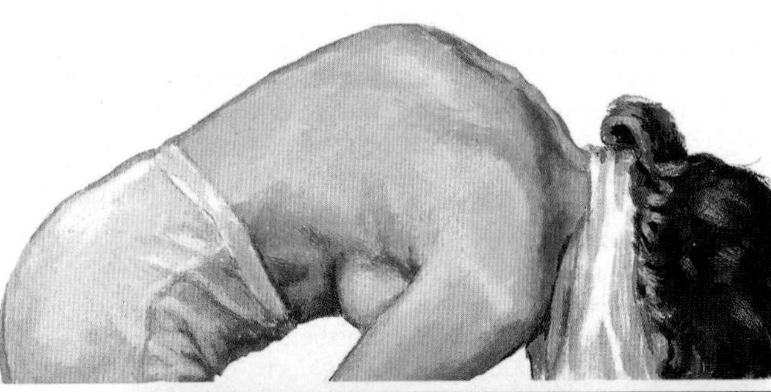

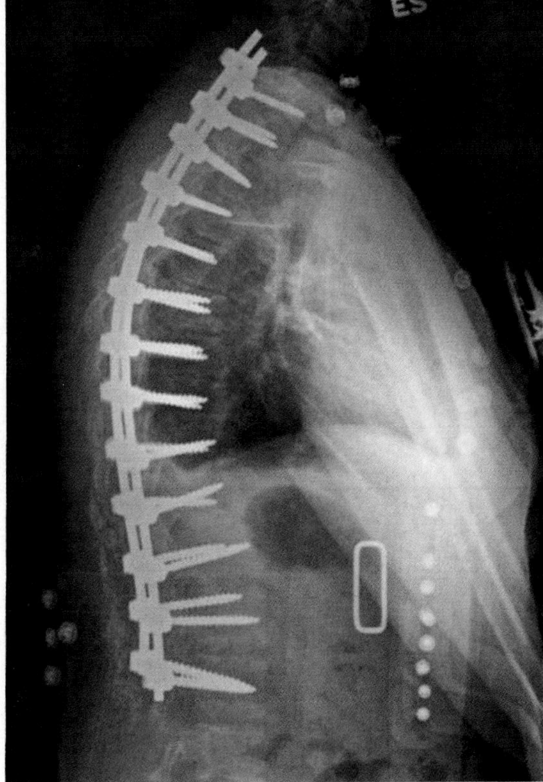

Lateral view following instrumented spinal fusion for Scheuermann kyphosis. Lumbar lordosis is diminished here by the postoperative brace, which is worn for 6 weeks after surgery.

CONGENITAL KYPHOSIS

Congenital kyphosis is due to the same embryologic failure of segmentation or formation of the vertebrae as congenital scoliosis. The direction of the curve (lateral or posterior) depends on the location of the spinal defect. Anterior defects cause kyphosis, and lateral defects cause scoliosis. A combined deformity, kyphoscoliosis, is common. In about 15% of patients, congenital deformities are associated with an anomaly of the neural elements (e.g., diastematomyelia, neurenteric cyst).

A kyphotic deformity that is secondary to failure of segmentation (congenital bar or block vertebrae) rarely causes neurologic deficits. However, a progressive kyphosis due to failure of formation may lead to paraplegia. In partial failure of formation (wedge vertebrae or hemivertebrae), neurologic deficits can occur whether the vertebral canal is in good alignment or dislocated.

Symmetric failure of formation (absent vertebrae), a rare defect, causes a pure angular kyphosis with a high risk (25%) of paraparesis. Asymmetric failure of formation commonly leads to formation of hemivertebrae and resultant kyphoscoliosis, most often in the thoracic or thoracolumbar spine. Although the alignment of the canal is usually maintained by the strong, intact posterior elements, kyphoscoliosis may be relentlessly progressive, often increasing 10 degrees per year. The risk of paraplegia is greatest when the apex of the curve is in the upper thoracic spine where there is less room for the spinal cord and the blood supply to the cord is most tenuous.

Partial failure of formation with vertebral canal dislocation (congenital dislocated spine) is characterized by a lack of continuity of the posterior elements of the vertebral canal, leading to instability and the risk of catastrophic neurologic loss from even minor trauma. Even if the injury does not occur, the curve progresses inexorably, producing a gradual loss of neurologic function. In some patients, the neurologic deficit is present at birth, the result of spinal cord compression rather than congenital malformations of the spinal cord.

Neurologic complications are common when the kyphosis or kyphoscoliosis is complicated by rotatory dislocation of the spine because the spinal cord is twisted over a very short segment. The hump, or kyphos, is abrupt and angular and the cord is fixed at the apex by the roots above and below, which are twisted in opposite directions.

Although functional impairment may be noted at birth or in early childhood, it occurs most commonly at the time of the adolescent growth spurt. Once present, the neurologic deficit gradually worsens. A sudden decline in neurologic function may result from minor trauma. Occurrence or worsening of spasticity in a child with kyphosis is an early sign of myelopathy and should prompt an evaluation leading to spinal fusion with anterior decompression of the spinal cord, if necessary. MRI has largely replaced CT myelography as the procedure of choice in the diagnosis of intraspinal defects. In infants and young children whose posterior elements are still cartilaginous, ultrasonography done by an experienced examiner is an excellent screening modality.

Treatment. Bracing and other nonoperative techniques have very limited application in the management of congenital kyphosis. Before significant kyphosis develops, spinal fusion may often be accomplished by the posterior approach alone. In the patient with a neurologic deficit secondary to either a congenital or a secondary kyphosis and a fixed deformity, anterior decompression of the vertebral canal is essential. If the curve is flexible, gradual traction may improve neurologic function but traction over a rigid kyphos is contraindicated.

About 10% of children with myelodysplasia have a variant of congenital kyphosis in the lumbar spine. The curves are frequently very large at birth and often lead to chronic ulceration of the gibbus. Kyphectomy at the time of sac closure may be necessary to achieve primary skin closure. In older children, kyphectomy with shortening of the lumbar spine and stabilization with instrumentation are often required.

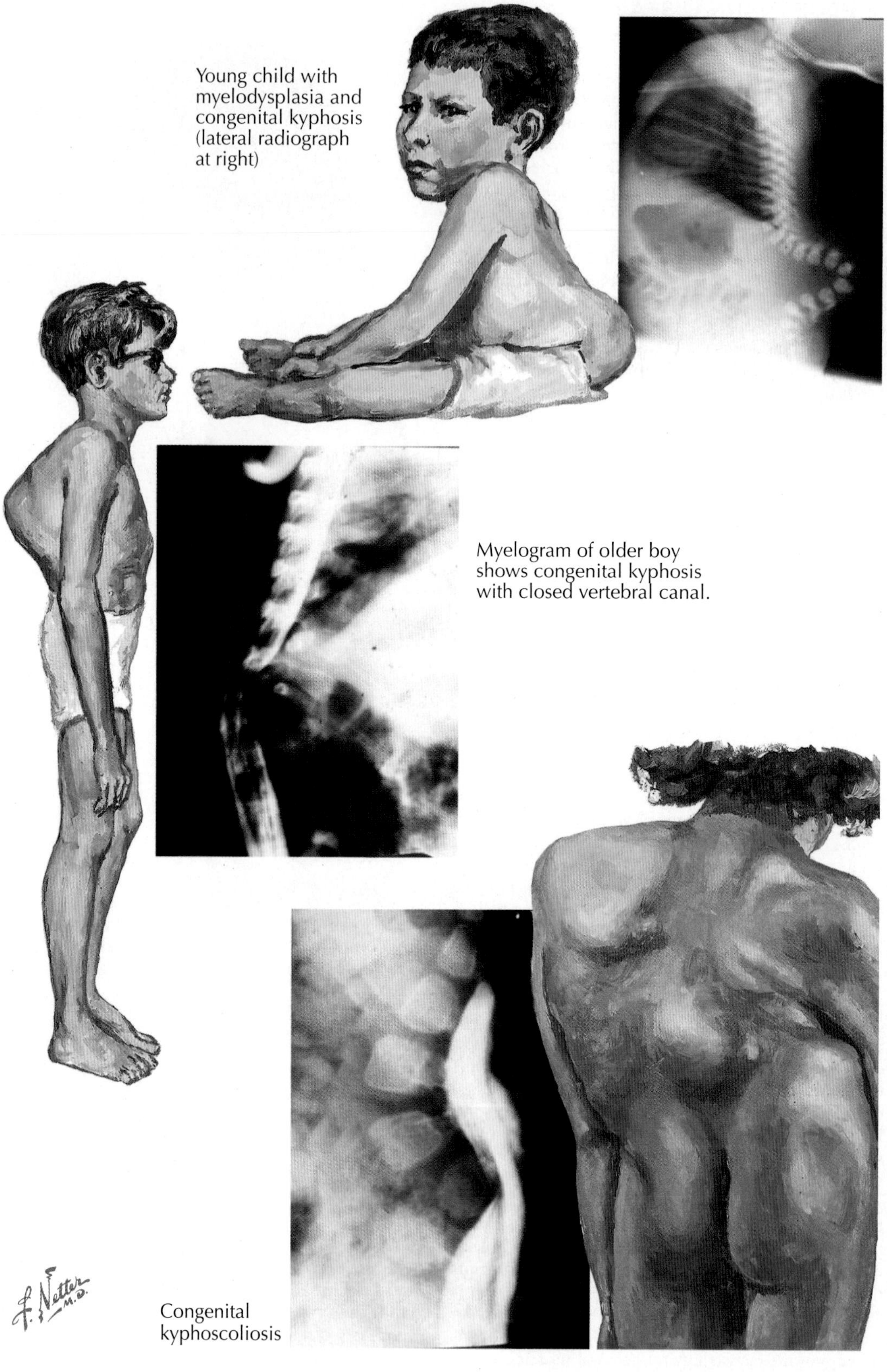

Young child with myelodysplasia and congenital kyphosis (lateral radiograph at right)

Myelogram of older boy shows congenital kyphosis with closed vertebral canal.

Congenital kyphoscoliosis

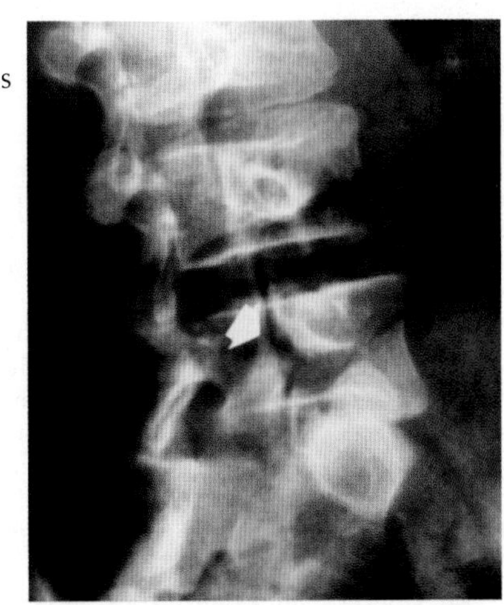

Spondylolysis without spondylolisthesis. Posterolateral view demonstrates formation of radiographic Scottie dog. On lateral radiograph, dog appears to be wearing a collar.

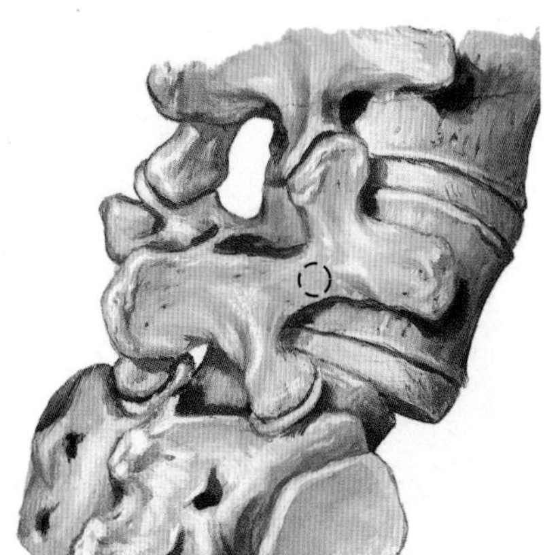

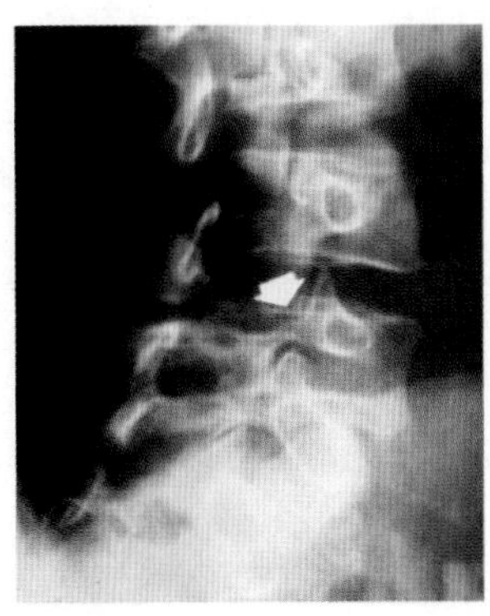

Dysplastic (congenital) spondylolisthesis. Luxation of L5 on sacrum. Dog's neck (isthmus) appears elongated.

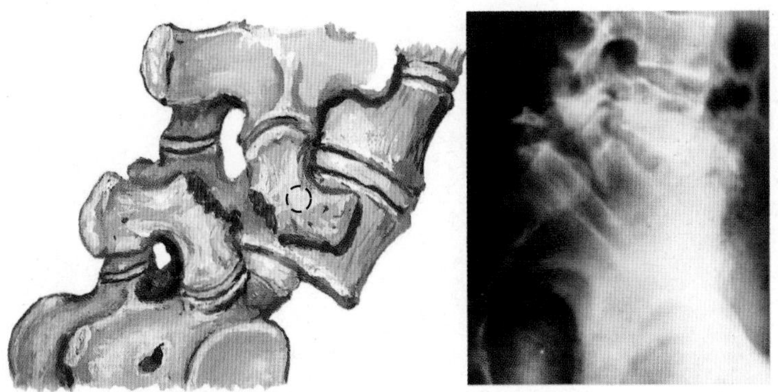

Isthmic-type spondylolisthesis. Anterior luxation of L5 on sacrum due to fracture of isthmus. Note that gap is wider and dog appears decapitated.

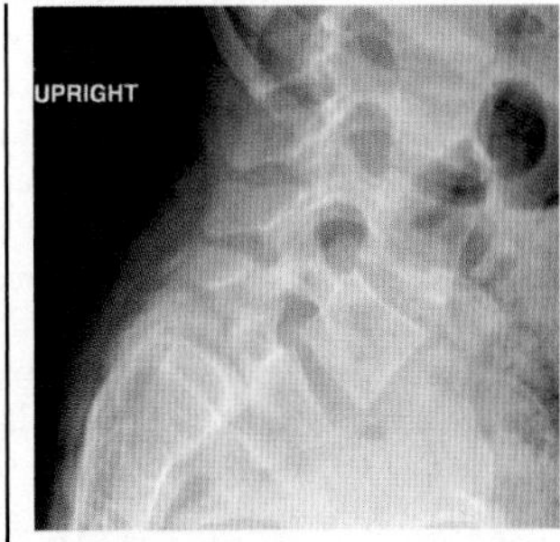

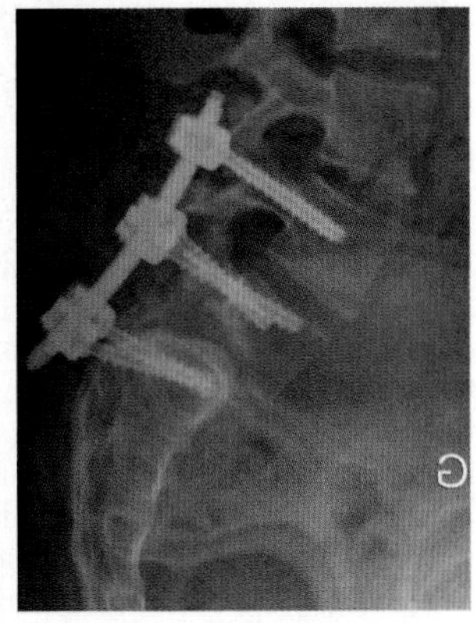

Preoperative (*top*) and postoperative (*bottom*) views of a spondylolisthesis reduced from a grade IV to a grade II slip. Pedicle screw fusion is from L4 to S1.

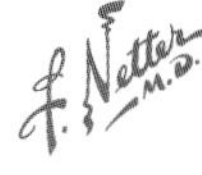

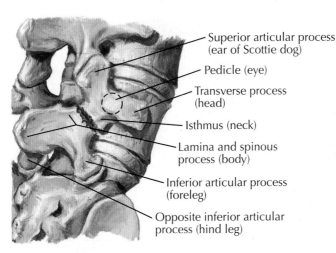

SPONDYLOLYSIS AND SPONDYLOLISTHESIS

Spondylolysis may represent a stress fracture of the pars interarticularis of the fifth lumbar vertebra. When the fracture allows L5 to slip forward on S1, it is called *isthmic spondylolisthesis.* Dysplastic, or congenital, spondylolisthesis, in contrast, is due to anomalous development of the posterior structures of the lumbosacral junction.

In children, spondylolysis rarely occurs before 5 years of age and is more common at age 7 or 8 years. Although a history of minor trauma is common, the injury is seldom severe. The onset of symptoms coincides closely with the adolescent growth spurt.

Lumbar lordosis is exacerbated by the normal hip flexion contractures of childhood. This posture focuses the force of weight bearing on the pars interarticularis, gradually leading to disruption. Shear stresses are greater on the pars interarticularis when the spine is extended and are further accentuated by lateral flexion of the extended spine.

Clinical Manifestations. Symptoms are relatively uncommon in children. Pain, when it occurs, is localized to the low back and, to a lesser extent, to the posterior buttocks and thighs. Symptoms are usually initiated and aggravated by repetitive and strenuous activity—particularly the flexion-extension of the spine common in rowing, gymnastics, and diving—and are decreased by rest or limitation of activity.

Palpation may elicit some tenderness in the low back, and there may be some splinting or guarding with restriction of side-to-side motion, particularly in acute conditions. Hamstring tightness and marked restriction of forward hip flexion are seen in 80% of symptomatic patients. Distortion of the pelvis and trunk may be clinically apparent in the late stages of spondylolisthesis.

Children, unlike adults, seldom have objective signs of nerve root compression such as motor weakness, reflex change, or sensory deficit and rarely have an associated disc protrusion. The examination must include a careful search for sacral anesthesia and bladder dysfunction.

Radiographic Findings. Large defects in the pars interarticularis (spondylolysis) are visible on nearly all radiographic views of the lumbar spine. However, if the spondylolysis is unilateral or not accompanied by spondylolisthesis, special techniques and oblique views of the lumbar spine may be needed.

In an acute injury, the gap in the pars interarticularis is narrow with irregular edges, whereas in the longstanding lesion, the edges are smooth and rounded. Bone scans may be needed to detect an early prespondylolytic stage (before fracture) in children. In dysplastic spondylolisthesis, the posterior facets appear to sublux and the pars interarticularis may become attenuated—like pulled taffy (the "greyhound" described by Hensinger).

In unilateral spondylolysis, the radiographic appearance of reactive sclerosis and hypertrophy of the contralateral pedicle and lamina may be confused with osteoid osteoma. This is an important concern because excision of a sclerotic pedicle associated with a contralateral spondylolysis may increase instability, leading to spondylolisthesis. Bone scans are not helpful in differentiating the two conditions.

Treatment. Spondylolysis usually responds well to conservative measures, restriction of some activities, and exercises for the back and abdominal muscles. Asymptomatic spondylolisthesis is more problematic because the risk of further slippage is difficult to determine. Symptomatic spondylolisthesis may require surgical stabilization of the spine. Surgery may entail an in situ fusion or reduction. Currently, most fusions are instrumented, which eliminates the need for a prolonged period of bracing.

MYELODYSPLASIA

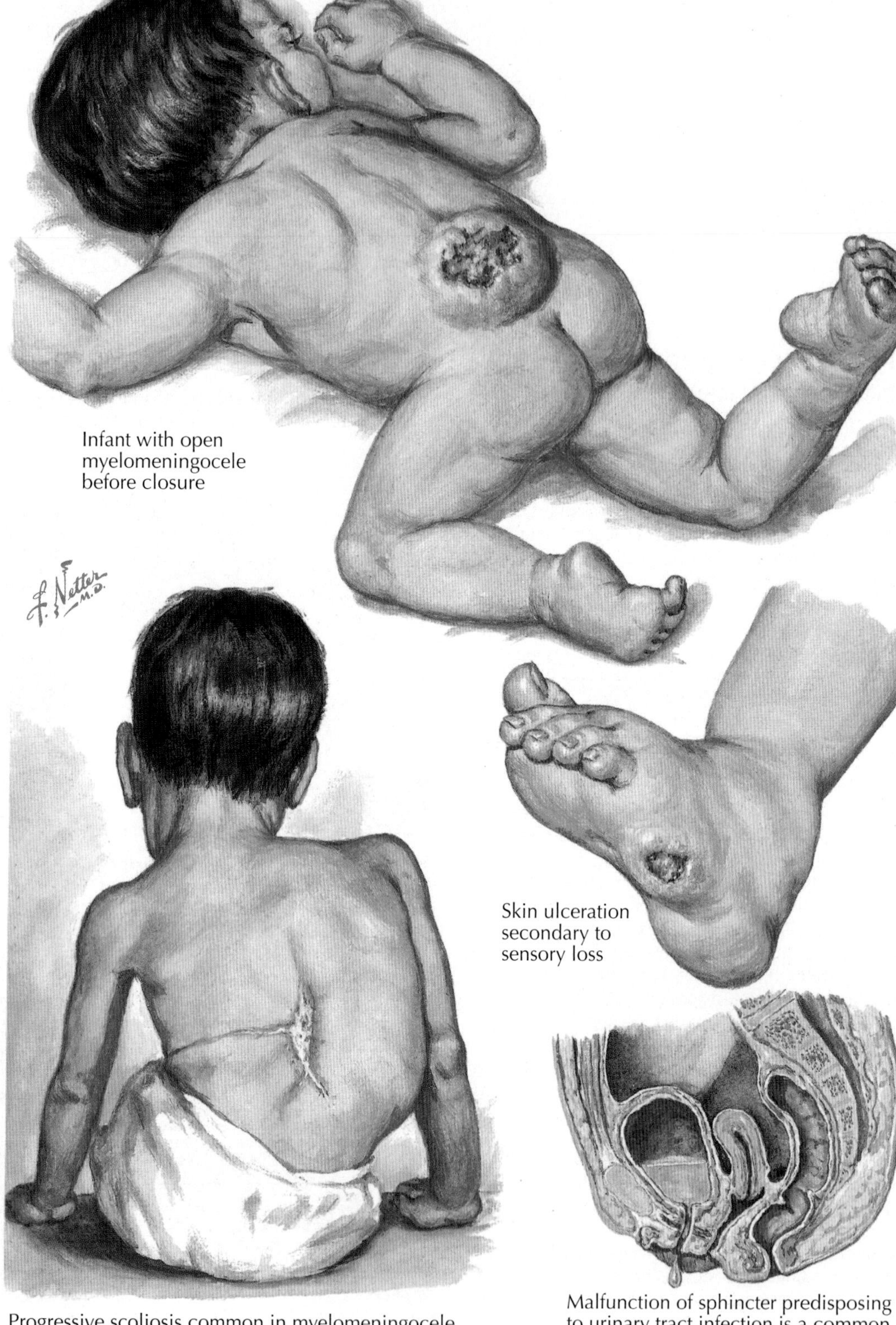

Infant with open myelomeningocele before closure

Skin ulceration secondary to sensory loss

Progressive scoliosis common in myelomeningocele

Malfunction of sphincter predisposing to urinary tract infection is a common complication.

The number of infants with myelodysplasia who survive infancy has increased dramatically in the past 30 years, and as clinical experience with these patients has increased, new principles and techniques of treatment have emerged.

Management of the patient with myelodysplasia requires a team approach. The team coordinator should visit the patient and family in the first days after birth and discuss the long-term implications of the patient's condition. The urologist, orthopedist, and neurosurgeon should conduct the initial evaluation, and physical therapy to improve and maintain joint motion should be started as soon as possible.

The clinical findings dictate the specific orthopedic procedures employed. The neurologic level of both motor and sensory function should be estimated. However, in newborns, it is often impossible to determine the exact level, and the findings vary depending on the examiner and the child's age. Because there is considerable variation from one side of the body to the other, each limb should be evaluated separately. The effects of muscle imbalance and presence of soft tissue contractures must be considered in the neurologic examination. Evaluation of the newborn should focus on determining which joints the child can control, and muscle strength can be assessed more accurately later.

The lesion generally follows anatomic lines; thus even in children with only mild involvement of the foot there may be significant weakness of the hip and the abductor muscles and increased tendency to late hip dislocation.

DEFORMITIES OF HIP

In an otherwise normal child, if the hips are dislocated but can be easily reduced, treatment is the same as that for congenital dislocation of the hip. If the hip has been dislocated early in fetal life (teratologic dislocation) and there are advanced adaptive changes of bone and soft tissue, reduction is not indicated. The primary goal is to produce a freely movable hip joint.

Contracted and/or spastic adductor muscles in conjunction with weak power of abductor muscles frequently lead to hip dislocation. If this imbalance is discovered early, intervention with physical therapy, bracing, or splinting can help prevent dislocation.

Many patients have contracture of the iliotibial band, which maintains the hip flexed, abducted, and externally rotated. Early and intensive physical therapy should be instituted to avoid a fixed deformity.

DEFORMITIES OF KNEE

The newborn with extension or flexion contractures should be treated with stretching exercises. A major goal of treatment is the ability to extend the knee and take advantage of the normal locking mechanism.

DEFORMITIES OF FOOT AND ANKLE

Both conservative and surgical management may be necessary to correct the position of deformed feet, increase suppleness, and allow proper shoe fit.

Cavovarus and equinovarus (clubfoot) should be corrected before the child learns to stand—before extensive adaptive and remodeling changes in both bone and soft tissue occur, making surgical intervention necessary. In the newborn period, calcaneovalgus with overpull of the anterior and paralysis of the posterior muscles (S1 distribution) often responds well to exercises, braces, or splints. Deformities such as vertical talus and stiff, rigid feet are less common.

DEFORMITIES OF SPINE

Although common in patients with myelodysplasia, spinal deformities are not usually a problem in the newborn period. However, congenital anomalies of the vertebrae occur in about 30% of affected children. In addition, 50% of patients eventually develop a curve in the otherwise normal-appearing vertebral bodies (developmental scoliosis).

Congenital kyphosis is unique to myelodysplasia and is of such magnitude that it can be recognized at birth. The kyphosis usually involves the entire lumbar spine from the thoracolumbar junction down, including the sacrum, with its apex at L2 or L3; there is usually complete paralysis below the level of the lesion. In the newborn, the size of the cutaneous defect and the rigidity and magnitude of the curve may make skin closure extremely difficult.

Lumbosacral Agenesis

Lumbosacral agenesis is a condition in which the sacrum and some of the lumbar vertebrae, or both, fail to develop. Although the etiology is not certain, it has been noted that 14% to 18% of affected patients have mothers with diabetes or a strong family history of diabetes.

Clinical Manifestations. The patient's appearance varies with the level of the vertebral lesion. Although partial sacral agenesis may not be noticeable, lumbar or complete sacral agenesis is a severe deformity.

The posture of the lower limbs has been likened to that of the "sitting Buddha" and is characterized by flexion-abduction contractures of the hips and severe knee flexion, with popliteal webbing; the feet are in equinovarus and tucked under the buttocks. Inspection of the back reveals a bony prominence, which is the last vertebral segment, and often gross motion between this and the pelvis. Flexion-extension may occur at the junction of the spine and pelvis rather than at the hips. When the patient sits unsupported, the pelvis rolls up under the thorax. Scoliosis, hemivertebrae, spina bifida, and meningocele are commonly associated spinal anomalies.

With low-level lesions, deformities of the foot and lower limb resemble those of resistant clubfoot or arthrogryposis. Children may be misdiagnosed for several years or until problems with toilet training call attention to the sacral anomalies. Although the clinical signs resemble those of arthrogryposis, patients with arthrogryposis have full sensation in the lower limbs, bowel and bladder control, and normal vertebral architecture.

The neurologic deficit is one of the most unusual features of this condition. Motor paralysis is profound, with no voluntary or reflex activity, and it corresponds anatomically within one level to what might be expected from vertebral loss. Even patients with the most severe involvement have sensation to the knees and spotty hypesthesia distally. Trophic ulceration of the feet is quite uncommon, suggesting at least protective sensation.

Bladder dysfunction is a consistent finding in all patients, even those with a relatively minor hemisacral defect, but the patterns of urinary function vary. Patients exhibit individual mixtures of upper and/or lower motor neuron disorders; perineal electromyography is necessary to obtain the correct diagnosis. Severe constipation with absence of the normal sensation of rectal distention is a common bowel abnormality.

The visceral anomalies are usually confined to the anogenital region (imperforate anus is the most common) and urinary tract (e.g., bladder dysfunction, hydronephrosis, vesical reflux and diverticulum, fused or absent kidney, exstrophy of the bladder, and hypospadias).

Radiographic Findings. A lesion at the level of the lumbar spine results in the complete absence of all vertebral development below it, including the sacrum and coccyx. However, lesions of the sacrum are less consistent, and, in about one-third of patients, the defect occurs on one side only. In lumbar or complete sacral agenesis there is usually no bony connection of the spine to the pelvis. The spinopelvic articulation should be examined with flexion-extension radiographs because its stability has important implications in treatment and rehabilitation.

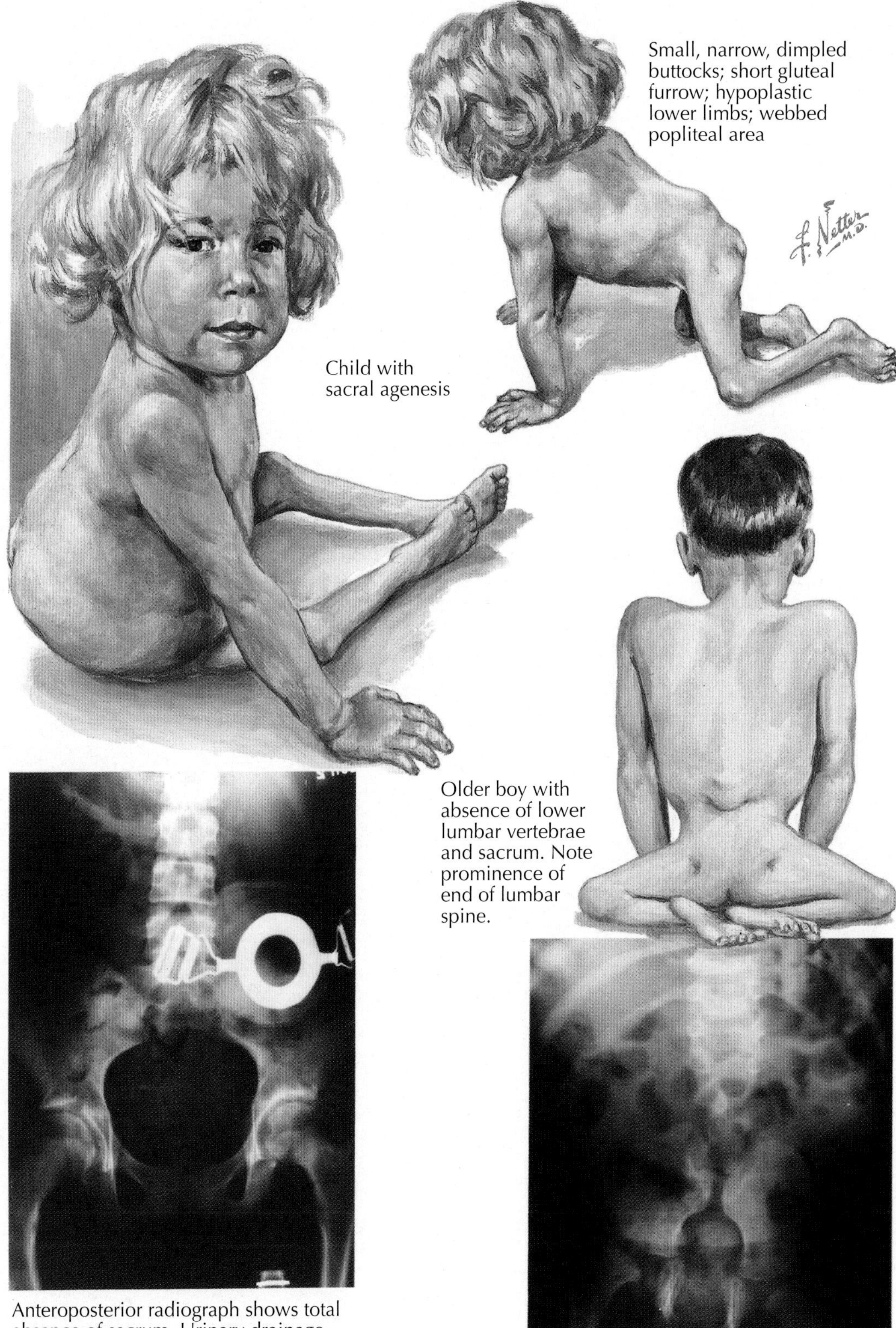
Small, narrow, dimpled buttocks; short gluteal furrow; hypoplastic lower limbs; webbed popliteal area
F. Netter M.D.
Child with sacral agenesis
Older boy with absence of lower lumbar vertebrae and sacrum. Note prominence of end of lumbar spine.

Anteroposterior radiograph shows total absence of sacrum. Urinary drainage bag visible.

Lumbosacral agenesis

Treatment. Treatment measures vary with the level of involvement, and the management plan, based on the following broad concepts, must be highly individualized.

If the sacropelvic ring is intact, the spinopelvic junction is usually stable, and the patient can walk with minimal or no brace support. Patients with significant deformities of only the feet and legs require vigorous correction, begun at birth, including serial plaster casts in conjunction with stretching and exercises to position the feet plantigrade and the knees in extension. Surgical release may be necessary if conservative measures are inadequate.

Because of the high incidence of associated defects that may lead to serious renal impairment, recognition and treatment of urinary abnormalities are an important part of management. Delay in diagnosis and treatment may lead to upper tract deterioration and severely limit therapeutic options.

PELVIS, HIP, AND THIGH

Superficial Veins and Cutaneous Nerves

SUPERFICIAL VEINS

Certain prominent veins, unaccompanied by arteries, are found in the subcutaneous tissue of the lower limb (Plate 2.1). The principal ones are the greater and lesser saphenous veins, which arise in the venous radicles in the feet and toes. Dorsal digital veins lie along the dorsal margins of each digit, uniting at the webs of the toes into short dorsal metatarsal veins that empty into the dorsal venous arch. There are also plantar digital veins, which drain into the dorsal metatarsal veins.

The *greater saphenous vein* continues the medial end of the dorsal venous arch and is the longest named vein of the body. It turns upward anterior to the medial malleolus at the ankle and, ascending immediately posterior to the medial margin of the tibia, passes the knee against the posterior border of the medial femoral condyle. In the thigh, the vein inclines anteriorly and lateralward; in the femoral triangle, it turns deeply through the saphenous opening to empty into the femoral vein. In the leg, the greater saphenous vein has tributaries from the heel of the foot, the front of the leg, and the calf. It also communicates with radicles of the lesser saphenous vein.

In the thigh, the greater saphenous vein also receives a large *accessory saphenous vein,* which collects the superficial radicles of the medial and posterior parts. Just before it turns through the saphenous opening, it receives the superficial external pudendal, superficial epigastric, and superficial circumflex iliac veins. On occasion, these veins pierce the cribriform fascia of the saphenous opening independently and empty directly into the femoral vein.

Valves in the greater saphenous vein vary from 10 to 20 in number and are more numerous in the leg than in the thigh. Perforating communications to deep veins pass through the deep fascia at all levels of the limb. Blood passes from superficial to deep through these communications, with valves in the communications determining the direction of drainage. In the leg, the greater saphenous vein is accompanied by a branch of the saphenous nerve; in the thigh, an anterior femoral cutaneous nerve lies next to it.

The *lesser saphenous vein,* continuing the lateral extension of the dorsal venous arch, receives lateral marginal veins in the foot and passes backward along the lateral border of the foot in company with the sural nerve. It then turns upward to ascend through the middle of the calf. The vein pierces the crural fascia, mostly in the middle third of the leg but frequently in the upper third, and ascends deep to or in a split of the deep fascia. It usually (75% of cases) terminates in the popliteal vein. The lesser saphenous vein has 6 to 12 valves. It communicates with radicles of the greater saphenous vein and also with deep veins of the leg. It frequently gives rise to a radicle, which communicates with the accessory saphenous vein. The lesser saphenous vein is accompanied by the sural nerve in the lower half of the leg; in its terminal course in the popliteal fossa, it has a close anatomic relationship to the tibial nerve.

The deep nerves of the lower limb are discussed separately (see Plates 2.5 to 2.7).

CUTANEOUS NERVES

Almost all of the cutaneous nerves of the lower limb originate from the lumbosacral plexus, which is formed from the ventral rami of the first lumbar to third sacral nerves (L1 to S3) (see Plates 2.5 to 2.7). However, the superior and middle cluneal nerves are lateral cutaneous branches of dorsal rami of certain of these nerves. The *superior cluneal nerves* are branches of the L1 to L3 nerves. They distribute to the skin of the gluteal region as far as the greater trochanter of the femur. The *middle cluneal nerves* are lateral branches of dorsal rami of S1 to S3 and provide cutaneous innervation to the skin over the back of the sacrum and adjacent gluteal region.

Iliac Crest Region

Certain lateral cutaneous branches of primarily abdominal nerves cross the crest of the ilium and distribute in the upper thigh. Thus the *lateral cutaneous branch of the subcostal nerve* (T12) distributes to the skin and subcutaneous tissue of the thigh to as low as the greater trochanter of the femur. The *lateral cutaneous branch of the iliohypogastric nerve* (L1) supplies the skin of the gluteal region posterior to the area of supply of the lateral cutaneous branch of the subcostal nerve. The ilioinguinal nerve of the lumbar plexus has a small femoral distribution through its *anterior scrotal* (or *anterior labial*) *branch* (L1). Twigs of this nerve reach the skin of the thigh adjacent to the scrotum (or labium majus). The *femoral branch of the genitofemoral nerve* (L1, L2) arises from the lumbar plexus to supply the skin over the femoral triangle.

Hip and Thigh

Anterior femoral cutaneous nerves (L2, L3) are multiple. They usually arise from the femoral nerve in the femoral triangle on the lateral surface of the femoral artery. Medially distributing representatives, the *medial femoral cutaneous nerves,* supply the skin and subcutaneous tissues in the distal two-thirds of the medial portion of the thigh. Other branches arising in the femoral triangle, the *intermediate femoral cutaneous nerves,* supply the skin of the distal three-fourths of the front of the thigh and extend to the front of the patella, where they assist in forming the patellar plexus.

The *lateral femoral cutaneous nerve* (L2, L3) is a direct branch of the lumbar plexus. It becomes subcutaneous about 10 cm below the anterior iliac spine and distributes to anterior and lateral aspects of the thigh. Its larger anterior distribution may reach the patellar plexus.

The *posterior femoral cutaneous nerve* (S1, S2, S3) from the sacral plexus descends in the posterior midline of the thigh deep to the fascia lata, giving off branches that pierce the fascia and distribute both medially and laterally. The nerve finally reaches the levels of the popliteal fossa and the upper calf. The posterior femoral cutaneous nerve, lying subgluteally alongside the sciatic nerve, gives rise to the *inferior cluneal nerve.* This nerve turns around the lower border of the gluteus maximus muscle and supplies the skin over the lower and lateral parts of the muscle.

A *perforating cutaneous nerve* (S2, S3) arises from the sacral plexus. It gets its name because it perforates the sacrotuberal ligament and the lower fibers of the gluteus maximus muscle and distributes to the skin over the medial part of the fold of the buttock.

The *obturator nerve* (L2, L3, L4) from the lumbar plexus is largely muscular in the thigh, but its anterior branch usually ends as a *cutaneous branch.* This is distributed to the skin of the distal third of the thigh on its medial surface.

Leg, Ankle, and Foot

The *saphenous nerve* (L3, L4) is the terminal branch of the femoral nerve, even though it arises in the femoral canal. It traverses the whole length of the adductor canal, at its lower end piercing the vastoadductor membrane to become superficial along with the saphenous branch of the descending genicular artery. It descends in the leg in company with the greater saphenous vein. An infrapatellar branch curves downward below the patella, forming the patellar plexus with terminals of the medial and lateral femoral cutaneous nerves. The saphenous nerve continues distally along the medial surface of the leg, distributing from there and finally reaching the posterior half of the dorsum and the medial side of the foot.

The *lateral sural cutaneous nerve* (L5, S1, S2) arises in the popliteal space from the common peroneal nerve. It distributes to the skin and subcutaneous connective tissue on the lateral part of the leg in its proximal two-thirds. The *peroneal communicating branch* is a small nerve that usually arises from the lateral sural cutaneous nerve in the popliteal space or over the lateral calf. It runs downward and medially to join the medial sural cutaneous nerve in the middle third of the leg to form the sural nerve.

The *medial sural cutaneous nerve* (S1, S2) arises from the tibial nerve in the popliteal fossa. It descends as far as the middle of the leg. Here, it is joined by the peroneal communicating nerve to form the sural nerve. The level of junction of these nerves is quite variable, and in about 20% of cases, they fail to unite; the peroneal communicating branch then distributes in the leg, and the medial sural cutaneous nerve supplies the heel and foot areas.

The *sural nerve* (S1, S2), formed as described earlier, usually becomes superficial at the middle of the length of the leg. It descends in company with the lesser saphenous vein, turning with it under the lateral malleolus onto the side of the foot. As the *lateral dorsal cutaneous nerve* of the foot, it is cutaneous to the lateral side of the foot, having previously given off *lateral calcaneal branches* to the ankle and heel. It extends to the little toe, has articular branches to the ankle and tarsal joints, and communicates with the intermediate dorsal cutaneous branch of the superficial peroneal nerve.

The *superficial peroneal nerve* (L4, L5, S1), a branch of the common peroneal nerve, descends to the distal third of the leg, where it almost immediately divides into two terminal branches. The *medial dorsal cutaneous nerve* supplies cutaneous twigs in the distal third of the leg and then, crossing the extensor retinaculum, divides over the dorsum of the foot into two or three branches for the supply of the dorsum and sides of the medial 2.5 toes. The *deep peroneal nerve* (L4, L5) has cutaneous terminals to the web and adjacent sides of the great and second toes; in this interval, the terminals of the medial dorsal cutaneous nerve merely communicate with the branches of the deep peroneal nerve.

The *intermediate dorsal cutaneous nerve* passes more laterally over the dorsum of the foot and divides into cutaneous branches to the lateral side of the ankle and the foot. It terminates in *dorsal digital branches* for the adjacent sides of the third and fourth and fourth and fifth toes. The more lateral branch communicates with the lateral dorsal cutaneous nerve. As in the fingers, the dorsal digital branches to the toes are smaller than the corresponding plantar digital nerves and distribute distalward only over the middle phalanges. The terminal segment of the toes is supplied by dorsal terminals of the plantar nerves.

The *tibial nerve* supplies the musculature of the back of the leg and continues into the foot behind the

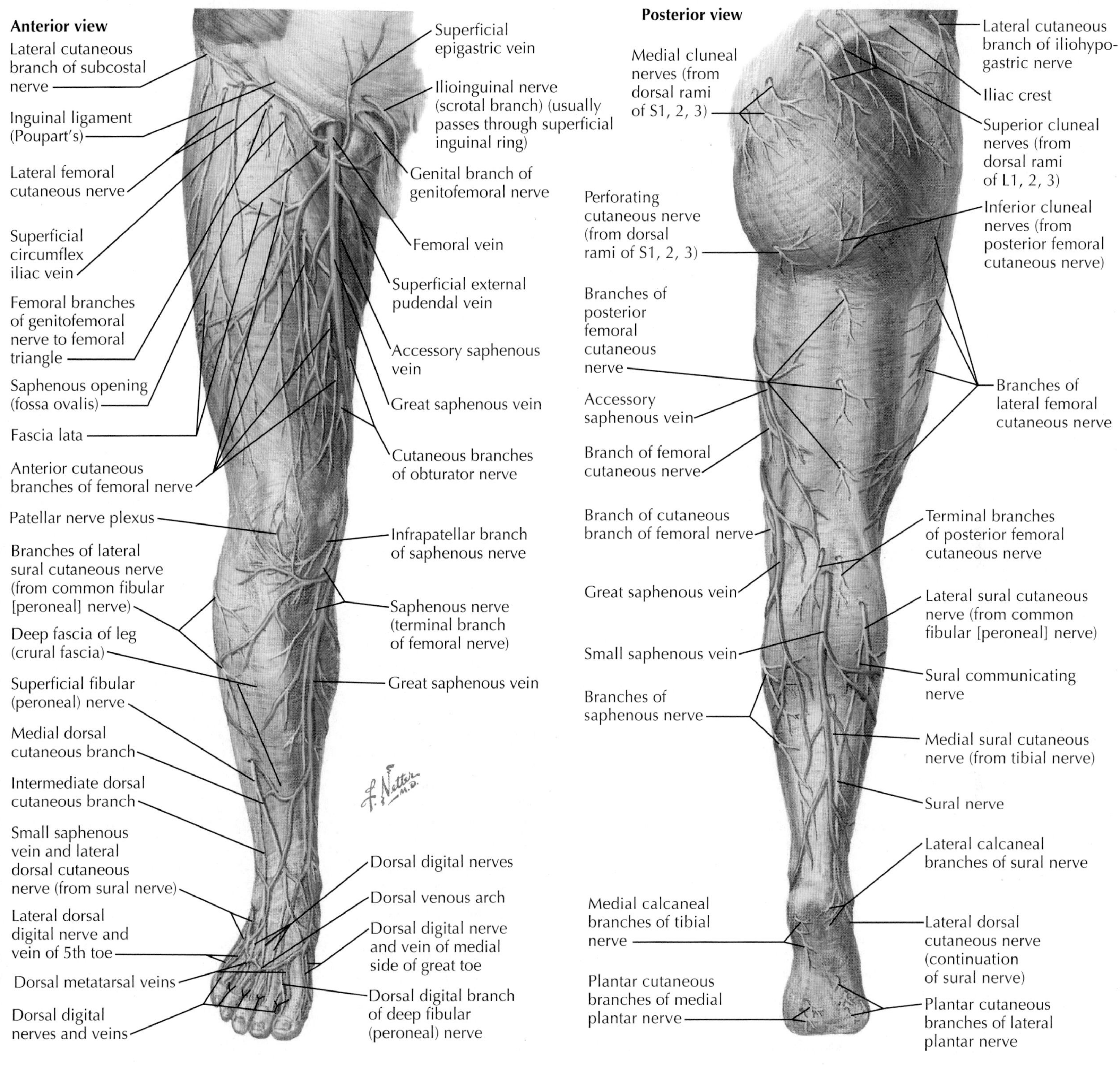

SUPERFICIAL VEINS AND CUTANEOUS NERVES (Continued)

medial malleolus. Its *medial calcaneal branches* (S1, S2) distribute to the heel and the posterior part of the sole of the foot. Derived from the tibial nerve deep to the abductor hallucis muscle are the medial and lateral plantar nerves. The *medial plantar nerve* (L4, L5) provides a *proper digital nerve* to the medial side of the great toe and three *common digital branches.* Each of the latter splits into two proper digital nerves, which supply the skin of the adjacent sides of digits I and II, II and III, and III and IV, respectively. The *lateral plantar nerve* (S1, S2) provides a common digital nerve, which also divides into proper digital nerves; two of them reach the adjacent sides of the fourth and fifth toes, and one reaches the lateral side of the little toe. The plantar digital nerves reach the whole plantar surface of the digits and also furnish small dorsal twigs for the nail bed and tip of each toe.

LUMBOSACRAL PLEXUS

NERVE SUPPLY

In describing the lower limb, the lumbosacral plexus may be said to be formed from the ventral rami of the first lumbar to third sacral nerves (L1 to S3), with a common small contribution from the 12th thoracic nerve (T12) (Plates 2.2 to 2.4). The lumbar portion of the plexus arises from the four upper lumbar nerves and gives rise to the iliohypogastric, ilioinguinal, genitofemoral, lateral femoral cutaneous, obturator, accessory obturator, and femoral nerves.

LUMBAR PLEXUS

As with the brachial plexus, the spinal nerves contributing to the lumbar plexus divide into anterior and posterior branches, but the plexus lacks some of the complexity of the brachial plexus, because the definitive nerves usually arise from combinations of looping contributions from adjacent spinal nerves. The lumbar plexus is formed deep to the psoas major muscle and lies anterior to the transverse processes of the lumbar vertebrae. Only the first two lumbar nerves contribute preganglionic sympathetic fibers to the sympathetic chain through white rami communicantes; all lumbar nerves receive postganglionic fibers through gray rami communicantes.

The *iliohypogastric nerve* arises from L1 together with a frequent contribution from T12. It emerges from the psoas major muscle at its lateral border and crosses the quadratus lumborum muscle to penetrate the transverse abdominal muscle near the iliac crest. This nerve, primarily motor to abdominal musculature, ends in an anterior cutaneous branch to the skin of the suprapubic region and a lateral cutaneous branch that crosses the iliac crest to distribute in the hip region. A lateral cutaneous branch of the subcostal nerve (T12) also supplies the upper thigh.

The *ilioinguinal nerve* from L1 has a similar course to the iliohypogastric nerve in the abdominal wall but enters the lateral end of the inguinal canal and accompanies the spermatic cord through that canal. Emerging at the superficial inguinal ring, it ends as the anterior scrotal (or anterior labial) nerve as a cutaneous nerve to the scrotum and adjacent area of the thigh. In about 35% of cases, the ilioinguinal nerve combines with the genitofemoral nerve in the abdomen, running with the latter on the surface of the psoas major muscle, but distributes finally in its typical cutaneous distribution.

The *genitofemoral nerve* arises by a union of branches from the anterior portions of L1 and L2. In the abdomen, it descends on the ventral surface of the psoas major muscle and then divides into genital and femoral branches. The genital branch innervates the cremaster muscle and gives twigs to the scrotum and adjacent thigh; the more medial femoral branch descends under the inguinal ligament on the surface of the external iliac artery to supply the skin of the femoral triangle.

The *lateral femoral cutaneous nerve* arises from the posterior branches of L2 and L3 (see Plate 2.5).

The *obturator nerve* is the largest nerve formed from the anterior divisions of the lumbar plexus, specifically from those of L2 to L4. The *accessory obturator nerve* is small and is present in only 9% of cases. (The obturator nerve is fully described in Plate 2.6.)

The *femoral nerve,* the largest branch of the lumbar plexus, is formed from the posterior branches of L2 to L4. Passing under the inguinal ligament, it shortly breaks up in the femoral triangle into its numerous branches. (This nerve is fully described in Plate 2.5.)

Muscular branches of the lumbar plexus distribute to the quadratus lumborum muscle (T12; L1, L2, L3

LUMBAR PLEXUS

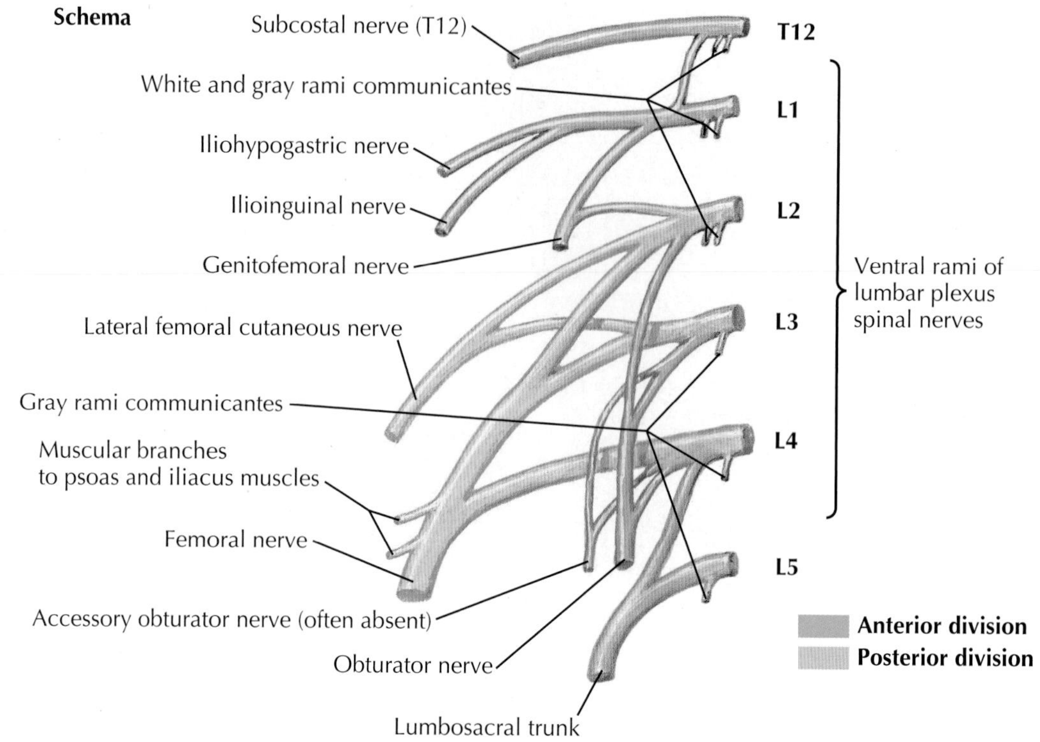

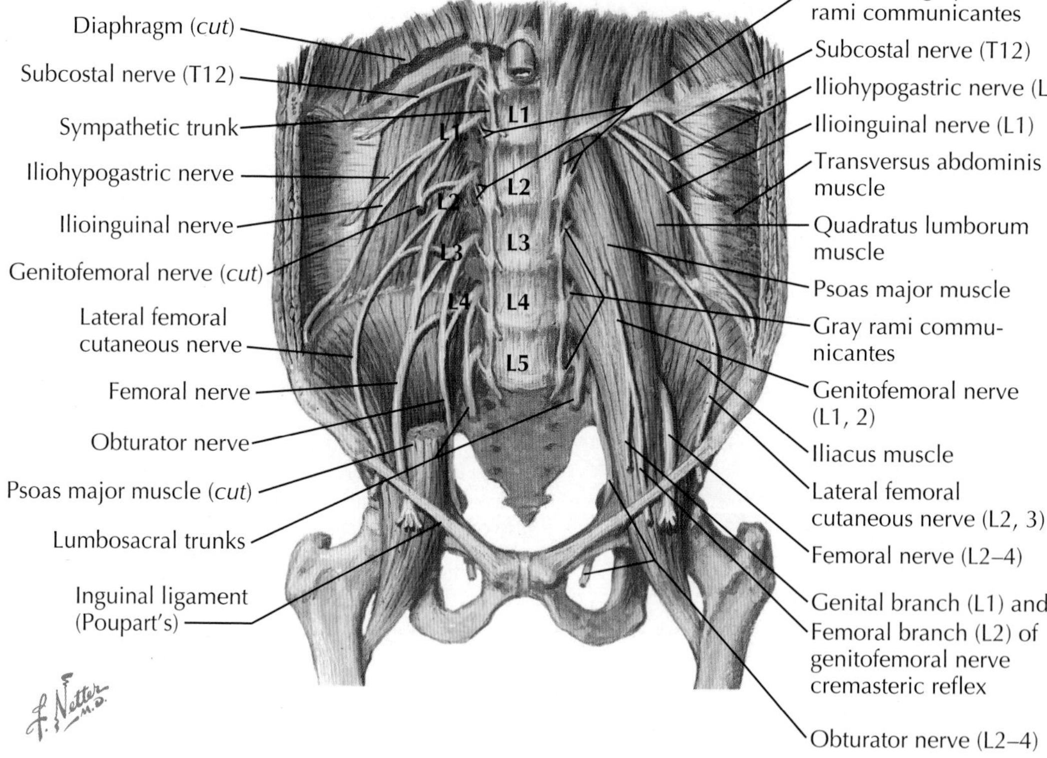

Lumbosacral Plexus (Continued)

[L4]), the psoas major muscle ([L1], L2, L3, L4), the psoas minor muscle (L1, L2), and the iliacus muscle (L2, L3, L4).

SACRAL PLEXUS

The sacral portion of the lumbosacral plexus, commonly designated the sacral plexus, is formed from the ventral rami of a part of the fourth lumbar nerve (L4) and the fifth lumbar and first, second, and third sacral nerves (L5; S1, S2, S3). The descending portion of L4 joins L5 over the ala of the sacrum to form the lumbosacral trunk, which then descends across the sacroiliac articulation to join the ventral ramus of S1. The lumbosacral trunk contains anterior and posterior branches of the ventral rami of L4 and L5. The ventral rami of S1, S2, S3 pass lateralward from the pelvic sacral foramina and divide into anterior and posterior branches in front of the piriformis muscle. The largest nerves of the sacral plexus are L5 and S1, and the superior gluteal artery usually leaves the pelvis by passing between them.

Converging toward the lower portion of the greater sciatic foramen, the plexus forms a broad triangular band, the apex of which passes through the foramen into the gluteal region. The pelvic splanchnic nerves, arising from the ventral rami of S2 to S4, represent the important sacral part of the craniosacral (parasympathetic) portion of the autonomic nervous system. They join the inferior hypogastric plexus and have a largely pelvic and perineal distribution. All of the nerves of the plexus receive gray rami communicantes from the sympathetic chain ganglia or trunk.

The principal nerve of the sacral plexus is the sciatic nerve (see Plate 2.7). It is composed of an anteriorly derived nerve, the tibial segment, and a nerve formed from posterior branches, the common peroneal nerve. These two nerves are usually combined in a single sheath, but in 10% of cases the two parts are separated in the greater sciatic foramen by all or part of the piriformis muscle. They are occasionally separate throughout the thigh. The nerves of the plexus and their sources are listed in tabular format in Plate 2.3.

NERVES OF GLUTEAL REGION

The *sciatic nerve* usually emerges from the pelvis at the lower border of the piriformis muscle and enters the thigh in the hollow between the ischial

Sacral and Coccygeal Plexuses

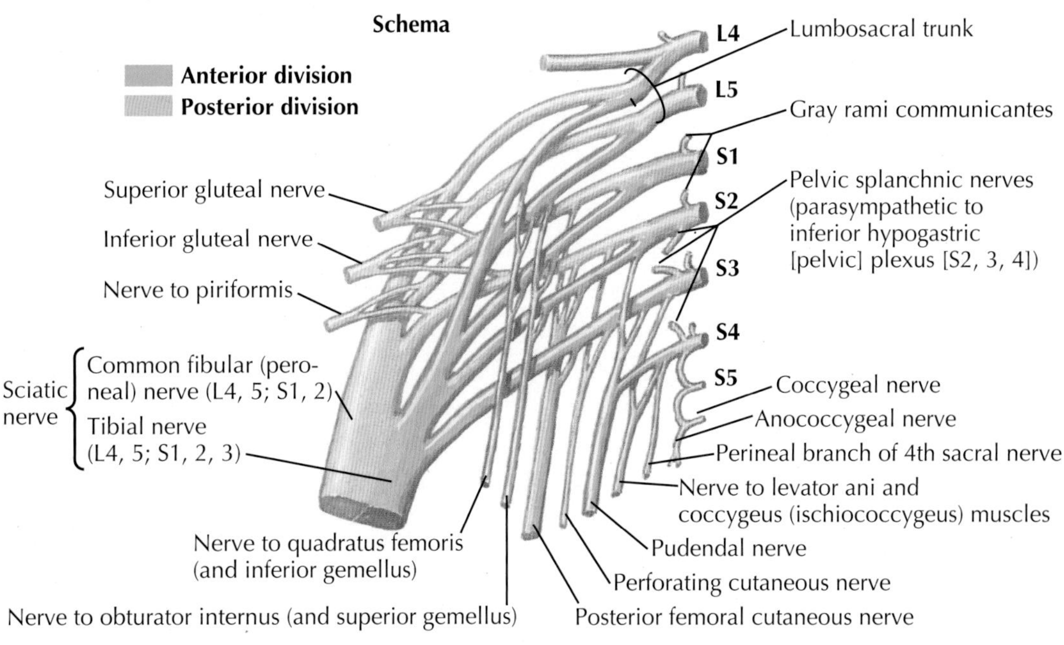

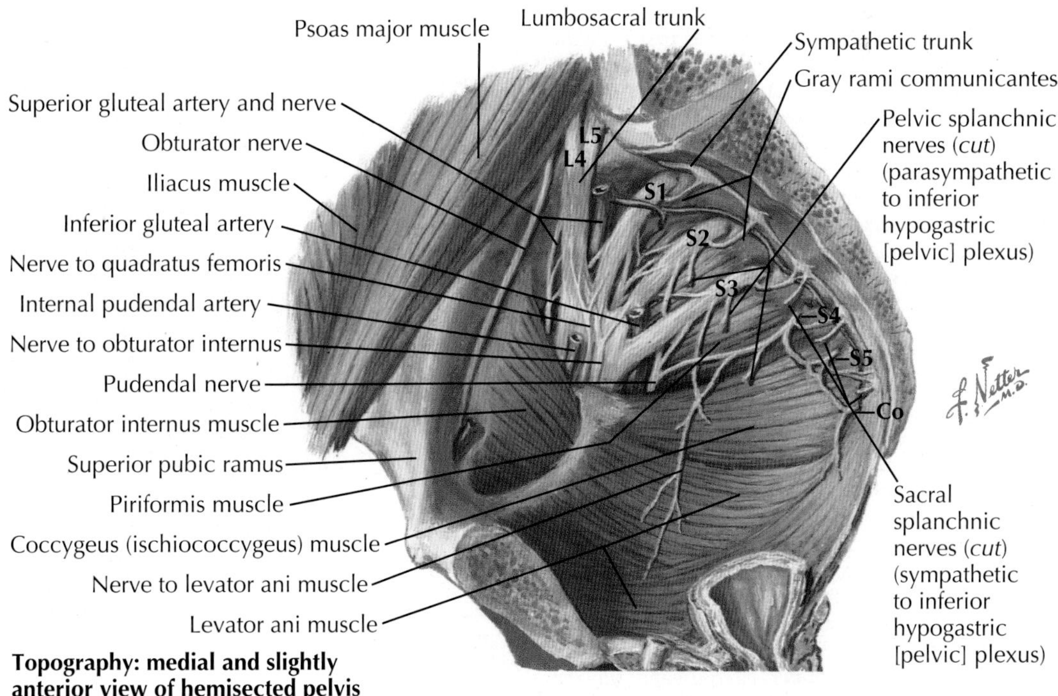

Topography: medial and slightly anterior view of hemisected pelvis

Nerves	Anterior Branches	Posterior Branches
Sciatic	Tibial — L4, 5; S1, 2, 3	Common peroneal — L4, 5; S1, 2
Muscular branches to piriformis, levator ani, coccygeus	S3, 4	S1, 2
Superior gluteal		L4, 5; S1
Inferior gluteal		L5; S1, 2
To quadratus femoris, inferior gemellus	L4, 5; S1	
To obturator internus, superior gemellus	L5; S1, 2	
Posterior femoral cutaneous	S2, 3	S1, 2
Perforating cutaneous		S2, 3

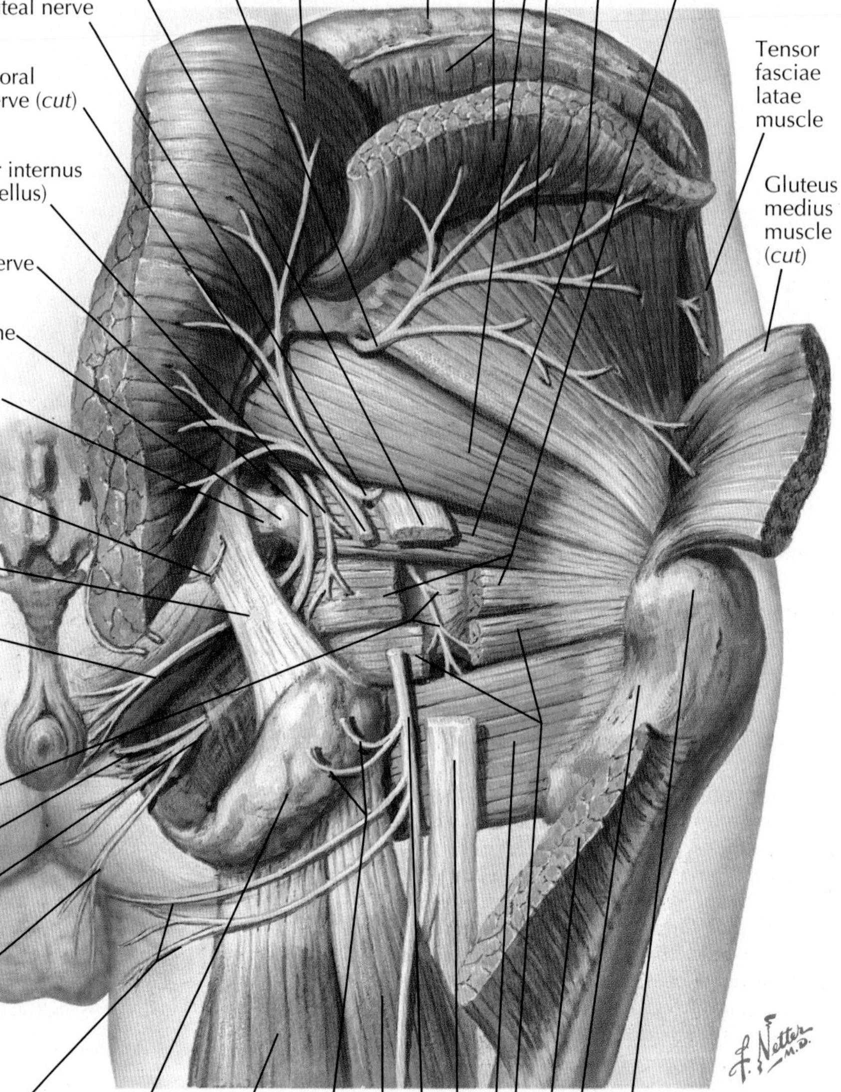

LUMBOSACRAL PLEXUS (Continued)

tuberosity and the greater trochanter of the femur (see Plate 2.7).

The *nerve to the piriformis muscle* may be represented by separate contributions from S1 and S2. Twigs arise from the dorsal aspect of these nerves and immediately enter the pelvic surface of the muscle. Muscular nerves to the levator ani and coccygeus muscles arise from the loop between the rami of S3 and S4 and descend to enter the pelvic surface of these muscles.

The *superior gluteal nerve,* from the posterior branches of L4, L5, and S1, passes from the pelvis above the piriformis muscle. Deep to the gluteus maximus and gluteus medius muscles, the nerve accompanies the superior gluteal vessels anteriorly over the surface of the gluteus minimus muscle. It supplies the gluteus medius and minimus muscles and, continuing beyond them, the tensor fasciae latae muscle.

The *inferior gluteal nerve,* formed from the posterior branches of L5 and S1, S2, passes from the pelvis below the piriformis muscle. It enters the deep surface of the gluteus maximus muscle, to which it is the sole supply.

The *nerve to the quadratus femoris* and *inferior gemellus muscles* is formed from the anterior branches of L4, L5, and S1. In the gluteal region, it is deep to the sciatic nerve and descends over the back of the ischium anterior to the gemellus muscles and the tendon of the internal obturator muscle. It provides articular branches to the hip joint and a branch to the inferior gemellus muscle and ends in the anterior surface of the quadratus femoris muscle.

The *nerve to the obturator internus* and *superior gemellus muscles* arises from anterior branches of L5 and S1, S2. In the gluteal region, it is inferomedial to the sciatic nerve and on the lateral side of the internal pudendal vessels. It crosses the superior gemellus muscle and supplies a small nerve to it. The remaining nerve to the obturator internus muscle crosses the ischial spine and enters the ischiorectal fossa through the lesser sciatic foramen. It ends in the perineal surface of the muscle.

The *posterior femoral cutaneous nerve* is a mixed nerve formed by posterior branches from S1 and S2 and anterior branches from S2 and S3; its cutaneous distributions are described on Plate 2.7. In the gluteal region, it lies alongside the sciatic nerve and descends in the midline of the thigh. It also provides perineal branches that are cutaneous in the perineum and the back of the scrotum.

The *perforating cutaneous nerve* arises from posterior branches of S2 and S3 and is associated at its origin with the lower roots of the posterior femoral cutaneous nerve. Its cutaneous distribution is described on Plate 2.7.

DERMATOMES OF LOWER LIMB

As in the upper limb, the serial order of distribution of lower limb nerves as seen in the lumbosacral plexus is retained in the cutaneous zones of appropriate nerves in the limb. The lumbar nerves have cutaneous terminals that distribute from above down and lateromedially. Sacral segments are restricted to the posterior aspect of the limb and the lateral side of the foot. The spiraling of nerve distribution is a consequence of the medial rotation of the lower limbs of almost 90 degrees that takes place in development, so that the future knees point ventrolaterally (see Plates 2.5 to 2.7). There is always an overlap of adjacent segments; therefore the lines of separation are indistinct.

Nerves of Thigh

FEMORAL NERVE

The femoral nerve (L2, L3, L4) is the largest branch of the lumbar plexus. It originates from the posterior divisions of the ventral rami of the second, third, and fourth lumbar nerves, passes inferolaterally through the psoas major muscle, and then runs in a groove between this muscle and the iliacus, which it supplies. It enters the thigh behind the inguinal ligament to lie lateral to the femoral vascular sheath in the femoral triangle. Twigs are given off to the hip and knee joints and adjacent vessels, and cutaneous branches are given off to anteromedial aspects of the lower limb.

Muscular branches supply the pectineus, sartorius, and quadriceps femoris muscles. The nerve to the pectineus muscle arises at the level of the inguinal ligament, whereas the branches to the sartorius muscle enter the upper two-thirds of the muscle, several arising in common with the anterior femoral cutaneous nerves. The branches to the quadriceps femoris muscle are arranged as illustrated, and those to the rectus femoris and vastus lateralis muscles enter the deep surfaces of the muscles. The branch to the vastus intermedius muscle enters its superficial surface and pierces the muscle to supply the underlying articularis genus muscle. The branch to the vastus medialis muscle runs in the adductor canal for a variable distance, on the lateral side of the femoral vessels and saphenous nerve, giving off successive branches to this muscle, some of which end in the vastus intermedius and articularis genus muscles.

The *anterior femoral cutaneous nerves* arise in the femoral triangle. All these branches pierce the fascia lata 8 to 10 cm distal to the inguinal ligament and descend to knee level, supplying the skin and fascia over the front and medial sides of the thigh.

The *saphenous nerve* is the largest and longest of the femoral branches. It arises at the femoral triangle and descends through it on the lateral side of the femoral vessels to enter the adductor canal. Here, it crosses the vessels obliquely to lie on their medial side in front of the lower end of the adductor magnus muscle. In the canal, the saphenous nerve communicates with branches of the anterior femoral cutaneous and obturator nerves to form the *subsartorial plexus.* At the lower end of the canal, it leaves the femoral vessels and gives off its *infrapatellar branch,* which curves around the posterior border of the sartorius muscle, pierces the fascia lata, and runs onward to supply the skin over the medial side and front of the knee and the patellar ligament. This branch assists offshoots from the anterior and lateral femoral cutaneous nerves in forming the *patellar plexus.*

The saphenous nerve continues its descent on the medial side of the knee, pierces the fascia lata between the tendons of the sartorius and gracilis muscles, courses downward on the medial side of the leg close to the greater saphenous vein, and gives off its *medial crural cutaneous branches.* In the lower leg, it subdivides terminally—the smaller branch follows the medial tibial border to the level of the ankle and the larger passes anterior to the medial malleolus to distribute to the skin and fascia on the medial side and dorsum of the foot.

Articular branches arising from the nerve to the rectus femoris muscle accompany the corresponding branches of the lateral femoral circumflex artery to the hip joint. Twigs from the branches to the vastus muscles and from the saphenous nerve supply the knee joint.

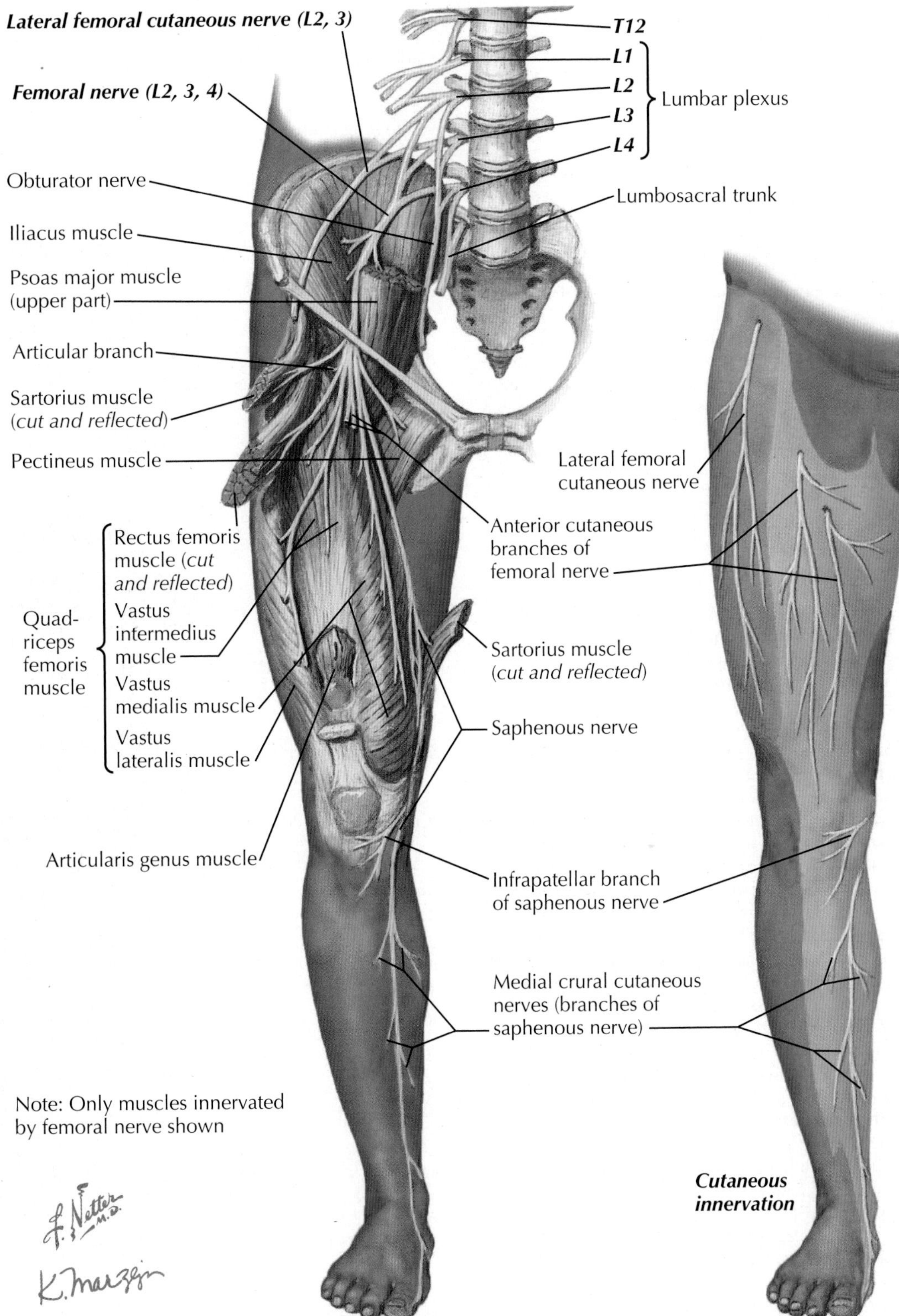

LATERAL FEMORAL CUTANEOUS NERVE

The lateral femoral cutaneous nerve (L2, L3) emerges from the lateral border of the psoas major muscle, passes obliquely over the iliacus muscle behind the parietal peritoneum and iliac fascia (which it supplies)

NERVES OF THIGH (Continued)

toward the anterior superior iliac spine, and enters the thigh by passing under or through the lateral end of the inguinal ligament (see Plate 2.5). The nerve then passes over or through the proximal part of the sartorius muscle and descends deep to the fascia lata. It gives off a number of small branches to the overlying skin before piercing the fascia about 10 cm below the inguinal ligament. The terminal branches of the lateral femoral cutaneous nerve supply the skin and fascia on the anterolateral surfaces of the thigh between the levels of the greater trochanter of the femur and the knee.

OBTURATOR NERVE

The obturator nerve (L2, L3, L4) supplies the obturator externus and adductor muscles of the thigh, gives filaments to the hip and knee joints, and has a variable cutaneous distribution to the medial sides of the thigh and leg.

The obturator nerve arises from the anterior divisions of the ventral rami of the second, third, and fourth lumbar nerves. The contribution from L2 is commonly the smallest and is sometimes absent. These roots unite within the posterior part of the psoas major muscle, forming a nerve that descends through the muscle to emerge from its medial border opposite the upper end of the sacroiliac joint. The obturator nerve runs outward and downward over the sacral ala and pelvic brim into the lesser pelvis, lying lateral to the ureter and internal iliac vessels. It then bends anteroinferiorly to follow the curvature of the lateral pelvic wall (anterior to the obturator vessels and lying on the obturator internus muscle) to reach the obturator groove at the upper part of the obturator foramen. The nerve passes through this groove and foramen to enter the thigh and divides into *anterior* and *posterior branches* shortly thereafter.

The *anterior branch* runs in front of the obturator externus and adductor brevis muscles and behind the pectineus and adductor longus muscles. Near its origin, it gives off an articular twig that enters the hip joint through the acetabular notch. Rarely, it supplies a branch to the pectineus muscle and sends muscular branches to the adductor longus, adductor gracilis, and adductor brevis muscles. The anterior branch finally divides into cutaneous, vascular, and communicating branches.

The *cutaneous branch* is inconstant. When present, it unites with branches of the saphenous and anterior femoral cutaneous nerves in the adductor canal to form the *subsartorial plexus* and assists in the innervation of the skin and fascia over the distal two-thirds of the medial side of the thigh. Infrequently, this branch is larger and passes between the adductor longus and gracilis muscles to descend behind the sartorius to the medial side of the knee and the adjacent part of the leg, where it assists the saphenous nerve in the cutaneous supply of those areas.

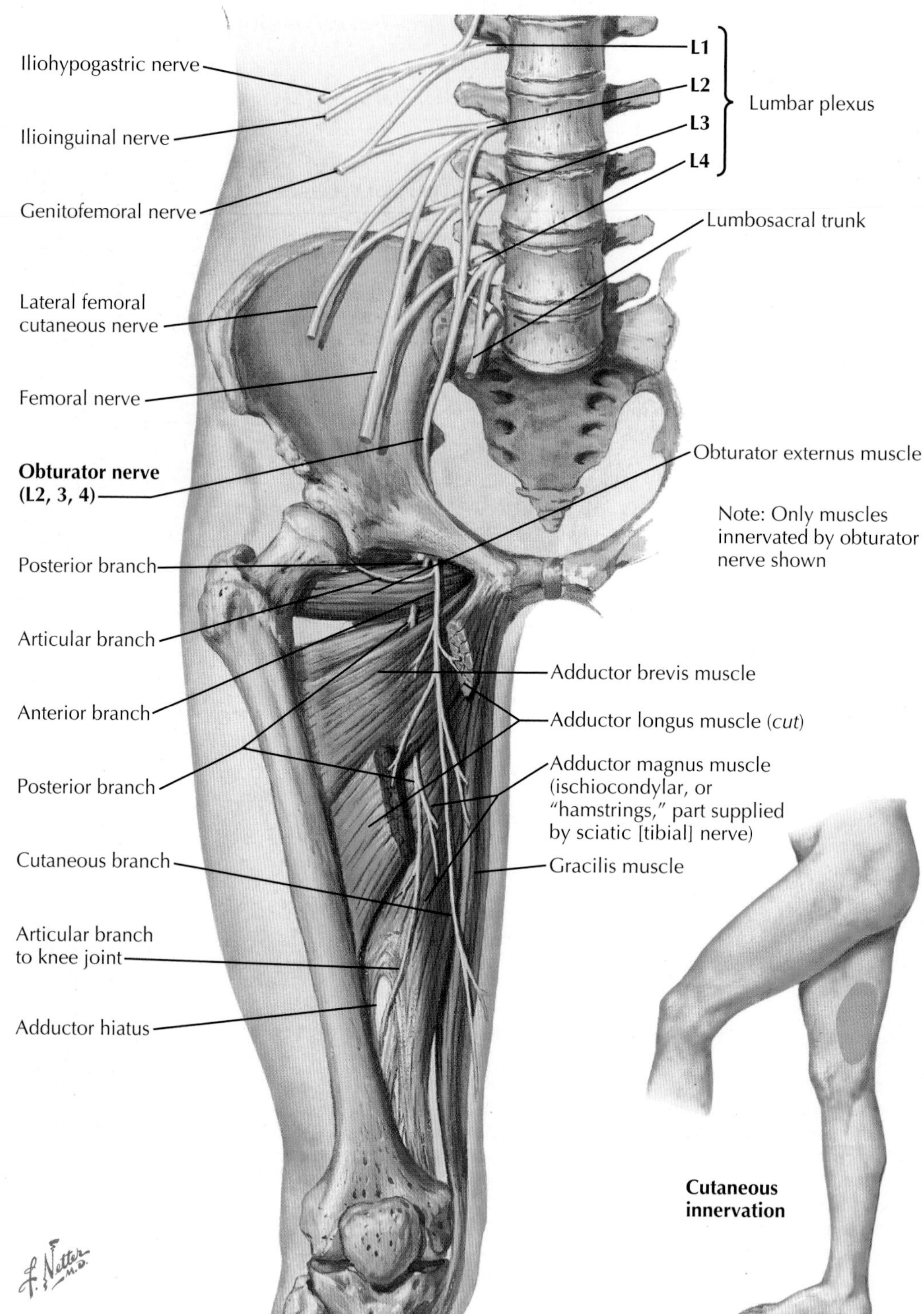

The *vascular branches* end in the femoral artery. Other fine *communicating branches* may link the obturator nerve with the anterior and posterior femoral cutaneous nerves and the inconstant accessory obturator nerve.

The *posterior branch* pierces the anterior part of the obturator externus muscle and supplies it. Thereafter, the nerve runs downward between the adductor brevis and adductor magnus muscles and splits into branches that are distributed to the upper (adductor) part of the adductor magnus and sometimes to the adductor brevis (especially if the latter does not receive a supply from the anterior branch of the obturator nerve). A slender branch emerges from the lower part of the adductor magnus, passes through the hiatus of the adductor canal together with the femoral artery, and then continues to the knee joint. The posterior branch contributes filaments to the femoral and popliteal vessels and ends by perforating the oblique popliteal ligament to supply the articular capsule, cruciate ligaments, and synovial membrane of the knee joint. The fibers to the capsule and ligaments are mostly of somatic origin, whereas those to the synovial membrane are mainly sympathetic.

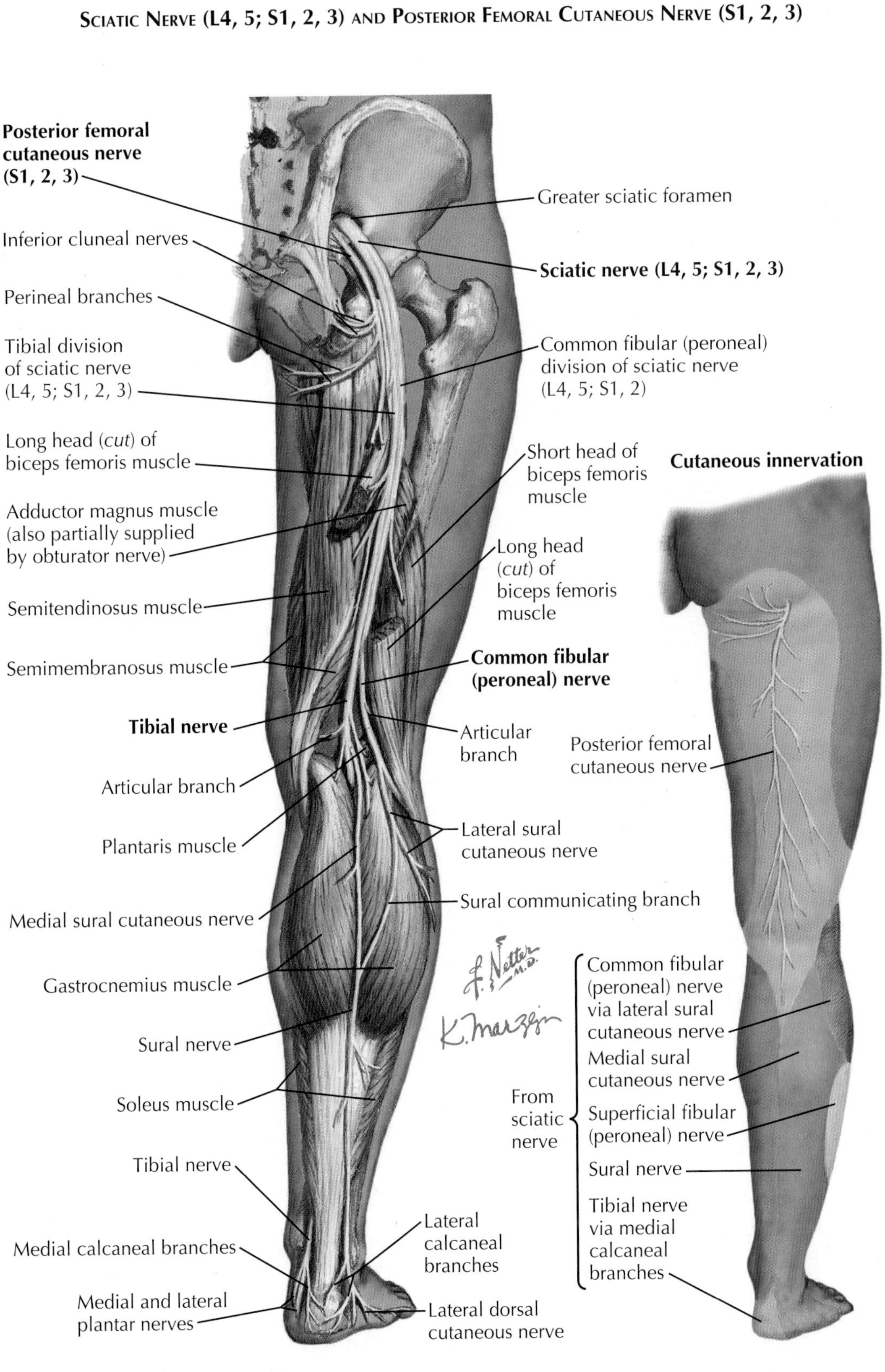

NERVES OF THIGH (Continued)

The *accessory obturator nerve* (L3, L4) is inconstant, small, and derived from the anterior divisions of the ventral rami of L3 and L4. It descends on the medial border of the psoas muscle and then crosses the superior pubic ramus to lie behind the pectineus muscle. It ends by helping to supply the pectineus but may also supply one twig to the hip joint and another twig that joins the anterior branch of the obturator nerve.

SCIATIC NERVE

The roots of the sciatic nerve (L4, L5; S1, S2, S3) arise from the ventral rami of the fourth lumbar to third sacral nerves and unite to form a single trunk that is ovoid in cross section and 16 to 20 mm wide in adults. In the lesser pelvis, the nerve lies anterior to the piriformis muscle, below which it enters the buttock through the greater sciatic foramen (in about 2% of individuals, the nerve pierces the piriformis). Next, the nerve inclines laterally beneath the gluteus maximus muscle, where it rests on the posterior surface of the ischium and the nerve to the quadratus femoris muscle. On its medial side, it is accompanied by the posterior femoral cutaneous nerve and by the inferior gluteal artery and its special branch to the nerve.

On reaching a point about midway between the ischial tuberosity and the greater trochanter of the femur, the nerve turns downward over the gemellus muscles, the obturator internus tendon, and the quadratus femoris muscle (which separate it from the hip joint) and leaves the buttock to enter the thigh beneath the lower border of the gluteus maximus muscle.

The sciatic nerve then descends near the middle of the back of the thigh, lying on the adductor magnus muscle and being crossed obliquely by the long head of the biceps femoris muscle. Just above the apex of the popliteal fossa, it is overlapped by the contiguous margins of the biceps femoris and semimembranosus muscles. In about 90% of cases the sciatic nerve divides into its terminal *tibial* and *common peroneal branches* near the apex of the popliteal fossa, whereas in 10% of cases the division occurs at higher levels. Rarely, the tibial and common peroneal nerves arise independently from the sacral plexus but pursue closely related courses until they reach the apex of the popliteal fossa.

In the buttock, the sciatic nerve supplies an *articular branch* to the hip, which perforates the posterior part of the joint capsule (see Plate 2.4). It may also supply *vascular filaments* to the inferior gluteal artery. (The entrance of the sciatic nerve and its variable relationship to the piriformis muscle are described in Plate 2.4.)

At levels below the quadratus femoris muscle, two branches of the tibial division of the sciatic nerve spring from its medial side to supply the so-called hamstring muscles of the thigh. The upper branch passes to the long head of the biceps femoris muscle and the upper portion of the semitendinosus; the lower branch innervates the lower portion of the semitendinosus and the semimembranosus muscles and the ischiocondylar portion of the adductor magnus muscle. The nerve to the short head of the biceps femoris muscle arises from the lateral side of the sciatic nerve (common peroneal division of the sciatic nerve) in the middle third of the thigh and enters the superficial surface of the muscle. From this nerve, an articular branch continues to the knee, providing proximal and distal branches that accompany the lateral superior genicular and lateral inferior genicular arteries to the knee joint.

The tibial and common peroneal nerves arise by a division of the sciatic nerve, usually at the upper limit of the popliteal fossa. The tibial nerve continues the vertical course of the sciatic nerve at the back of the knee and into the leg. The common peroneal nerve follows the tendon of the biceps femoris muscle along the upper lateral margin of the popliteal space and into the leg, curving forward around the neck of the fibula.

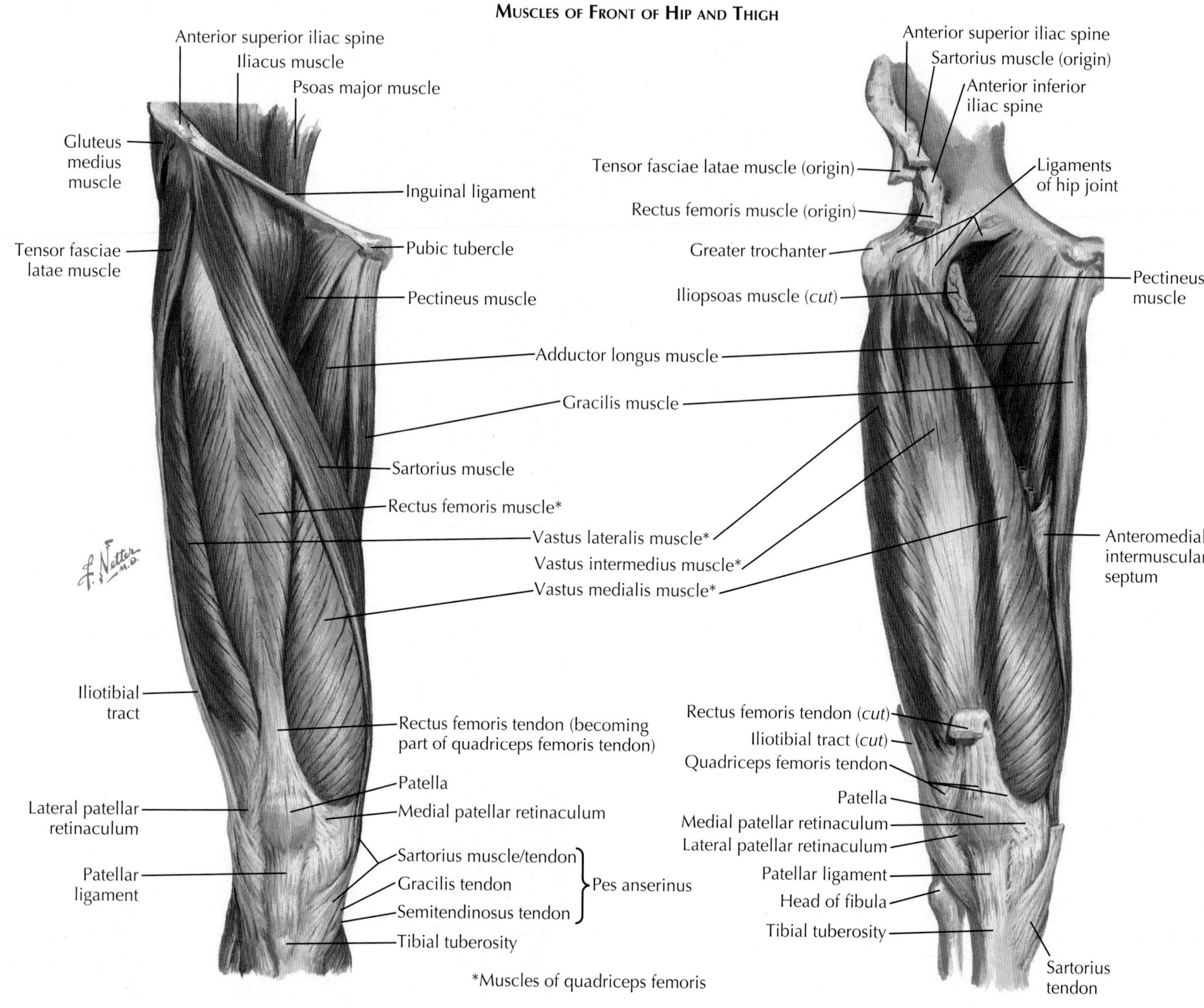

Fasciae and Muscles of Hip and Thigh

The region of the hip and thigh extends from the iliac crest to the knee. The upper portion is the hip, which is limited generally by the level of the greater trochanter of the femur. The subcutaneous connective tissue contains a considerable amount of fat, especially in the gluteal region. The subcutaneous tissue here is continuous with the similar layer of the lower abdomen, and the membranous layer of the latter region continues beyond the inguinal ligament to become attached to the fascia lata a short distance beyond the ligament. The layer attaches medially to the pubic tubercle and laterally to the iliac crest. It also attaches to the margins of the saphenous opening and fills the opening itself with the *cribriform fascia,* a subcutaneous connective tissue perforated for the passage of the greater saphenous vein and other blood and lymphatic vessels.

Fascia Lata

The fascia lata is the uppermost division of a complete stocking-like investment of the soft parts of the limb (see Plate 2.9). Below the knee, this investment is represented by the crural fascia and the plantar and dorsal fasciae of the foot. The fascia lata is strong, thicker where it has tendinous contributions and thinner in the gluteal region. It has a complete bony attachment to the pelvis at the pubic crest and symphysis, the ischiopubic ramus, and the tuberosity of the ischium. From here, an attachment to the sacrotuberal ligament carries it to the dorsum of the coccyx and the sacrum. It continues to the posterior superior iliac spine and along the external lip of the iliac crest to the anterior superior iliac spine, the inguinal ligament, and the pubic tubercle. Here, a deep lamina follows the pecten of the pubis behind the femoral vein.

The *gluteal aponeurosis* lies between the iliac crest and the superior border of the gluteus maximus muscle, which provides part of the origin of the gluteus medius. A strong lateral band, the *iliotibial tract,* arises from the tubercle of the iliac crest and serves as a tendon of the tensor fasciae latae muscle and as part of the tendon of the gluteus maximus muscle. The tract ends at the knee, where it reinforces the capsule of the knee joint and attaches to the condyle of the tibia.

The lateral and medial intermuscular septa unite the fascia lata to the periosteum of the femur and separate the muscles of the posterior and anterior compartments

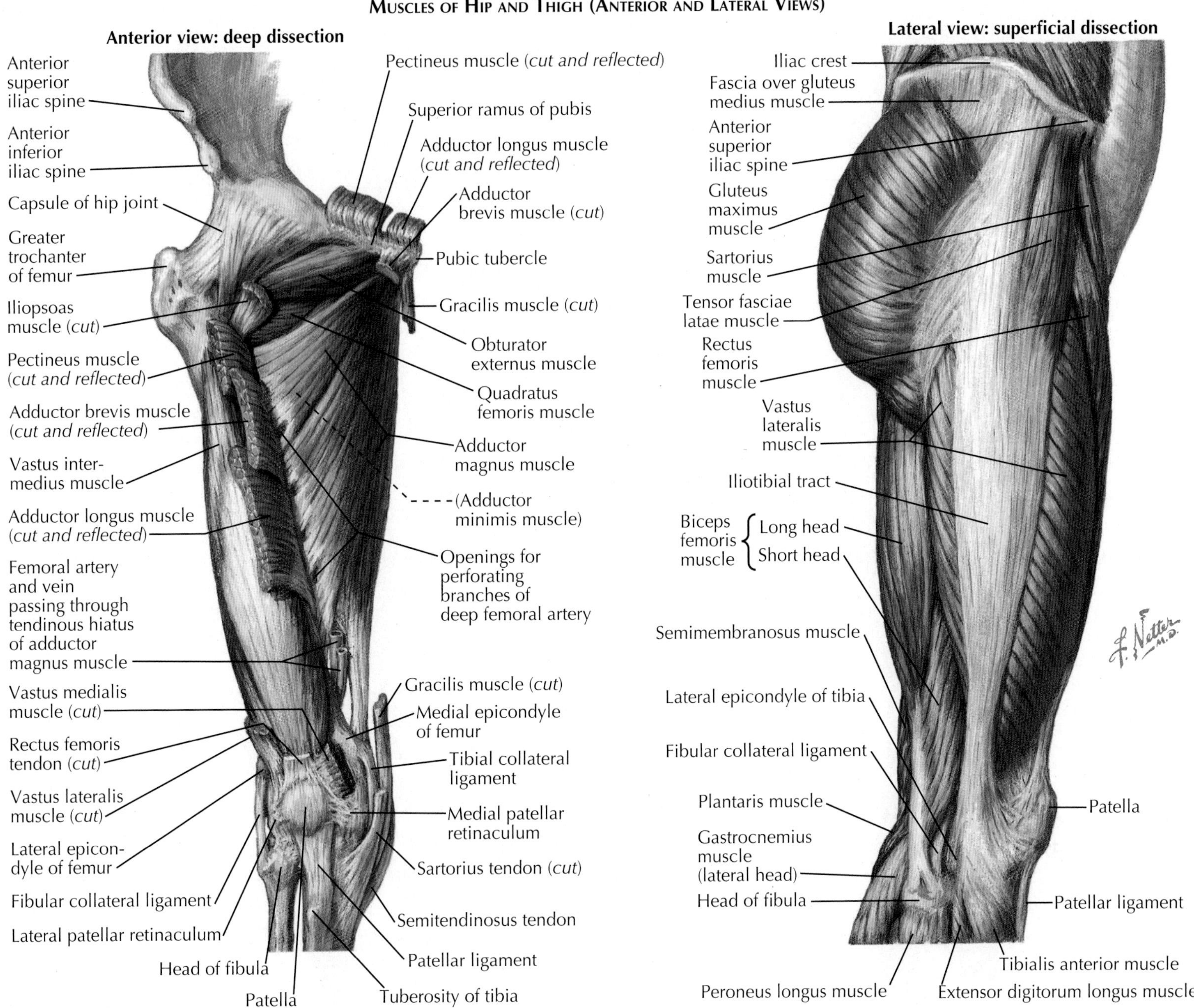

Fasciae and Muscles of Hip and Thigh (Continued)

and the muscles of the medial and anterior groups. The medial intermuscular septum splits to enclose the sartorius muscle and helps to form the adductor canal (see Plate 2.8). The iliotibial tract attaches deeply to the lateral intermuscular septum.

At the *saphenous opening*, a superficial sheet of fascia lata continues along the inguinal ligament to the pubic tubercle, whereas a deep lamina attaches to the pecten of the pubis.

Muscles

The muscles of the hip and thigh are divided into four groups: anterior, medial, posterior, and lateral femoral muscles (see Plates 2.8 to 2.10). Additionally, the psoas major and iliacus muscles, although located for the most part and arising within the lower abdomen, insert into the thigh (lesser trochanter of femur) and have their principal action as flexors of the thigh. In systematizing the femoral muscles, it is useful to note that muscles arising from the pubis and ischium are preaxial and are innervated by nerves derived from the anterior branches of the lumbosacral plexus, namely, the obturator or tibial nerves; however, muscles arising from the ilium or femur are postaxial and are innervated by either the femoral or common peroneal nerves of posterior branch derivation. The anterior group muscles are all postaxial in classification and innervation, and the medial group muscles are preaxial. The posterior and lateral groups contain muscles of both types.

Anterior Femoral Muscles

The anterior femoral muscles are the sartorius, quadriceps femoris (combined rectus femoris and vastus muscles), and the articularis genus muscles (see Plate 2.8).

The *sartorius* is the longest muscle in the body. Ribbon-like in form, it arises from the anterior superior spine of the ilium and from the notch just below the spine. It is diagonally placed, ending on the medial side of the leg. Its insertion is into the medial surface of the tibia, below the tuberosity and nearly as far forward as the crest. In this insertion, it is associated with the tendons of the gracilis and semitendinosus muscles in the *pes anserinus,* which is separated from the tibia by a bursa. Contraction of the sartorius produces flexion, abduction, and lateral rotation of the thigh. It also flexes the leg because its tendon passes behind the transverse axis of the knee. The sartorius

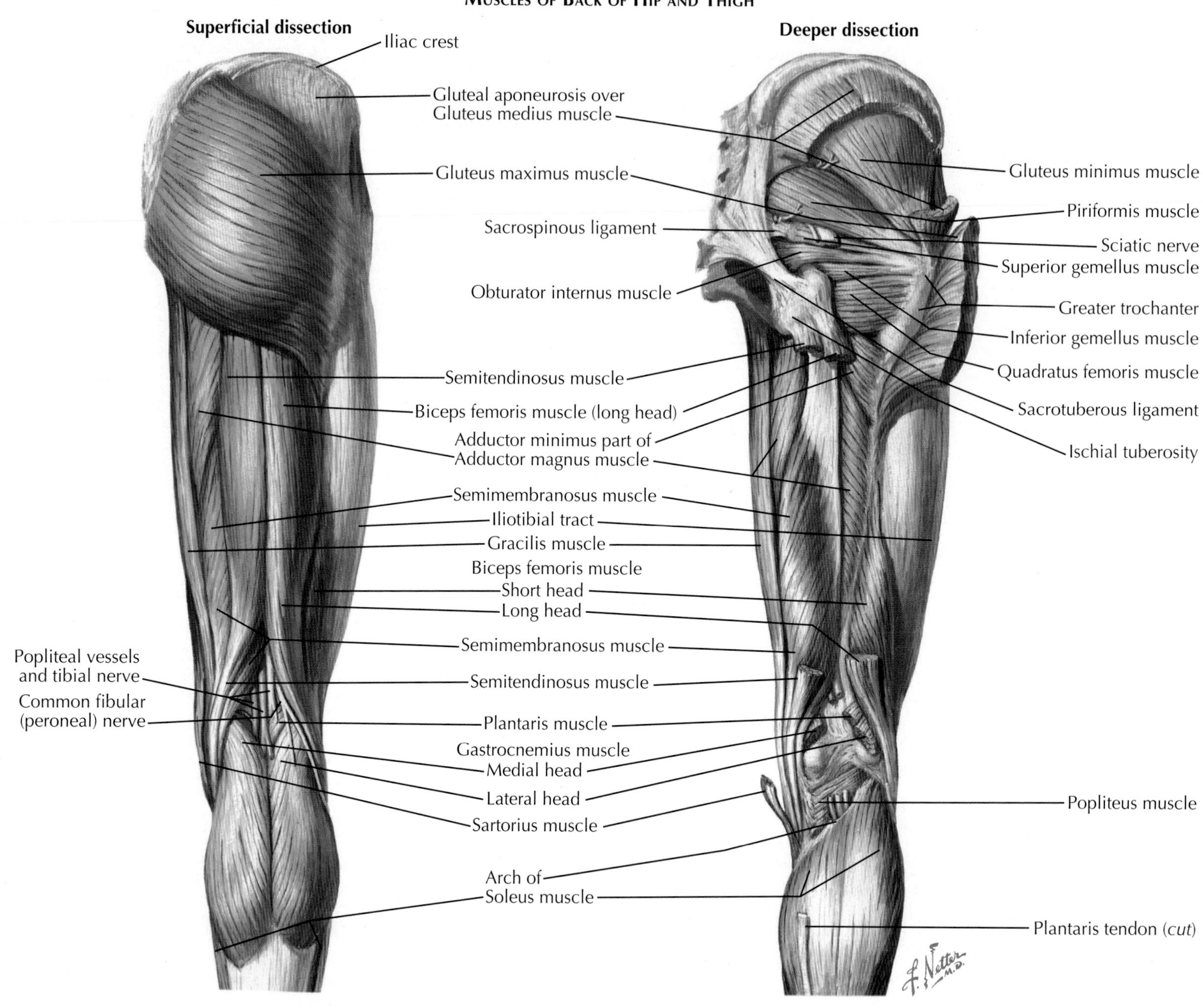

Fasciae and Muscles of Hip and Thigh (Continued)

forms the lateral border of the femoral triangle in the upper third of the thigh; in the middle third, it forms the roof of the adductor canal. The femoral nerve innervates the sartorius muscle by two branches, with nerve fibers from L2 and L3.

The four parts of the *quadriceps femoris muscle* arise separately but end in closely related parts of the tibia—the tuberosity and condyles. The *rectus femoris muscle,* as its name implies, runs straight down the thigh. Somewhat fusiform in shape, its superficial fibers have a bipennate arrangement. The muscle arises by two tendons. The straight head takes origin from the anterior inferior spine of the ilium; the reflected head arises from the groove above the acetabulum. These tendons unite at an acute angle and continue into a central aponeurosis that is expanded downward into the muscle. From this, the muscle fibers arise, turn around its margin, and end in the tendon of insertion. The latter broadens to attach to the proximal border of the patella and spreads over its surface to the tuberosity of the tibia (patellar ligament). Two branches of the femoral nerve with fibers from L3 and L4 innervate the muscle.

The *vastus lateralis muscle* is the largest component of the quadriceps femoris muscle. It arises from the femur by a broad aponeurosis attached to the upper part of the intertrochanteric line, the anterior and inferior borders of the greater trochanter, the gluteal tuberosity, the immediately adjacent portion of the lateral lip of the linea aspera, and the lateral intermuscular septum throughout its length. This aponeurosis covers the superior portion of the muscle, and from its deep surface, many muscle fibers take origin. The tendon of the vastus lateralis muscle inserts into the superolateral border of the patella and the lateral condyle of the tibia. The large branch of the femoral nerve (L3, L4) to the vastus lateralis muscle accompanies the descending branch of the lateral circumflex femoral artery.

The *vastus medialis muscle* arises from the whole extent of the medial lip of the linea aspera, the distal half of the intertrochanteric line, and the medial intermuscular septum. The aponeurotic fibers of origin adhere to the tendons of insertion of the adductor longus and adductor magnus muscles. The fibers are directed downward and forward toward the knee. The aponeurotic tendon inserts into the tendon of the rectus femoris, the superomedial border of the patella, and the

Fasciae and Muscles of Hip and Thigh (Continued)

medial condyle of the tibia. Two branches of the femoral nerve (L3, L4) supply this muscle.

The *vastus intermedius muscle* arises from the shaft of the femur, from the lower half of the lateral lip of the linea aspera, and from the lateral intermuscular septum. Its fibers end in a superficial aponeurosis, which blends with the deep surface of the tendons of the rectus femoris and with the vastus medialis and vastus lateralis muscles. The vastus intermedius is innervated superficially by a branch of the femoral nerve (L3, L4) and also by the upper nerve to the vastus medialis.

The four parts of the quadriceps femoris muscle converge on the patella, which is regarded as a sesamoid developed in its tendon. The *patellar ligament* is the terminal part of the tendinous insertion of the quadriceps femoris muscle. It ends in the tuberosity of the tibia. The *suprapatellar bursa* intervenes between the quadriceps femoris tendon and the lower end of the femur and communicates freely with the cavity of the knee joint. A deep *infrapatellar bursa* lies between the patellar ligament (just above its insertion) and the tibia. *Medial* and *lateral patellar retinacula* insert into the condyles of the tibia.

The quadriceps femoris muscle is the great extensor of the leg at the knee, with all parts of the muscle contributing to this action. The line of traction, which is along the axis of the femur, is not directly in line with the tibia. Thus there is a tendency to displace the patella lateralward as the muscle contracts. The numerous low, almost horizontal fibers of the vastus medialis muscle counter this displacing force. The rectus femoris muscle also acts in flexion of the thigh at the hip. Its two almost right-angled tendons of origin combine to serve the full range of flexion action. Initially in line with the rest of the muscle, the straight tendon becomes less effective as the thigh is flexed, but as this tendon loses its effectiveness, the flexed thigh becomes more and more in line with the reflected tendon, and thus its attachment becomes the optimal site for traction. The quadriceps muscles are generally uncontracted in relaxed standing.

The *articularis genus muscle* consists of a number of small muscular bundles that arise from the lower fourth of the front of the femur. Lying deep to the vastus intermedius muscle, these bundles insert into the upper part of the synovial membrane of the knee joint.

Medial Femoral Muscles

The medial femoral muscles are the gracilis, pectineus, adductor longus, adductor brevis, adductor magnus, and obturator externus muscles (see Plate 2.8).

The *gracilis muscle* is long and slender and is superficially placed on the medial aspect of the thigh. Its thin tendon arises along the pubic symphysis and the inferior ramus of the pubis. Its tapered tendon inserts into the upper part of the shaft of the tibia as part of the pes anserinus, lying between the tendons of the sartorius and semitendinosus muscles. A bursa deep to the tendon separates it from the tibial collateral ligament. The gracilis muscle adducts the thigh and assists in flexion

Bony Attachments of Muscles of Hip and Thigh: Anterior View

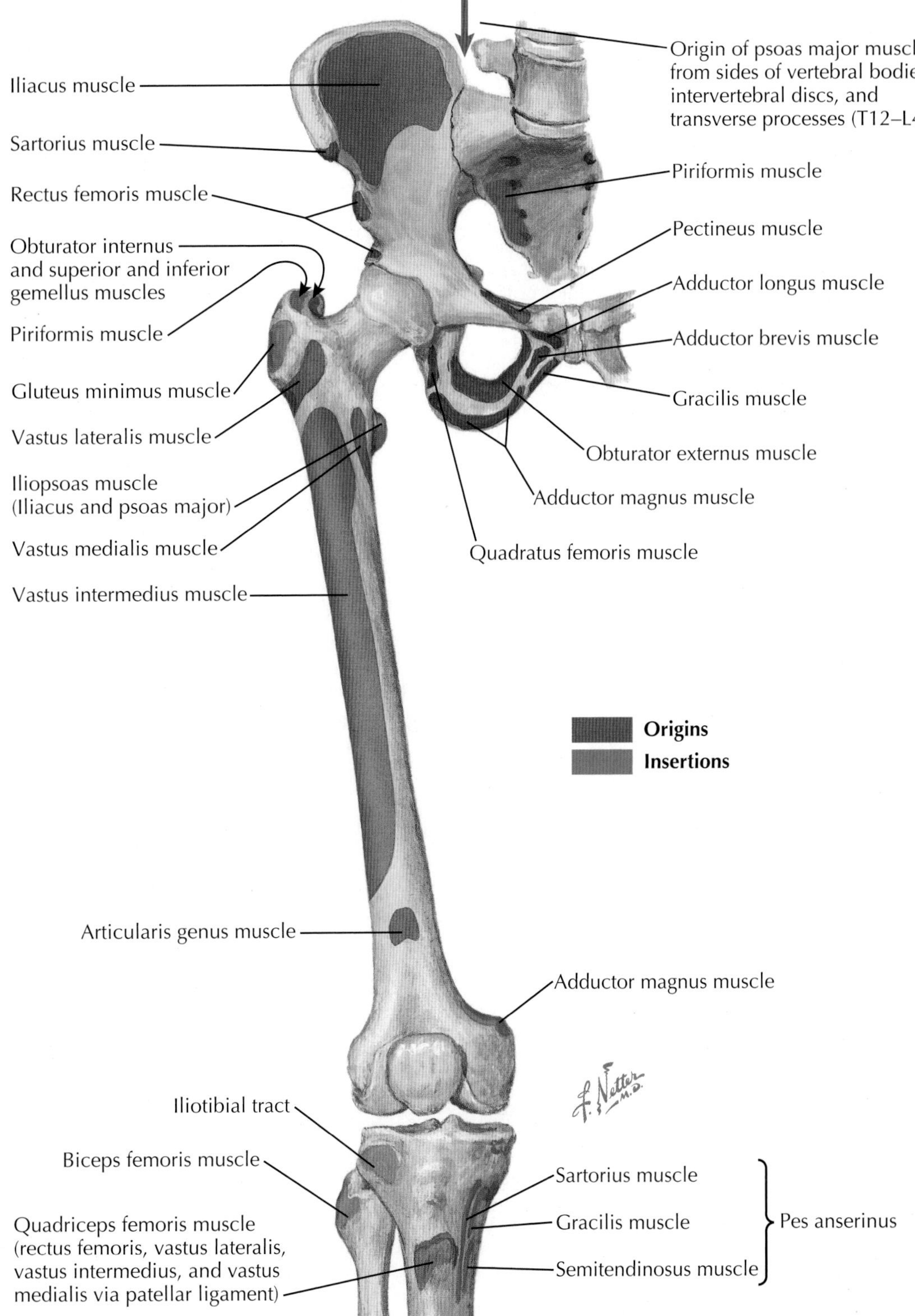

of the leg at the knee. It also participates in flexion and medial rotation of the thigh at the hip. The gracilis muscle is innervated by a branch of the anterior division of the obturator nerve (L2, L3).

The *pectineus muscle* is flat and quadrangular and forms the medial part of the floor of the femoral triangle. It arises from the pecten of the pubis and the surface of the bone below the pecten, between the iliopubic eminence laterally and the pubic tubercle medially. The fibers of the muscle pass downward, backward, and lateralward and insert by a 5-cm-wide tendon into the pectineal line of the femur. The muscle adducts, rotates medially, and assists in flexion of the thigh. It is supplied by a branch of the femoral nerve, which enters the lateral portion of the muscle, and also by the accessory obturator nerve, when this is present. There are variable divisions of the muscle into ventromedial and dorsolateral portions.

The *adductor longus muscle* lies in the same plane as the pectineus and forms the medial boundary of the

FASCIAE AND MUSCLES OF HIP AND THIGH (Continued)

femoral triangle. It arises in a flat, narrow tendon from the medial portion of the superior ramus of the pubis. It expands into a broad, triangular muscular belly and inserts by a thin tendon into the middle third of the medial lip of the linea aspera of the femur, between the tendons of the vastus medialis and the adductor magnus muscles. The adductor longus muscle adducts the thigh and assists in its flexion and medial rotation. Its nerve, a branch of the anterior division of the obturator nerve (L2, L3), reaches it on the deep surface of its middle third.

The *adductor brevis muscle* is deep to the pectineus and adductor longus muscles. It is an adductor of the thigh and, to a lesser degree, assists in its flexion and medial rotation. The adductor brevis has a narrow origin from the inferior pubic ramus, between the origins of the gracilis and obturator externus muscles. Its muscular fibers fan out to end in an aponeurosis that inserts into the lower two-thirds of the pectineal line of the femur and the upper half of the medial lip of the linea aspera. Branches of the anterior division of the obturator nerve (L2, L3) enter the middle third of the muscle near its proximal border. Its tendon is pierced by perforating branches of the deep femoral artery and their accompanying veins.

The *adductor magnus muscle* is the largest muscle of the medial femoral group. It is triangular and actually consists of a combination of two muscles that have different innervations. The muscle arises from the lower part of the inferior pubic ramus, the ramus of the ischium, and the ischial tuberosity. Its muscular fibers fan out to the whole length of the linea aspera of the femur; the upper fibers are horizontal and the lower fibers are vertical. The upper horizontal fibers, sometimes designated as the adductor minimus muscle, insert into the medial side of the gluteal ridge and the uppermost part of the linea aspera of the femur. Below this, the aponeurosis of insertion ends in the whole length of the medial lip of the linea aspera and the supracondylar line of the femur.

The most medial and posterior portion of the muscle, its ischiocondylar portion, arises from the ischial tuberosity and forms a round tendon that ends in the adductor tubercle of the medial epicondyle of the femur. The upper anterior portion of the muscle is a strong adductor and assists in flexion and medial rotation of the thigh. It is innervated by the posterior division of the obturator nerve (L3, L4). The *ischiocondylar portion* of the muscle is one of the hamstring muscles of the back of the thigh. Its particular action is to extend the thigh and rotate it; it is innervated on its dorsal surface by a branch from the tibial division of the sciatic nerve (L4, S1).

In the lower third of the thigh, aponeurotic fibers spread lateralward from the rounded tendon of the adductor magnus muscle toward the vastus medialis muscle and end in the medial intermuscular septum. This strong *vastoadductor membrane* covers the distal end of the adductor canal and may be pierced for the passage of the saphenous nerve and the descending genicular artery and vein. Farther, the aponeurosis of insertion of the adductor magnus muscle is pierced adjacent to the femur by four openings for the passage of the perforating branches of the deep femoral artery and accompanying veins. Finally, a large gap exists between the lower end of the aponeurosis and the tendon to the adductor tubercle. Through this *adductor hiatus,* the femoral vessels pass back and down into the popliteal space, where they become the popliteal vessels.

The *obturator externus muscle* arises from the external aspect of the superior and inferior rami of the pubis and the ramus of the ischium and from the external surface of the obturator membrane. Its tendon passes across the back of the neck of the femur and the capsule of the hip joint to insert in the trochanteric fossa of the femur. The synovial membrane of the hip joint acts as a bursa separating the tendon from the neck of the femur. This muscle is a lateral rotator of the thigh. It is supplied by a branch of the obturator nerve (L3, L4).

BONY ATTACHMENTS OF MUSCLES OF HIP AND THIGH: POSTERIOR VIEW

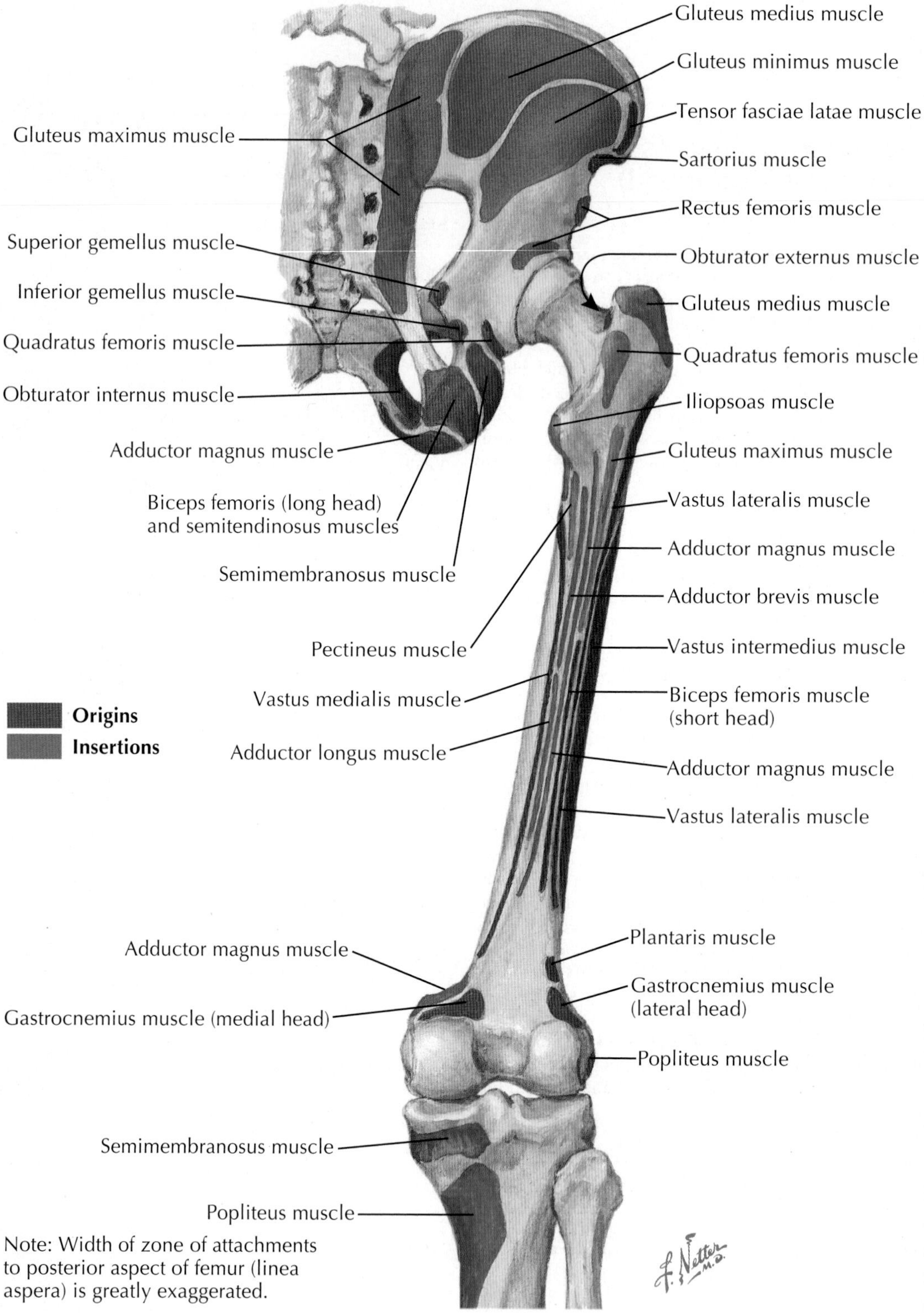

Note: Width of zone of attachments to posterior aspect of femur (linea aspera) is greatly exaggerated.

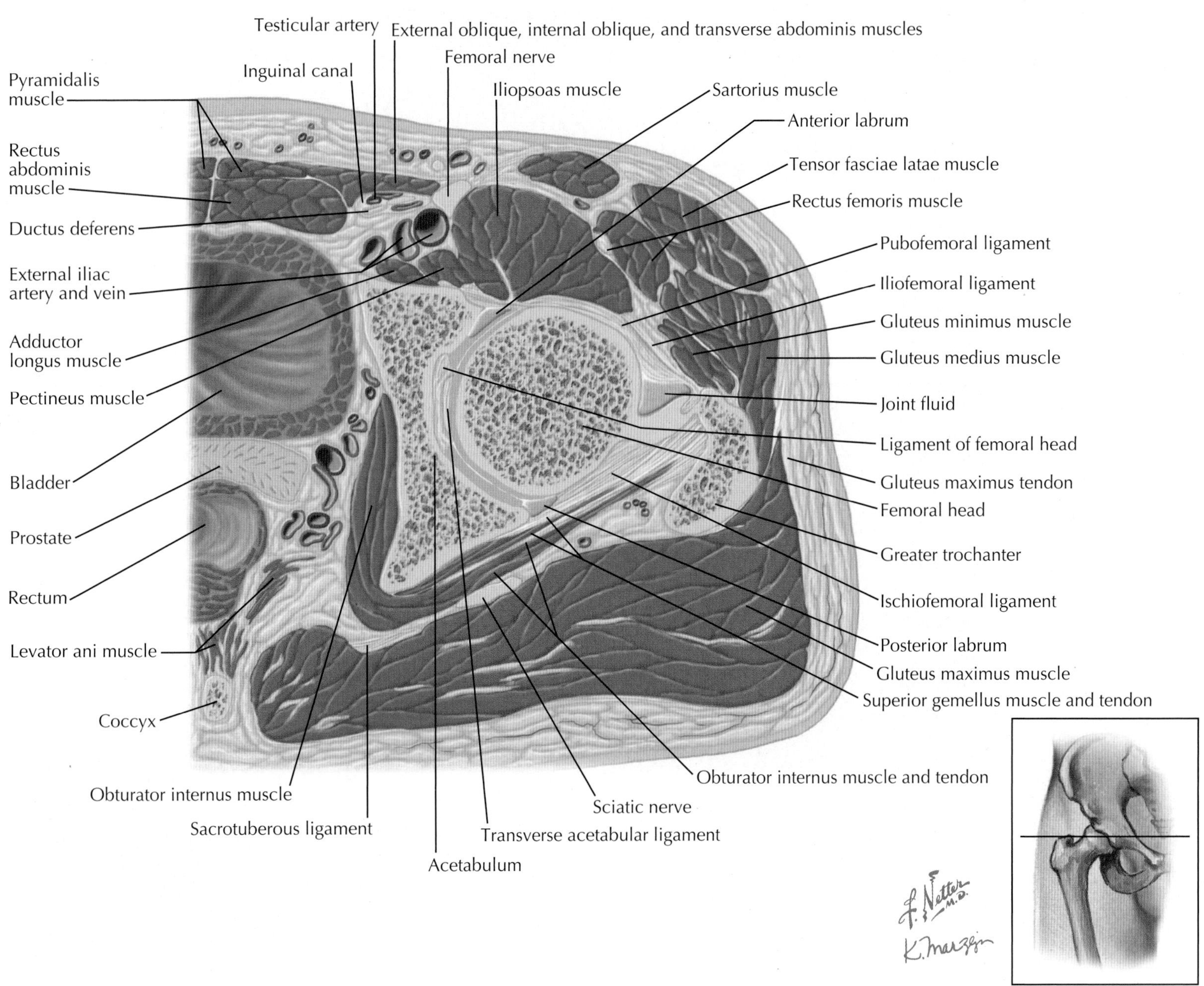

Fasciae and Muscles of Hip and Thigh (Continued)

POSTERIOR FEMORAL MUSCLES

The posterior femoral muscles compose the hamstring group, which includes the semitendinosus, semimembranosus, biceps femoris muscles, and the ischiocondylar portion of the adductor magnus (see Plate 2.10).

The *semitendinosus muscle* is aptly named, because about half its length is tendinous. It arises from the lower and medial impression on the tuberosity of the ischium in common with the long head of the biceps femoris muscle. The semitendinosus tendon forms the medial margin of the popliteal space at the knee; it then curves around the medial condyle of the tibia and inserts as part of the pes anserinus into the upper part of the medial surface of the tibia. It is separated from the tibial collateral ligament by a bursa. Two branches of the tibial division of the sciatic nerve (L4, L5, S1, S2) usually reach this muscle.

The *semimembranosus muscle* arises by a long, flat tendon (or membrane) from the upper and outer impression on the tuberosity of the ischium. The muscular belly begins about halfway down the thigh. The insertion of the muscle at the knee is rather complex. It ends mainly in the horizontal groove on the posteromedial aspect of the medial condyle of the tibia, but a prominent reflection from here forms the oblique popliteal ligament of the knee joint capsule. Other fibers extend from the tendon to the tibial collateral ligament and onto the fascia of the popliteus muscle. The semimembranosus muscle is innervated by a branch of the tibial division of the sciatic nerve arising in common with the lower nerve to the semitendinosus muscle.

The *biceps femoris muscle* is a secondary combination of one preaxial muscle, the long head, and one postaxial muscle, the short head. The long head arises in combination with the semitendinosus muscle from the lower and medial impression of the ischial tuberosity and the lower part of the sacrotuberal ligament. The short head arises from the lateral lip of the linea aspera of the femur, the proximal two-thirds of the supracondylar line, and the lateral intermuscular septum. The muscle fibers of the short head join the tendon of the long head to form the heavy round tendon that forms the lateral margin of the popliteal fossa.

At the knee, the tendon divides around the fibular collateral ligament and ends on the lateral aspect of the head of the fibula, the lateral condyle of the tibia, and in

CROSS-SECTIONAL ANATOMY OF HIP: CORONAL VIEW

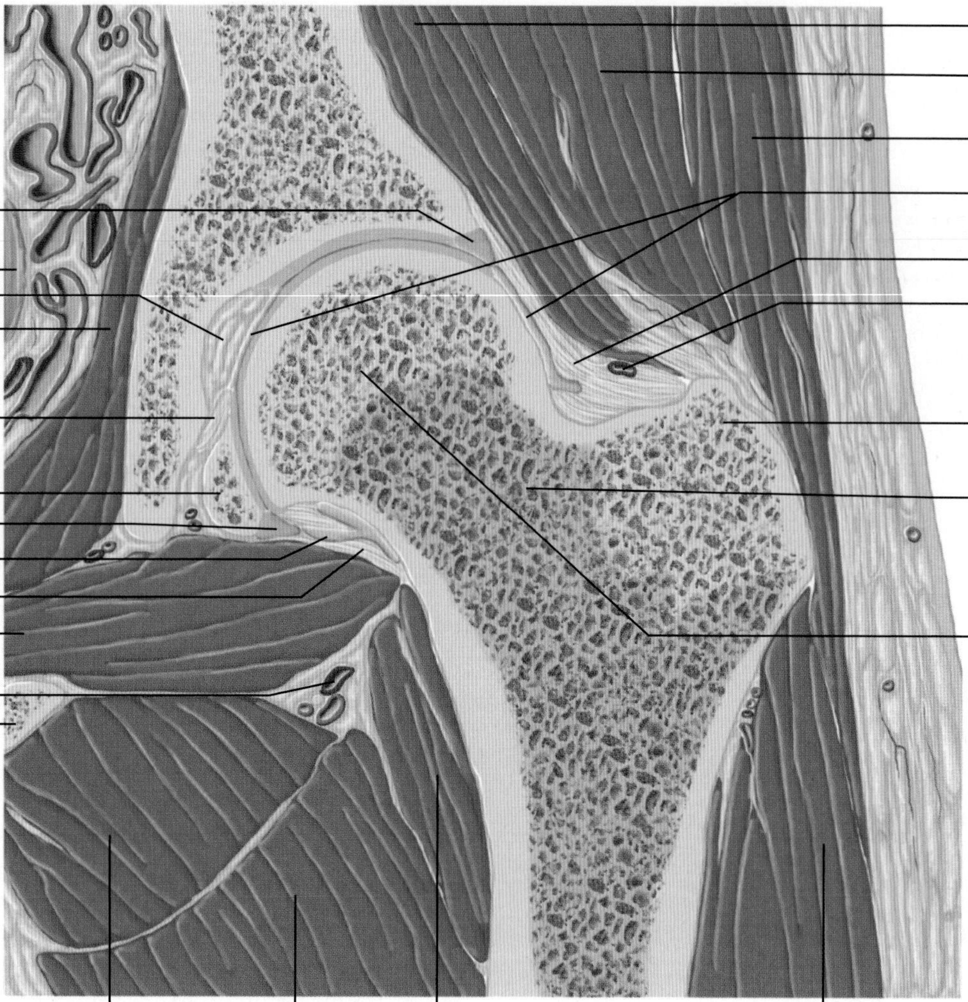

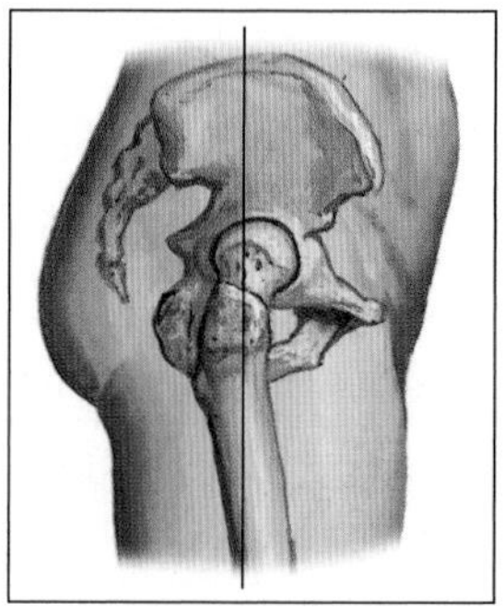

FASCIAE AND MUSCLES OF HIP AND THIGH (Continued)

the deep fascia of the lateral aspect of the leg. As a combination of two muscles of differing origins, the two heads are differently innervated. The long head usually receives two branches of the tibial division of the sciatic nerve (S1, S2, S3), one to the upper third and one to the middle third of the muscle. The nerve to the short head is a branch of the common peroneal division of the sciatic nerve (L5, S1, S2), which enters the superficial surface of the muscle.

The hamstring muscles flex the leg and extend the thigh. Their ligamentous, or protective, action at the hip joint is important. In the usual movement, flexion and extension are carried out together, and maximal excursion at one joint carries the limitation of less than maximal excursion at the other. There is also minimal rotary action, with the "semi" muscles rotating the flexed leg medially and the biceps femoris muscle rotating it laterally.

LATERAL FEMORAL MUSCLES

The lateral femoral muscles lie largely in the hip region. They are the gluteus maximus, gluteus medius, gluteus minimus, tensor fasciae latae, piriformis, obturator internus, superior gemellus, inferior gemellus, and quadratus femoris muscles (see Plates 2.10 and 2.13).

The *gluteus maximus muscle* is a heavy, coarsely fasciculated muscle, superficially situated in the buttock. It is quadrilateral, and its fasciculi are directed downward and outward. The muscle arises from the posterior gluteal line of the ilium and the area of the bone above and behind it, the posterior surface of the sacrum and coccyx, the sacrotuberal ligament, and the gluteal aponeurosis overlying the gluteus medius muscle. The larger upper portion and the superficial fibers of the lower portion insert into the iliotibial tract of the fascia lata; the deeper fibers of the lower portion reach the gluteal tuberosity of the femur and the lateral intermuscular septum.

The upper portion of the muscle is separated from the greater trochanter of the femur by the large trochanteric bursa. Other bursae separate the tendon of the muscle from the origin of the vastus lateralis muscle (of the quadriceps femoris muscle) and the lower portion of the muscle from the ischial tuberosity. The gluteus maximus is distinctly a muscle of the erect posture but becomes active only under conditions of effort. It is a powerful extensor of the thigh and, acting from its insertion, equally an extensor of the trunk. It is a strong lateral rotator, and its superior fibers come into play in forcible abduction of the thigh. Its insertion into the iliotibial tract may promote stability of the femur on the tibia, but the extensive blending of this tract with the lateral intermuscular septum would prevent significant action of the muscle on the tibia. The inferior gluteal nerve (L5, S1, S2) is the sole supply of this muscle.

The *gluteus medius muscle* lies largely anterior to the gluteus maximus under the strong vertical fibers of the gluteal aponeurosis but also partly underlies the gluteus maximus. It arises from the external surface of the ilium between the anterior and posterior gluteal lines and from the gluteal aponeurosis. Its flattened tendon

Fasciae and Muscles of Hip and Thigh (Continued)

inserts into the posterosuperior angle of the greater trochanter of the femur and into a diagonal ridge on its lateral surface. A bursa separates the tendon from the trochanter proximal to its insertion.

The *gluteus minimus muscle* underlies the gluteus medius, arising from the ilium between its anterior gluteal and inferior gluteal lines. Its insertion is onto the anterosuperior angle of the greater trochanter, with a bursa intervening between the tendon and the medial part of the anterior surface of the trochanter. The gluteus medius and minimus muscles abduct the femur and rotate the thigh medialward. These are important functions in walking, because when one foot is raised off the ground, the gluteus muscles, holding the pelvic bone of the other side down toward the greater trochanter, prevent the collapse of the pelvis on its unsupported side. The same muscles, by their rotary action, swing the pelvis forward as the step is taken. Both muscles are innervated by the superior gluteal nerve (L4, L5, S1), accompanied by branches of the superior gluteal vessels between the two muscles.

The *tensor fasciae latae muscle* is fusiform and is enclosed between two layers of the fascia lata. It arises from the anterior part of the external lip of the iliac crest, the outer surface of the anterior superior spine of the ilium, and the notch below the spine. The muscle inserts into the iliotibial tract, which blends into both layers of its investing fascia. The tensor fasciae latae muscle assists in flexion, abduction, and medial rotation (weakly) of the thigh. It probably aids in stabilizing the femur on the tibia, although the long, strong connection of the iliotibial tract with the lateral intermuscular septum must make direct action at the knee minimal. The superior gluteal nerve ends in the tensor fasciae latae, together with an inferior branch of the superior gluteal artery.

The *piriformis muscle* arises within the pelvis from the front of the sacrum between the first to fourth sacral foramina. It passes through the greater sciatic foramen to insert onto the upper border of the greater trochanter of the femur. It is a lateral rotator of the thigh and assists in abduction. Its nerves are one or two branches from S1 and S2.

The *obturator internus muscle* arises from the entire bony margin of the obturator foramen (except the obturator groove), the inner surface of the obturator membrane, and the pelvic surface of the coxal bone behind and above the obturator foramen. The fibers of the muscle converge to pass through the lesser sciatic foramen, where it is separated from the bone of the lesser sciatic notch and then, running horizontally, ends in the medial surface of the greater trochanter of the femur above the trochanteric fossa. The muscle is a lateral rotator of the thigh and has some abduction capability. Its nerve (L5, S1, S2) also supplies the superior gemellus muscle. The tendon of the obturator internus muscle receives the superior gemellus tendon along its superior border and superficial surface and the inferior gemellus tendon along its inferior margin.

Cross-Sectional Anatomy of Thigh

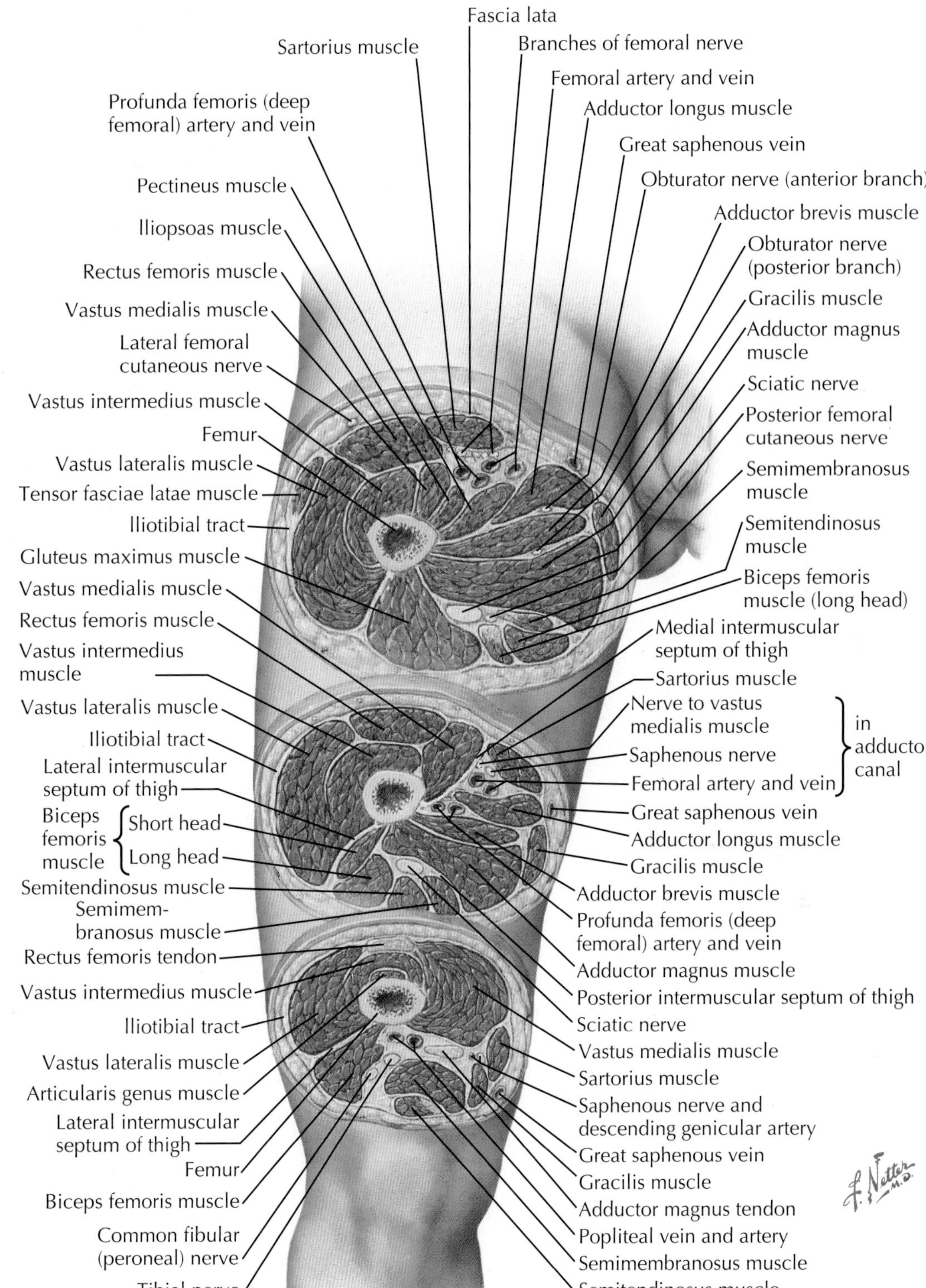

The *superior* and *inferior gemellus muscles* are small, tapered muscles that lie parallel to the tendon of the internal obturator; the superior gemellus muscle above the tendon arises from the ischial spine, and the inferior gemellus muscle below the tendon arises from the ischial tuberosity. Accessories of the internal obturator muscle, the gemellus muscles have the same action. The nerve to the superior gemellus muscle comes from that to the internal obturator muscle; the nerve to the inferior gemellus is in common with the nerve to the quadratus femoris muscle.

The *quadratus femoris muscle* is thick and quadrilateral and is located below the inferior gemellus muscle. It arises from the upper part of the lateral border of the ischial tuberosity and inserts on the quadrate line of the femur, which extends downward from the intertrochanteric crest. This muscle is a strong lateral rotator of the thigh. Its nerve supply is from L4, L5, and S1.

ARTERIES AND NERVES OF THIGH: ANTERIOR VIEWS

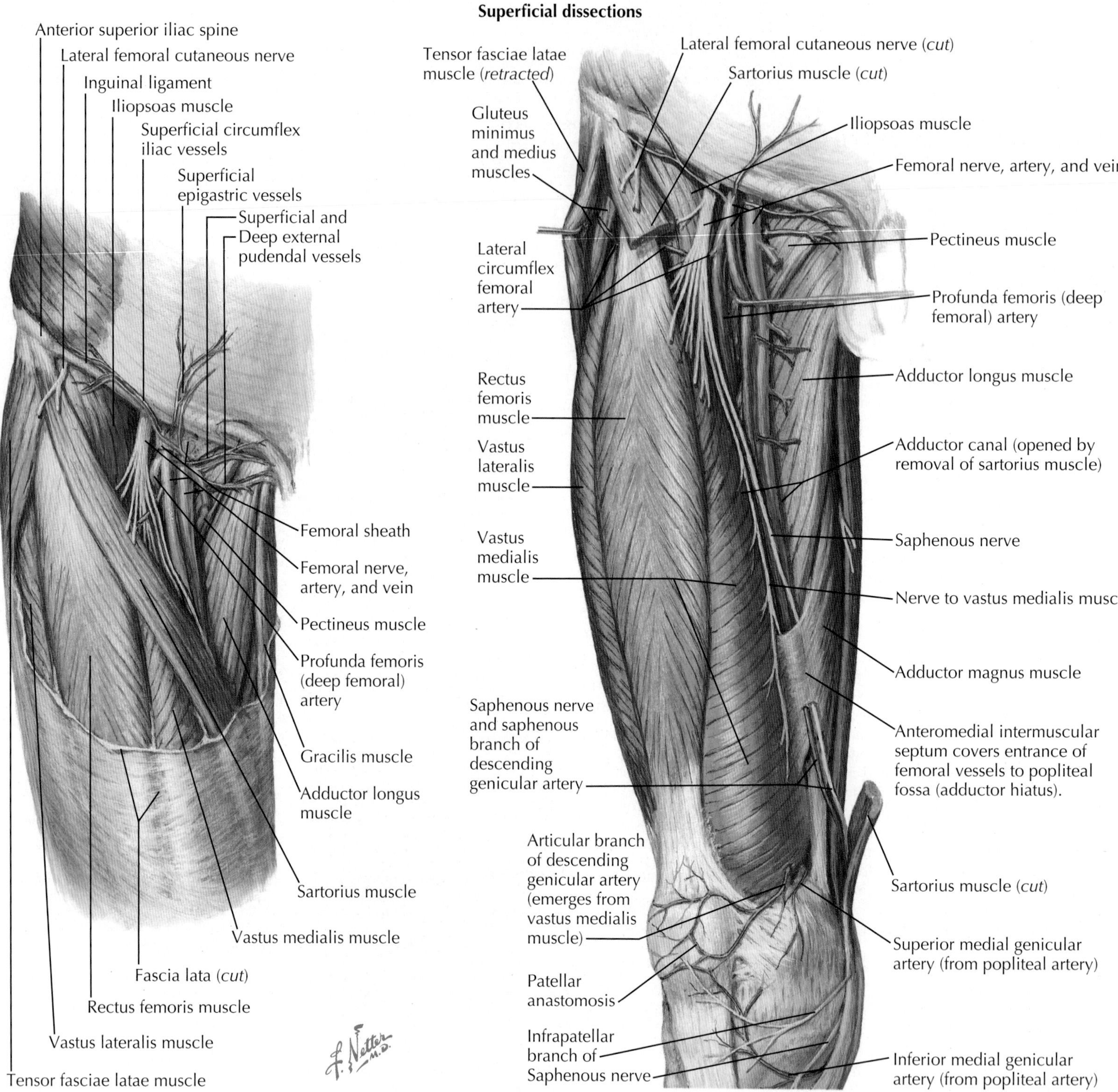

BLOOD SUPPLY OF THIGH

ARTERIES

The femoral, obturator, superior gluteal, and inferior gluteal arteries supply the thigh. The former two distribute principally anteriorly; the latter two distribute in the hip region. The femoral artery is the continuation of the external iliac artery. It distributes largely in the femoral triangle and descends through the mid regions of the thigh in the adductor canal.

The *femoral triangle* is a subfascial space in the upper third of the thigh. It is bound by the inguinal ligament above and by the sartorius muscle laterally and the adductor longus muscle medially. The apex of the triangle lies downward; it is formed by the crossing of the sartorius muscle over the adductor longus. The floor of the triangle is also muscular. The borders of the iliopsoas and pectineus muscles bound a deep groove in the floor, and, here, the medial circumflex femoral artery passes to the back of the thigh. The femoral artery enters the adductor canal at the apex of the triangle. The femoral vein lies on the pectineus muscle, medial to the femoral artery; here, it receives the greater saphenous vein. The femoral nerve descends under the inguinal ligament in the groove between the iliacus and psoas major muscles. In the triangle, it divides into most of its muscular and cutaneous branches; only the saphenous nerve and one of the nerves to the vastus medialis muscle continue into the adductor canal.

The femoral artery and vein are covered by the *femoral sheath* for about 3 cm beyond the inguinal ligament. Here, the extraperitoneal connective tissue of the abdomen extends between the vessels and

Blood Supply of Thigh (Continued)

forms three compartments—a lateral one for the artery, a middle one for the vein, and a medial one for one or more deep inguinal lymph nodes and fat. The medial compartment is known as the *femoral canal,* and its abdominal opening is the *femoral ring.*

The *adductor canal* conducts the femoral vessels and one or two nerves through the middle third of the thigh. It begins about 15 cm below the inguinal ligament at the crossing of the sartorius muscle over the adductor longus muscle and ends at the upper limit of the adductor hiatus, a separation in the tendinous insertion of the adductor magnus muscle that allows the femoral vessels to reach the back of the knee. The canal occupies the middle third of the thigh, and its termination is marked medially by a strong fascial band from the vastus medialis to the adductor magnus muscles—the vastoadductor membrane. As the femoral vessels pass behind the femur to become the popliteal artery and vein, this membrane is perforated by the saphenous nerve and the descending genicular artery.

Branches of the femoral artery are the superficial epigastric, superficial circumflex iliac, superficial external pudendal, deep external pudendal, deep femoral, and descending genicular arteries. The first four branches are primarily related to the lower abdominal wall and the perineum.

The *deep femoral artery,* the largest branch, arises from the lateral side of the femoral artery about 5 cm below the inguinal ligament. It sinks deeply into the thigh as it descends, lying behind the femoral artery and vein on the medial side of the femur. It crosses the tendon of the adductor brevis muscle and, at its lower border, passes deep to the tendon of the adductor longus muscle. In the lower third of the thigh, the deep femoral artery ends as the fourth perforating artery. In the femoral triangle, this artery gives rise to the medial and lateral circumflex femoral arteries and muscular branches; in the adductor canal, it provides three perforating branches.

The *medial circumflex femoral artery* springs from the medial and posterior aspect of the deep femoral artery. Its course is deep into the femoral triangle, between the pectineus and iliopsoas muscles and under the neck of the femur to the back of the thigh. Deep to the adductor brevis muscle, an acetabular branch enters the hip joint beneath the transverse ligament of the acetabulum. Several muscular branches supply the adductor brevis and adductor magnus muscles, one distributing with the obturator nerve. Anterior to the quadratus femoris muscle, the artery divides into an ascending branch to the trochanteric fossa of the femur and a descending branch to the hamstring muscles beyond the ischial tuberosity.

The *lateral circumflex femoral artery* arises from the lateral side of the deep femoral artery, passes lateralward deep to the sartorius and the rectus femoris muscles, and divides into anterior, transverse, and descending branches. The ascending branch passes upward beneath the tensor fasciae latae muscle and anastomoses with terminals of the superior gluteal artery. The small transverse branch enters the vastus lateralis muscle, winds around the femur below its greater trochanter, and anastomoses on the back of the thigh with the medial circumflex femoral, inferior gluteal, and first perforating arteries (cruciate anastomosis). An articular artery for the hip joint may arise from either branch. The descending branch passes on the vastus lateralis muscle, accompanied by a branch of the femoral nerve to this muscle, and anastomoses with the descending genicular branch of the femoral artery and the lateral superior genicular branch of the popliteal artery.

The *perforating arteries* are usually three in number and arise from the posterior surface of the deep femoral artery. They pass directly against the linea aspera of the femur and pierce the tendons of the adductor muscles to reach the muscles of the posterior compartment of the thigh. The first perforating artery passes immediately below the pectineus and through the middle of the tendon of the adductor brevis muscle; the second, after giving off a nutrient artery to the femur, through its lower 3 or 4 cm; and the third, just below the lowest part of the adductor brevis. The deep femoral artery ends as the fourth perforating artery, which pierces the adductor magnus muscle and largely ends in the short head of the biceps femoris muscle. These vessels anastomose with all the vessels of the back of the thigh.

Arteries and Nerves of Thigh: Deep Dissection (Anterior View)

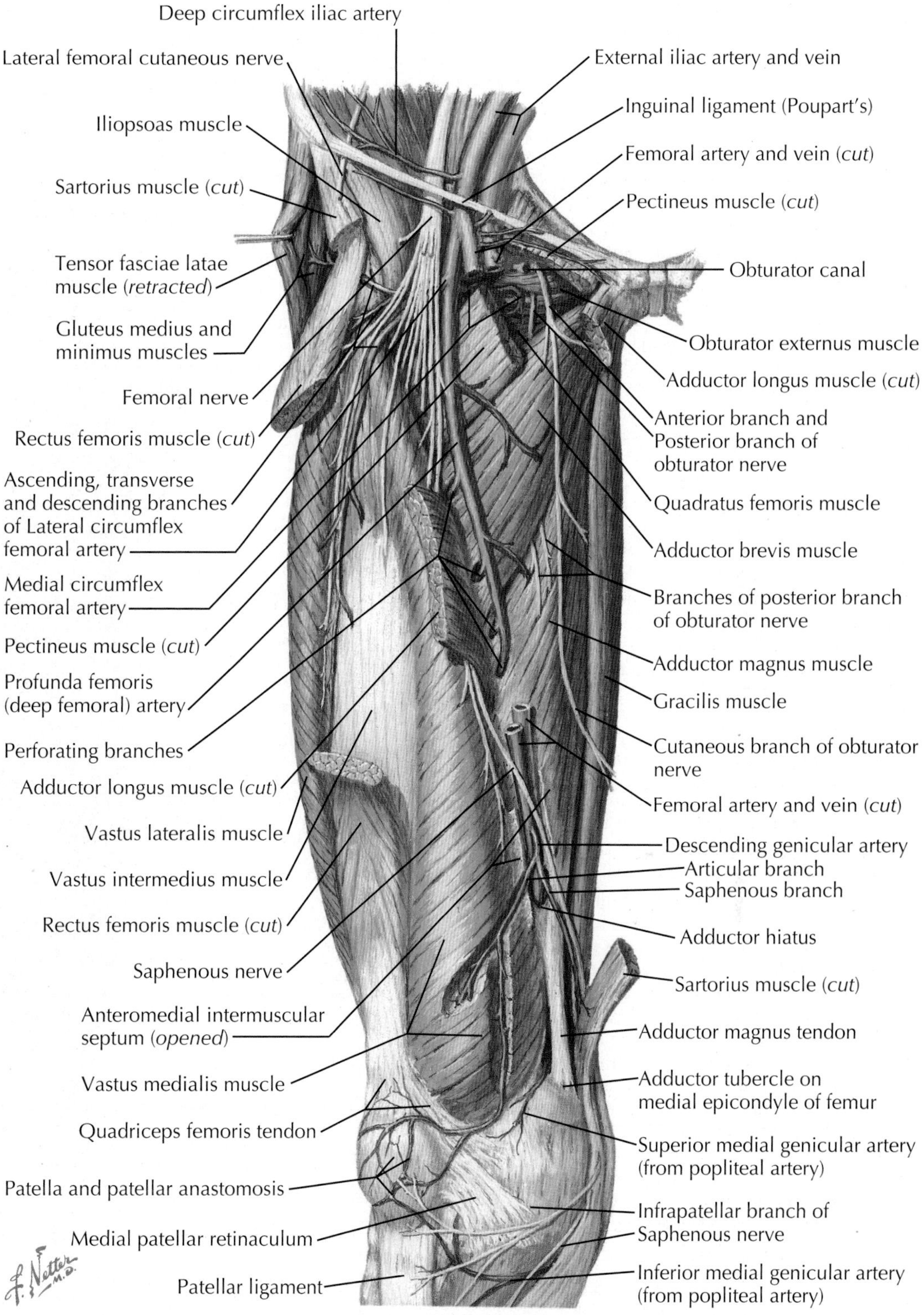

Arteries and Nerves of Thigh: Deep Dissection (Posterior View)

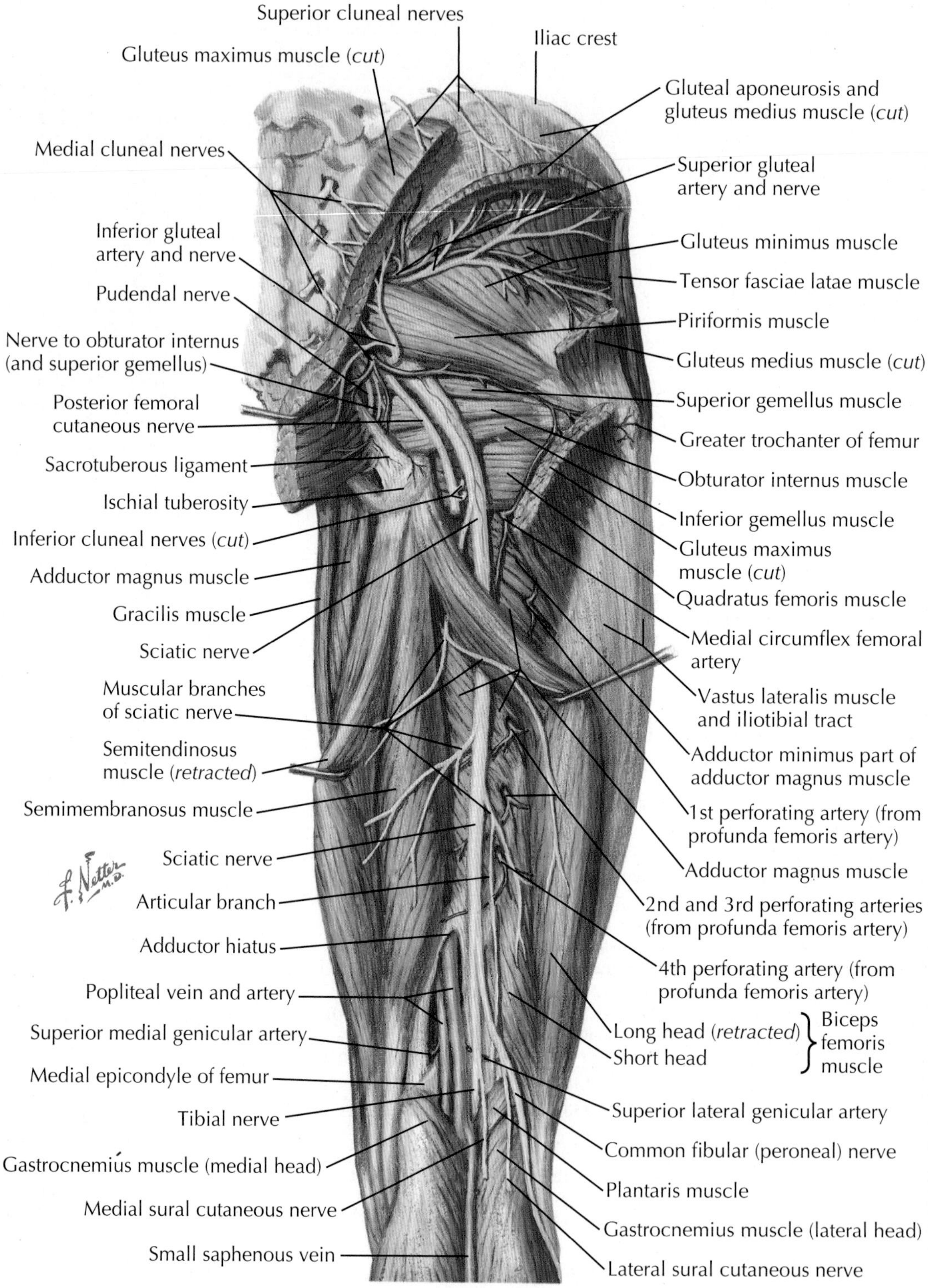

Blood Supply of Thigh (Continued)

The *descending genicular artery* arises from the femoral artery just before the latter passes through the adductor hiatus and immediately divides into saphenous and articular branches. The *saphenous branch* pierces the vastoadductor membrane and descends between the tendons of the gracilis and sartorius muscles in company with the saphenous nerve, supplying the skin and superficial tissues in the upper medial part of the leg. The *articular branch* descends in the substance of the vastus medialis muscle to the medial side of the knee. It supplies the vastus medialis muscle, and a branch passes lateralward over the patellar surface to anastomose with all other arteries at the knee joint.

The *obturator artery* is a branch of the internal iliac artery. It leaves the pelvis via the obturator canal and immediately divides into anterior and posterior branches. These supply the obturator externus and obturator internus muscles and give branches to the adductor brevis and adductor magnus muscles. The posterior branch gives off an *acetabular artery,* which enters the hip joint through the acetabular notch and provides the small artery of the capitis femoris ligament.

The *superior* and *inferior gluteal arteries* are branches of the internal iliac artery. Although arising within the pelvis, they exit immediately into the gluteal region of the thigh. The *superior gluteal artery* emerges above the piriformis muscle and there divides into a superficial branch to the gluteus maximus muscle and a deep branch to the intermuscular plane between the gluteus medius and gluteus minimus muscles. An upper radicle of this branch supplies the gluteus medius, gluteus minimus, and tensor fasciae latae muscles and reaches as far as the anterior superior iliac spine. A lower radicle is directed toward the greater trochanter of the femur and supplies the gluteal muscles and the hip joint.

The *inferior gluteal artery* leaves the pelvis below the piriformis muscle and provides large muscular branches to the gluteus maximus muscle and muscles arising from the ischial tuberosity. Small branches pass medially as far as the skin over the coccyx. An anastomotic branch descends across the short lateral rotator muscles of the hip and contributes to the cruciate anastomosis of the back of the thigh. Cutaneous branches accompany radicles of the posterior femoral cutaneous nerve, and an accompanying artery of the sciatic nerve descends on the surface of that nerve. The inferior gluteal artery is long and slender and may reach as far as the lower part of the thigh. It is developmentally the major artery of the lower limb.

VEINS

In general, the veins of the hip and thigh are venae comitantes of the arteries. The superior and inferior gluteal veins and the obturator vein enter the pelvis with their corresponding arteries; they are tributary to the internal iliac vein. The femoral vein is posterior to the femoral artery at the adductor hiatus but medial to it as it passes under the inguinal ligament to become the external iliac vein. The femoral vein contains two or three bicuspid valves; one is just inferior to the junction with the deep femoral vein, and one is at the level of the inguinal ligament. The superficial circumflex iliac, superficial epigastric, and superficial external pudendal veins enter the greater saphenous and not the femoral vein, and the deep external pudendal vein is usually the highest tributary of the femoral vein. The venae comitantes of the descending genicular artery may enter the lower end of the femoral vein or may end in this vessel at the femoral triangle.

The deep femoral vein enters the femoral vein at a much less regular level than that characterizing the origin of the deep femoral artery (about 8 cm below the inguinal ligament). The perforating veins on the back of the thigh help form a long anastomotic channel, which is formed by interconnections and connections with tributaries of the popliteal vein below and the inferior gluteal vein above. In three-fourths of cases, the medial and lateral circumflex femoral veins empty into the femoral vein rather than into the deep femoral vein and their widespread radicles anastomose with many other veins of the thigh.

Bones and Ligaments at Hip

FEMUR

The femur is the longest and strongest bone in the body, comprising a shaft and two irregular extremities that articulate at the hip and knee joints.

The superior extremity of the bone has a nearly spheric *head* mounted on an angulated neck, and prominent trochanters provide for muscular attachments. The head is smooth, with an articular surface that is largest above and anteriorly; this is interrupted medially by a depression, the fovea capitis femoris, into which attaches the capitis femoris ligament.

The *neck* is about 5 cm long and forms an angle with the shaft, which varies in the normal person from 115 to 140 degrees. It is compressed anteroposteriorly and contains a large number of prominent pits for the entrance of blood vessels.

The *greater trochanter* is the bony prominence of the hip. It is palpable 12 to 14 cm below the iliac crest, is large and square, and marks the upper end of the shaft of the femur. Its large quadrilateral surface is divided by an oblique ridge running from the posterosuperior to its anteroinferior angles. In front and above the ridge there is a triangular surface (which may be smooth) for a bursa. Below and behind the ridge the bone is also smooth. Its posterior rounded border bounds the trochanteric fossa and continues downward as the intertrochanteric crest. The trochanteric fossa is a deep pit on the internal aspect of the trochanter.

The *lesser trochanter* is a blunt, conical projection at the junction of the inferior border of the neck with the shaft of the femur. The trochanters are joined behind by the intertrochanteric crest. On the anterior surface of the femur, the junction of the neck and shaft is also ridged. This is the intertrochanteric line, which provides attachment for the capsule of the hip joint across the front of the bone and continues as a spiral line, winding backward to blend into the medial lip of the linea aspera.

The *shaft* of the bone is fairly uniform in caliber but broadens slightly at its extremities. It is bowed forward and its surface is smooth, except for the thickened ridge along its posterior surface, the linea aspera. This is especially prominent in the middle third of the bone, where lateral and medial lips are developed. Superiorly, the lateral lip blends with the prominent gluteal tuberosity; an intermediate lip extends as the pectineal line to the posterior border of the lesser trochanter, and the medial lip continues as the spiral line. The nutrient foramen of the femur, directed upward, is located on the linea aspera.

The *inferior extremity* of the femur is broadened about threefold for the knee joint. Its surfaces, except at the sides, are articular—two oblong *condyles* for articulation with the tibia are separated by an intercondylar fossa and united anteriorly by the patellar surface. The wheel-like condyles are also curved from side to side. The intercondylar fossa is especially deep posteriorly and is separated by a ridge from the popliteal surface of the femur above. The medial condyle is longer than the lateral condyle. The condyles rest on the horizontal condyles of the tibia, and the shaft of the femur inclines downward and inward.

OSTEOLOGY OF THE FEMUR

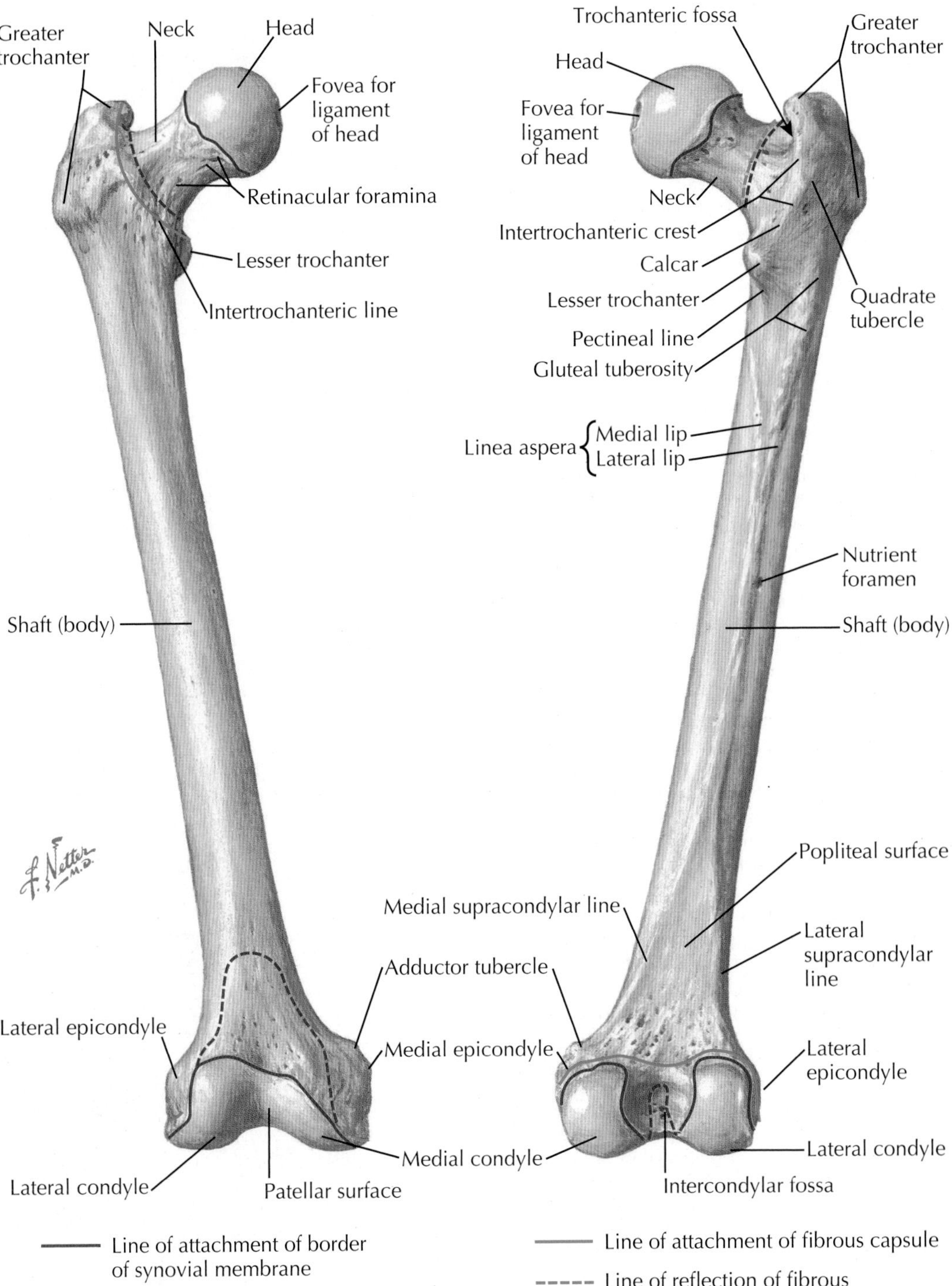

The *epicondyles* bulge above and within the curvatures of the condyles. The medial epicondyle is the more prominent, giving attachment to the tibial collateral ligament of the knee joint. It bears on its upper surface a pointed projection, the adductor tubercle. The lateral epicondyle gives rise to the fibular collateral ligament. A groove below the epicondyle borders the articular margin.

The femur is *ossified* from five centers: one for the shaft, one each for the head and inferior extremity, and one for each trochanter. The shaft is ossified at birth; ossification extends into the neck after birth. The center for the inferior extremity of the bone appears during the ninth month of fetal life; that for the head appears during the first year. The center in the greater trochanter appears during ages 3 to 5; that for the lesser trochanter appears at age 9 or 10 years. The epiphyses for the head and trochanters fuse with the shaft at ages 14 to 17 years; those at the knee fuse with the shaft at about age 17.5 years in boys but by age 15 years in girls.

BONES AND LIGAMENTS AT HIP (Continued)

HIP JOINT

Movements of the hip joint are flexion-extension, abduction-adduction, and medial and lateral rotation. Circumduction is also allowed.

The hip joint, a synovial ball-and-socket joint, consists of the articulation of the globular head of the femur in the cup-like acetabulum of the coxal bone. Compared with the shoulder joint, it has greater stability and some decrease in freedom of movement. The head forms about two-thirds of a sphere and is covered by articular cartilage, thickest above and thinning to an irregular line of termination at the junction of the head and neck. The acetabulum of the coxal bone exhibits a horseshoe-shaped articular surface arching around the acetabular fossa. The articular fossa lodges a mass of fat covered by synovial membrane; the transverse ligament of the acetabulum closes the fossa below. An acetabular labrum attaches to the bony rim and to the ligament. Its thin, free edge cups around the head of the femur and holds it firmly.

The *articular capsule* of the joint is strong. It is attached to the bony rim of the acetabulum above and to the transverse ligament of the acetabulum inferiorly. On the femur, it is attached anteriorly to the intertrochanteric line and to the junction of the neck of the femur and its trochanters. Behind, the capsule has an arched free border, covering only two-thirds of the neck of the femur distally. Most of the fibers of the capsule are longitudinal, running from the coxal bone to the femur, but some deeper fibers run circularly. These zona orbicularis fibers are most marked in the posterior part of the capsule; they help hold the head of the femur in the acetabulum.

Three ligaments, as thickenings of the capsule, add strength. The very strong *iliofemoral ligament* lies on the anterior surface of the capsule, in the form of an inverted Y. Its stem is attached to the lower part of the anterior inferior iliac spine, with the diverging bands attaching below to the whole length of the intertrochanteric line. The iliofemoral ligament becomes taut in full extension of the femur and thus helps to maintain erect posture, because in this position the body's weight tends to roll the pelvis backward on the femoral heads. The *pubofemoral ligament* is applied to the medial and inferior part of the capsule. Arising from the pubic part of the acetabulum and the obturator crest of the superior ramus of the pubis, this ligament reaches the underside of the neck of the femur and the iliofemoral ligament. The ligament becomes taut in extension and also limits abduction. The articular capsule is thinnest between the iliofemoral and pubofemoral ligaments but is crossed here by the robust iliopsoas tendon. The *iliopectineal bursa* lies between this tendon and the capsule. The *ischiofemoral ligament* forms the posterior margin of the capsule. It arises from the ischial portion of the acetabulum and spirals lateralward and upward, ending in the superior part of the femoral neck. The *capitis femoris ligament,* about 3.5 cm long, is intracapsular, arising from the two margins of the acetabular notch and the lower border of the transverse acetabular ligament and ending in the fossa of the head of the femur. It becomes taut in adduction of the femur.

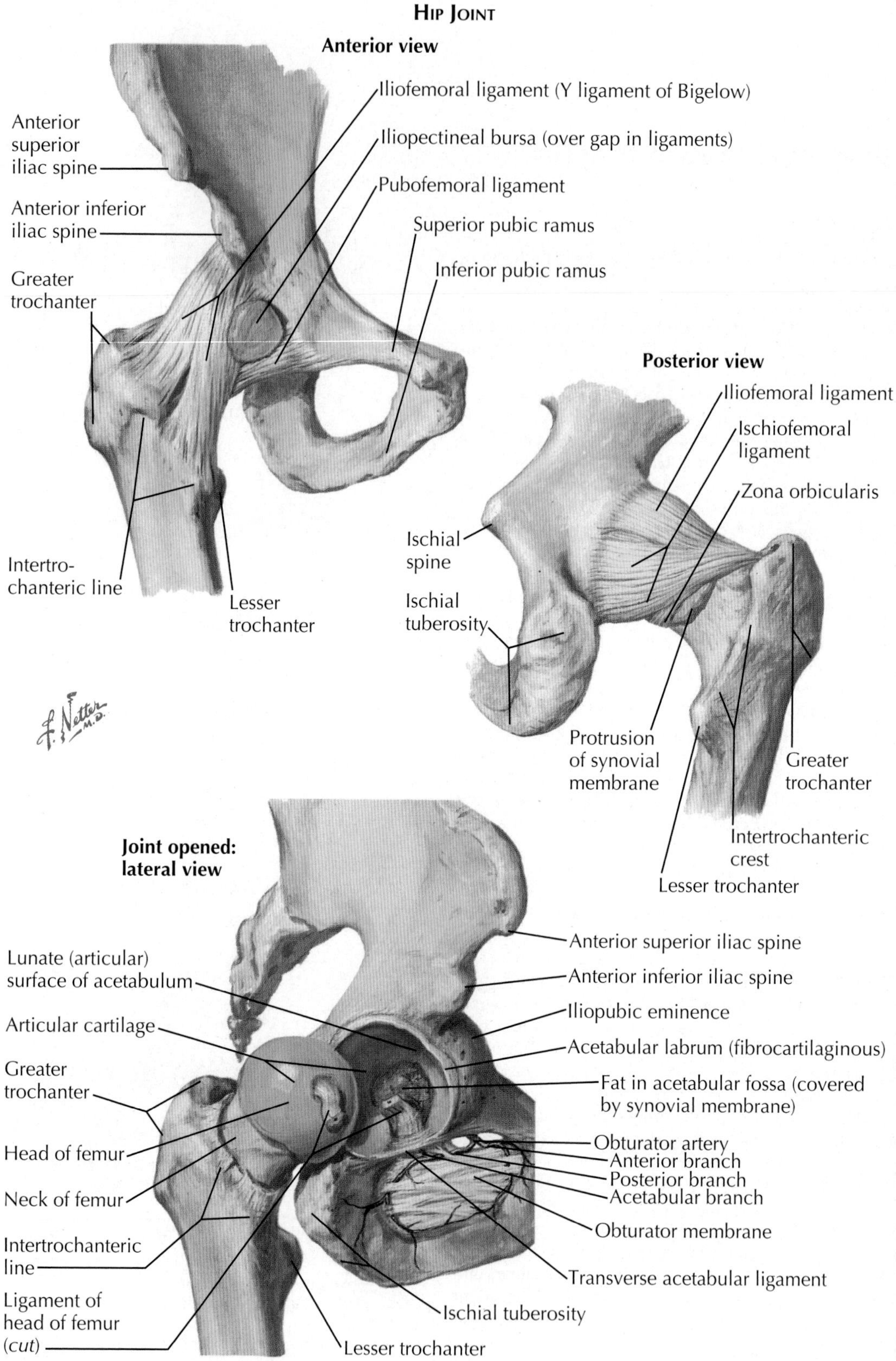

The *synovial membrane* of the hip joint lines the articular capsule, covers the acetabular labrum, and is extended, sleeve-like, over the ligament of the head of the femur. The membrane covers the fat of the acetabular notch and is reflected back along the femoral neck at the femoral attachment of the capsule. Blood vessels to the head and neck of the femur course under these synovial reflections.

The *arteries* of the hip joint are branches of the medial and lateral circumflex femoral arteries, the deep branch of the superior gluteal artery, and the inferior gluteal artery. The posterior branch of the obturator artery provides a significant portion of the blood supply of the femoral head. *Nerve supply* to the hip joint is derived from the nerves supplying the quadratus femoris and rectus femoris muscles, the anterior division of the obturator nerve (rarely also from the accessory obturator nerve), and the superior gluteal nerve.

Measurement of hip flexion/extension

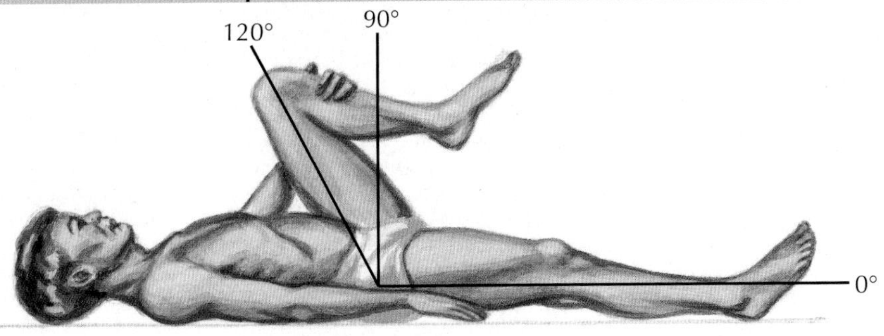

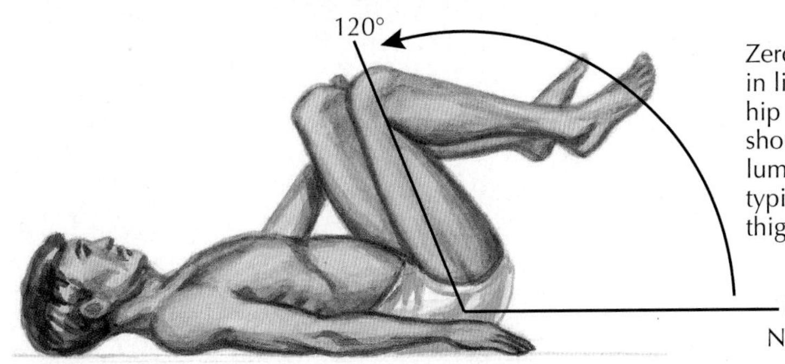

Zero starting position is the thigh in line with the trunk. In measuring hip extension, the contralateral limb should be held in flexion to eliminate lumbar spine motion. Hip flexion is typically measured by bringing both thighs into flexion.

Thomas test

Positive Thomas test indicates a hip flexion contracture: the affected hip cannot be extended to the neutral position.

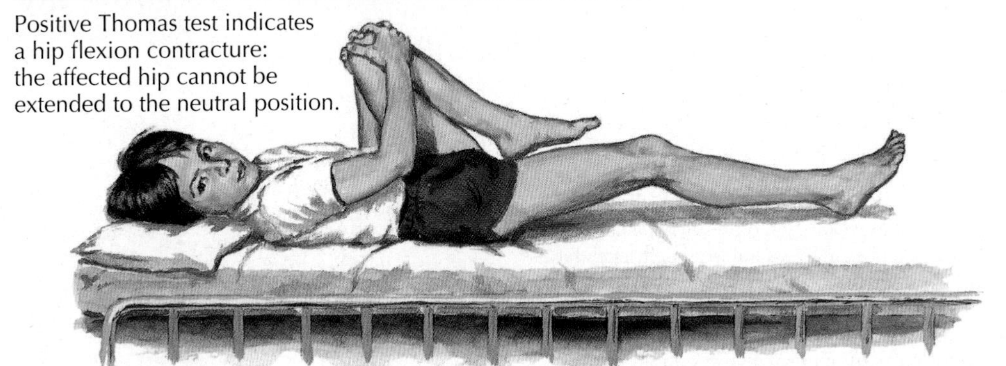

Trendelenburg test

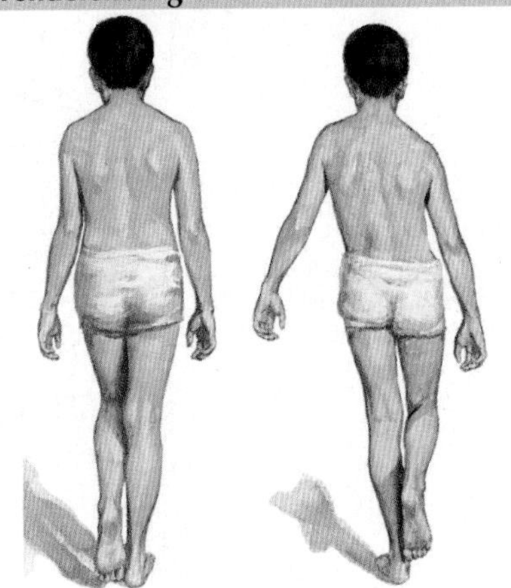

Left: patient demonstrates negative Trendelenburg test of normal right hip. *Right:* positive test of involved left hip. When weight is on affected side, normal hip drops, indicating weakness of left gluteus medius muscle. Trunk shifts left as patient attempts to decrease biochemical stresses across involved hip and thereby maintain balance.

F. Netter M.D.
JOHN A.CRAIG—AD

Physical Examination

Physical examination of the hip is initiated with observation of the patient. Specific note is made of body habitus. Gait is evaluated directly, looking for a Trendelenburg or antalgic gait that favors the affected side. Both gait patterns are associated with intraarticular and extraarticular hip pathologic processes.

The patient is then placed supine on an examination table, and landmarks are palpated. These landmarks include the anterior superior iliac spine, iliac crest, pubic symphysis, pubic tubercles, and proximal adductor tendons. The abdomen may also be palpated in this position if there is concern about any abdominal disorder.

Range of motion of the hips is then evaluated. This may be also examined combined with the upright and prone position based on the preference of the examiner. First checked is hip flexion, followed by internal and external rotation with the hip flexed to 90 degrees. In full extension, the hip is taken into adduction as well as abduction. Straight-leg hip flexion can also be evaluated for hamstring tightness or radicular low back pain. Deficits or painful ranges are noted compared with the contralateral/unaffected side. Specific tests for the hip joint in this position include the anterior impingement test (flexion/adduction/internal rotation), which is commonly painful in the face of labral tears or osteoarthritis. The hip may also to be placed in the figure-4 position, looking for pain or a loss of motion that may also indicate intraarticular findings. Straight-leg raising is performed to evaluate hip flexion strength in the supine position. Resisted adduction is also tested in the supine position to evaluate strength and integrity of the adductors.

The patient is then placed in the lateral decubitus position, and both the affected and nonpainful side are evaluated. Palpation is begun over the greater trochanter (trochanteric bursa posterior/superiorly), the gluteus medius/minimus tendons just proximal to the tip of the trochanter, and the piriformis tendon at the proximal/posterior aspect of the trochanter just posterior to the abductor musculature. The iliotibial band is checked for tightness with the Ober test. Hip abduction strength is evaluated with the hip held in the abducted position against resistance.

A prone examination is then completed. Examination of the hamstrings is best completed in this position, as well as palpation of the ischial tuberosity and proximal hamstring insertion and muscle bellies. Hamstring strength is tested with resisted knee flexion at 90 and 45 degrees. The Thomas test is useful to look for hip flexion contracture while the patient is in this position.

Completion of the hip examination is then done in the upright position. Palpation of the posterior iliac crest and posterior superior iliac spine/sacroiliac joint is completed at this point. This position also allows for palpation of the midline and paraspinal lumbar spine. Hip flexion strength in this position isolates the iliopsoas unit.

The joint proximal (lumbar spine) and distal (knee) are also evaluated for completeness and to rule out referred pain. This may also be inferred from good history taking.

Radiographic Classification of Proximal Femoral Focal Deficiency

Type A
Femoral head and adequate acetabulum present. At maturity, ossification centers of femoral head, neck, and trochanter fuse and resulting unit is sharply abducted, causing greater trochanter to impinge on ilium. At junction of this unit with high-riding, short femoral shaft, pseudarthrosis is usually present.

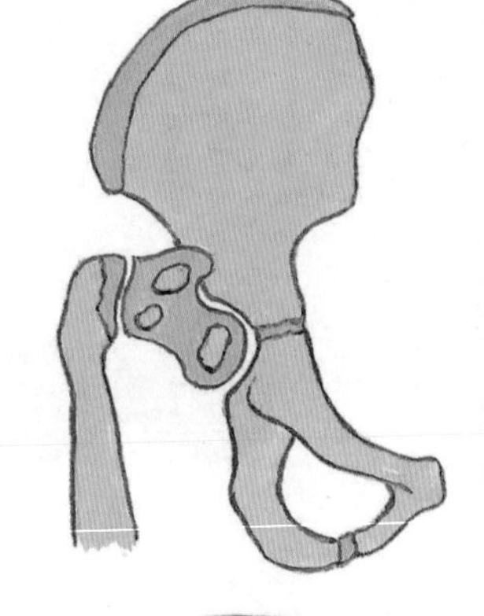

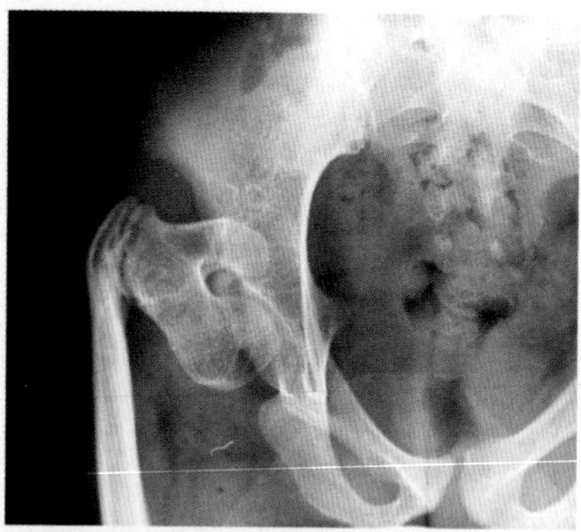

Type B
Femoral head and acetabulum present but trochanter never ossifies; no continuity between femoral head and high-riding shaft. Ossific tuft at proximal end of shaft probably represents vestigial trochanter.

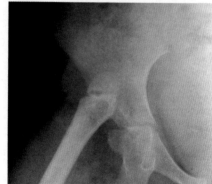

Type C
Femoral head absent or not ossified; acetabulum dysplastic. Femoral shaft is very short and displaced laterally and superiorly.

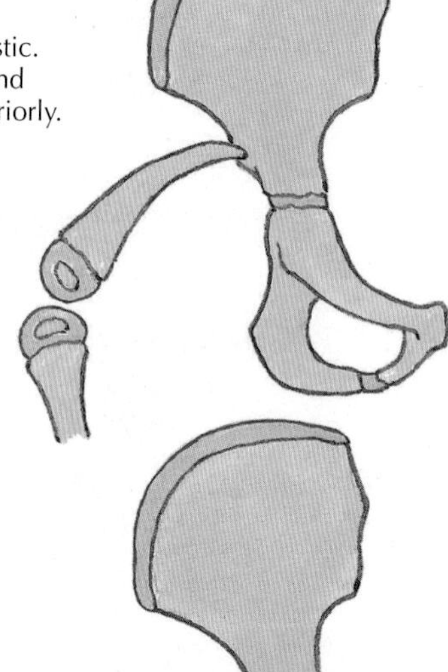

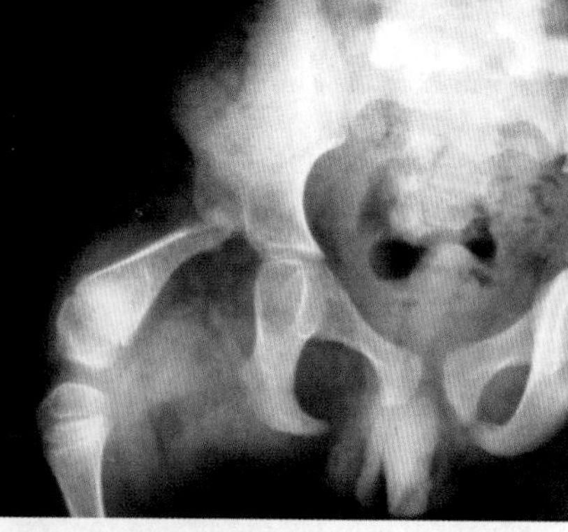

Type D
Acetabulum and femoral head absent. Femoral shortening severe. Proximal end of femoral shaft rides low; no ossific tuft. Often bilateral.

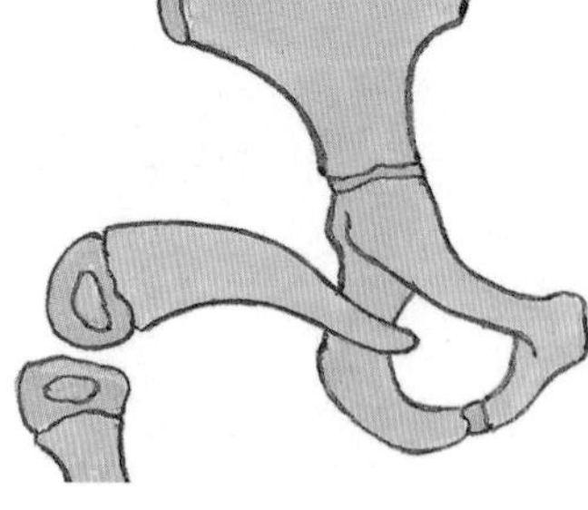

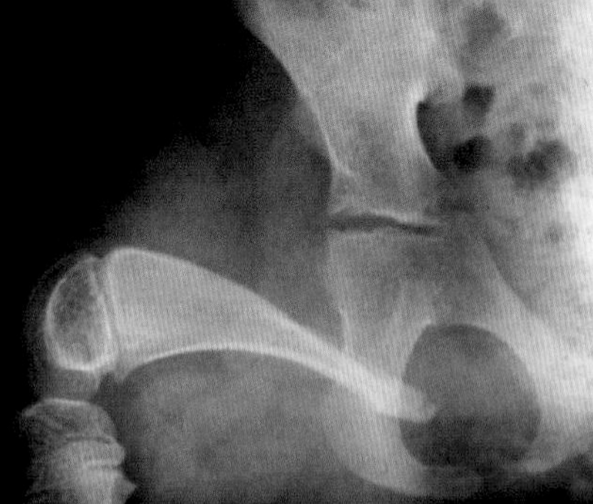

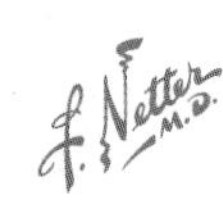

Proximal Femoral Focal Deficiency

Proximal femoral focal deficiency is a randomly occurring congenital abnormality of the proximal femur and hip joint. It is usually unilateral and, in 68% of patients, is accompanied by fibular hemimelia on the ipsilateral side. About 50% of affected patients have skeletal abnormalities of other limbs as well. Based on results of a large radiographic survey, proximal femoral focal deficiency has been classified into four types, according to the type and severity of the femoral and acetabular defects.

Clinical Manifestations. Regardless of the extent of the anatomic defect, the clinical manifestations of proximal femoral focal deficiency are quite consistent (see Plate 2.23). The affected limb is held in varying degrees of flexion, abduction, and external rotation at the hip. The femoral segment of the limb is much shorter than the normal femur. In the patient with concomitant fibular hemimelia, the sole of the foot on the affected side is usually level with the knee joint on the unaffected side. Soft tissue contracture about the hip and some flexion contracture in the knee are also evident.

These deformities result in a number of biomechanical problems: (1) leg length discrepancy, (2) malrotation, (3) inadequacy of the proximal musculature, and (4) instability of the hip joint.

In patients with unilateral involvement, the unequal leg lengths obviously hinder bipedal ambulation. In patients with bilateral involvement, symmetric leg length discrepancy results in a striking disproportionate dwarfism.

Radiographic Findings. The radiographic appearance of proximal femoral focal deficiency varies considerably according to the extent of the anatomic defects. The major diagnostic problem is differentiating proximal femoral focal deficiency types A and B from congenital short femur associated with coxa vara (see Plate 2.24). For both conditions, radiographs taken in infancy are difficult to interpret. If the diagnosis is uncertain, treatment should be postponed until the specific deformity is conclusively demonstrated on serial radiographs.

Treatment. In formulating a management plan for this complex deformity, it is important to establish early realistic goals for rehabilitation. The primary aim is to facilitate bipedal ambulation. Although correction of the flexion, abduction, and external rotation of the hip is desirable, it is not always possible. Both nonsurgical and surgical methods are used to help compensate for instability of the hip joint and inadequacy of the hip musculature.

In the past, crutches were the only aid for patients with unilateral involvement, and persons with disproportionate dwarfism simply ambulated on their own malformed lower limbs. Later, orthoses such as shoe lifts were devised to compensate for leg length discrepancy and allow some degree of unassisted ambulation. More recently, nonstandard prostheses have been designed that better equalize limb lengths and improve gait. In some patients, amputation facilitates the application and improves the comfort of these prostheses.

Three general treatment options are available for patients with unilateral involvement. The first is to fabricate a prosthesis that fits around the deformity. The

Proximal Femoral Focal Deficiency

design of the device is limited only by the ingenuity of the prosthetist. The second option is to consider the deformity as a homologue of an above-knee amputation and to devise the equivalent of an above-knee prosthesis that accommodates the deformity. The third option is to consider the deformity as the equivalent of a below-knee amputation and to design a suitable prosthesis.

Treatment of the deformity as an above-knee amputation is facilitated by removing the foot. The surgical procedure, which consists of ankle disarticulation and Syme-type closure with the heel flap, produces a suitable end-bearing stump.

If the deformity is treated as a below-knee amputation, surgical conversion is necessary. A 180-degree Van Nes rotational osteotomy of the tibia is performed so that the retained ankle joint functions as a knee joint and the remaining foot becomes the below-knee residual limb.

The patient with a bilateral condition—whose primary problem is disproportionate dwarfism—should be treated with bilateral extension prostheses that fit around the deformities. The prostheses, which are lengthened as needed to establish peer height, make the patient a precarious "stilt walker." Many patients learn to ambulate quite competently on these stilts with the assistance of a cane or crutches.

Conversion of bilateral deformities to above-knee or below-knee amputations is not recommended because patients with bilateral involvement can ambulate without assistance. Bilateral Syme amputations and rotational osteotomies may rob the patient of this ability.

When the deformity is treated as a below-knee or above-knee amputation, surgical stabilization of the hip improves gait characteristics. However, establishing a stable valgus relationship between the head of the femur and the diaphysis is possible only in types A and B, which have a competent acetabulum, a femoral head that eventually ossifies, and a congruent relationship between the femoral head and the acetabulum. Thus hip reconstruction is indicated in types A and B only. Other surgical modalities to promote a more stable hip (e.g., fusing the femur to the ilium and using the knee joint as a hip joint) have not improved patient rehabilitation.

Arthrodesis of the knee is useful in selected patients. If a unilateral deformity is converted to an end-bearing, above-knee stump, knee arthrodesis overcomes any residual knee flexion deformity. This technique is also beneficial in a unilateral deformity considered as a below-knee amputation. Thus if the rotational osteotomy is successful, the child may be fitted with a standard below-knee prosthesis that is secured with a thigh corset (and knee joints), without the need to use other types of auxiliary suspension such as a suction socket.

CONGENITAL SHORT FEMUR WITH COXA VARA

Congenital short femur is classified into three distinct types: (1) miniaturization of the femur without other deformity, (2) miniaturization of the femur with coxa vara, and (3) miniaturization with lateral bowing or angulation of the femur (see Plate 2.24).

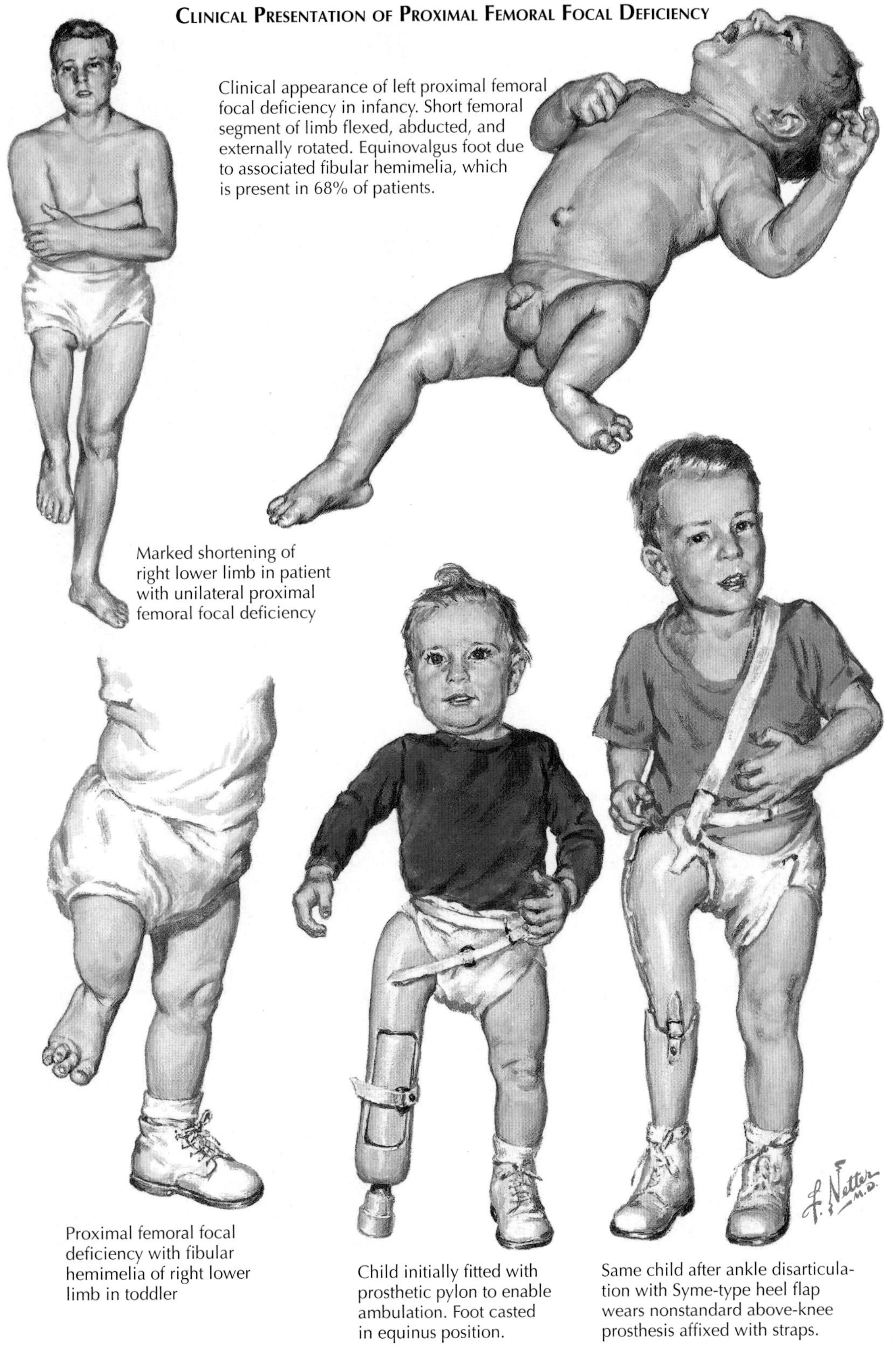

Clinical Presentation of Proximal Femoral Focal Deficiency

Clinical appearance of left proximal femoral focal deficiency in infancy. Short femoral segment of limb flexed, abducted, and externally rotated. Equinovalgus foot due to associated fibular hemimelia, which is present in 68% of patients.

Marked shortening of right lower limb in patient with unilateral proximal femoral focal deficiency

Proximal femoral focal deficiency with fibular hemimelia of right lower limb in toddler

Child initially fitted with prosthetic pylon to enable ambulation. Foot casted in equinus position.

Same child after ankle disarticulation with Syme-type heel flap wears nonstandard above-knee prosthesis affixed with straps.

F. Netter M.D.

Congenital Short Femur with Coxa Vara

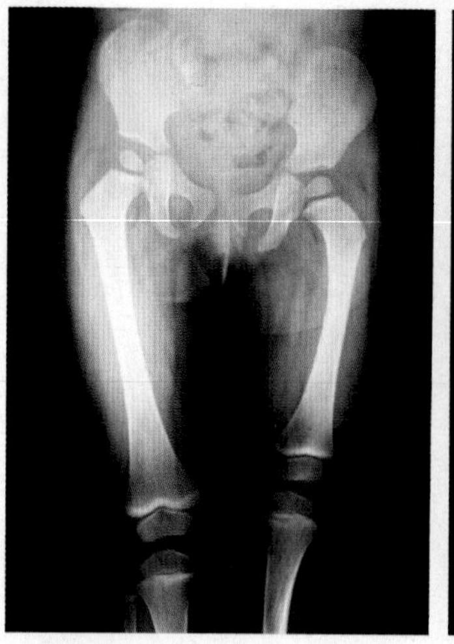
Miniaturization of femur with no deformity

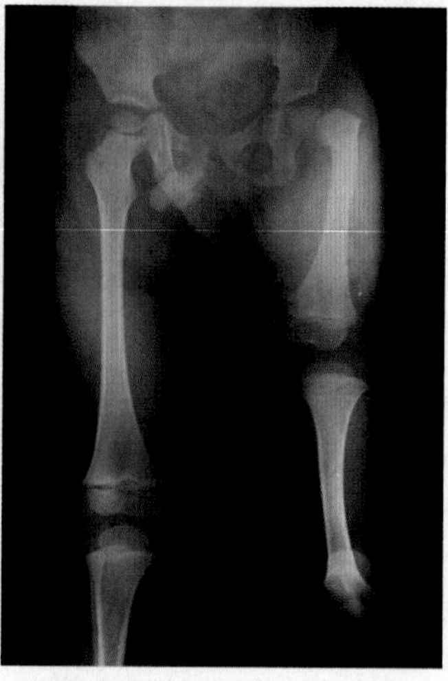
Miniaturization of femur with associated coxa vara

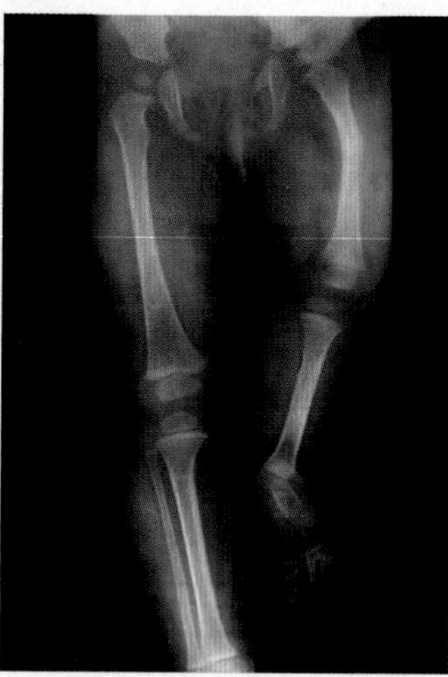
Miniaturization of femur with lateral bowing or angulation

Proximal Femoral Focal Deficiency

Coxa vara is an abnormality of the proximal femur characterized by a neck-diaphysis angle of less than 120 degrees. Causes are multiple. Although it is often congenital, it may also result from a metabolic aberration or trauma. Coxa vara is associated with several types of generalized skeletal abnormalities and often accompanies congenital short femur.

Clinical Manifestations. Leg length discrepancy is the major deformity in short femur with coxa vara. Unlike proximal femoral focal deficiency, there is no flexion, abduction, and external rotation deformity of the hip. However, fibular hemimelia with a moderately severe valgus deformity of the ankle may also be present on the affected side, exacerbating the leg length discrepancy.

Radiographic Findings. Radiographs of congenital short femur with associated coxa vara usually show the proximal end of the femoral diaphysis in bony continuity with the femoral head and neck, and the proximal end of the femur does not ride above the Hilgenreiner line. On the other hand, in proximal femoral focal deficiency types A and B, the proximal femur usually rides above the superior rim of the acetabulum; this finding is a useful factor in the differential diagnosis (see Plate 2.22).

Treatment. Management of a deformity of this magnitude requires a team of specialists, including a physician interested in such problems, an experienced prosthetist, and a skilled physical therapist, to collectively evaluate the problem and select the most appropriate treatment modalities. It is most important to describe to the patient and the family the overall management plan that will result in maximal function.

Coxa vara should be treated as soon as the diagnosis is certain. The primary goal is to establish a stable valgus relationship between the diaphysis and the head and neck of the femur. Subtrochanteric osteotomy is performed to produce a position of maximum valgus, not simply to restore the neck-diaphysis angle to greater than 120 degrees. (This procedure is not appropriate for proximal femoral focal deficiency.) Any incompetence of the acetabulum on the affected side should be treated with appropriate hip reconstruction techniques.

Treatment of the combined deformities of short femur and coxa vara varies. Because the major defect is leg length discrepancy primarily owing to the short femur and concomitant fibular hemimelia, it is usually difficult to equalize the levels of the knees. Shoe lifts to accommodate for the unequal limb lengths are successful in some patients. The Syme amputation, which produces an end-bearing below-knee stump, permits the use of a below-knee prosthesis; in many patients, this result is both more cosmetic and possibly more functional than a simple shoe lift with or without an orthotic device. Some children with stable hips and knees may be candidates for leg-lengthening procedures.

The use of shoe lifts and conversion to a below-knee amputation does not equalize the levels of the knees, however. This can be accomplished by an end-bearing above-knee amputation. In this procedure, a portion of the tibia is fused to the femur and the amputation is done at a level that matches the contralateral normal knee joint.

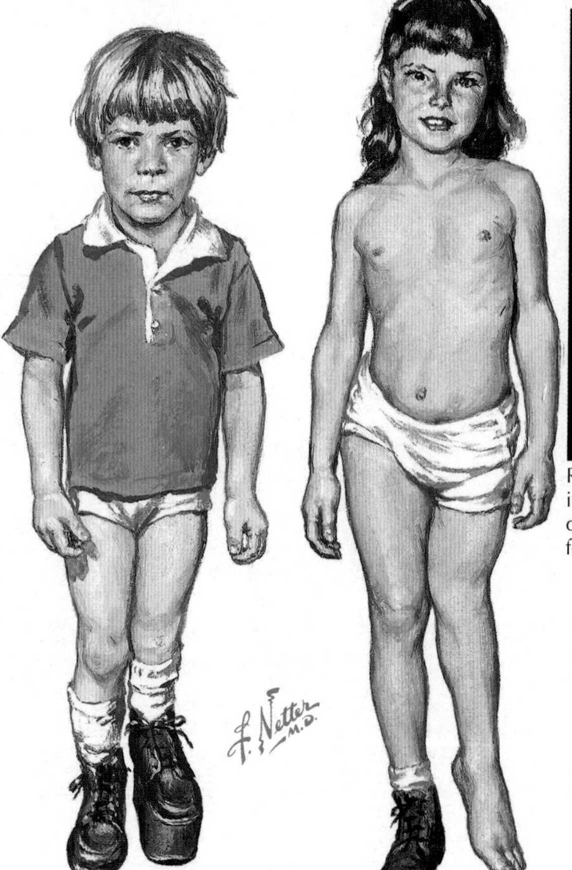

Boy wears built-up boot to compensate for moderate congenital short left femur.

Girl with congenital short left femur with associated coxa vara

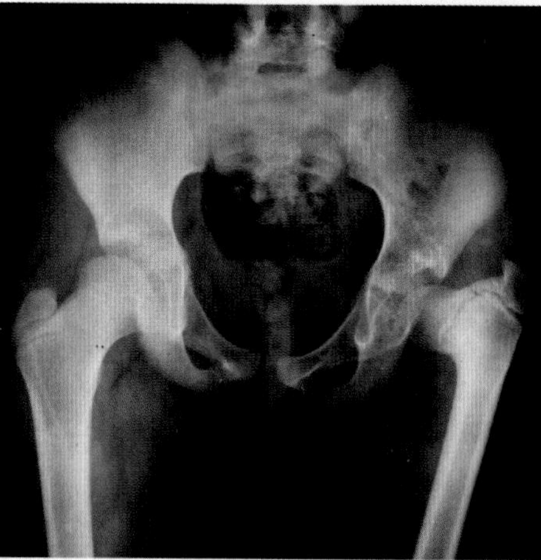
Radiograph shows congenital coxa vara. Defect in inferior part of femoral neck causes varus deformity to develop between head and neck of femur.

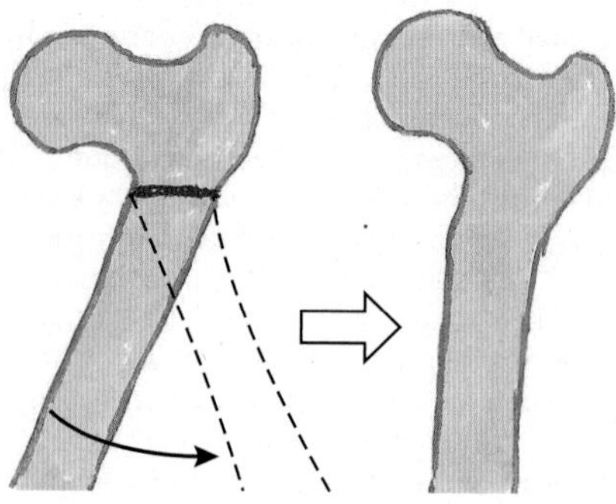
Principle of subtrochanteric abduction osteotomy for coxa vara

Recognition of Developmental Dislocation of the Hip

Ortolani (reduction) test. With baby relaxed and content on firm surface, hips and knees are fixed to 90 degrees. Hips are examined one at a time. Examiner grasps baby's thigh with middle finger over greater trochanter and lifts thigh to bring femoral head from its dislocated posterior position to opposite the acetabulum. Simultaneously, with thigh gently abducted, femoral head is reduced into acetabulum. In positive finding, examiner senses reduction by palpable, nearly audible "clunk."

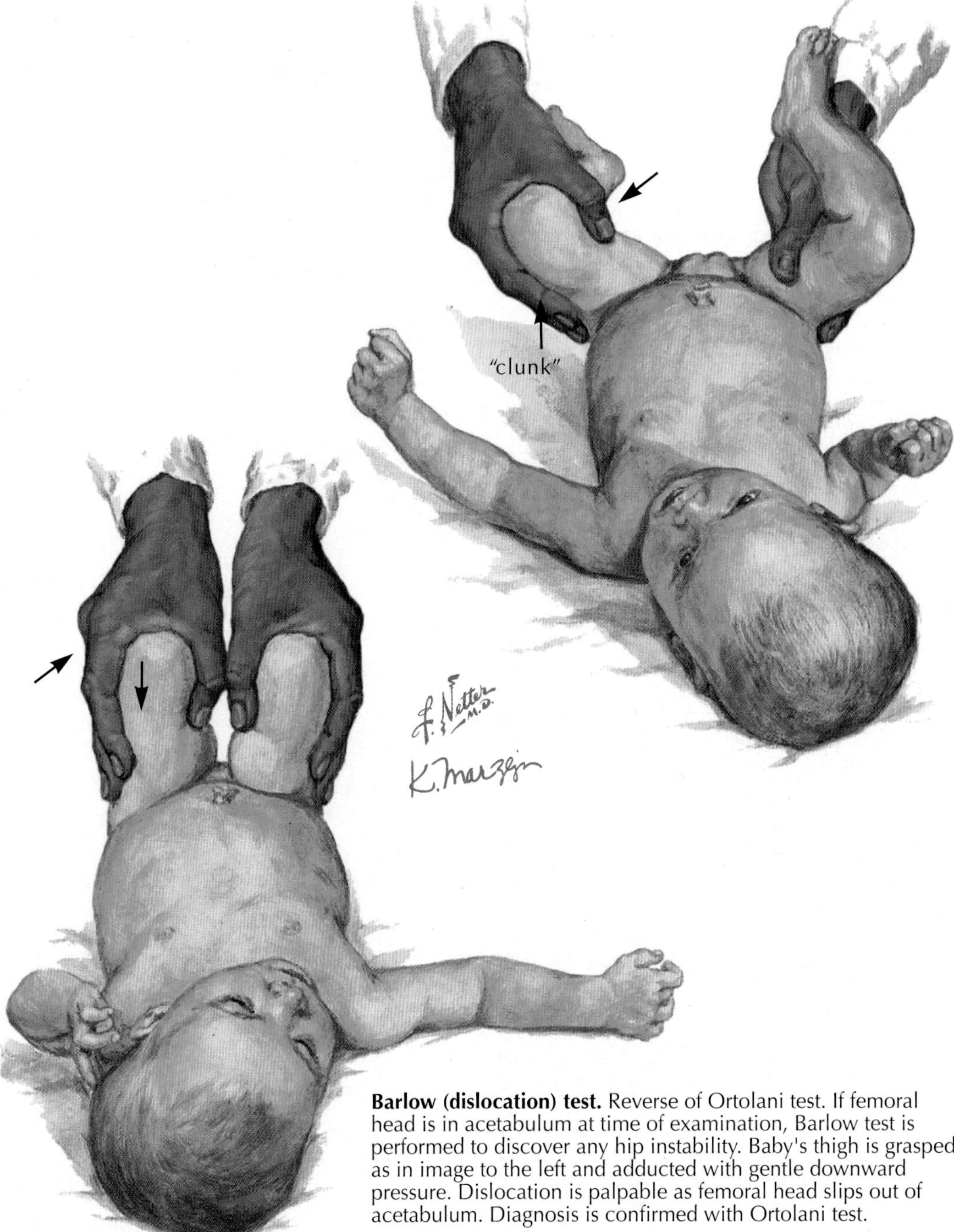

Barlow (dislocation) test. Reverse of Ortolani test. If femoral head is in acetabulum at time of examination, Barlow test is performed to discover any hip instability. Baby's thigh is grasped as in image to the left and adducted with gentle downward pressure. Dislocation is palpable as femoral head slips out of acetabulum. Diagnosis is confirmed with Ortolani test.

Developmental Dislocation of the Hip

Methods for the early detection of developmental dislocation of the hip (DDH) have been reported for nearly 100 years. The first screening program in the United States was described and initiated in the 1930s. After World War II, extensive screening programs in the United States, Sweden, and England resulted in the early identification and, ultimately, simple, effective, and safe treatment protocols.

In the United States approximately 10 in 1000 infants are born with DDH. As a result of screening programs, 96% of these children have normal hip function. The longer the dislocation goes untreated, the more difficult it is to obtain a satisfactory result. Routine screening for this entity should be an integral part of newborn well-child care.

ETIOLOGIC FACTORS

The etiology of DDH remains multifactorial. Mechanical and physiologic properties of both the mother and infant have been implicated, combining to produce instability and dislocation.

The age at onset of instability affects the severity of the condition. The typical developmental dislocation develops just before delivery in an otherwise normal infant. At birth, the clinical findings are often subtle and radiographs are usually normal. In contrast, if the dislocation occurs early in gestation, the clinical and radiographic findings are more severe, with advanced adaptive changes in the femoral head and pelvis. This is often termed teratologic dislocation and is typically found in patients with underlying conditions such as arthrogryposis, chromosomal abnormalities, and other severe congenital anomalies such as spina bifida and lumbosacral agenesis. Teratologic dislocations occur in less than 2% of patients with DDH.

MECHANICAL FACTORS

Mechanical factors most likely occur in the last trimester of pregnancy. All have the effect of restricting intrauterine space for the fetus, also termed packaging. Roughly 60% of infants with DDH are firstborns, suggesting that the tight unstretched uterus and abdominal wall may inhibit fetal movement. It is believed that the fetal pelvis becomes trapped within the maternal pelvis, preventing the normal flexion of the fetal hip and knee.

Breech presentation also plays a significant role in DDH. From 30% to 50% of affected children are delivered in breech presentation. When the knees are extended in the frank breech position, excessive hamstring stretch contributes further to hip laxity and instability. DDH is seen more frequently in children with congenital knee dislocation or recurvatum, as well as other packaging phenomena such as metatarsus adductus and congenital muscular torticollis.

The left hip is more commonly involved than the right in theory because the left hip is trapped against the maternal sacrum in the most frequent presenting position—left occiput anterior. The maternal sacrum forces the left hip into flexion and adduction, contributing to instability and potentially dislocation. In this position, the femoral head is covered more by the joint capsule than the acetabulum proper.

HORMONAL FACTORS

Maternal estrogens and other hormones that affect relaxation of the pelvis immediately before delivery also affect the fetal hip. Their presence may lead to

DEVELOPMENTAL DISLOCATION OF THE HIP (Continued)

temporary laxity in the hip joint in the fetus and newborn. Studies suggest that the female infant is more affected by these hormones, which may explain the higher incidence of DDH (6:1) in females.

Up to 20% of cases are deemed familial. This may be due to an inborn or possibly an inherited error of estrogen metabolism and may explain the higher rates of familial disease in Northern Italians, Scandinavians, and some Navajo tribes.

POSTNATAL ENVIRONMENTAL FACTORS

In the first months of life, normal hip position is that of abduction and flexion. In cultures in which swaddling of infants places the hips in positions of extension and adduction, there is a 10-fold increase in DDH rates. The practice of holding the child by the feet in the newborn period places the hips in extension and should be avoided.

PATHOGENIC FACTORS

The pathogenesis of a typical developmentally dislocated hip is probably quite simple. Near the time of delivery, the joint capsule is likely distended and elastic. After delivery, the femoral head is free to move about the distended lax capsule and can come in and out of the acetabulum freely. In newborns, the femoral head can often be easily reduced to the normal position. At this stage, the soft tissue structures and joint surfaces are essentially normal and therefore the capacity to develop a normal hip exists. Therefore, for a stable hip to develop, the femoral head needs to stay in contact with the acetabulum as the joint capsule loses its laxity and returns to a normal configuration. However, if the dislocation is allowed to persist, the capsule, joint, and other soft tissues go through a series of adaptive changes. This makes the dislocation more difficult to reduce, and the chance of obtaining a satisfactory long-term result becomes increasingly difficult to achieve.

It has been demonstrated that the stimulus for development of a normal acetabulum is the presence of a normal femoral head within the acetabulum. Conversely, a normal femoral head will develop if it is contained within a normal acetabulum. Because the infant grows so rapidly in the first year of life (tripling in size in the first 12 months), there is tremendous remodeling potential in this period to convert pathologic changes to normal anatomy.

CLINICAL FINDINGS IN DEVELOPMENTAL DISLOCATION OF THE HIP
(If untreated, signs become more obvious with growth and weight bearing.)

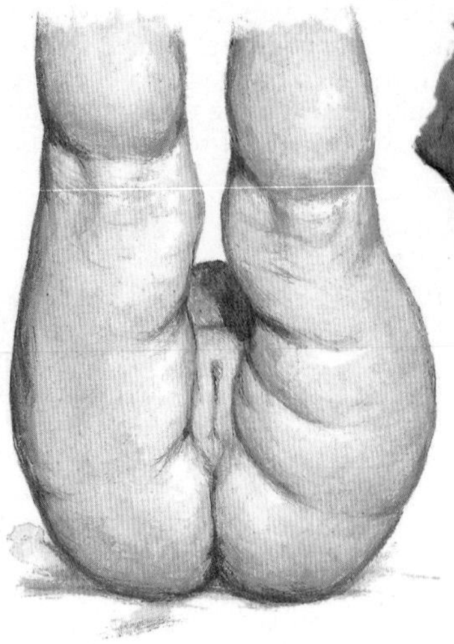

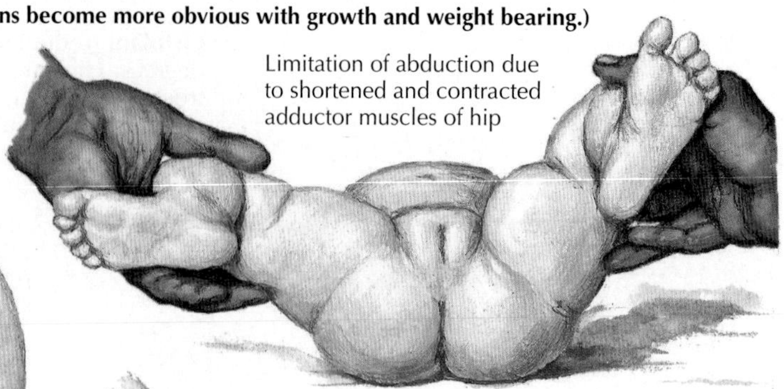

Limitation of abduction due to shortened and contracted adductor muscles of hip

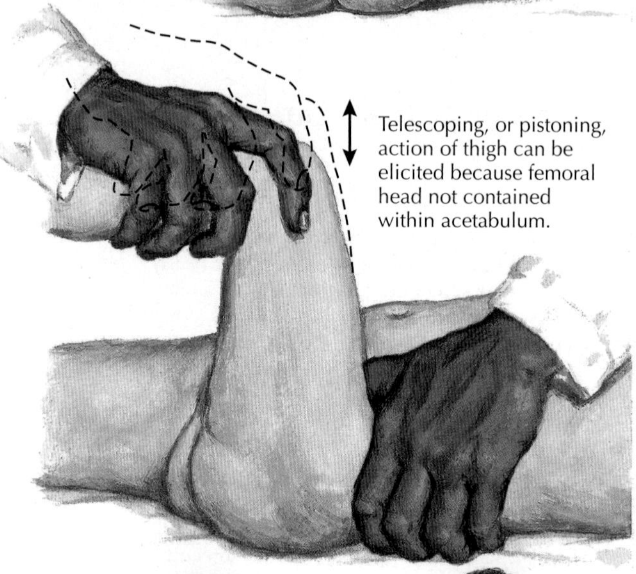

Shortening of thigh with bunching up of soft tissues and accentuation of skin folds

Telescoping, or pistoning, action of thigh can be elicited because femoral head not contained within acetabulum.

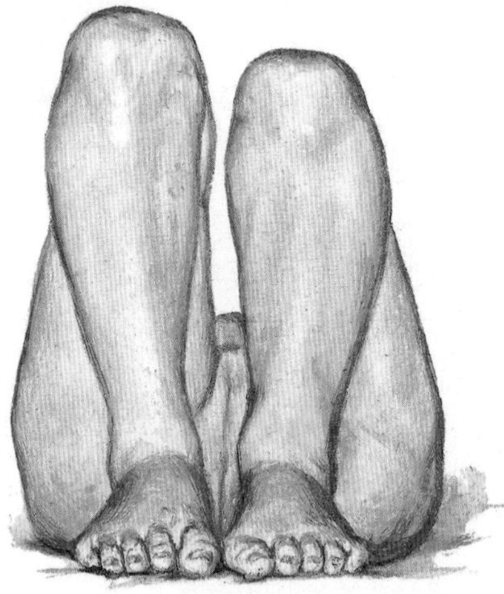

Allis or Galeazzi sign.
With knees and hips flexed, knee on affected side is lower because femoral head lies posterior to acetabulum in this position.

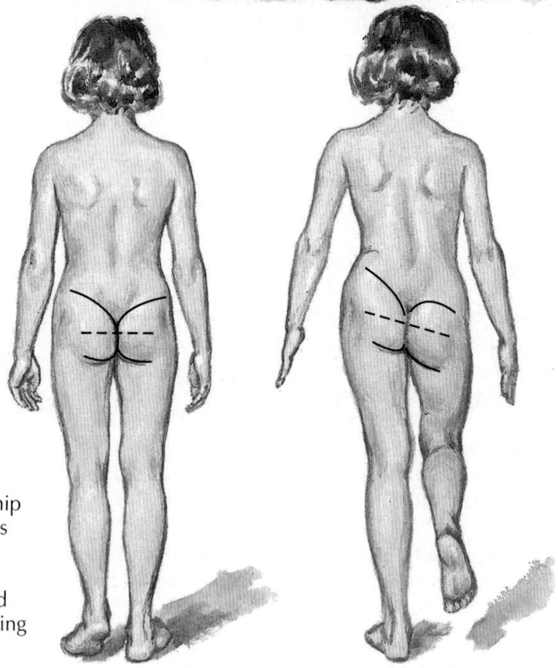

Trendelenburg test.
Left: Child with congenital dislocation of hip stands on both feet; hips and brim of pelvis are approximately level, except for slight shortening of thigh on affected left side.
Right: Child stands with weight on affected side; normal right hip drops down, indicating weakness of abductor muscles of left hip.

F. Netter M.D.
K. Marzen

If the dislocation is not treated, the initially simple problem becomes more complex. Persistent dislocation is met with normal muscle forces causing proximal and lateral migration of the femoral head. The iliopsoas, adductors, and hamstrings do not exist at their normal resting length and become contracted. The acetabulum becomes dysplastic (more shallow) without the stimulus of the femoral head. Fibrofatty tissue termed *pulvinar* develops within the joint. The ligamentum teres becomes thickened, and the transverse acetabular ligament becomes taut and migrates superiorly into the joint. The joint capsule balloons anteriorly and becomes redundant. The tight iliopsoas tendon compresses the joint capsule, trapping the femoral head outside the acetabulum and blocking reduction of the joint. This creates an hourglass configuration of the joint space. Undue pressure on the labrum causes it to enlarge and sometimes invert into the joint, preventing reduction, and thus it is termed an *inverted limbus.*

Developmental Dislocation of the Hip (Continued)

The chronically dislocated femoral head eventually becomes misshapen and flattened as it articulates with the outer table of the pelvis. The normal femoral rotation is blocked, and the femoral head and neck stay in a position of relative anteversion and valgus.

EXAMINATION OF THE NEONATE AND INFANT

The examination procedures described by Ortolani and Barlow are the most reliable methods of making the diagnosis of DDH in the neonate (see Plate 2.25). The Ortolani test is a test of hip reduction. If the infant's hip is dislocated, it can be reduced with this maneuver, which is also termed an Ortolani-positive hip. The Barlow test demonstrates the reverse. Gentle flexion and adduction of the infant's hip produces a painless clunk of dislocation, indicating an unstable joint. Over time, if instability is allowed to persist, these findings disappear and the only reliable finding is limited abduction.

Based on the variability of the clinical findings, there exists a spectrum of disease in DDH. The least severe form is simple dysplasia with stable hip joints, followed by a Barlow-positive hip (reduced but dislocatable), then an Ortolani-positive hip (dislocated but reducible), and finally teratologic or irreducible hips. This spectrum is best illustrated during the neonatal period.

CLINICAL MANIFESTATIONS IN OLDER CHILDREN

The findings of DDH become more obvious as children grow. The surrounding soft tissue and bone gradually adapt to the abnormal position of the femoral head. With time, it becomes increasingly difficult to reduce the femoral head into the acetabulum, and the Ortolani test ultimately becomes negative, with the femoral head remaining trapped outside the acetabulum. All major muscle groups about the hip become contracted. Most apparent are the adductors, which manifest clinically as decreased abduction of the affected hip. The thigh is relatively shortened and the skin and subcutaneous tissue bunch up, producing asymmetry in the thigh skin folds on occasion. With a unilateral dislocation, when the patient is supine and the hips and knees are flexed, the knees are not at the same level (positive Allis or Galeazzi sign). The femur can be moved freely up and down, which is described as pistoning or telescoping.

Radiologic Diagnosis of Developmental Dislocation of the Hip

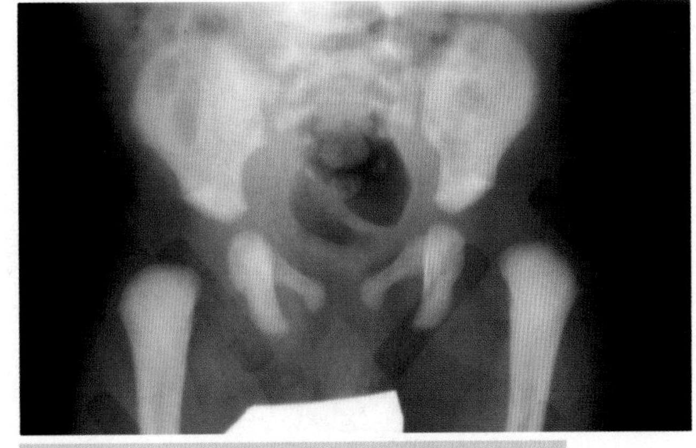

Radiograph of pelvis and hips of 4-day-old infant with congenital dislocation of left hip appears normal. Routine radiographs are seldom diagnostic in first month of life.

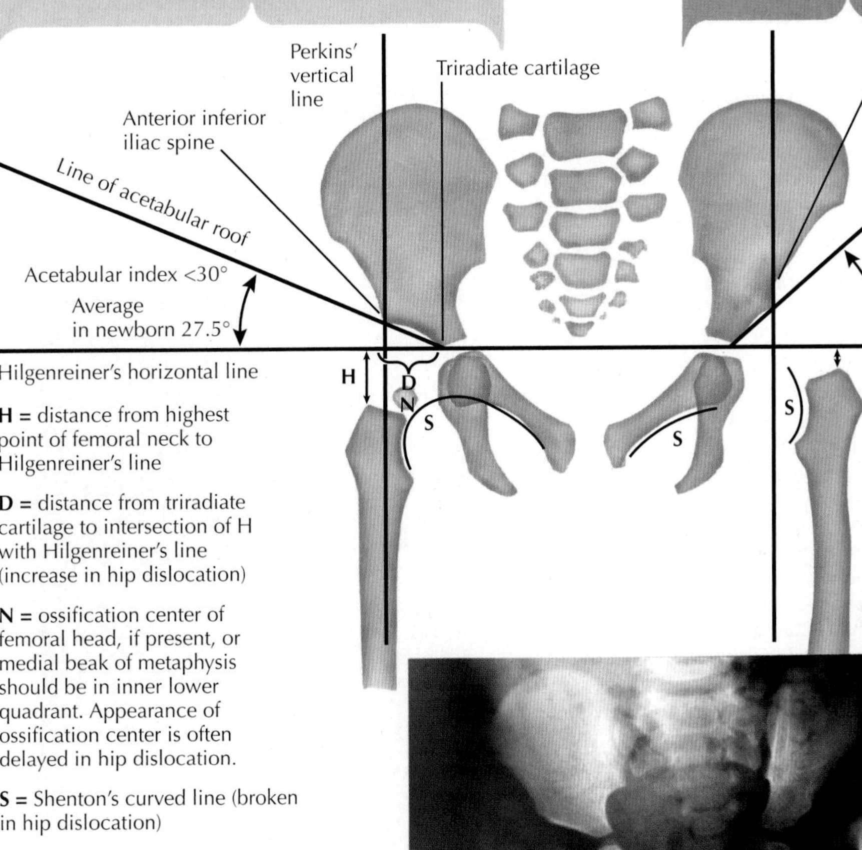
Normal
Hip dislocation
Perkins' vertical line
Triradiate cartilage
False acetabulum
Anterior inferior iliac spine
Line of acetabular roof
Acetabular index <30°
Average in newborn 27.5°
>30°
Hilgenreiner's horizontal line
H
D
N
S
H = distance from highest point of femoral neck to Hilgenreiner's line
D = distance from triradiate cartilage to intersection of H with Hilgenreiner's line (increase in hip dislocation)
N = ossification center of femoral head, if present, or medial beak of metaphysis should be in inner lower quadrant. Appearance of ossification center is often delayed in hip dislocation.
S = Shenton's curved line (broken in hip dislocation)
H shortened; femoral neck may be above Hilgenreiner's line.
F. Netter M.D.

Radiograph of 15-month-old child with congenital dislocation of left hip reveals classic signs: increase in acetabular index (acetabular dysplasia), lateral and proximal displacement of femoral neck, development of false acetabulum, broken Shenton's line, and delayed ossification of femoral head.

The child walks with a limp, owing to relative limb shortening and pelvic tilt due to abductor weakness. The Trendelenburg test can be used to assess abductor weakness. When both hips are dislocated, the perineal space is widened and the trochanters appear more prominent than normal. There is hyperlordosis of the lumbar spine, and the child walks with a waddling gait.

RADIOGRAPHIC EVALUATION

Selective screening imaging in children with suspected disease is the most reliable and cost-effective measure to diagnose and treat DDH in an efficient manner. Ultrasound examination can provide an accurate assessment of the femoral and acetabular anatomy and is superior to radiographs in the first 3 to 4 months of life. Higher false-positive results are seen in ultrasound

Adaptive Changes in Dislocated Hip That Interfere With Reduction

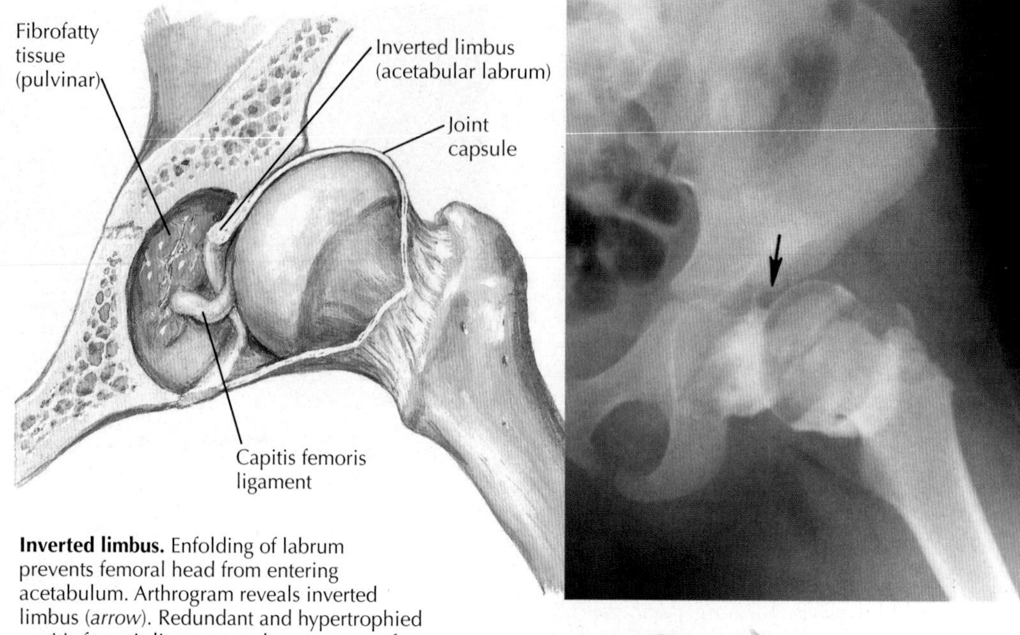

Inverted limbus. Enfolding of labrum prevents femoral head from entering acetabulum. Arthrogram reveals inverted limbus (*arrow*). Redundant and hypertrophied capitis femoris ligament and contracture of transverse acetabular ligament may also hinder reduction.

Iliopsoas tendon

Hourglass configuration of joint space. Arthrogram reveals typical bilocular appearance due to stretching and narrowing of joint capsule. Iliopsoas tendon further constricts isthmus of capsule.

Developmental Dislocation of the Hip (Continued)

examinations earlier than 4 weeks of life due to immaturity. Ultrasound can also provide a dynamic assessment of hip stability because the Ortolani and Barlow tests can be applied while visualized with ultrasound. The true percentage of acetabular coverage of the femoral head can be quantified.

Plain radiographs (anteroposterior [AP] and frog-leg views) become more useful after 4 to 5 months of life once the femoral epiphysis begins to ossify. Characteristic findings of DDH include (1) proximal and lateral migration of the femoral head/neck on the ilium; (2) a shallow, incompletely developed acetabulum; (3) development of a false acetabulum; and (4) delayed ossification of the proximal femoral ossific nucleus. A useful method of assessing infantile hips involves a system of lines on the AP pelvis radiograph. Accurate positioning of the child for the radiograph is critical. The legs must be extended and the hips in neutral rotation. These are most helpful when unilateral disease is present because there is a normal comparison on the same film.

In the older child, contrast arthrography may be helpful to visualize articular changes. It is seldom indicated as a sole imaging modality but rather used in conjunction with treatments such as closed reduction and assessing the adequacy of reduction.

The goal of treatment remains to return the femoral head to its normal position within the acetabulum and to keep it there to allow appropriate development. In the infant younger than the age of 6 months, closed reduction can usually be accomplished and is almost always accompanied by an adductor tenotomy to maintain reduction in a cast. In older children, gentle closed reduction becomes more difficult, and more invasive measures are needed to achieve the goal of a stable reduction.

TREATMENT PROTOCOL

Closed Reduction With Bracing

In a large number of children, hip instability noted at birth spontaneously resolves in a few weeks. Simple positioning and close clinical and radiographic follow-up are all that is typically needed in these cases. The newborn with documented more severe instability (Ortolani-positive hips) should be placed in some type of restraint device, typically a Pavlik harness. The reduction should be maintained for several weeks.

Although there are many devices that have historically been employed to maintain reduction of the unstable newborn hip (e.g., double diapers, Ilfeld splint, Von Rosen splint, Frejka pillow), the current choice remains the Pavlik harness. It provides the proper restraints with a shoulder harness, foot cuffs, and straps that tether the limbs at customizable degrees of flexion and abduction. Velcro closures make the harness simple to apply and remove for bathing.

The harness is applied loosely with the straps maintaining reduction of the hip in a position of around (no greater than) 100 degrees of flexion and limiting adduction such that the knees cannot touch when brought to midline. This zone can be adjusted based on the stability of the hip. Care must be taken to avoid excessive flexion or abduction, because they can result in femoral nerve neurapraxia and avascular necrosis, respectively. Once the device is properly applied, ultrasonography is used to confirm reduction. Follow-up ultrasound examinations in the harness can also be used for monitoring as well as radiographs after 4 months of age.

DEVELOPMENTAL DISLOCATION OF THE HIP (Continued)

The advantages of the Pavlik harness are several. It allows for spontaneous hip motion within the limits of stability. It also prevents extension of the hip and knee, which predisposes hips to instability. The infant can remain in the harness for essentially all care except bathing, and the risk of avascular necrosis remains very low because there is no forced abduction. The duration of treatment is typically related to patient age at onset of treatment.

Closed Reduction Under Anesthesia

For patients who do not respond to conservative treatment with a Pavlik harness or who are closer to 6 months of age when diagnosed with a dislocated hip, closed reduction of the hip is typically achieved with the patient under general anesthesia. The soft tissue contractures and adaptive changes make it such that the hip cannot spontaneously reduce. Gentle flexion and abduction of the hip is applied. The reduced hip must then be maintained in a comfortable and normal physiologic position of flexion and abduction. This position is critical. It must avoid excessive stress to the joint yet also keep the femoral head from redislocating. Ninety degrees of flexion with moderate abduction is the ideal position, referred to by Salter as the "human position." Tension on the hip can be lessened with a percutaneous adductor tenotomy, which is utilized in a majority of such cases. Once a closed reduction under anesthesia is accomplished, the hip is immobilized in a spica cast for about 3 months. Radiographs with or without an arthrogram should demonstrate the femoral head and neck directed toward the triradiate cartilage. Before cast immobilization, the safe zone of Ramsey is determined. This is defined as the range of motion within which the hip remains reduced. The safe zone can, and in most cases should, be increased with a percutaneous adductor tenotomy.

Open Reduction

If an adequate closed reduction is unable to be achieved and maintained, open reduction should be considered.

Medial (Adductor) Approach

This approach is typically used in patients younger than the age of 12 months. Although age is an important consideration for this approach, perhaps more important is patient size. The larger the child, the farther away the femoral head is from the medial-based incision and hence the more difficult it becomes to accomplish reduction through this approach.

DEVICE FOR TREATMENT OF CLINICALLY REDUCIBLE DISLOCATION OF HIP

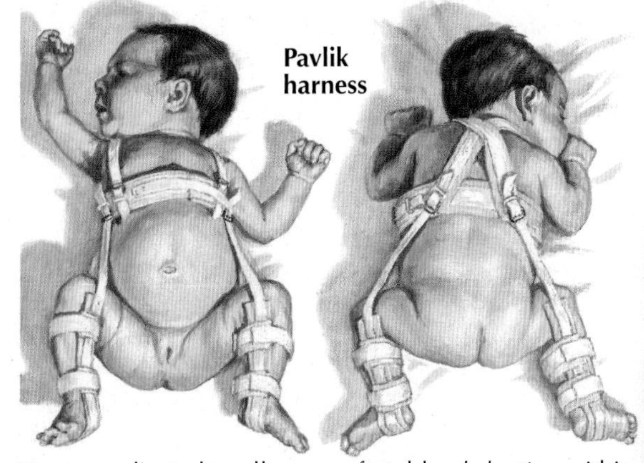

Harness adjusted to allow comfortable *abduction* within safe zone. Forced abduction beyond this limit may lead to avascular necrosis of femoral head. Posterior strap serves as checkrein to prevent hip from *adducting* to point of redislocation.

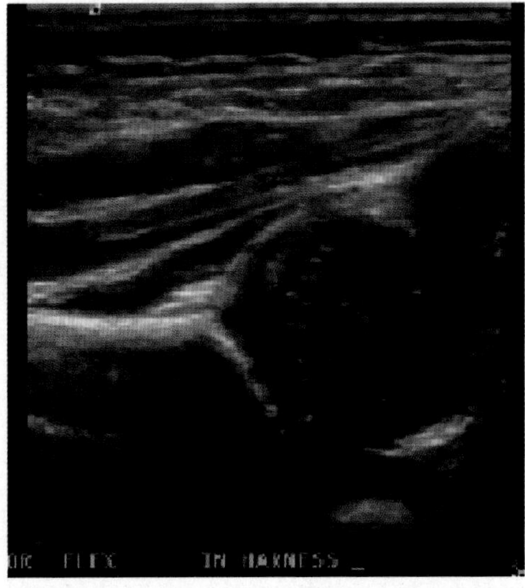

Coronal ultrasonogram of an infant hip. Ultrasound examination provides excellent detail of the largely cartilaginous femoral head and acetabulum. Dynamic examination can also be performed to assess stability. The examination can also be performed while the child is in a Pavlik harness if necessary.

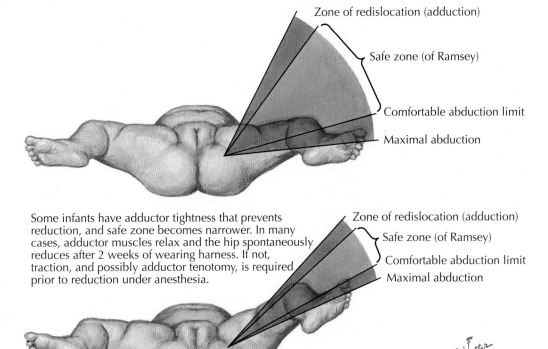

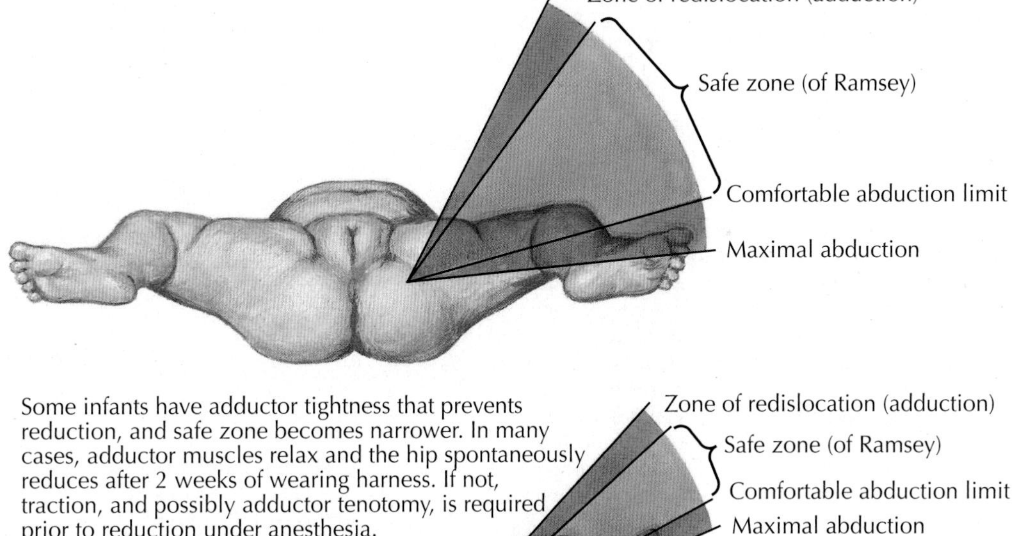

Some infants have adductor tightness that prevents reduction, and safe zone becomes narrower. In many cases, adductor muscles relax and the hip spontaneously reduces after 2 weeks of wearing harness. If not, traction, and possibly adductor tenotomy, is required prior to reduction under anesthesia.

The medial approach allows direct access to the contracted portion of the capsule but does not permit visualization or access to the redundant capsule for plication to prevent redislocation. The medial femoral circumflex artery is at risk in this approach and lies in close proximity to the psoas tendon.

The hip capsule is identified and opened, and the femoral head is reduced. Anatomic obstacles to reduction, such as the pulvinar, may need to be excised to permit reduction. An inverted limbus can be mobilized if necessary, and a taut transverse acetabular ligament can be incised if necessary to permit reduction. Once the hip is reduced, capsular closure is not necessary.

After wound closure, the child is immobilized in a bilateral hip spica cast. The cast is carefully molded about the trochanter to maintain reduction and prevent redislocation into the redundant capsule. Excessive abduction force should not be used.

DEVELOPMENTAL DISLOCATION OF THE HIP (Continued)

Anterolateral Approach

In older and larger children, the femoral head cannot be adequately accessed via a medial approach. The anterolateral approach is utilized for these cases. An oblique incision ("bikini line incision") just distal to and along the course of the iliac crest allows access and provides an excellent cosmetic result. As with the medial approach, the intraarticular obstacles to reduction are removed and the hip is reduced. The redundant portion of the capsule is excised and plicated to add stability to the reduction. A postoperative spica cast is applied to support the reduction. If the position of the hip alone does not provide enough stability, the quality of the reduction/capsulorrhaphy should be reassessed.

After open reduction, children younger than the age of 2 can wear a postoperative hip abduction orthosis until acetabular remodeling has occurred. In older children with less remodeling potential, pelvic osteotomy can be performed to improve the acetabular anatomy. The Salter innominate osteotomy provides additional anterior and lateral coverage, which is deficient in patients with DDH. Derotational osteotomies of the proximal femur can also be performed to better position the femoral head in the acetabulum. Femoral shortening osteotomy is frequently used to decrease tension on the reduction. These bony procedures can be used at the time of open reduction if deemed necessary by the surgeon.

COMPLICATIONS OF TREATMENT

Avascular Necrosis of the Femoral Head

Forcing the hip into extreme and unusual positions can have severe consequences, the most devastating of which is avascular necrosis of the femoral head. Compromise of the blood supply to the femoral head for even a short time can produce complete death of the femoral head. Redislocation of the hip can be problematic but can ultimately be corrected. Extreme leg positions to maintain a reduction must be avoided.

Several points regarding the femoral head blood supply and reduction of the femoral head have been described by Ogden. In the newborn, both the lateral and medial circumflex femoral arteries supply the femoral head. Contributions from the lateral circumflex regress by age 5 to 6 months. The medial femoral circumflex artery residing on the posterior femoral neck becomes the predominant blood supply to the femoral head. Interruption of the medial circumflex in the newborn may have little effect on the femoral head, but in the child older than 6 months, it can produce devastating necrosis of the entire femoral head. This has a profound effect on the developing proximal femur.

Earlier rates of avascular necrosis after closed reduction of the hip were unacceptably high. It is postulated that forced wide abduction places pressure on the medial femoral circumflex artery with contact from the limbus and other posterior structures, occluding the primary vessel to the femoral head. The vessel can also be compressed along its tortuous course by the iliopsoas tendon against the inferior pubic ramus as well as the pectineus-adductor group. Surgical release of these muscles lessens the tension on the reduction and reduces compression on the critical blood supply to the femoral head, reducing the rate of avascular necrosis.

BLOOD SUPPLY TO FEMORAL HEAD IN INFANCY (AFTER OGDEN)

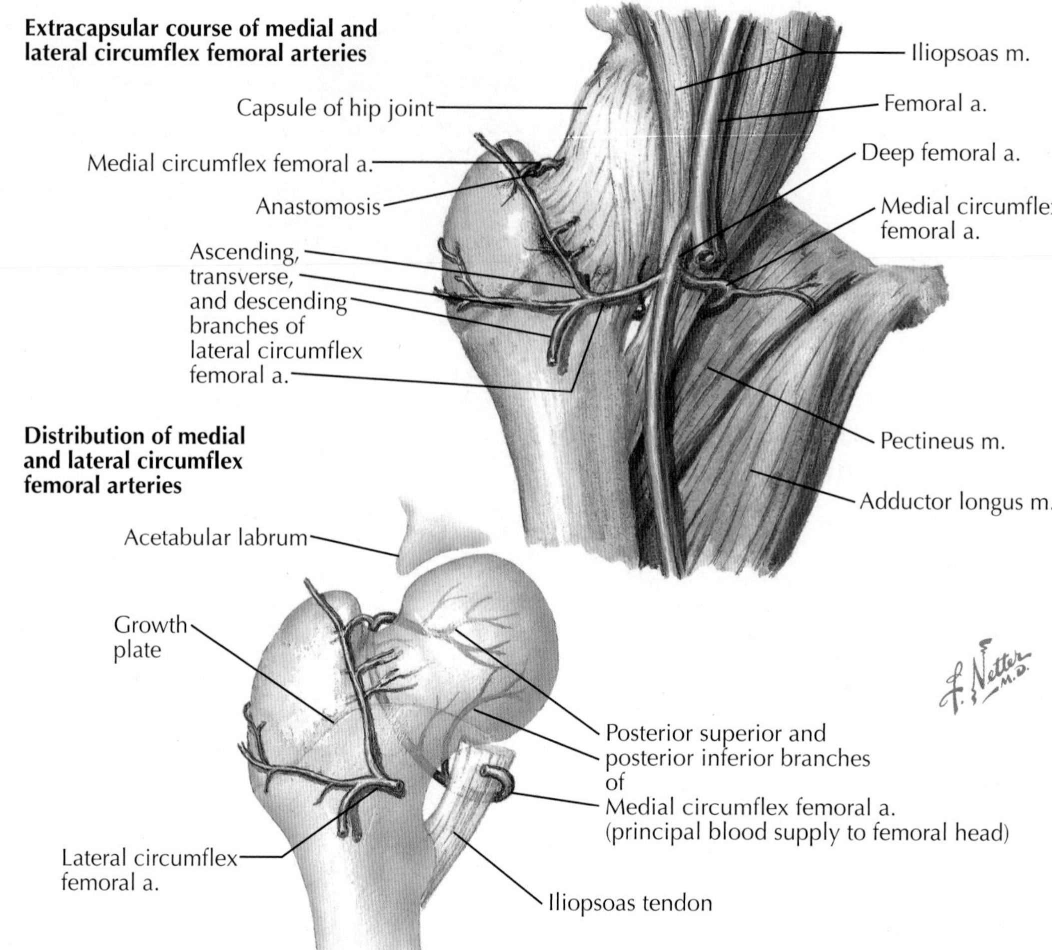

Compression of medial circumflex femoral artery in extreme abduction, internal rotation, and flexion

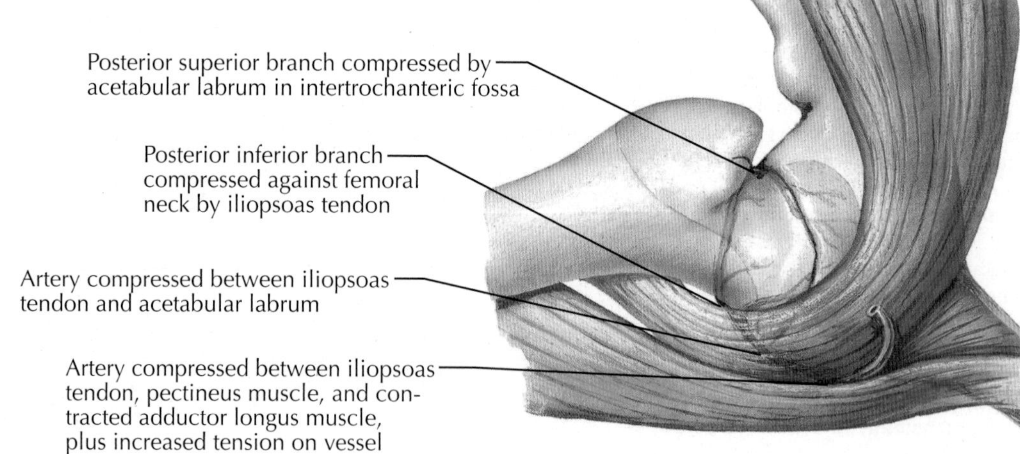

LEGG-CALVÉ-PERTHES DISEASE

Legg-Calvé-Perthes disease is defined as idiopathic avascular necrosis of the epiphysis of the femoral head (capital femoral epiphysis) and its associated complications in a growing child. It is a common but poorly understood hip disorder.

The disease develops more often in boys than girls (4 or 5:1). It can occur between 2 and 12 years of age (mean age, 7 years), and, when the involvement is bilateral, the changes usually appear in one hip at least 1 year earlier than in the other. If the child is older than 12 years at the time of clinical onset, the disorder is not considered true Legg-Calvé-Perthes disease but rather adolescent avascular necrosis, which has a poor prognosis similar to that of the adult form.

PREDISPOSING FACTORS

Genetic Aspects

The incidence of Legg-Calvé-Perthes disease is 1% to 20% higher in families of involved children, although there is no consistent pattern of inheritance. Studies in England have indicated that affected children are more likely than unaffected children to have low birth weight, abnormal birth presentation (breech and transverse presentations), and older parents. The disease is also more prevalent in later-born children (particularly the third to the sixth child).

The disorder occurs more frequently in Asian, Eskimo, and Central European populations, whereas the incidence is decreased in Black, Australian Aborigine, American Indian, and Polynesian populations.

The English studies have also demonstrated a higher than normal incidence of minor congenital genitourinary anomalies (e.g., renal abnormalities, inguinal hernias, and undescended testes) in affected children as well as in their first-degree relatives.

Abnormal Growth and Development

Legg-Calvé-Perthes disease may be a manifestation of an unknown systemic disorder rather than an isolated abnormality of the hip joint. The bone age of affected children is typically 1 to 3 years lower than their chronologic age. As a consequence, affected children are usually shorter than their peers, and the shortness of stature, although slight, persists into adulthood.

Disproportionate growth, abnormalities in skeletal growth and maturation, and elevated serum levels of somatomedin have been demonstrated. Affected children are typically smaller in all dimensions except head circumference, and their limbs have disproportionately small distal segments. The relationship between growth abnormalities, serum somatomedin, and ischemia of the epiphysis of the femoral head remains obscure. However, these findings support the concept of an underlying systemic disorder.

Environmental Factors

Although the effect of environment on the incidence is not clear, a large number of affected children in England are from lower socioeconomic groups. Whether this reflects dietary or environmental influences or a combination is not clear. In addition, there may be a geographic factor at play, as the incidence of disease is higher in far northern or southern latitudes and much lower near equatorial regions. The reason for this is unknown.

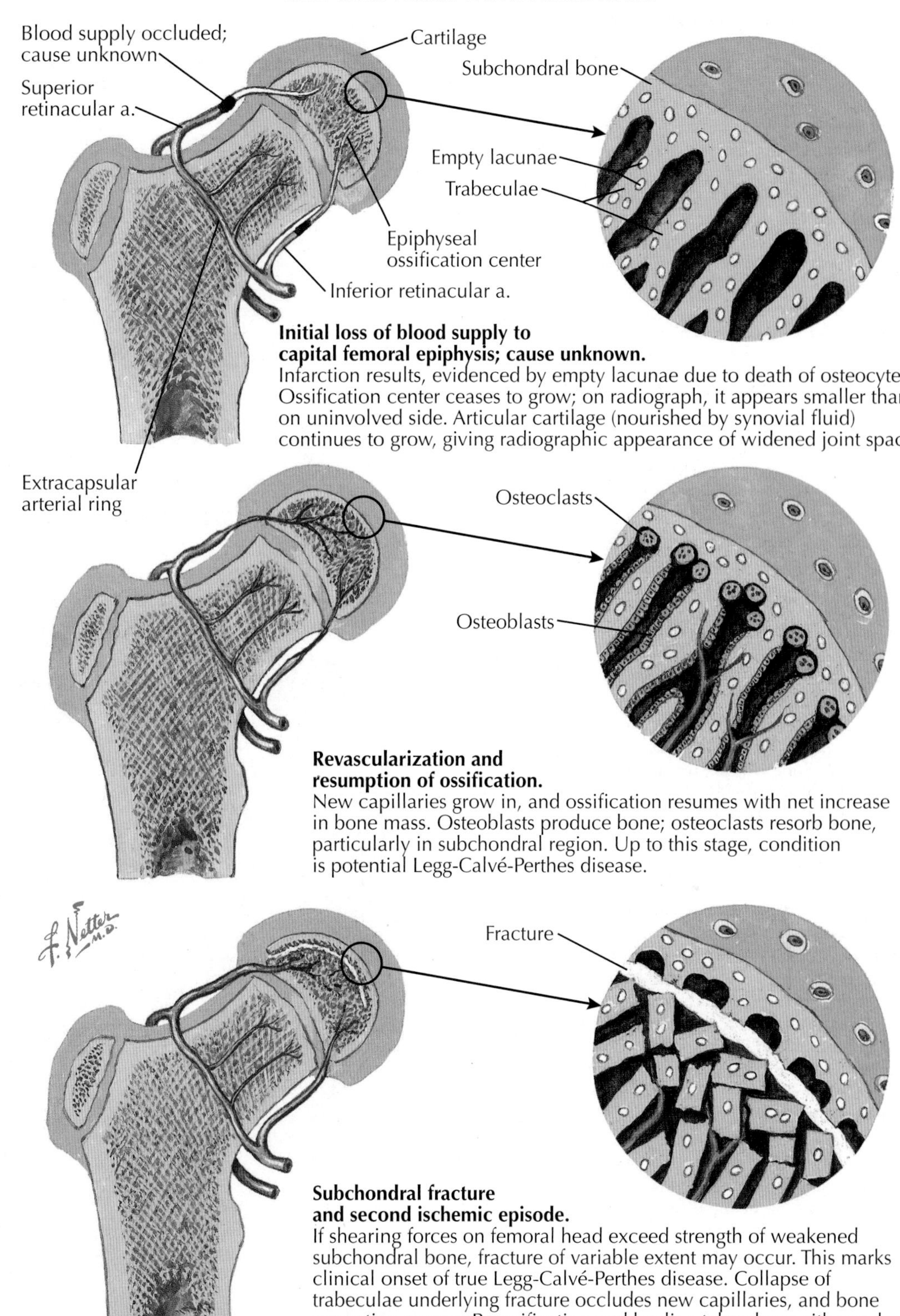

LEGG-CALVÉ-PERTHES DISEASE: PATHOGENESIS
Blood supply occluded; cause unknown
Cartilage
Subchondral bone
Superior retinacular a.
Empty lacunae
Trabeculae
Epiphyseal ossification center
Inferior retinacular a.
Initial loss of blood supply to capital femoral epiphysis; cause unknown.
Infarction results, evidenced by empty lacunae due to death of osteocytes. Ossification center ceases to grow; on radiograph, it appears smaller than on uninvolved side. Articular cartilage (nourished by synovial fluid) continues to grow, giving radiographic appearance of widened joint space.
Extracapsular arterial ring
Osteoclasts
Osteoblasts
Revascularization and resumption of ossification.
New capillaries grow in, and ossification resumes with net increase in bone mass. Osteoblasts produce bone; osteoclasts resorb bone, particularly in subchondral region. Up to this stage, condition is potential Legg-Calvé-Perthes disease.
F. Netter M.D.
Fracture
Subchondral fracture and second ischemic episode.
If shearing forces on femoral head exceed strength of weakened subchondral bone, fracture of variable extent may occur. This marks clinical onset of true Legg-Calvé-Perthes disease. Collapse of trabeculae underlying fracture occludes new capillaries, and bone resorption occurs. Reossification and healing take place with good or poor functional result.

ETIOLOGY AND PATHOGENESIS

The etiology of Legg-Calvé-Perthes disease is not yet understood, but it is accepted that the avascular necrosis is due to an interruption of the blood supply to the epiphysis of the femoral head, especially the contributions from the superior and inferior retinacular arteries. Current etiologic theories include trauma to the retinacular vessels, vascular occlusion secondary to increased intracapsular pressure from acute transient synovitis, venous obstruction with secondary intraepiphyseal thrombosis, vascular irregularities (congenital or developmental), and increased blood viscosity resulting in stasis and decreased blood flow.

Although the cause remains unclear, numerous studies have delineated the pathogenesis of Legg-Calvé-Perthes disease. Initially, an ischemic episode of unknown etiology occurs, rendering most, if not all, of the epiphysis avascular. Endochondral ossification in

LEGG-CALVÉ-PERTHES DISEASE (Continued)

the preosseous epiphyseal cartilage and growth plate ceases temporarily, while the articular cartilage, which is nourished by synovial fluid, continues to grow. This results in the radiographic appearance of a widened medial cartilage (joint) space and a smaller ossification center in the involved hip. This is the first radiographic manifestation, and it precedes any change in the density of the epiphysis. At this stage, the marrow space of the epiphysis is necrotic.

Revascularization of the structurally intact but avascular epiphysis occurs from the periphery as new capillaries recanalize the previous vascular channels. Resumption of endochondral ossification within the epiphysis begins peripherally and progresses centrally. With the ingrowth of capillaries, osteoclasts and osteoblasts cover the surface of the avascular subchondral cortical bone and the central trabecular bone. New bone is deposited on the avascular bone, producing a net increase in bone mass per unit area; this accounts for the increased density of the epiphysis that is apparent on radiographs taken in early stages of the disease.

The deposition of new trabecular bone and resorption of avascular bone occur simultaneously. In the subchondral area, bone resorption exceeds new bone formation. A critical point is reached during resorption when the subchondral area becomes biomechanically weak and therefore susceptible to a pathologic fracture. Up to this point, the disease process is clinically silent and asymptomatic. The continuation of this "potential" form of Legg-Calvé-Perthes disease or the development of the "true" form depends on whether a subchondral fracture occurs.

In the *potential form* of the disease, a subchondral fracture does not occur because the stresses and shearing forces acting on the revascularized epiphysis of the femoral head do not exceed the strength of the weakened subchondral area. The reossification process continues uninterrupted, with ultimate resumption of normal growth and development. Thus there is no epiphyseal resorption, no extrusion or subluxation of the femoral head, and no potential for deformity. The child remains asymptomatic and retains good range of motion in the hip joint. The subchondral area eventually regains its normal strength and stability, and a "head-within-a-head" is visible on radiographs. The head-within-a-head represents a growth arrest line that outlines the ossification center at the time of the initial infarction.

In the *true form* of the disease, the strength of the weakened subchondral area is exceeded and a pathologic subchondral fracture occurs (see Plate 2.31). The magnitude of stress or trauma necessary to produce such a fracture is difficult to quantitate and appears to vary with both the degree of preexisting weakness and the applied shearing forces. In most cases, the fracture seems to result from normal vigorous activity rather than from a specific injury. The painful subchondral fracture heralds the clinical onset of true Legg-Calvé-Perthes disease, and only the true form produces the typical clinical and radiographic features and requires 2 to 4 years, or even longer, for complete healing to occur.

Changes in Epiphysis

The subchondral fracture characteristically begins in the anterolateral aspect of the epiphysis near the growth plate because this area receives the greatest concentration of stress during weight bearing. The pathologic fracture extends superiorly and posteriorly until it reaches areas where the strength of the remaining subchondral bone exceeds the shearing forces acting on the femoral head. There is minimal, if any, extension of the subchondral fracture after the initial fracture. The reasons for this are not clear, but it is thought that the resulting pain causes the child to be less active, thereby reducing the stress on the femoral head.

The revascularized trabecular bone beneath the subchondral fracture undergoes a second episode of local ischemia secondary to trabecular collapse and occlusion of the ingrowing capillaries. This second ischemic episode, mechanical in origin, involves either part or all of the epiphysis, depending on the extent of the subchondral fracture. The structural stability of the epiphysis is lost; the ingrowth of new capillaries is impeded by the obliteration of the vascular channels and the presence

LEGG-CALVÉ-PERTHES DISEASE: PHYSICAL EXAMINATION

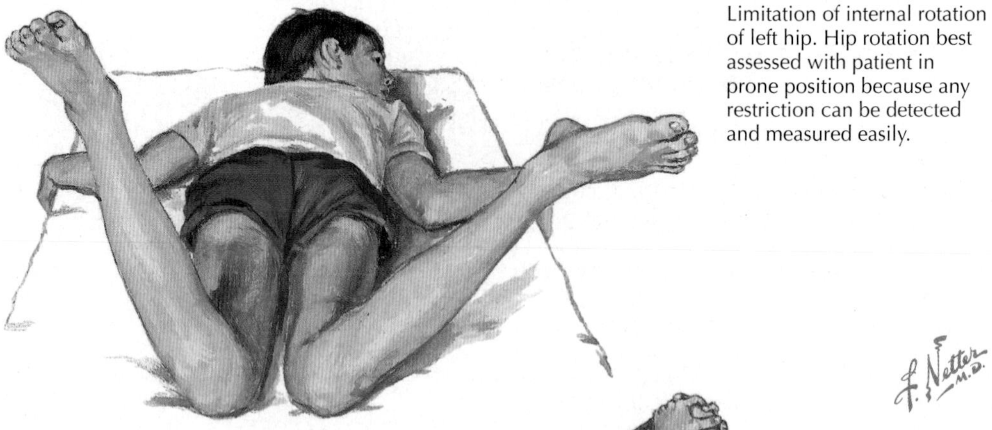

Limitation of internal rotation of left hip. Hip rotation best assessed with patient in prone position because any restriction can be detected and measured easily.

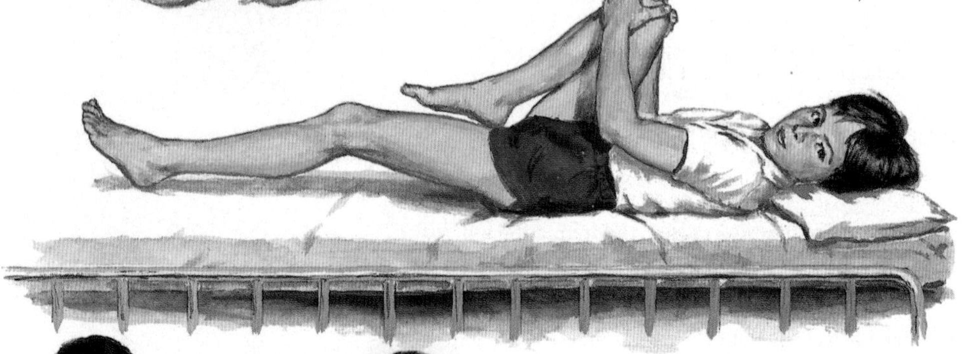

Thomas sign.
Hip flexion contracture determined with patient supine. Unaffected hip flexed only until lumbar spine is flat against examining table. Affected hip cannot be fully extended, and angle of flexion is recorded. A 15-degree flexion contracture of hip is typical of Legg-Calvé-Perthes disease.

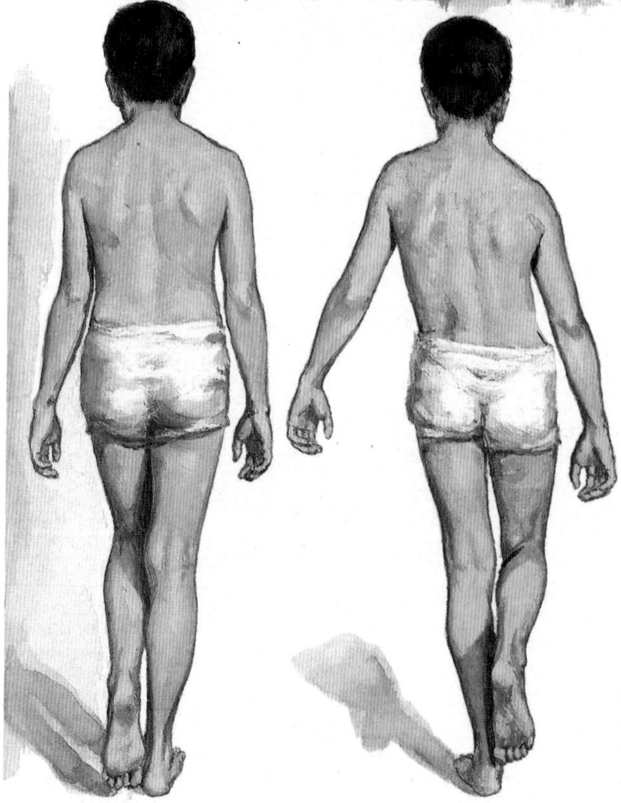

Trendelenburg test.
Left: Patient demonstrates negative Trendelenburg test of normal right hip. *Right:* Positive test of involved left hip. When weight is on affected side, normal hip drops, indicating weakness of left gluteus medius muscle. Trunk shifts left as patient attempts to decrease biomechanical stresses across involved hip and thereby maintain balance.

LEGG-CALVÉ-PERTHES DISEASE (Continued)

of fractured bone (both cortical and trabecular) and marrow debris. Consequently, the entire area is slowly revascularized, with resorption of the fibro-osseous tissue, by a process termed *creeping substitution.* In this reparative process, the avascular bone is slowly resorbed from the periphery of the area of the second infarction and replaced by vascular fibrous tissue that, in turn, is eventually replaced by primary trabecular bone.

During the process of creeping substitution, the femoral head, although not soft in the physical sense, can be molded into a round or flat shape by the forces acting on it. This remodeling property, or biologic plasticity, lasts until subchondral reossification begins. Potential deformities may be caused by the different rates of growth happening simultaneously within the femoral head—areas not undergoing resorption grow faster than the involved area. The combined factors of pressure and asymmetric growth result in a potential for extrusion and subluxation of the femoral head and eventual deformity. Thus true Legg-Calvé-Perthes disease is actually a complication of avascular necrosis.

Secondary alterations in the growth plate and metaphysis also occur and can lead to further disturbances in endochondral ossification and growth in the proximal femur.

Changes in Growth Plate

Because the blood supply to the growth plate comes from the epiphyseal side, the two ischemic episodes also produce ischemic changes in the growth plate. The chondrocyte columns become distorted with some loss of their cellular components; they do not undergo normal ossification, which results in an excess of calcified cartilage in the primary trabecular bone.

Changes in Metaphysis

Four types of metaphyseal changes have been noted: presence of adipose tissue, osteolytic lesions (well-circumscribed areas of fibrocartilage), disorganized ossification, and extrusion of the growth plate. Whereas only adipose tissue changes are detected early in the disease, osteolytic lesions are seen in the later stages. When these fibrocartilaginous lesions are in contact with the growth plate, the normal architecture of the growth plate is lost and the lesions appear on radiographs as cysts. In the areas without osteolytic lesions, ossification is disorganized and bars, or columns, of unossified cartilage appear to "stream" or "flow" down into the metaphysis. Necrosis of bone is not seen in the metaphysis. In some severely deformed femoral heads, the growth plate extrudes down the sides of the femoral neck.

The changes in the growth plate and metaphysis ultimately alter the growth in length of the proximal femur and produce the short, thick femoral neck (coxa breva) and enlarged (coxa magna) and flattened (coxa plana) femoral head typically seen in Legg-Calvé-Perthes disease. The greater trochanter, being uninvolved, continues to grow and may eventually rise above the level of the femoral head. The combination of a short femoral neck and a high greater trochanter is considered "functional" coxa vara. The performance of the hip abductor (gluteus medius) muscles is disturbed, with a resultant limp or Trendelenburg gait and a positive Trendelenburg test (see Plate 2.32). The short femoral neck also produces a limb length discrepancy of 1 to 2 cm.

LEGG-CALVÉ-PERTHES DISEASE: PHYSICAL EXAMINATION (CONTINUED)

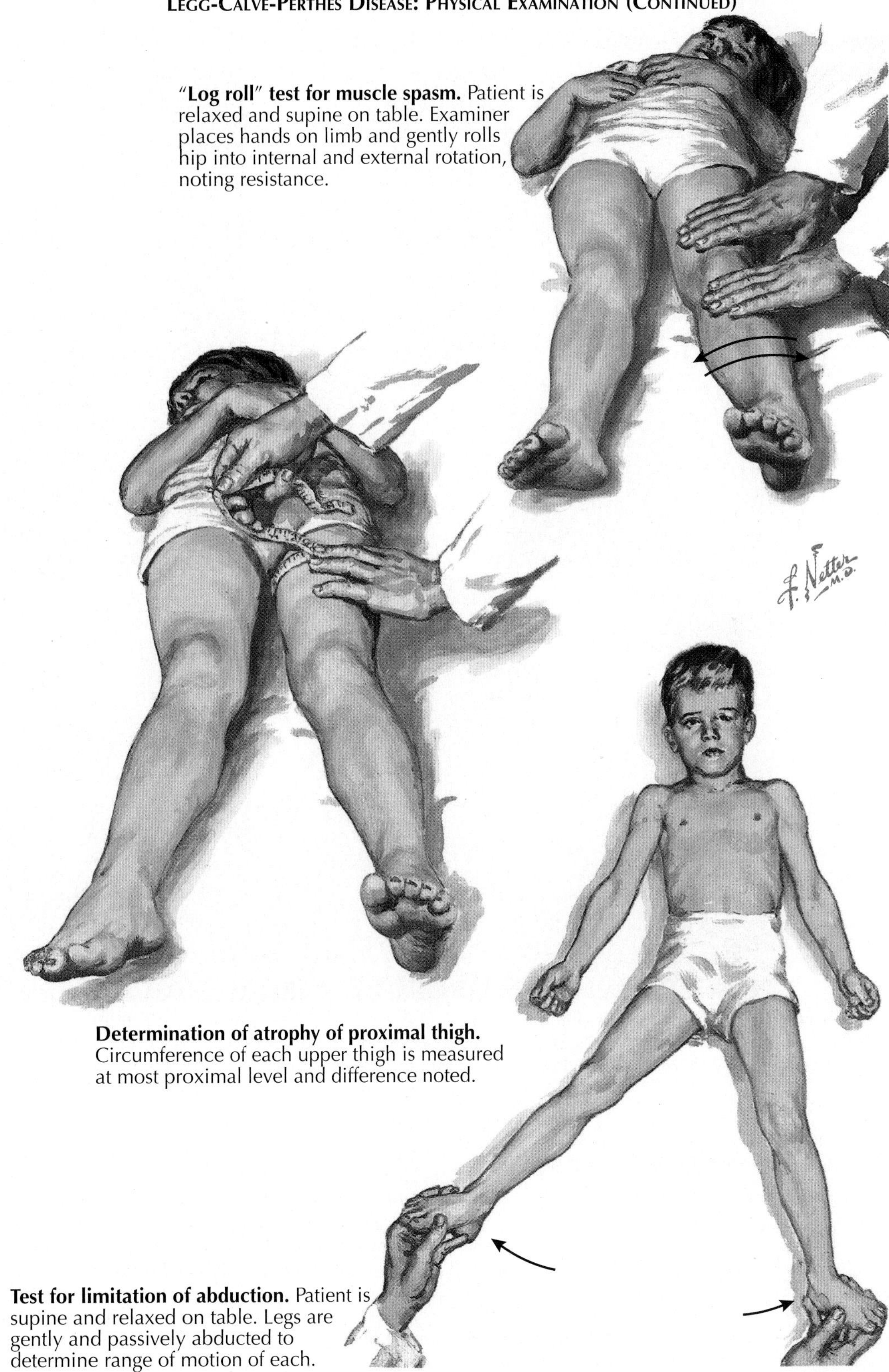

"Log roll" test for muscle spasm. Patient is relaxed and supine on table. Examiner places hands on limb and gently rolls hip into internal and external rotation, noting resistance.

Determination of atrophy of proximal thigh. Circumference of each upper thigh is measured at most proximal level and difference noted.

Test for limitation of abduction. Patient is supine and relaxed on table. Legs are gently and passively abducted to determine range of motion of each.

CLINICAL MANIFESTATIONS

The pertinent early findings include antalgic gait, muscle spasm and restricted hip motion, atrophy of the proximal thigh, and short stature. A small percentage of children have a history of trauma that is usually mild. Nevertheless, such trauma may be sufficient to produce the pathologic subchondral fracture.

Initial symptoms are mild and intermittent pain in the anterior thigh, a limp, or both. Although many children do not report pain, on close questioning most admit to mild pain either in the anterior thigh or the knee. The onset of pain may be acute or insidious. Referred pain from the hip to the anterior thigh or knee must be considered. Because the child's initial symptoms are typically mild, parents frequently do not seek medical attention for several weeks after clinical onset, or longer.

Stages of Legg-Calvé-Perthes Disease

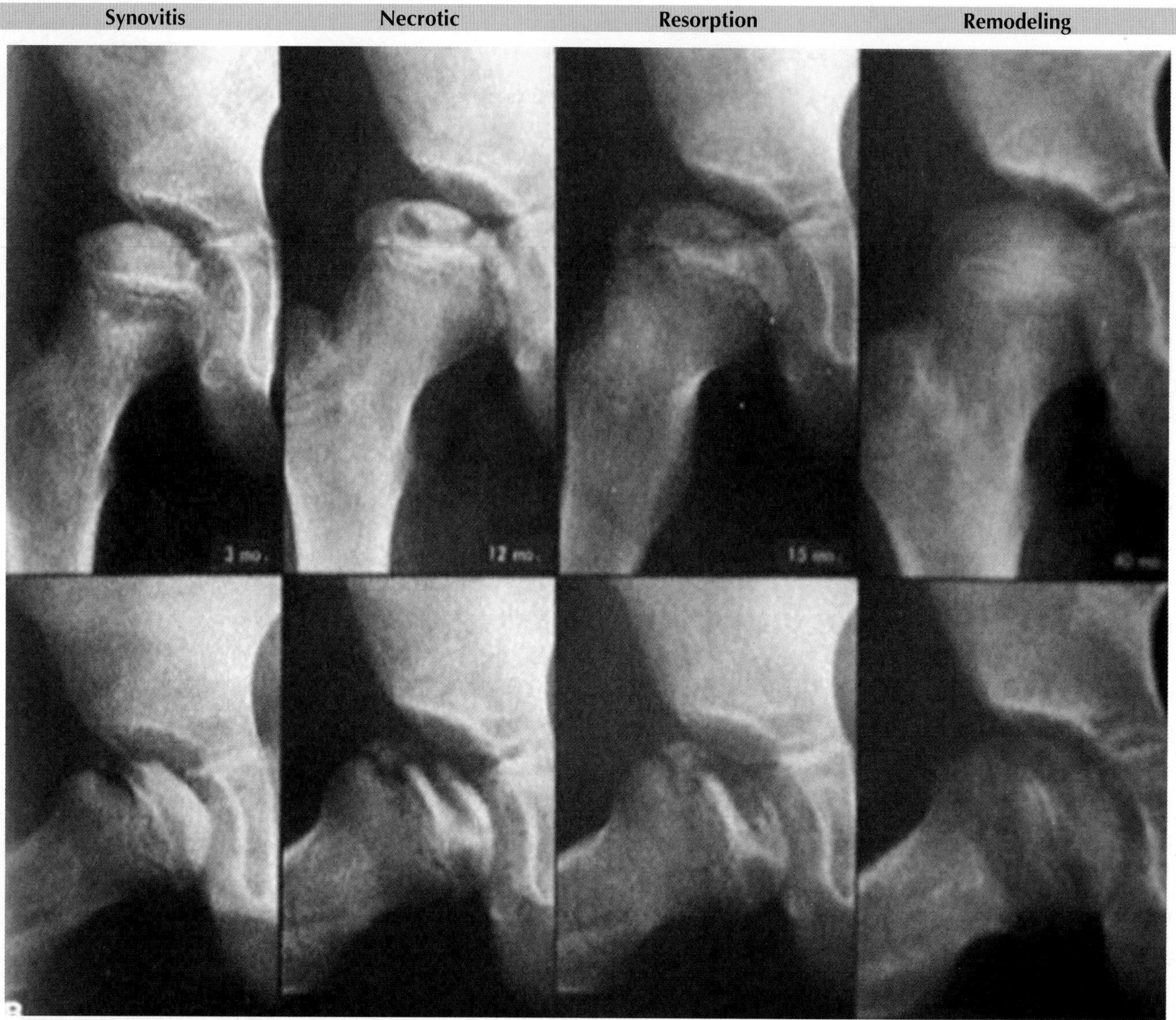

Anteroposterior and frog-leg lateral radiographic appearance of a child's right hip illustrating the various stages of the Legg-Calvé-Perthes disease process. *Left to right,* Synovitis/growth arrest stage, necrotic/subchondral fracture stage, resorption stage, and reossification/remodeling stage. A fifth stage (healed) is present once the disease process is complete and the residual sphericity of the femoral head can be assessed.

Legg-Calvé-Perthes Disease (Continued)

Antalgic gait is noted when the patient shortens the time of weight bearing on the involved limb during walking to reduce discomfort. Pain from the irritable hip can also cause reflex inhibition of the hip abductor muscles with a resultant positive Trendelenburg test, a common early sign (see Plate 2.32).

Muscle spasm is best detected by the "log roll" test, a painless test that reveals any guarding or muscle spasm (secondary to irritability of the hip joint), especially when the involved limb is rolled inward (see Plate 2.33). Once the child's confidence is gained, the hip can usually be examined more thoroughly to determine the complete range of motion. Mild limitation of motion, particularly abduction and internal rotation, is the typical finding. This may be best elucidated by noting asymmetry in both abduction and internal rotation. There may also be limitation of extension, as evidenced by a mild hip flexion contracture (Thomas sign), as well as deep tenderness over the anterior aspect of the hip.

Disuse atrophy of the proximal thigh muscles is a consequence of prolonged hip irritability and the resultant limitation of motion. The atrophic thigh is usually 2 to 3 cm smaller, especially during the early symptomatic phases. As the symptoms subside, the atrophy resolves.

Short stature due to delayed bone age is another typical finding in affected children. The patient's bone age can be determined with the Greulich and Pyle atlas.

Results of laboratory tests are normal, except for an occasionally abnormal erythrocyte sedimentation rate, which may be slightly elevated (30–40 mm/hr).

RADIOGRAPHIC EVALUATION

Routine radiographic assessment is essential for diagnosis and for determining progression of the disease, sphericity of the femoral head, possibility of epiphyseal extrusion or collapse, and response to treatment. Arthrography is a useful adjunct, especially in the setting of the operating room to best define the true sphericity, or lack thereof, of the femoral head. Magnetic resonance imaging (MRI) can also be helpful in rare cases, and radionuclide bone scanning currently plays a very limited role.

The entire disease process can usually be assessed from plain AP and Lauenstein frog-leg radiographs of the pelvis (both hips). Extrusion and subluxation of the femoral head can be measured on these radiographs using the Wiberg center-edge angle. An extrusion index developed by Green and associates has been demonstrated to be prognostically significant. Sphericity of the femoral head in the reossification and healed stages is currently best determined by the Mose circle criteria. In this technique, a transparent template with concentric circles at 2-mm intervals, placed on both AP and frog-leg radiographs, is centered over the femoral head to measure both the sphericity and diameter of the femoral head. If the sphericity is equal in both projections, the hip is rated "good." A variance of up to 2 mm is rated "fair," whereas a variance of 3 mm or more is rated "poor." The good and fair ratings are considered satisfactory results, whereas poor ratings are unsatisfactory. Sphericity may improve with growth

Legg-Calvé-Perthes Disease (Continued)

and development if the healed femoral head remains well contained in the acetabulum.

Computerized methods are being investigated to allow better objective quantification of hip joint architecture and for plotting changes in configuration that occur with time.

Early in the resorption stage, arthrography may be required to assess the sphericity of the articular surface of the femoral head. The contour of the partially resorbed ossification center of the epiphysis may not reflect the contour of the articular surface, and range of motion in the hip is usually the best indicator of potential femoral head deformity. Only "questionable" hips require arthrography.

Bone scans have largely been replaced by MRI. MRI is helpful in defining epiphyseal infarction and the contours of the femoral head, both of which are prognostically significant. Like radionuclide bone scans, MRI does not correlate with the extent of epiphyseal involvement.

STAGES OF DISEASE

Radiographic evaluation has determined five distinct stages of Legg-Calvé-Perthes disease, which represent a continuum of the disease process.

Growth Arrest

This stage occurs immediately after the initial ischemic episode in the femoral head, when endochondral ossification of the preosseous cartilage ceases. During this avascular phase, which may last 6 to 12 months, there is a slight but progressive difference in the size (height and width) of the involved epiphysis and that of the opposite normal hip. The joint space also appears to be wider because of the continued growth of the articular cartilage. These relatively small differences (1–3 mm) are visible and measurable on an AP radiograph of the pelvis. Toward the end of this stage, epiphyseal density increases. During this stage, which is only potential Legg-Calvé-Perthes disease, the disease is clinically silent and asymptomatic.

Subchondral Fracture

The subchondral fracture initiates true Legg-Calvé-Perthes disease. Radiographic visibility of the fracture varies with the age of the patient at clinical onset and the extent of epiphyseal involvement. The duration varies from an average of 3 months in children 4 years of age or younger to 8.5 months in children 10 years or older.

Resorption

In this stage, also called fragmentation or necrosis, the necrotic bone beneath the subchondral fracture is gradually and irregularly resorbed. This process produces the radiographic appearance of fragmentation because the bone is resorbed and replaced by vascular fibrous tissue (creeping substitution) and later by primary bone. The resorption phase lasts 6 to 12 months and is longest when there is extensive epiphyseal involvement or when the child is 10 years of age or older at clinical onset. This phase is usually complete 12 to 17 months after clinical onset.

Reossification

During the healing, or reossification, stage, ossification of the primary bone begins irregularly in the subchondral area and progresses centrally. Eventually, the newly formed areas of bone coalesce and the epiphysis progressively regains its normal strength. Reossification takes 6 to 24 months.

Healed Stage

The healed, or residual, stage signals the complete ossification of the epiphysis of the femoral head, with or without residual deformity.

CLASSIFICATION

There have been many classification systems developed to describe the disease process. Most systems, such as the Catterall and Salter-Thompson classification systems, are helpful retrospectively but have little prognostic value. The lateral pillar classification system is currently the most widely used and valuable classification system because it has been shown to have some prognostic significance.

Legg-Calvé-Perthes Disease: Lateral Pillar Classification

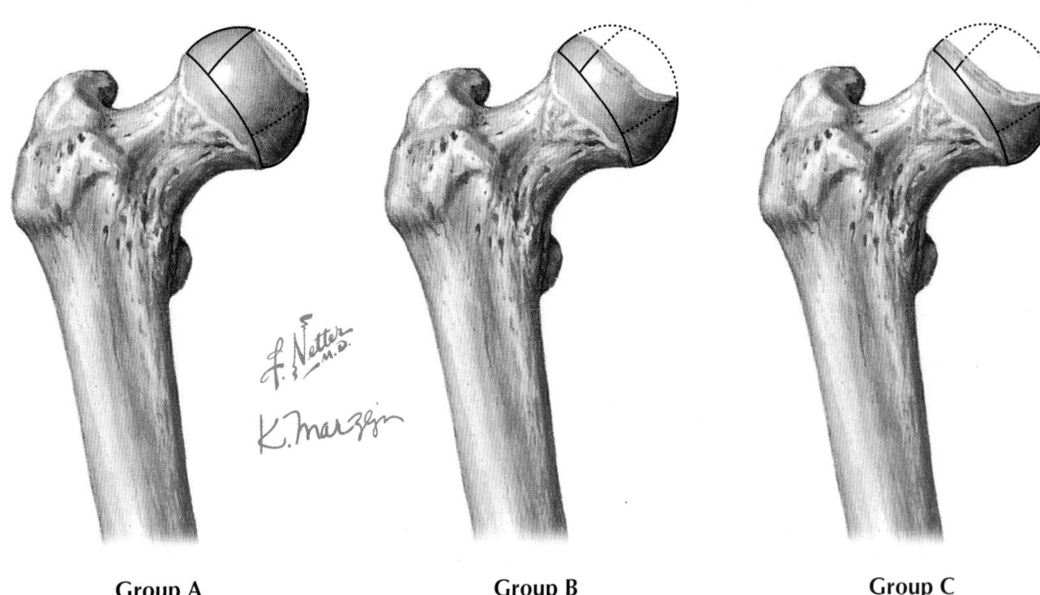

The lateral pillar classification of Legg-Calvé-Perthes disease. Hips in group A retain full height of the lateral pillar on AP radiographs. In group B hips, the lateral pillar shows some loss of height but retains at least 50% of its original height. Group C hips show collapse of the lateral pillar to less than 50% of original height.

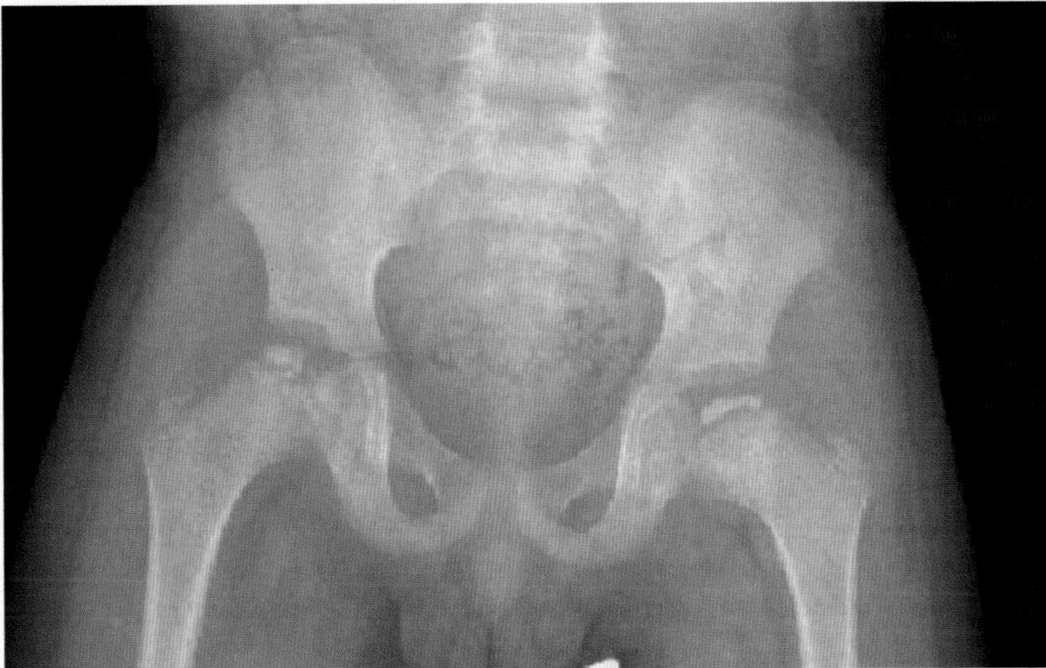

AP pelvis radiograph of a 6-year-old boy with a highly unusual case of Legg-Calvé-Perthes disease in both hips. The right hip is a lateral pillar group B hip, and the left is a lateral pillar group C hip. Note that the hips are in different stages of the disease process, which is typically the case with bilateral involvement.

LEGG-CALVÉ-PERTHES DISEASE (Continued)

The lateral pillar classification system developed by Hering and colleagues separates diseased hips into three groups (A, B, and C) on the basis of the remaining height of the lateral third of the femoral head epiphysis. Group A hips have maintenance of 100% of the lateral pillar height. These have the best prognosis long term and are least likely to extrude. Group B hips have decreased lateral pillar height but have at least 50% of the lateral pillar height remaining. Group C hips have less than 50% of the lateral pillar height remaining and have an almost uniformly poor prognosis.

PROGNOSIS

The short-term prognosis for patients with Legg-Calvé-Perthes disease focuses on femoral head deformity at the completion of the healing stage. The long-term prognosis involves the potential for secondary osteoarthritis of the hip in adulthood.

Deformity of Femoral Head

The ultimate goal of treatment is a spherical femoral head at the completion of growth. Six factors determine the potential for femoral head deformity.

1. *Sex of patient.* In general, the outcome is less favorable in girls than in boys. Involvement of the femoral head is often more extensive in girls; and because they mature earlier than boys, there is less remaining skeletal growth from the time of clinical onset and consequently less opportunity for epiphyseal remodeling.
2. *Age at clinical onset.* The older the child at clinical onset, the less favorable the prognosis, particularly in children 10 years of age and older. This may also be related to the reduced remaining skeletal growth and potential for femoral head remodeling in older children.
3. *Extent of epiphyseal involvement.* More extensive involvement is correlated with a poorer prognosis.
4. *Containment of femoral head.* Extrusion, subluxation, or asymmetric growth of the femoral head increases the stress concentrated on it during weight bearing. The ability to maintain the femoral head within the acetabulum with appropriate treatment is a significant factor for a favorable prognosis.
5. *Persistent loss of motion.* This is usually due to either muscle spasm (adductors or iliopsoas muscle), muscle contractures, anterolateral extrusion or subluxation of the femoral head, or a combination thereof. The loss of motion prevents adequate remodeling of the femoral head by the acetabulum.
6. *Premature closure of the growth plate.* When involvement of the epiphysis is extensive (lateral pillar group C), the growth plate may be sufficiently damaged to cause premature closure. This can result in asymmetric growth and inadequate remodeling that contributes to femoral head deformity, greater trochanteric overgrowth (functional coxa vara), and a limb length discrepancy.

Late Degenerative Osteoarthritis

The incidence of late degenerative osteoarthritis depends on residual deformity of the femoral head and the patient's age at clinical onset. The risk is directly correlated with the extent of residual deformity. Three types of congruency between the femoral head and the acetabulum have been classified: spherical congruency, aspherical congruency, and aspherical incongruency. Spherical congruency is not associated with osteoarthritis, whereas aspherical congruency predisposes to mild-to-moderate osteoarthritis in late adulthood. Patients with aspherical incongruency usually develop degenerative osteoarthritis before age 50 years.

Studies also show that the incidence of osteoarthritis of the hip in adults with deformed femoral heads is negligible in patients age 5 years or younger at the time of clinical onset, 38% in patients 6 to 9 years, and 100% in patients 10 years or older. Aspherical incongruency, a predisposing factor for osteoarthritis, is also more likely to develop in children who are older at the time of clinical onset.

LEGG-CALVÉ-PERTHES DISEASE: CONSERVATIVE MANAGEMENT

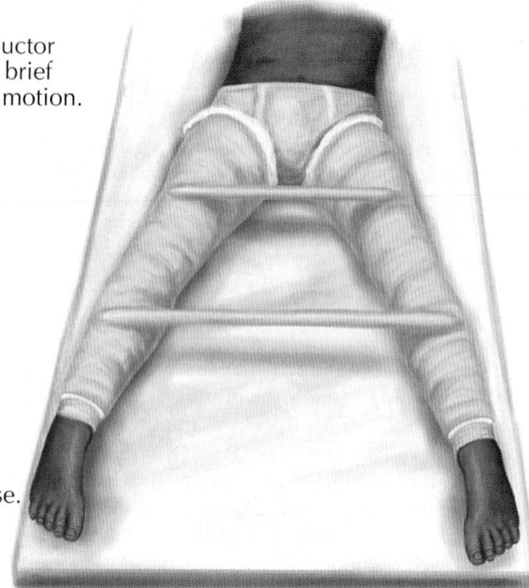

Child in Petrie cast following adductor tenotomy. Cast immobilization is brief (weeks) to improve and maintain motion.

Arthrogram of a child with Legg-Calvé-Perthes disease. Images are taken in AP (*top left*), frog-leg lateral (*top right*), abduction internal rotation (*bottom left*), and adduction (*bottom right*). Note the flattening of the femoral head on the AP view. The abduction internal rotation view demonstrates the containability of the hip.

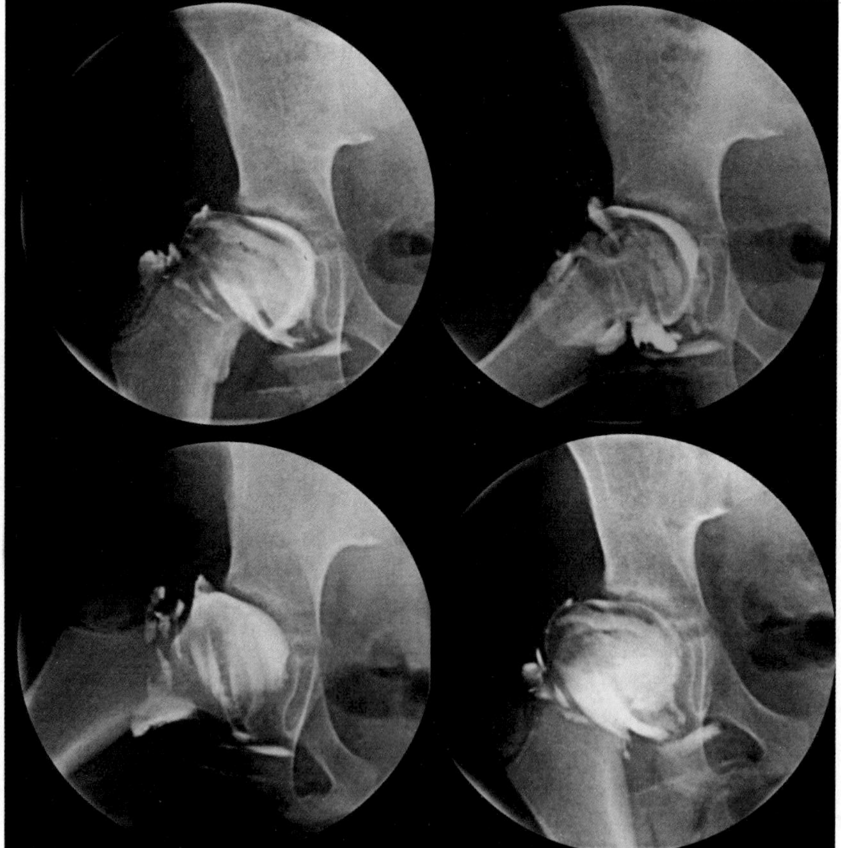

LEGG-CALVÉ-PERTHES DISEASE (Continued)

Thus of the two significant factors in the long-term prognosis, only femoral head deformity may be preventable, or at least altered, by appropriate treatment.

TREATMENT

The only justification for treatment is prevention of femoral head deformity and secondary osteoarthritis. When indicated, treatment should interfere as little as possible with the child's psychologic and physical development.

The four basic goals of treatment are to eliminate hip irritability, restore and maintain a good range of hip motion, prevent femoral head extrusion and subluxation, and attain a spheric femoral head on healing.

Elimination of Hip Irritability

After the subchondral fracture, the synovium becomes inflamed and the hip irritable. The associated pain and muscle spasm lead to the restriction of motion followed by muscle contractures, especially of the adductor and iliopsoas muscles, and possible anterolateral extrusion or subluxation of the femoral head. Elimination of this irritability is always the first objective and is usually accomplished by rest and scheduled antiinflammatory medications. Non–weight bearing for brief periods may also help the symptoms of irritability, and crutches or other aids can be helpful if the child is able to use them.

Restoration and Maintenance of Motion

Generally, satisfactory range of motion in the hip returns as the hip irritability is eliminated, although residual stiffness may persist in some children. Physical therapy with passive and active range-of-motion exercises helps to restore motion, but gentle progressive abduction traction, especially at night, is occasionally required. To maintain hip motion, a program consisting of abduction and internal rotation stretching exercises may be helpful.

Regardless of the sphericity of the femoral head, almost all children with lateral pillar group C involvement show a slight but persistent loss of abduction and internal rotation due to mild coxa magna.

Prevention of Femoral Head Collapse

Extrusion or subluxation of the femoral head increases the risk of epiphyseal collapse and subsequent deformity. Radiographic evidence of extrusion is therefore a poor prognostic factor and an indication for treatment.

Attainment of Spheric Femoral Head

This goal requires a full understanding of the pathogenesis and prognostic factors associated with deformity of the femoral head as well as the appropriate management techniques.

FEMORAL VARUS DEROTATIONAL OSTEOTOMY

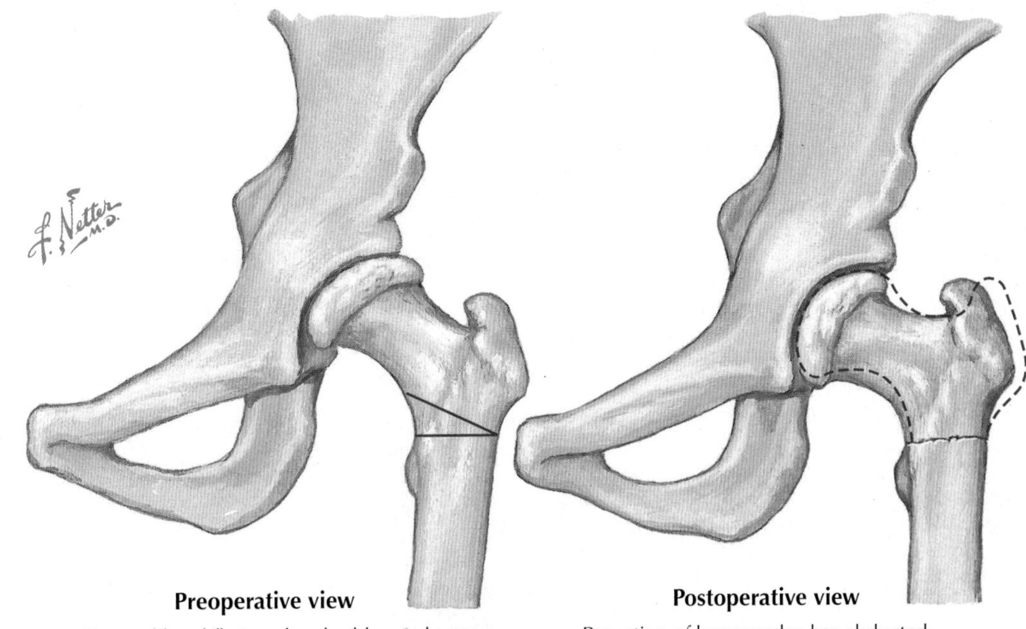

Preoperative view

Femoral head flattened and subluxated, protruding well outside lateral margin of acetabulum. Red lines indicate proposed osteotomy and wedge of bone to be resected.

Postoperative view

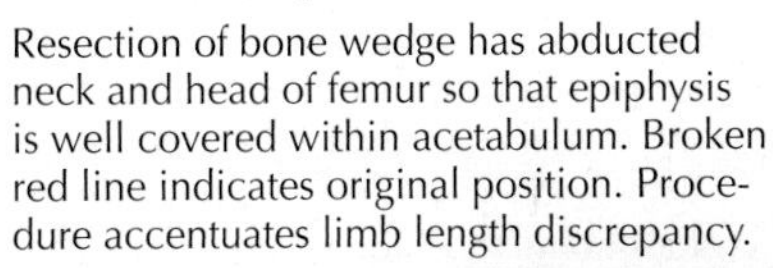

Resection of bone wedge has abducted neck and head of femur so that epiphysis is well covered within acetabulum. Broken red line indicates original position. Procedure accentuates limb length discrepancy.

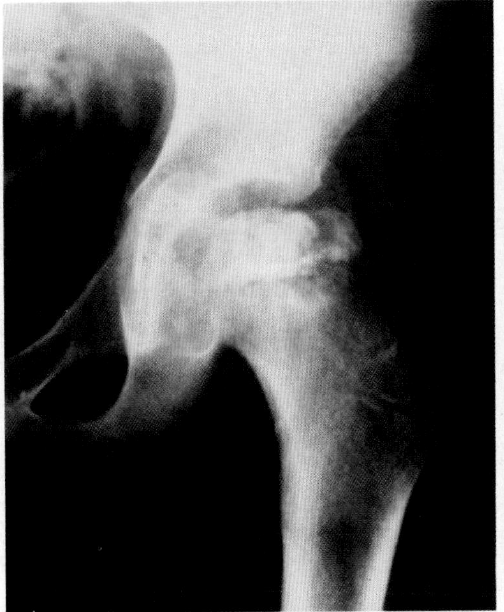

AP radiograph of 8-year-old boy shows Catterall group 2 (Salter-Thompson group A) involvement in left hip. Subluxation with lateral margin of acetabulum directly over area of resorption. Lateral margin of femoral head no longer provides support.

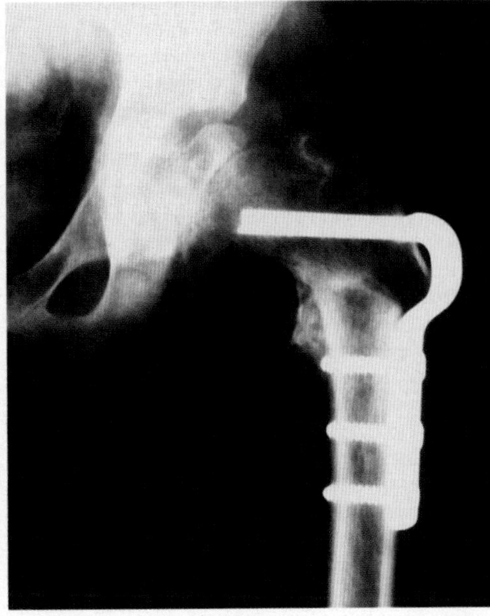

Three months after varus derotational osteotomy. AP radiograph shows subluxation corrected; lateral margin of femoral head within acetabulum and again provides support.

CONCEPTS OF CONTAINMENT

Until the 1960s, treatment for Legg-Calvé-Perthes disease was complete and prolonged bed rest—with or without traction or abduction of the involved limb—and the use of so-called weight-relieving devices. All affected children were treated, and treatment often lasted 2 to 4 years. Containment techniques have been devised to permit weight bearing while redirecting the compressive forces on the femoral head to assist in the healing and remodeling process. The currently accepted forms of management range from observation to surgery.

Observation

Appropriate treatment of all children who are younger than 6 years at clinical onset regardless of the extent of epiphyseal involvement is by observation only, provided there is no limitation of hip motion and no subluxation. Observation is also appropriate for children age 6 years or older with lateral pillar group A and some lateral pillar group B involvement who have a good range of hip motion and no radiographic evidence of femoral head extrusion or collapse.

Intermittent Symptomatic Treatment

Temporary or periodic bed rest and abduction stretching exercises can be used in conjunction with observation. Hip irritability with a temporary decrease in motion

LEGG-CALVÉ-PERTHES DISEASE (Continued)

often recurs during the subchondral fracture and resorption phases. If these symptoms persist and there is no radiographic evidence of femoral head extrusion, rest and protected weight bearing for 1 to 2 weeks sometimes may be necessary. Two or three recurrent episodes of irritability may indicate the need for a short period (1–2 months) of nonsurgical containment to decrease the risk of extrusion. Radiographs should be taken at 2- to 4-month intervals to ensure that the irritability is not due to early deformity of the femoral head.

Definitive Early Treatment

Nonsurgical or surgical containment of the femoral head early in the disease is indicated in children 6 years of age or older at clinical onset—possibly in girls age 5 years or older—who have lateral pillar group B or B/C border involvement or when femoral head extrusion is seen on the weight-bearing AP radiograph. Studies have shown that patients with lateral pillar group C changes have unfavorable outcomes even with surgical intervention, especially in the older child; therefore many advocate for no surgical treatment for these patients.

Use of containment techniques requires a good-to-full range of hip motion (especially abduction), no residual irritability, and a round or almost round femoral head. Containment methods, whether nonsurgical or surgical, appear to increase satisfactory results (mostly good and fair) by 16% to 20% compared with no treatment or natural history.

Nonsurgical containment refers to the use of abduction casts (Petrie) or occasionally an orthosis to abduct the involved limb and redirect the femoral head within the acetabulum (see Plate 2.36). The Petrie cast fixes the lower limbs in 30 to 40 degrees of abduction with an approximate 5-degree internal rotation. The cast provides continuous containment because it cannot be removed by either the child or the parents. Disadvantages include stiffness of the knee and ankle joints with adaptive articular changes, significant restriction in ambulation, frequent need for change and repair, and excessive weight. Petrie casts are now reserved for management after surgical adductor lengthening to improve and maintain motion in abduction, therefore "containing" the joint.

Abduction braces are lighter and less cumbersome than casts, but they are quite expensive. Also, because they are removable, compliance may not be consistent. Their use is now largely historical because purely nonoperative treatment has been shown to not be beneficial. The Atlanta Scottish Rite Children's Hospital brace and Salter stirrup provided temporary nonsurgical containment.

Surgical containment has three major advantages: (1) the period of restriction is less than 2 months, after which the child may gradually return to full activity; (2) the femoral head containment is permanent; and (3) the permanent improvement in containment continues to enhance remodeling of the healed femoral head long after the active phase of disease is over. Surgery does not alter the length of the disease process or provide a cure, but it does provide satisfactory results in the great majority of patients.

Treatment with femoral varus derotational osteotomy usually involves a varus angulation of the proximal femur, with or without rotation, to redirect the femoral head into the acetabulum (see Plate 2.37). The varus angulation should be no greater than 110 degrees but should allow containment of the epiphysis of the femoral head within a vertical (Perkin's) line drawn on the radiograph at the lateral margin of the acetabulum; some surgeons also recommend 10 to 15 degrees of internal rotation of the proximal segment. The osteotomy is usually held securely with threaded screws and a side plate or blade plate. Femoral osteotomy, although a technically less demanding procedure than innominate osteotomy, produces some inherent problems, mainly the increase in limb length discrepancy, potential coxa vara, and Trendelenburg gait. In addition, the metal fixation device should be removed and there is a small risk of fracture of the proximal femur through the screw holes after plate removal. The limb shortening associated with femoral osteotomy usually resolves in younger children and in patients who achieve satisfactory results.

INNOMINATE OSTEOTOMY

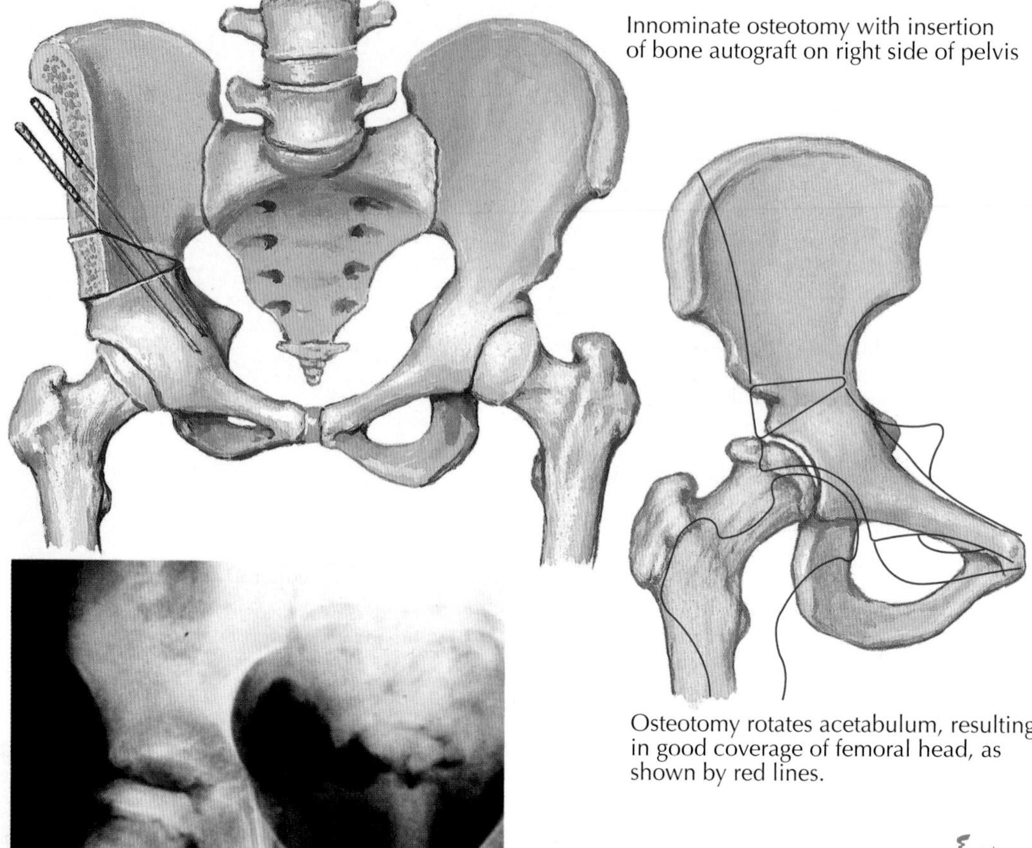
Innominate osteotomy with insertion of bone autograft on right side of pelvis
Osteotomy rotates acetabulum, resulting in good coverage of femoral head, as shown by red lines.
F. Netter M.D.

Preoperative anteroposterior radiograph shows flattening and protrusion of femoral head.

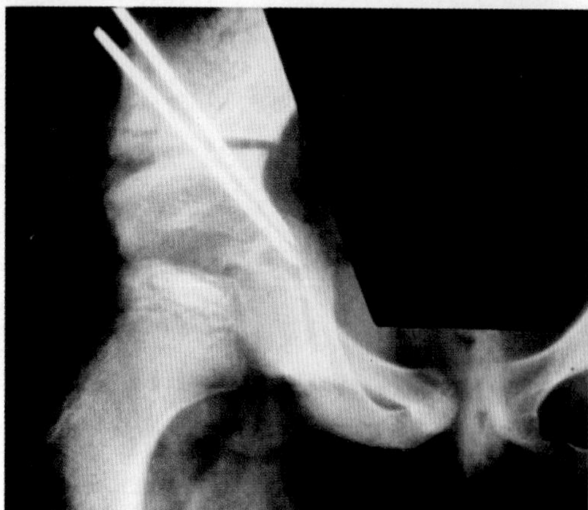

Good coverage of femoral head 6 weeks after innominate osteotomy

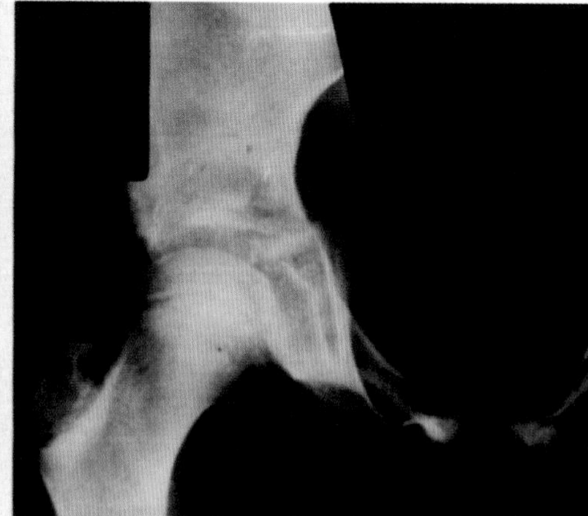

Healed, spherical femoral head (pins removed), 3 years after surgery

LEGG-CALVÉ-PERTHES DISEASE (Continued)

In 1962, Salter began to treat older children with more severe forms of the disease with an innominate osteotomy (see Plate 2.38), which is a technically more difficult procedure than femoral osteotomy. However, its advantages include better anterior and lateral coverage of the femoral head, no further shortening of the femoral neck (coxa breva), no increase in limb length discrepancy (it actually lengthens the lower limb by about 1 cm), and improvement of the Trendelenburg gait. Also, removal of fixation devices is easier and there is no risk of fracture of the proximal femur. The Salter innominate osteotomy can be combined with a proximal femoral osteotomy for additional containment and is frequently used in patients with moderate disease. The triple innominate osteotomy has also been used for containment, typically in patients who have more severe disease. Although even more technically demanding than the Salter innominate osteotomy, the triple innominate osteotomy provides significantly more containment when needed, without the disadvantages of the proximal femoral procedure (varus, limp, and Trendelenburg gait, and need for implant removal).

Late Surgical Management for Deformity

If a significant deformity prevents reduction of the femoral head into the acetabulum or remodeling after treatment with standard containment methods, an alternative must be considered. Several surgical procedures at least partially correct the various existing deformities, thereby alleviating the associated symptoms. These are salvage procedures that can alleviate symptoms but do not favorably alter the natural history of the disease.

Proximal femoral valgus osteotomy is employed when the radiograph demonstrates that hip joint congruency is better when the extended hip is adducted. The biomechanics of the hip joint are improved by this procedure in which the greater trochanter is moved distally as well as laterally, thus enhancing the strength of the abductor muscles as well as increasing the range of abduction of the lower limb.

Premature closure of the epiphysis of the femoral head can occur in advanced forms of the disease, resulting in shortening of the femoral neck and progressive overgrowth of the greater trochanter. Advancing the greater trochanter distally and laterally relieves muscle pain and decreases or eliminates the characteristic Trendelenburg gait. Lateral displacement of the greater trochanter can also decrease the pressure between the femoral head and the acetabulum and may minimize the risk of late degenerative osteoarthritis.

In addition to the proximal femoral valgus osteotomy, a *Chiari osteotomy* or *shelf osteotomy* may produce improved coverage of the femoral head and reduction of symptoms. Again, these are salvage procedures that are designed to reduce the short-term symptoms but unfortunately do not seem to alter the natural history of severe Legg-Calvé-Perthes disease, which ultimately leads to early arthrosis of the joint.

Late Surgical Management for Degenerative Osteoarthritis

Significant degenerative osteoarthritis in adults is usually managed by total hip replacement.

The prognosis for children with Legg-Calvé-Perthes disease is much better now than in the past. Active treatment is not always required, and many patients need only careful observation or intermittent symptomatic treatment. A variety of nonsurgical and surgical containment techniques are available that produce equally good long-term results. When surgical treatment is required, it restricts the child for a relatively short period of time, thus reducing the potential for psychologic problems.

Further studies will concentrate more on the etiology of Legg-Calvé-Perthes disease as well as on pharmacologic treatment options. Several animal studies in recent years have shown potential promise in bisphosphonate and bone morphogenic protein therapy, yet more research will be needed to determine the clinical efficacy and safety of these drugs in the treatment of Legg-Calvé-Perthes disease. Only greater understanding of the disease can provide the means for eliminating it or significantly altering its course.

INNOMINATE OSTEOTOMY (CONTINUED)

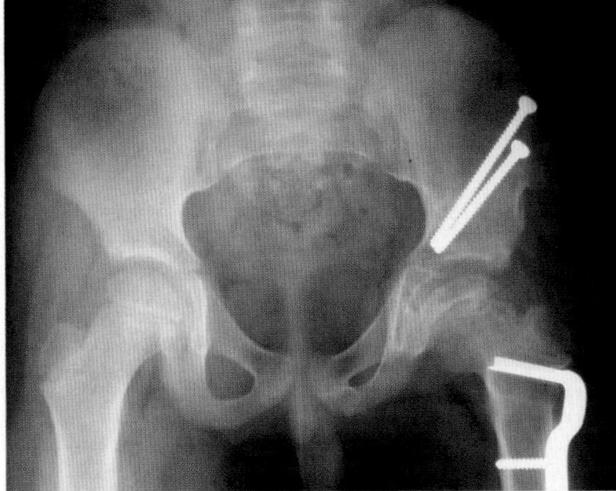

AP pelvis radiograph of an 8-year-old child 1 year after Salter innominate osteotomy in combination with femoral varus osteotomy. The femoral head is contained nicely, and femoral head remains spherical.

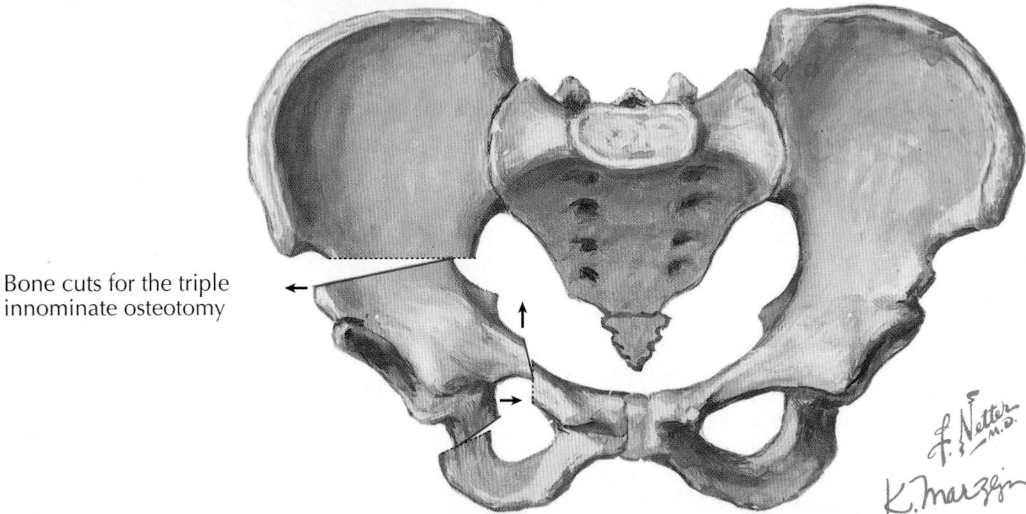

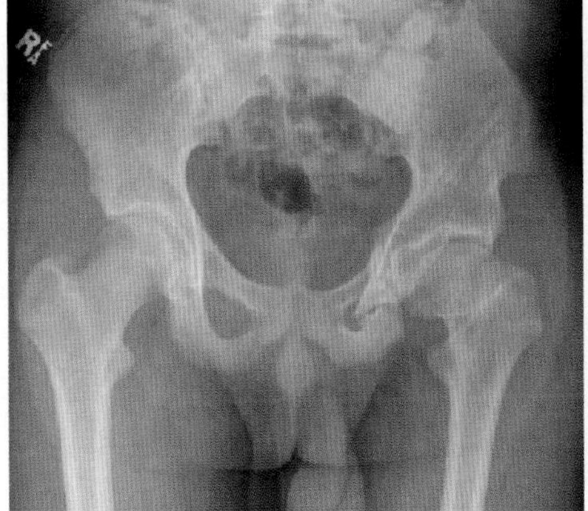

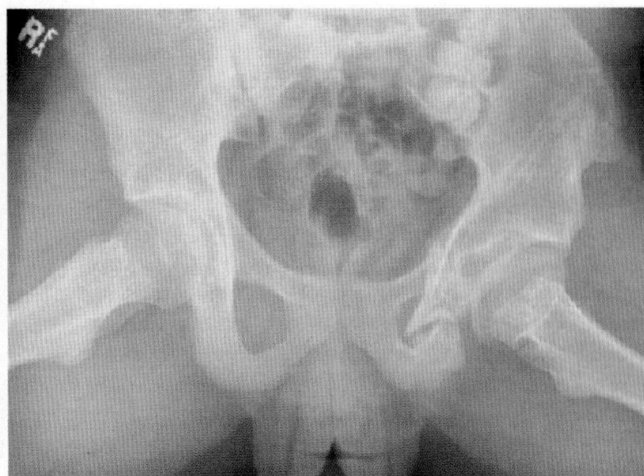

AP and frog-leg lateral views of the pelvis of a 12-year-old boy 5 years after triple innominate osteotomy for Legg-Calvé-Perthes disease of the left hip (lateral pillar group B/C border at presentation). The femoral head was contained and remains aspherically congruent. Note the ischial osteotomy fibrous union that remains asymptomatic.

Slipped Capital Femoral Epiphysis

Slipped capital femoral epiphysis (SCFE) refers to the displacement of the epiphysis of the femoral head. It occurs most commonly in boys 10 to 17 years of age (average age at onset is 12 years). The initial examination reveals bilateral involvement in about one-third of patients, but patients with unilateral involvement do have a risk of a subsequent slip on the contralateral side depending on patient age and etiology of the slip.

The etiology of SCFE is unclear, although various traumatic, inflammatory, and endocrine factors have been proposed. For example, the position of the growth plate of the proximal femur normally changes from horizontal to oblique during preadolescence and adolescence. Thus the weight increase that occurs during the adolescent growth spurt puts extra strain on the growth plate.

The disorder is often accompanied by rapid growth and is sometimes associated with adiposogenital dystrophy, a condition characterized by obesity and deficient gonadal development. These findings suggest an endocrine basis for the skeletal problem. The major complications of SCFE are avascular necrosis, chondrolysis, femoroacetabular impingement, and, later, degenerative osteoarthritis.

Clinical Manifestations. The severity and onset of symptoms reflect the three categories of SCFE. Most common is the stable slip (>90% of cases), which causes persistent pain referable to the hip or distal medial thigh and often as far as the knee. These patients are still able to weight-bear either with or without assistive devices. In some patients, the pain is restricted to the area of the vastus medialis muscle and the slip itself is overlooked. Limp, pain, and loss of hip motion are the other usual presenting manifestations. The most important diagnostic finding is the loss of internal rotation. This is easily detected on examination because, as the hip is flexed, it rolls into external rotation and abduction (termed *obligate external rotation*); restricted internal rotation becomes more pronounced as the slip increases.

An *unstable slip* (<5% of patients) produces the sudden onset of pain severe enough to prevent weight bearing even with aids. Patients usually report minimal or no previous symptoms. There may or may not be a traumatic inciting event.

Patients with a third type of slip first experience a persistent aching in the hip, thigh, or knee and sometimes a limp that is the result of a stable slip. Subsequent trauma—even minor—may cause an unstable slip superimposed on the chronic slip. The unstable slip is heralded by sudden, severe pain.

Radiographic Findings. SCFE produces classic radiographic features. In the earliest stages, there is a widening of the epiphyseal line (representing the growth plate). An AP radiograph of a normal hip shows the epiphysis of the femoral head projecting above and lateral to the superior border of the femoral neck. A slip must be suspected if a straight (Klein) line drawn up the lateral surface of the femoral neck does not touch the femoral head. Because the AP view does not always reveal the initial slip, which is usually posterior, a frog-leg radiograph is essential for the diagnosis.

A three-grade classification of slipped capital femoral epiphysis is helpful in the radiographic evaluation. Grade I refers to displacement of the epiphysis up to one-third the width of the femoral neck. Grade II represents a slip greater than one-third but less than one-half of the width of the neck. Grade III includes slips of greater than one-half of the width of the neck. The most common radiographic measurement of slip severity is the Southwick slip angle. This is the angle between the femoral shaft and a line perpendicular to the femoral epiphysis on the frog-leg radiograph; this is subtracted from the measurement of the normal hip (or 10 is subtracted if both hips are involved). Slips are then graded as mild (0–30 degrees), moderate (30–60 degrees), or severe (>60 degrees). More severe slips have been shown to have a worse prognosis.

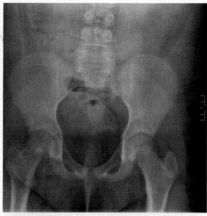

Physical Examination and Classification of Slipped Capital Femoral Epiphysis

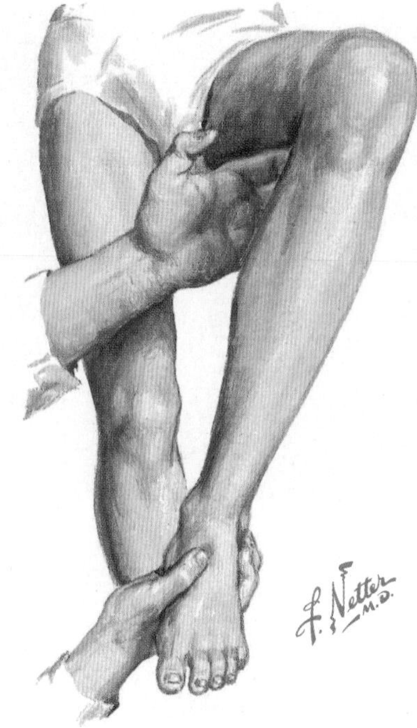

Best diagnostic in physical examination. With patient supine, as thigh is flexed it rolls into external rotation and abduction.

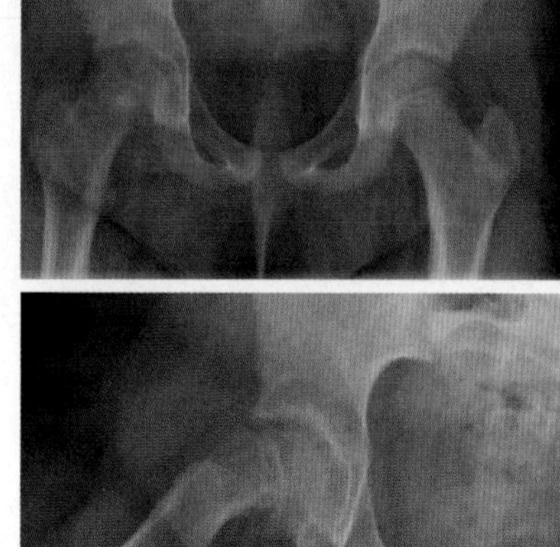

Slipped capital femoral epiphysis may present as subtle initial radiographic findings on an AP pelvis radiograph as the slip typically occurs in the sagittal plane. Frog-leg lateral radiographs are always indicated when this disorder is suspected.

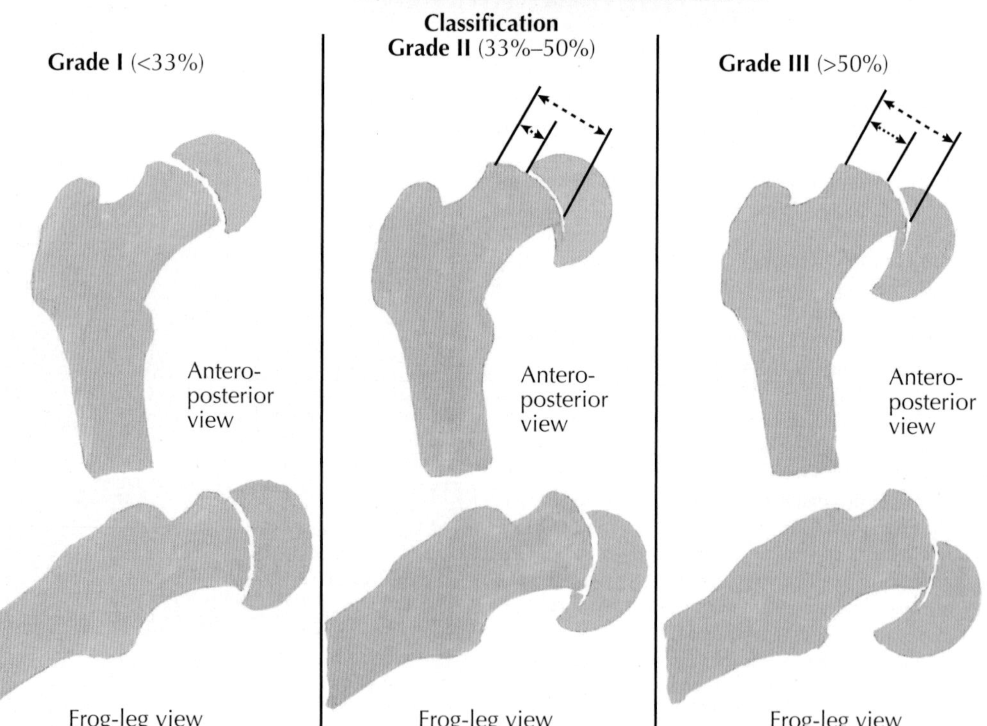

Slipped Capital Femoral Epiphysis (Continued)

Treatment. The primary goals of treatment are to stop displacement and keep the proximal femoral deformity to a minimum while maintaining a close to normal range of hip motion and to delay the onset of osteoarthritis.

Stable Slip. Bed rest and urgent in situ fixation is the gold standard for treatment of the stable slip. Placement of a single partially threaded cannulated screw under image intensification is the most advocated and simplest technique with the lowest complication rate. Postoperatively, patients can bear weight as tolerated with aids as needed for comfort for around 4 to 6 weeks' time. They can then progress to activities as tolerated. Symptoms usually resolve soon after screw stabilization of the physis.

Radiographic follow-up is necessary to ensure physeal closure (usually between 9 and 12 months postoperatively) and for surveillance of complications (avascular necrosis) and contralateral disease.

Unstable Slip. Urgent in situ fixation of the slip with one to two partially or fully threaded screws remains the gold standard of treatment for an unstable slip. Forceful attempts at reduction should not be attempted because they may lead to avascular necrosis of the femoral head, which is a greater threat to the hip than incomplete reduction. However, many argue to perform a gentle reduction maneuver prior to pinning to help improve deformity. Urgent surgical dislocation with visualization of the femoral head vasculature has been advocated by some authors to treat the unstable slip, especially with severe deformity. It is much more invasive and technically demanding but can provide near-normalization of the proximal femoral anatomy with a similar risk of avascular necrosis as from the deformity itself.

Incorrect placement of screws is the most common error in surgical management. Because of the minor but real risk of segmented avascular necrosis, screws are placed to avoid the weight-bearing area of the femoral head. The best possible construct is a single screw placed across the proximal femoral physis such that the tip of the screw lies in the center of the femoral head in both the AP and lateral radiograph. Five threads should cross the physis if possible to avoid the epiphysis growing off the physis.

In a grade III slip, visible on both AP and frog-leg radiographs, the epiphysis and metaphysis overlap only 25% of the width of the femoral neck, leaving very little room for a screw to cross from the femoral neck to the head. Screw placement through the anterior aspect of the base of the neck and directing them posteromedially allows them to engage the head without leaving the bone. This technique is applicable to slips of any grade. Care must be taken in more severe slips to avoid leaving the head of the screw in a position too anterior that creates impingement on the acetabulum.

Pinning is the initial treatment of choice for all grades of slip. After closure of the growth plate, reconstructive procedures such as intertrochanteric osteotomy may be performed if needed. Osteotomy of the femoral neck is never indicated because it often leads to avascular necrosis. The modified Dunn procedure is also advocated by some, either in the setting of severe, acute slip or as an option for severe residual deformity. This procedure involves a trochanteric osteotomy for surgical hip dislocation, followed by mobilization of the femoral epiphysis and resection of reactive metaphyseal callus. Femoral osteoplasty may also help late symptoms after physeal closure. This can be accomplished through a surgical dislocation with either a mini-open or arthroscopic approach.

Chondrolysis. Treatment comprises traction, range-of-motion exercises, and use of antiinflammatory medications, which help decrease joint reaction and increase hip motion. After resolution, range-of-motion exercises and walking with a crutch should be continued for a prolonged period. After the initial loss of articular cartilage, there may be a gradual improvement in the joint space and hip movement may improve slightly. Fortunately, chondrolysis has been seen far less frequently since the advent of intraoperative fluoroscopy because inadvertent pin or screw penetration of the joint is the most likely cause.

Pin Fixation in Slipped Capital Femoral Epiphysis

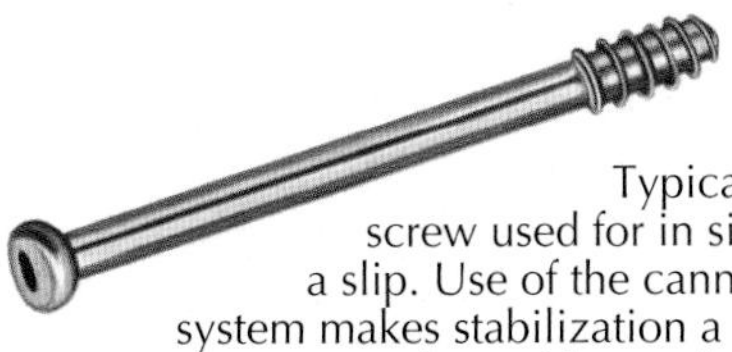

Typical cannulated screw used for in situ fixation of a slip. Use of the cannulated screw system makes stabilization a percutaneous procedure with very low morbidity.

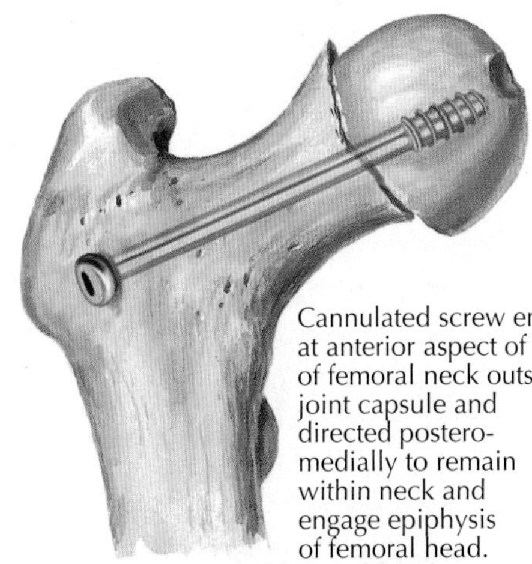

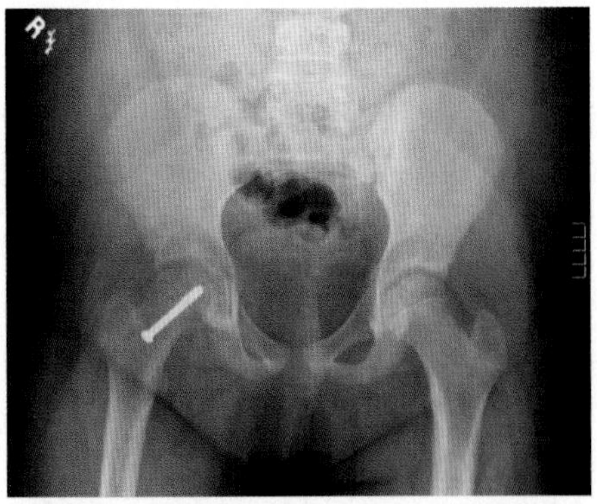

Cannulated screw enters at anterior aspect of base of femoral neck outside joint capsule and directed posteromedially to remain within neck and engage epiphysis of femoral head.

AP pelvis radiograph of a 10-year-old girl following in situ screw fixation of a right slip.

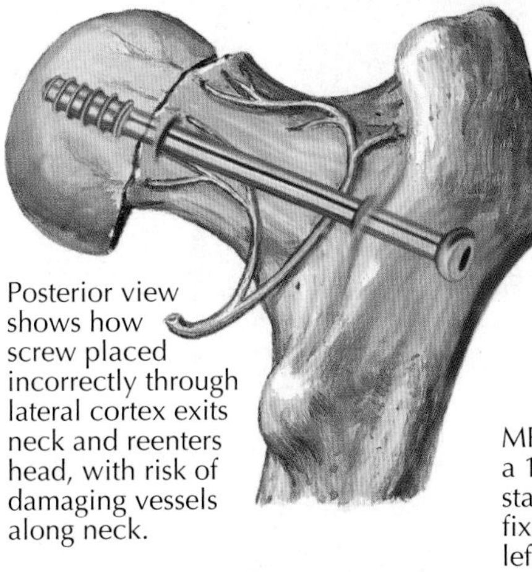

Posterior view shows how screw placed incorrectly through lateral cortex exits neck and reenters head, with risk of damaging vessels along neck.

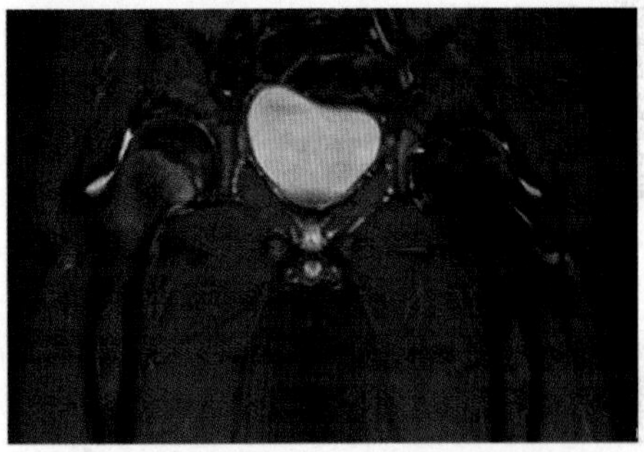

MR image of a 13-year-old boy status post in situ fixation of the left hip (metallic artifact signifies screw) with left hip pain and a limp similar to his contralateral hip. Initial radiographs of the right hip were normal. MRI reveals signal changes about the physis signifying a very early slip, which was treated with in situ fixation.

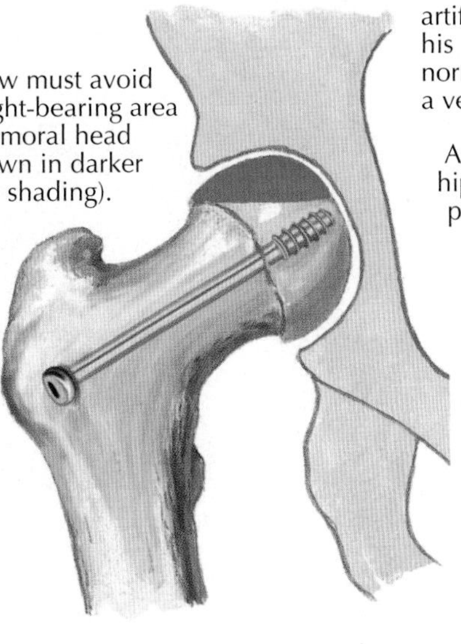

Screw must avoid weight-bearing area of femoral head (shown in darker blue shading).

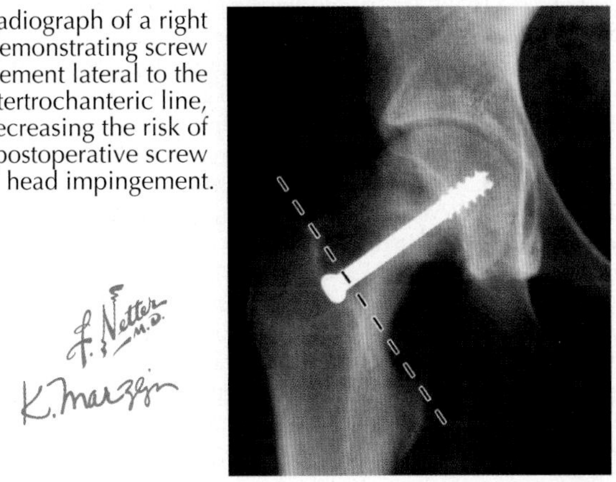

AP radiograph of a right hip demonstrating screw placement lateral to the intertrochanteric line, decreasing the risk of postoperative screw head impingement.

F. Netter M.D.
K. Marzen

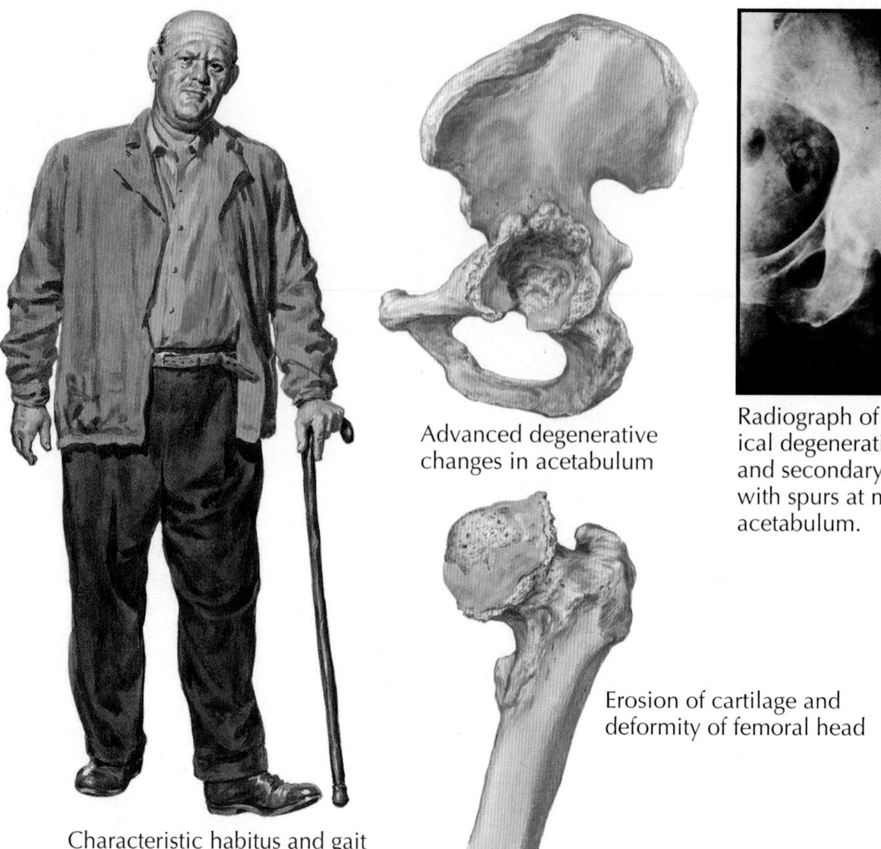

Hip Joint Involvement in Osteoarthritis

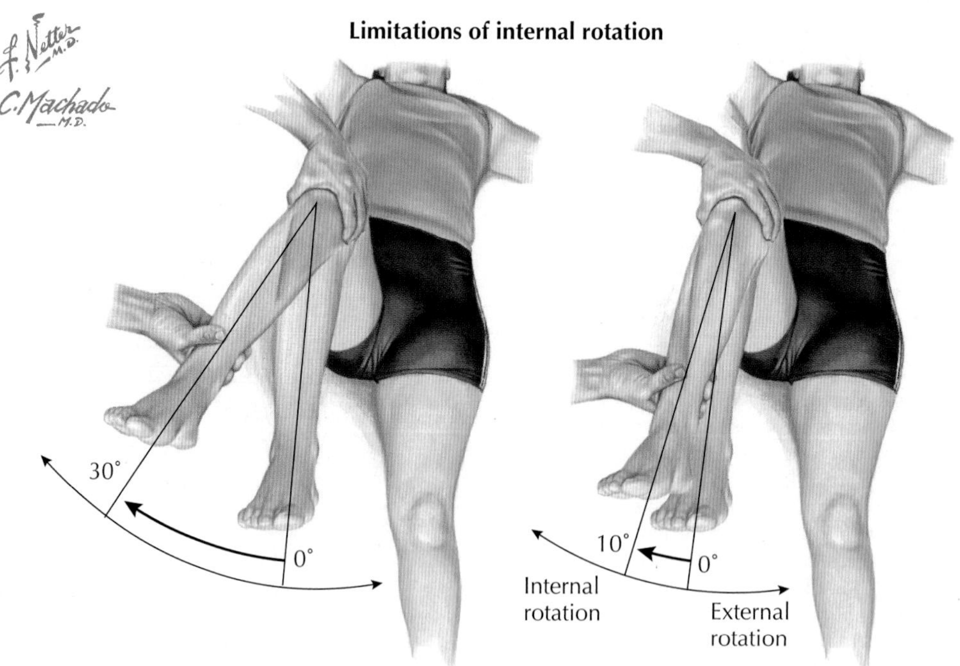

Loss of internal rotation with hip flexed is a sensitive and easy test of hip arthritis.

Osteoarthritis (OA) of the hip is a common problem in the United States and worldwide. As many as one in four Americans may experience OA in their lifetime. With the continued growth of the elderly population in the United States and the desire for these patients to continue an active lifestyle, OA is a growing medical and economic concern. Appropriate management of OA, both medically and surgically, requires the physician to be able to accurately diagnose the condition.

The typical patient with primary OA of the hip presents in middle age or later. Difficulty with gait and walking distances is often a common chief complaint. Pain can vary in location and severity, although groin pain is the classic location. Pain typically worsens with increased activity and is relieved with rest. Often, patients report accompanied stiffness in the affected joint, especially after periods of inactivity. Stiffness that is alleviated by movement is common in the early stages of OA. As the OA progresses to the more severe stages, pain may be present even at rest or at night. Other common complaints include some limitations in the ability to perform activities of daily living. Loss of flexion and internal rotation of the hip may make putting on shoes and socks difficult, for example.

The differential diagnosis of hip OA can be wide. Some such examples include avascular necrosis of the femoral head, which would closely mimic the symptoms of OA. Trochanteric bursitis often presents as localized lateral hip pain reproduced by palpation. Lumbar stenosis may cause radicular pain that radiates to the groin. Lumbar back pain often presents as pain localized to the buttock. Finally tumors of the lumbar spine, pelvis, or upper thigh may cause pain in this general region.

Radiographs usually confirm the diagnosis the diagnosis of OA. Joint space narrowing, sclerosis, and osteophyte formation are the hallmark features of OA. Occasionally, the etiology of hip pain cannot be elucidated, even after history, physical examination, and radiographs. In these cases, MRI of the hip or a diagnostic hip injection under fluoroscopic guidance can assist in the diagnosis.

Treatment of OA of the hip needs to be individualized to the particular patient. Conditions such as gastric ulcers, cardiac disease, and renal disease, as well as patient expectations, must be considered. Nonoperative treatment includes patient education, acetaminophen or nonsteroidal antiinflammatory drugs (NSAIDs), physical therapy for muscle strengthening, activity modification, and the use of ambulatory aids. Patients who have severe pain unresponsive to nonoperative treatment are candidates for total hip arthroplasty. Total hip arthroplasty often dramatically reduces pain and improves function, but the decision to proceed has to be made with the understanding of the risks involved.

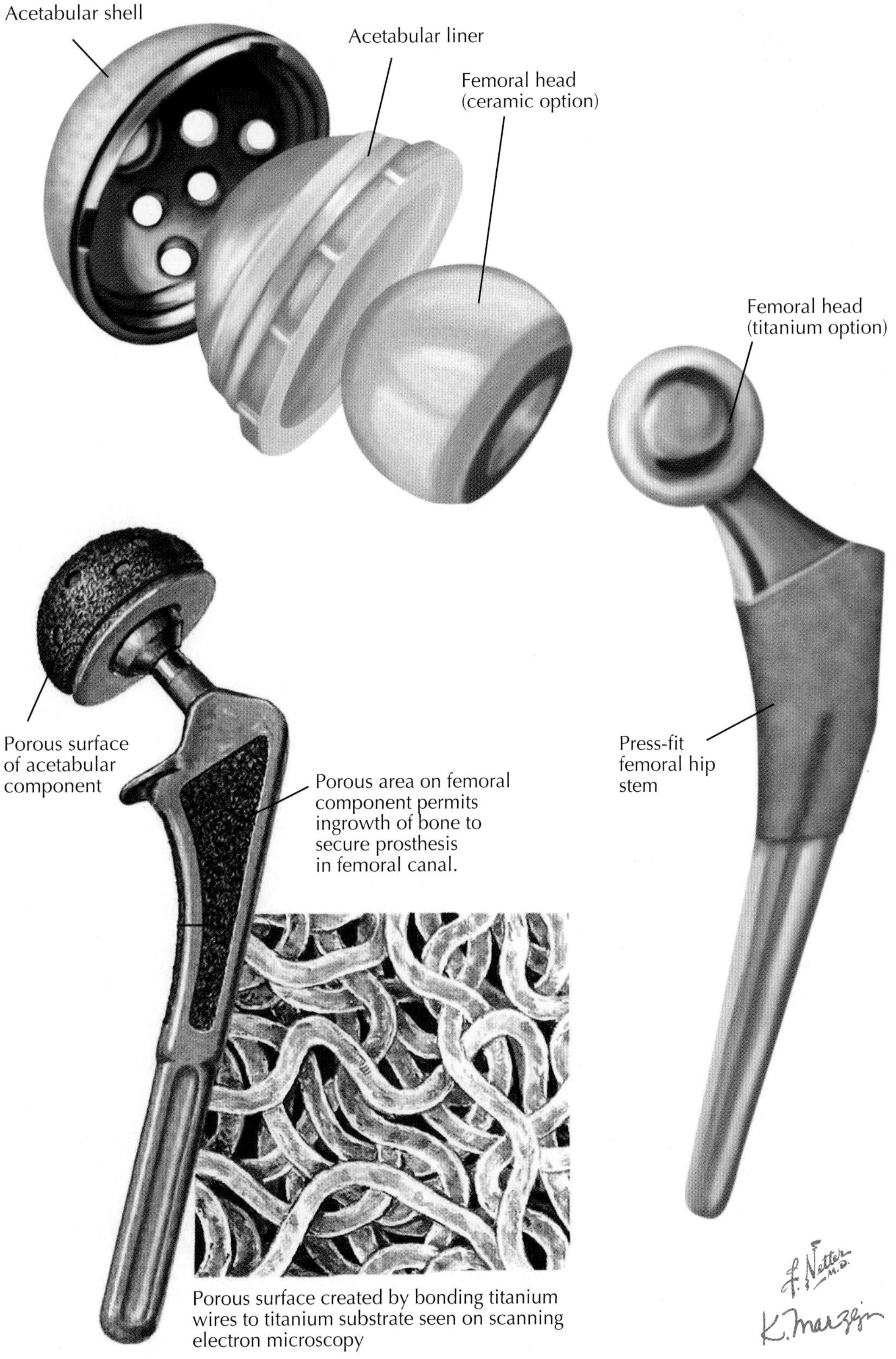

Porous surface created by bonding titanium wires to titanium substrate seen on scanning electron microscopy

Total Hip Replacement: Prostheses

Arthroplasty, or surgical reconstruction of the joints, has revolutionized the treatment of crippling diseases such as osteoarthritis and rheumatoid arthritis, which destroy the joint's smooth cartilage surfaces and lead to painful, decreased motion. Relief of pain and improved hip function are dramatic advantages of reconstruction procedures. Hip arthroplasty benefits not only the older patient; total hip replacement and other procedures using prostheses also now permit young and middle-aged patients with congenital, developmental, arthritic, traumatic, malignant, or metabolic hip disorders to lead active and productive lives.

Treatment with a total hip prosthesis must always be weighed against nonsurgical treatment and other more conservative surgical procedures that do not sacrifice as much bone. Appropriate selection of patients is essential.

Hip prostheses must function under high mechanical loads for many years, and the strength of materials used is critical. The technique of total hip replacement began as an improvement on the placement of molds or films between degenerated joint surfaces (interpositional arthroplasty). In 1923 Smith-Petersen used a Pyrex cup to cover and reshape an arthritic femoral head in a technique called mold arthroplasty. This brittle cup broke under stress, but the technique led to the development of interpositional molds made of a stronger material, Vitallium, a noncorrosive and relatively inert cobalt-chromium alloy.

In the early 1960s, Sir John Charnley developed the technique of low-friction total hip arthroplasty, which is still the standard against which all newer variations must be measured. From his work, two important principles have stood the test of time and govern all subsequent modifications. The first is the principle of low friction; that is, a bearing of a highly polished metal alloy against ultra-high-molecular-weight polyethylene. The second is the principle of rigid fixation of components to bone. For the first, he advocated a small-diameter (22.25 mm) bearing and, for the second, the use of methyl methacrylate (acrylic) cement to act as a grouting material by forming an interlocking mechanical bond with the trabecular bone.

Femoral and acetabular components are made in a variety of sizes, and it is possible to mix and match femoral stems with acetabular cups of different systems. All new implants have detachable heads that allow adjustment of the neck length of the prosthesis, making it much easier to correct and equalize leg length.

New designs in total hip prostheses include implants that do not require acrylic cement for fixation to bone. The metal backing of the acetabular cup and the sides of the femoral stem have pores allowing the ingrowth of bone trabeculae to produce a "biologic fixation" of prosthesis to bone. However, because good bone quality is needed for implant stability and maximal bone ingrowth, this type of prosthesis is not indicated for all patients.

Newer prostheses are currently in use that allow for faster and more complete bony ingrowth. The surface has a higher porosity and pore sizes that are more similar to normal trabecular bone. These devices have the potential to increase the longevity of total hip replacement; however, long-term data are not yet available.

TRABECULAR BONE AND TRABECULAR METAL SLIDE

In the United States, porous ingrowth prosthetic implant total hip arthroplasty is the gold standard. Cemented prostheses are currently used only in the elderly or in patients with poor bone quality.

Total Hip Replacement: Steps 1 to 3

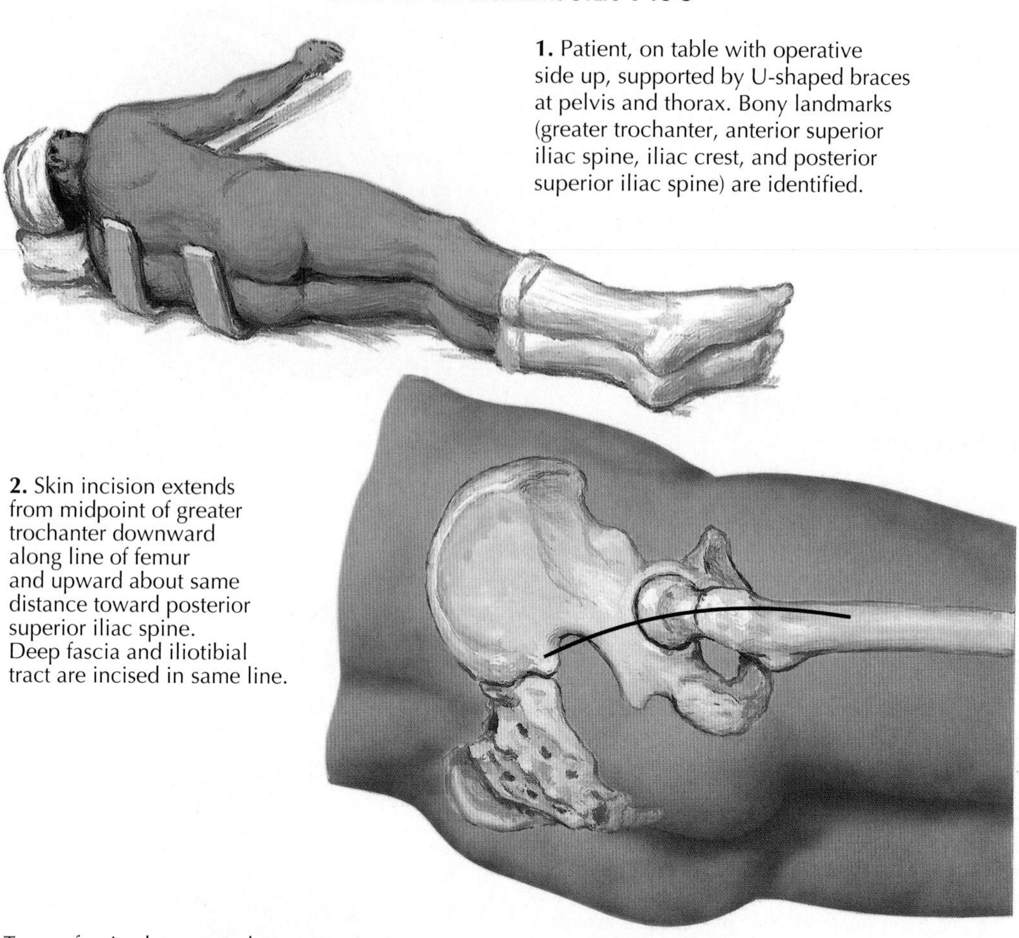

1. Patient, on table with operative side up, supported by U-shaped braces at pelvis and thorax. Bony landmarks (greater trochanter, anterior superior iliac spine, iliac crest, and posterior superior iliac spine) are identified.

2. Skin incision extends from midpoint of greater trochanter downward along line of femur and upward about same distance toward posterior superior iliac spine. Deep fascia and iliotibial tract are incised in same line.

Tensor fasciae latae muscle
Iliotibial tract
Vastus lateralis muscle
Gluteus medius muscle
Iliac crest
Gluteus maximus muscle
Piriformis muscle
Sciatic nerve
Quadratus femoris muscle
Inferior gemellus muscle
Obturator internus muscle
Superior gemellus muscle
Short external rotator muscles

3. Fibers of gluteus maximus muscle separated by blunt dissection, its femoral insertion partially detached. Piriformis and short external rotator muscles are exposed with care to avoid sciatic nerve (usually obscured by fat).

Total Hip Replacement: Technique

The procedure for total hip replacement begins with preoperative planning, which includes a complete medical work-up of the patient to identify any existing health problems. A rheumatologist or internist often works with the orthopedic surgeon in planning the appropriate medical therapy. The rehabilitation program should also be thoroughly discussed with the patient.

The goal of preoperative planning is to create a graphic representation of a joint that will provide optimal function. The biomechanical principles that govern movement, weight bearing, and impact must be observed. The prosthetic components must be selected carefully to maximize fit and function for each individual.

Lateral and AP radiographs are taken to determine the bony anatomy and the size of the femoral canal. Then clear plastic templates of each prosthesis are placed on the radiographs to choose the correct size. At this time, any existing deformities must be taken into consideration. Many patients have a limb length discrepancy, usually a shortening of the painful limb, owing to superior displacement of the femoral head resulting from destruction of the joint space. This can be corrected with resection of the femur at the appropriate level and use of an implant with the proper neck length. If a flexion contracture of the hip exists, a more extensive dissection of the soft tissues is necessary.

The acetabulum must be evaluated for dysplasia or deficiency; in such cases, reconstruction with bone grafts, screws, or special devices is carried out (see Plate 2.49). Custom-designed implants are required if standard-sized implants are inadequate. Patients with congenital dislocation of the hip may need extra-small implants with special angles of the femoral neck. Long-stemmed prostheses are often needed to extend past fracture sites or defect sites in the femur. If a cementless implant is used, it must fit tightly into the femoral canal and pelvis.

One of the disadvantages of the posterior approach is a historically higher rate of dislocation. However, with newer techniques—larger-diameter femoral heads and capsular repair before skin closure—this has largely been mitigated.

Total Hip Replacement: Steps 4 to 8

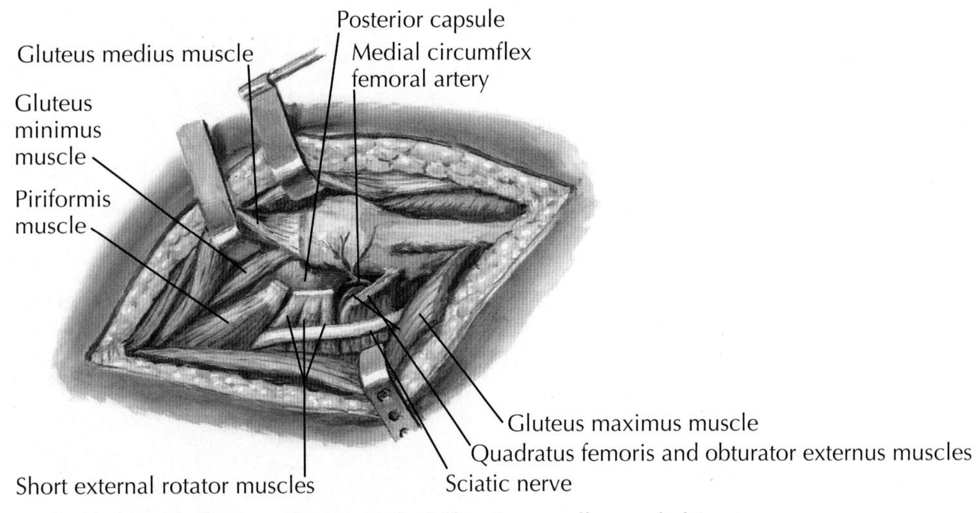

4. Gluteus medius muscle retracted; piriformis, gemellus, and obturator internus muscles divided close to their insertion into greater trochanter. Quadratus femoris and obturator externus muscles partially or totally detached. Medial circumflex femoral artery identified and cauterized.

F. Netter M.D.
K. Marzen

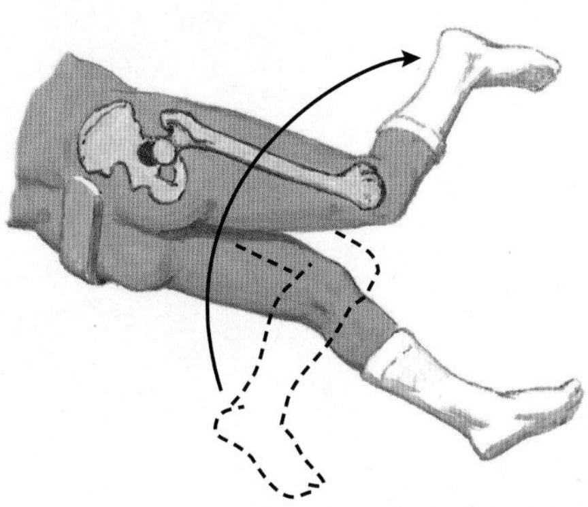

5. T-shaped incision made in joint capsule with care to protect sciatic nerve. Hip dislocated by full internal rotation of limb in flexion and adduction.

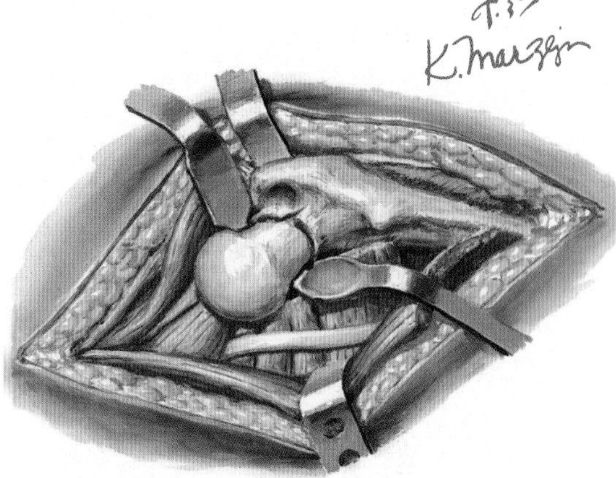

6. Fully exposed femoral head and neck are supported with superior and inferior retractors.

7. Line for cutting femoral neck determined by placing trial prosthesis on femur and matching its center of rotation with that of femoral head. Femur marked with osteotome at distal margin of prosthetic collar.

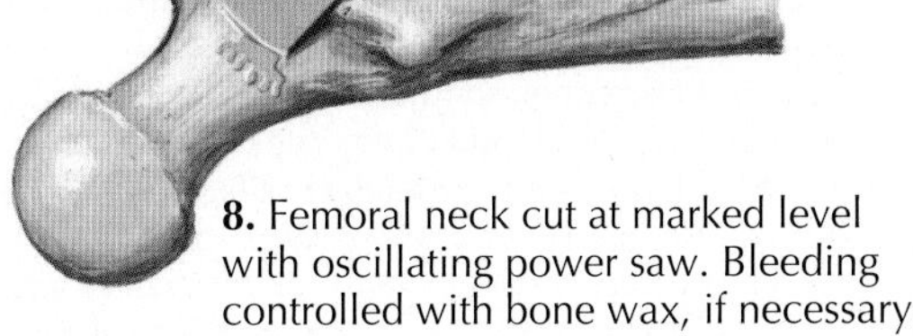

8. Femoral neck cut at marked level with oscillating power saw. Bleeding controlled with bone wax, if necessary.

Total Hip Replacement: Technique (Continued)

The direct lateral approach is another common approach to hip replacement. In this approach, the abductors are split to gain access to the hip joint. This historically allowed for a lower rate of dislocation but with a higher rate of Trendelenburg gait after the surgery because the abductors are violated.

A mini anterior approach to the hip has become more popular. This approach is a true muscle-sparing approach. Proponents of this approach state that because no muscles are cut, patients recover more quickly from their total hip arthroplasty. However, this has not yet been proven in clinical studies.

PREPARATION

The patient is placed in the lateral decubitus position (supine if an anterior approach is used). A number of anatomic exposures can be used for total hip replacement, each of which has advantages and disadvantages. The posterior, or modified Moore, approach is commonly used for reconstruction of osteoarthritic hips. It allows quick and safe access to the joint without interfering with the abductor mechanism.

The limb is prepared with iodine solution and draped to allow free movement. The bony landmarks are marked on the skin. The anterior and posterior superior iliac spine, greater trochanter, iliac crest, and shaft of the femur are all palpable.

INCISION

A typical incision is centered on the greater trochanter and curves gently posteriorly, in line proximally with the fibers of the gluteus maximus muscle (see Plate 2.44). Distally, the incision overlies the femoral shaft. An incision is made in the fascia lata and the fascia over the gluteus maximus muscle. The fibers of the gluteus maximus muscle are separated proximally by blunt incision, without denervating the muscle. Care must be taken to protect the underlying sciatic nerve. The hip is internally rotated, and the piriformis tendon is identified.

TOTAL HIP REPLACEMENT: STEPS 9 TO 12

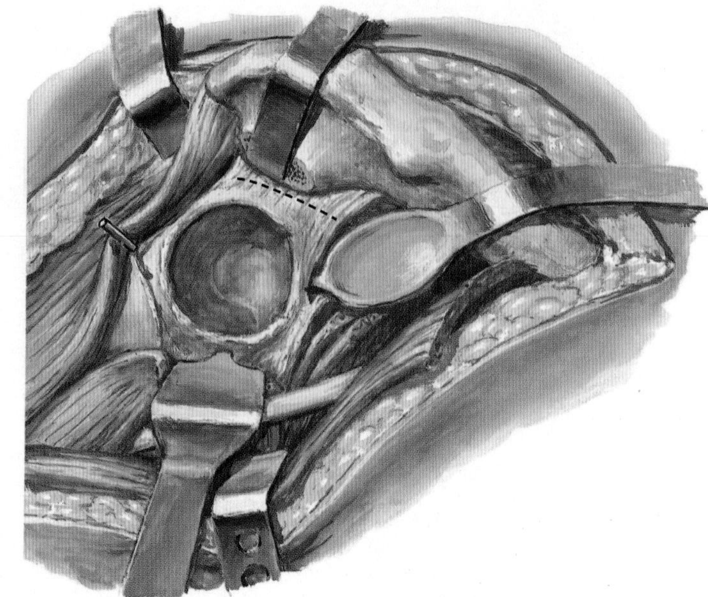

9. To expose acetabulum, femur with cut neck retracted anteriorly. Gluteus medius and minimis muscles retracted with pin. Posterior capsule and short external rotator muscles retracted with spiked retractor; inferior retractor placed under transverse acetabular ligament. Anterior capsule may also be cut to increase exposure.

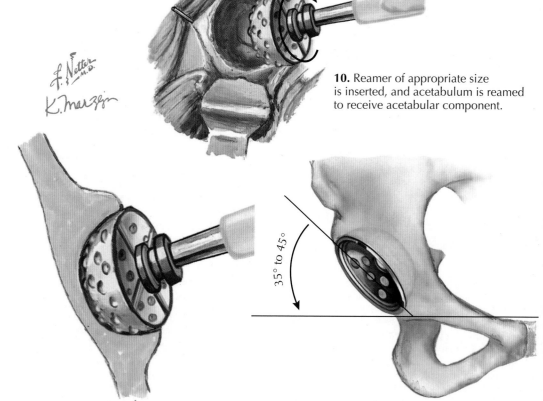

10. Reamer of appropriate size is inserted, and acetabulum is reamed to receive acetabular component.

11. Reamers of increasing size are used to enlarge acetabulum to fit acetabular cup of preselected size.

35° to 45°

12. Final position of cup is 35- to 45-degree lateral inclination and 15-degree anteversion.

TOTAL HIP REPLACEMENT: TECHNIQUE (Continued)

DISLOCATION OF HIP AND FEMORAL TRANSECTION

A retractor is passed above the piriformis and beneath the gluteus medius and minimus muscles to delineate the superior hip capsule; another is placed deeply at the proximal border of the quadratus femoris muscle to outline the inferior joint capsule (see Plate 2.45). The piriformis and short external rotator muscles are removed from their insertions into the trochanter and stripped back to expose the posterior hip capsule, which is incised.

An anterior capsulotomy is optional. It facilitates exposure of the acetabulum and improves mobility of the femur and is desirable when the hip deformity is severe or exposure is inhibited for other reasons. In such cases, it may be helpful to expose its femoral insertion in the interval between the tensor fasciae latae and the gluteus medius muscles before making the posterior exposure.

An alternative approach is to remove the greater trochanter and reflect the attached gluteus maximus and minimus muscles superiorly for better exposure of the acetabulum. The trochanter and attached abductor muscles are turned back and held with Steinmann pins placed in the ilium, and the superolateral capsule is reflected.

After capsulotomy, the hip is ready for dislocation; it is flexed, internally rotated, and adducted to bring the femoral head and acetabulum into view. The limb is kept in internal rotation, and the insertions of the quadratus femoris muscle and the inferior capsule are incised and reflected so that the lesser trochanter can be visualized. The psoas tendon is identified but not cut. The surgeon is now ready to plan the femoral neck osteotomy.

The trial prosthesis is laid on the femur to check that the implant's center of rotation coincides with that of the femoral head. Existing deformities of the head and neck should be corrected. Measurements upward from the lesser trochanter should be recorded for use in determining the level of the osteotomy, the desired level of the center of motion of the prosthetic femoral head,

Total Hip Replacement: Steps 13 to 18

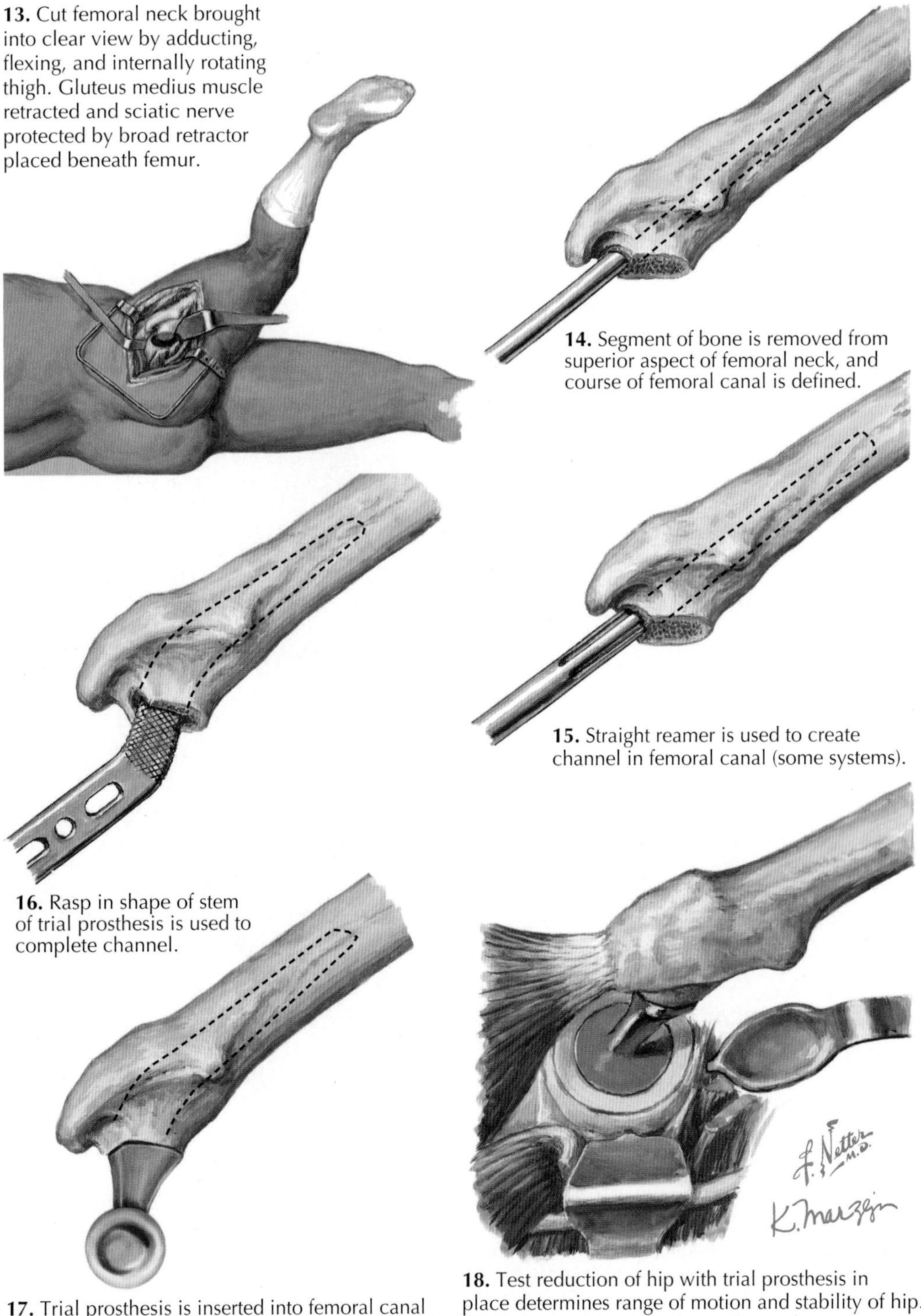

13. Cut femoral neck brought into clear view by adducting, flexing, and internally rotating thigh. Gluteus medius muscle retracted and sciatic nerve protected by broad retractor placed beneath femur.

14. Segment of bone is removed from superior aspect of femoral neck, and course of femoral canal is defined.

15. Straight reamer is used to create channel in femoral canal (some systems).

16. Rasp in shape of stem of trial prosthesis is used to complete channel.

17. Trial prosthesis is inserted into femoral canal to ensure fit (its collar flush with cut surface of femoral neck).

18. Test reduction of hip with trial prosthesis in place determines range of motion and stability of hip. If joint is too tight or too loose, femoral component with shorter or longer neck required.

Total Hip Replacement: Technique (Continued)

and the degree of offset. The transection line is marked on the neck of the femur, and a smooth cut is made with an oscillating saw.

ACETABULAR COMPONENT

The femur is retracted anteriorly to expose the acetabulum (see Plate 2.46). Unrestricted exposure of the acetabulum is the key to easy reaming and positioning of the prosthesis. Further exposure is obtained by placing a retractor posteriorly into the ischium (which also protects the sciatic nerve from injury during reaming) and another retractor inferiorly beneath the transverse acetabular ligament. The acetabulum is reamed in a medial direction to remove osteophytes and to define the true medial wall. Larger reamers are then used until the appropriate size is obtained. Trial acetabular cups are inserted, and the one with the best fit is selected. The trial cup must be positioned in the proper degrees of anteversion and of lateral inclination with the horizontal plane. Generally, the lateral inclination should be 35 to 45 degrees and anteversion should be 15 to 30 degrees. A porous ingrowth component of the appropriate size is then impacted into the acetabulum. Generally, the size of the acetabular component is 1 to 2 mm larger than the last reamer used, so that a "press fit" is obtained. One or two screws may optionally be placed to help the initial stability of the new socket.

Acetabular Options

Various bearing options are available for the acetabular component. The most common option is one made of ultra-high-molecular-weight polyethylene. Historically, hip prostheses utilizing this material would last for 10 to 15 years. However, currently the ultra-high-molecular-weight polyethylene is being irradiated to crosslink the polyethylene. This makes the material much more wear resistant, especially when a femoral head made of ceramic is used.

The final option is metal acetabular liner. This has the lowest wear rate of any available material today. However, there is a catastrophic risk of ceramic fracture. Should this occur, revision surgery is necessary. Another disadvantage is squeaking of the hip. This is an uncommon occurrence (with a rate of 1%–8%) but can sometimes be quite loud. Patients who develop this complication may desire revision if the squeaking is audible.

TOTAL HIP REPLACEMENT: STEPS 19 AND 20

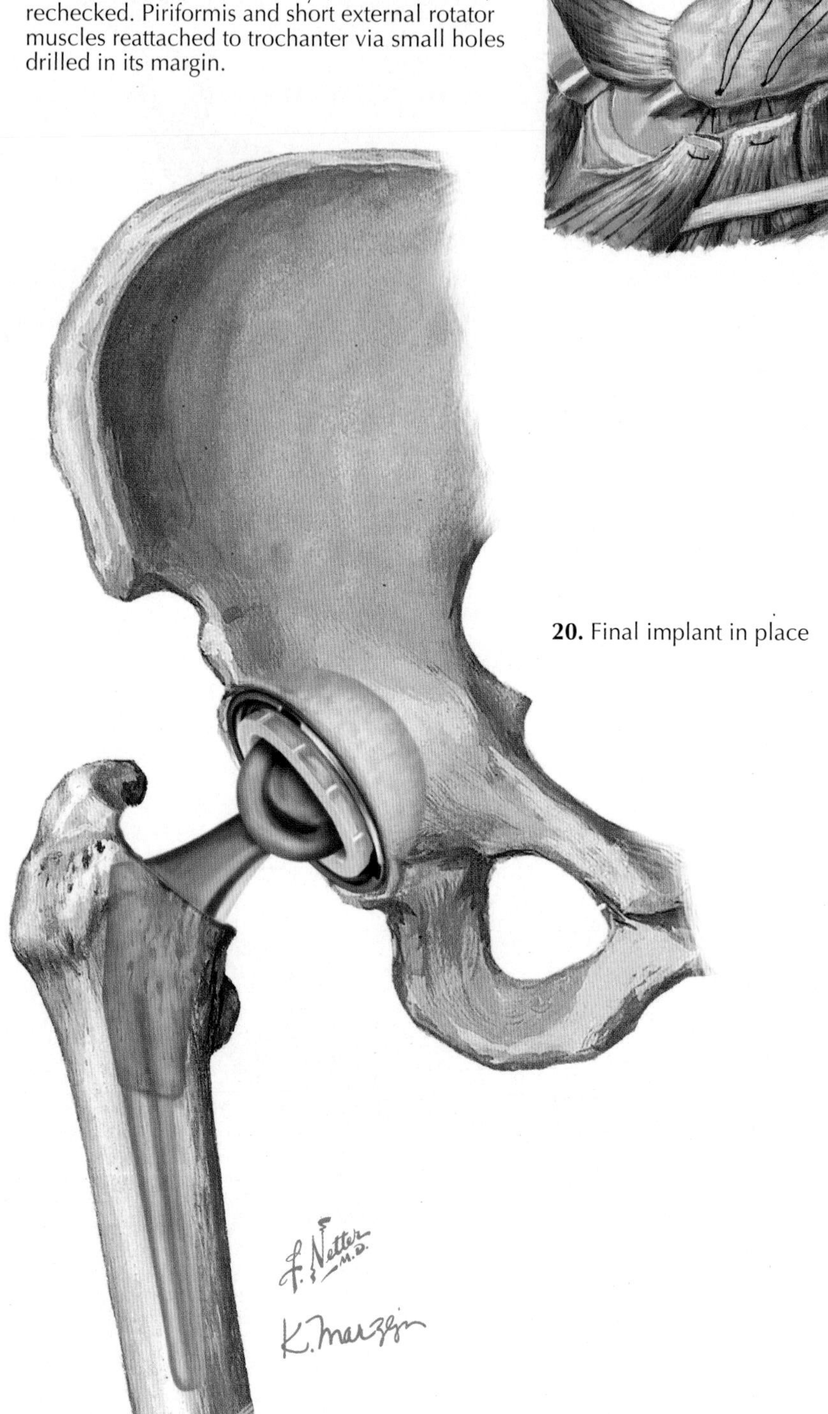

19. Acetabular cup irrigated, and prosthetic head reduced into it. Joint mobility (in all directions) rechecked. Piriformis and short external rotator muscles reattached to trochanter via small holes drilled in its margin.

20. Final implant in place

TOTAL HIP REPLACEMENT: TECHNIQUE (Continued)

FEMORAL COMPONENT

A broad retractor is placed beneath the femoral neck to bring it into clear view (see Plate 2.47). During reaming of the femoral canal, the leg is placed so that proper anteversion and valgus positioning of the stem can be achieved. The thigh is flexed, internally rotated, and adducted to achieve the best exposure of the femoral canal; a canal-finding instrument is inserted to determine the correct direction. Straight reamers and then rasps are used to shape the femoral canal. A trial prosthesis is placed in the femur, and the hip is temporarily reduced. Range of motion is tested, noting hip stability at the extremes of motion. If dislocation occurs too easily, either component may be incorrectly positioned. If soft tissue laxity contributes to instability, an implant with a longer neck may be needed.

After stable movement is demonstrated, the trial component is removed and the final implant is placed. If a cemented stem is used, a canal plug is inserted in the femur about 2 cm beyond the implant stem. This allows pressurization of the cement and prevents its flow to the distal femur. The femoral canal is again irrigated to wash out blood and debris and dried while the second batch of cement is mixed.

Cement is injected into the femoral canal and then pressurized; more cement is added and then again pressurized. The implant is then inserted and correctly aligned in a neutral or slightly valgus position in the medial-lateral plane and kept in place until the cement polymerizes. Extruded cement is removed. After the wound is irrigated, the hip is reduced and once again tested for a stable full range of motion.

The posterior capsule, piriformis muscle, and conjoined tendon of the short external rotator muscles are reattached in the trochanter through drill holes. The gluteus maximus tendon is repaired with interrupted sutures if it has been released. If a trochanteric osteotomy has been done, the trochanter fragment is replaced and secured with wires. Abductor muscle tension can be increased, if desired, by advancing the bone fragment. The deep fascia lata and gluteus maximus fascia are closed with interrupted sutures, the skin is closed with clips or a continuous monofilament suture, and a sterile dressing is applied.

Dysplastic Acetabulum and Protrusio Acetabuli

Dysplastic Acetabulum

Preoperative view

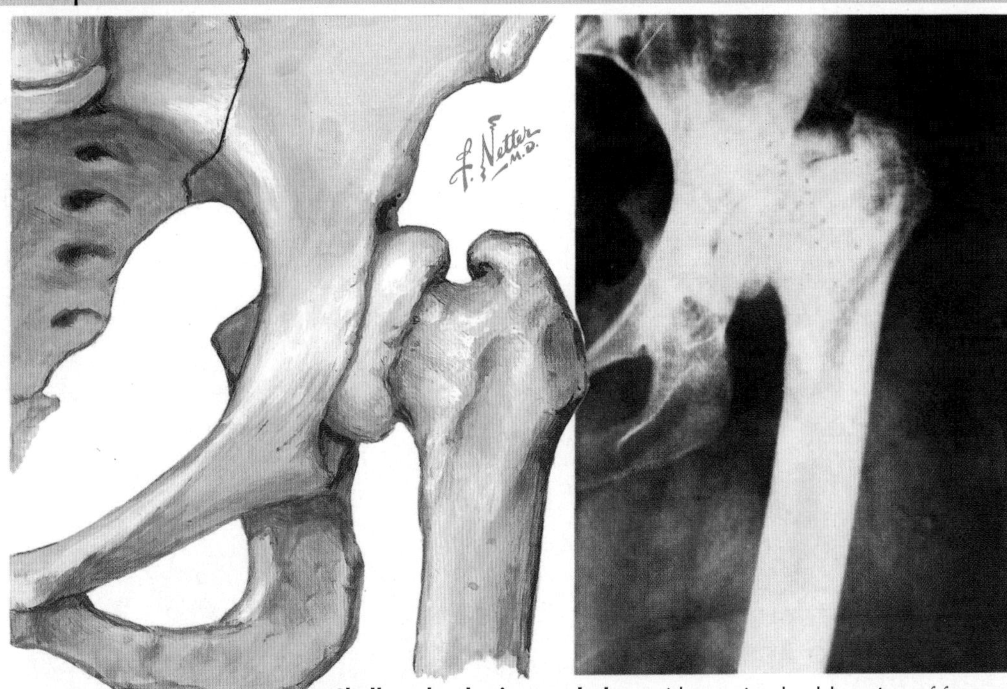

Shallow dysplastic acetabulum with proximal subluxation of femoral head and superolateral deficiency of acetabulum

Postoperative view

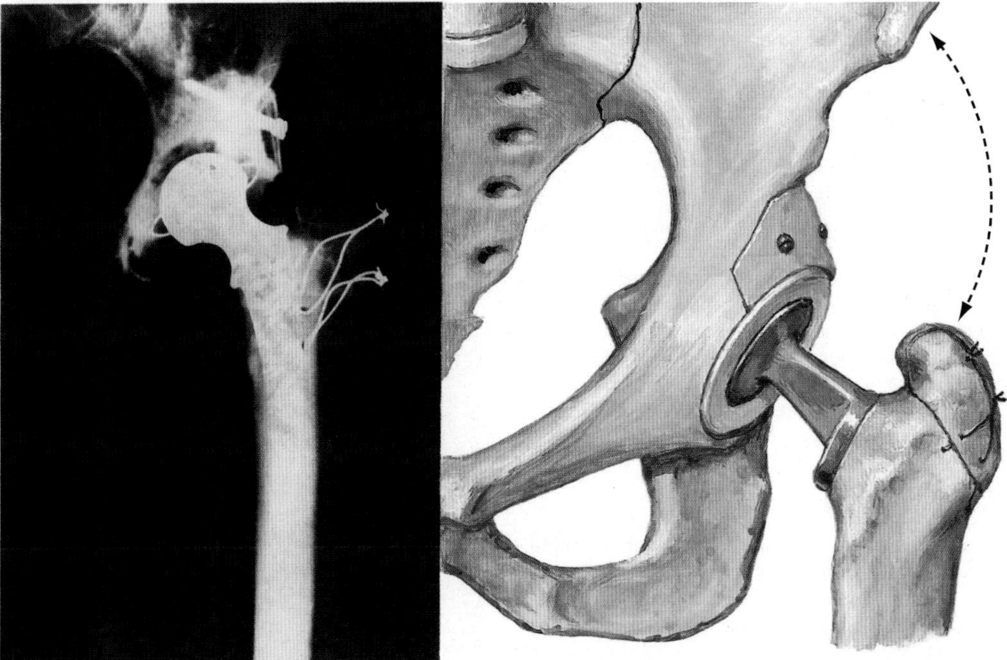

Total hip replacement with reinforcement of superior acetabulum with bone graft from excised femoral head. Bone graft held in place with screws. Limb slightly lengthened and tension in abductor muscle mass increased.

Reconstruction of the dysplastic or deficient acetabulum presents a particularly difficult surgical challenge because the anatomic landmarks commonly used as reference points may not be in their normal positions. Portions of the bony circumference of the acetabulum may be deficient as a result of old fractures or congenital dysplasia. For example, in a long-standing posterior fracture dislocation of the hip, the posterior wall of the acetabulum is usually severely deficient; in congenital dislocation of the hip, the acetabulum is shallow and poorly developed. If the femoral head has been dislocated for many years, it articulates with the iliac wing in a pseudoacetabulum. The true acetabulum is stunted, small, and shallow, but its anatomic configuration is usually preserved and identifiable once the contracted overlying inferior capsule is reflected.

DYSPLASTIC ACETABULUM

Dysplasia of the acetabulum is often seen without actual dislocation of the femoral head. Usually, the acetabulum is shallow and the femur is displaced laterally. The superolateral wall, or roof, of the acetabulum is deficient and must be reconstructed with a bone graft before it can support an acetabular prosthetic component.

Total hip replacement in the patient with congenital hip dislocation is extremely difficult. Because the acetabulum may be deficient in bone mass and the proximal femur malformed, as is common, modular prostheses are sometimes required.

Treatment. A bone graft is often used to reinforce the superior acetabulum; it can be fashioned from the resected femoral head. The bone graft is fixed to the ilium with screws and then reamed to receive a small acetabular component, with the pubic bone and ischium used as anterior and posterior landmarks to avoid excessive reaming. Modular femoral components with varying angles and neck lengths can be used to achieve a near-normal abductor lever arm.

After a failed total hip replacement, bone autografts or allografts may also be used to reconstruct an acetabulum that is deficient in bone mass. After thorough removal of the loose acetabular component, bone mass deficiencies are repaired. A new acetabular component, often made with trabecular metal, is then impacted and secured with screws. Segmental defects are preferably reconstructed with trabecular metal augments. Cavitational defects, on the other hand, may be filled with allografts, usually best impacted into the cavity in the form of chips. A smooth surface can be created by reaming in reverse.

MEDIAL WALL DEFECT

Another common site of bone mass deficiency is the medial wall, or floor, of the acetabulum. Often discovered during revision surgery, this problem is frequently related to the first procedure, during which the medial wall was perforated. This condition is also seen in inflammatory arthritis.

Treatment. Medial wall deficits have been classified by size into three types: minor (diameter <1 cm), intermediate (diameter <3 cm), and major (diameter >3 cm).

PROTRUSIO ACETABULI

Bilateral primary protrusio acetabuli. Bone of acetabular floor is thin and protrudes into pelvis, resulting in medial displacement of femoral head and restriction of hip motion.

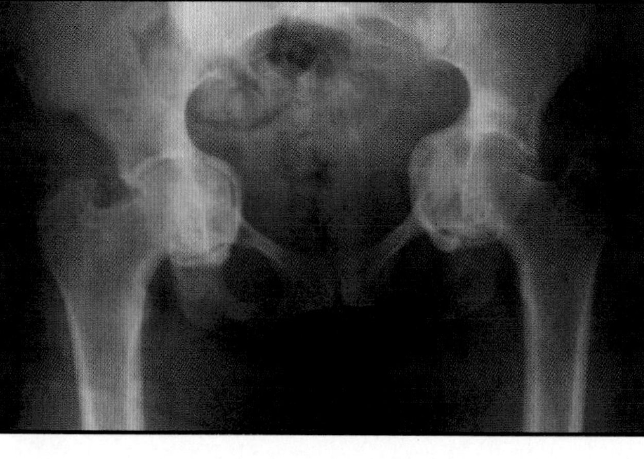

Bone graft
Cement
Acetabular prosthesis
Femoral prosthesis

Acetabular floors augmented with bone grafts from excised femoral heads; total hip reconstruction completed. Right acetabulum reinforced with bone graft held in place with screws.

DYSPLASTIC ACETABULUM AND PROTRUSIO ACETABULI (Continued)

All deficits are repaired surgically with one of three types of bone grafts. *Bulk bone* is used to reconstruct major deficits. For example, a large plug is fashioned from a resected femoral head and used to fill a medial wall defect. Screws may be added to further stabilize the graft, and a hemispheric depression can be reamed in the graft. *Chips of trabecular bone* are harvested and used as packing material to fill small deficits, cysts, and cracks. *Pulverized bone* (from reaming or a bone mill) can be made into a soft, paste-like consistency and finger packed into small deficits.

Bulky pieces of bone allograft maintain their structural integrity and may be variously replaced by host living bone through a process called *creeping substitution;* the trabeculae in the bone allograft act as a "trellis" for the ingrowth of live bone. Cementing into a bone graft is possible as long as the host bone–bone graft interface is adequate and intimate.

PROTRUSIO ACETABULI

As a result of any disease that causes bone resorption, the pelvic bones become osteoporotic and soft and the medial wall of the acetabulum may be gradually displaced medially. Bone remodeling in response to applied load causes varying degrees of superomedial protrusion of the femoral head. Protrusio acetabuli occurs when the femoral head is displaced past the ilioischial line in the pelvis. Other conditions that can cause progressive protrusion of the acetabulum are osteomalacia, rickets, Paget disease of bone, and infections. Central dislocation of the femur due to trauma can also heal with a protrusion deformity. Arthrokatadysis (Otto pelvis) is a rare idiopathic form of severe bilateral protrusio acetabuli most often seen in adolescent females. Metastatic carcinoma to the pelvis can lead to pathologic fractures, which result in a protrusion deformity.

Primary manifestations of protrusio acetabuli are thigh pain and decreased range of motion. Lateral and rotatory movements are particularly inhibited by the impingement of the femoral neck against the acetabular labrum, or rim. A classification of protrusion deformities distinguishes cases with an intact medial wall from those with a perforated medial wall. Third-degree protrusio acetabuli is the most severe, occurring when the medial displacement is greater than 5 mm, and is coupled with penetration of the medial wall. Protrusio acetabuli prosthetica occurs when a hip prosthesis is gradually displaced through the soft bone of the medial wall.

Treatment. Like medial wall defects, protrusio acetabuli is treated with various types of bone grafts to reinforce areas deficient in bone mass to ensure that prosthetic components remain in the correct anatomic positions.

If there is enough anterior and posterior wall remaining, a cementless socket is impacted in place with cancellous bone graft behind it. If severe deficiencies are present, an antiprotrusio cage may be placed over the top of the cementless socket. This cage rests on the ilium and ischium, thereby transferring the load from the hip to the intact pelvis.

Total Hip Replacement: Complications

Although many complications may follow total hip replacement, their incidence is fortunately low. The most common postoperative complications are deep venous thrombosis (DVT), neurologic complications, loosening of prosthetic component, dislocation, fracture, and infection.

The usual risks associated with general anesthesia and stress after any surgical procedure must be discussed with the patient. Because there may be significant blood loss during this procedure, replacement blood must be available. Transient hypotension, an uncommon intraoperative problem specific to hip replacement, occurs in some patients after the compression of cement into the femoral canal. The etiology of this phenomenon is still unclear, but it is theorized that a small amount of unpolymerized monomer in the cement may cause vasodilation or perhaps the increased pressure in the femoral canal causes fat embolization. Adequate blood volume must be maintained, and rapid infusion of fluids may be required to restabilize the blood pressure.

Deep Venous Thrombosis

Although not unique to total hip replacement, DVT is unusually common in this type of surgery, occurring in 30% to 50% of cases. Most clots are small and asymptomatic and form in the small veins of the lower limb. Thrombosis of the femoral and iliac veins should be treated early with anticoagulants to minimize the risk of pulmonary embolism. At present, ultrasound is the most common test to screen for DVT, although routine screening is not recommended. Pulmonary embolism serious enough to cause death occurs in a very small percentage of patients, and postoperative treatment with aspirin, low-molecular-weight heparin, or oral warfarin is therefore recommended. Evaluation of arterial blood gases is required if the patient becomes confused or develops inspiratory chest pain. Although ventilation, perfusion scans, and chest computed tomography (CT) can help rule out a significant pulmonary embolism, angiography is the only definitive test. Fat embolism syndrome from disruption of the femoral bone marrow is rare.

Loosening of Femoral Component

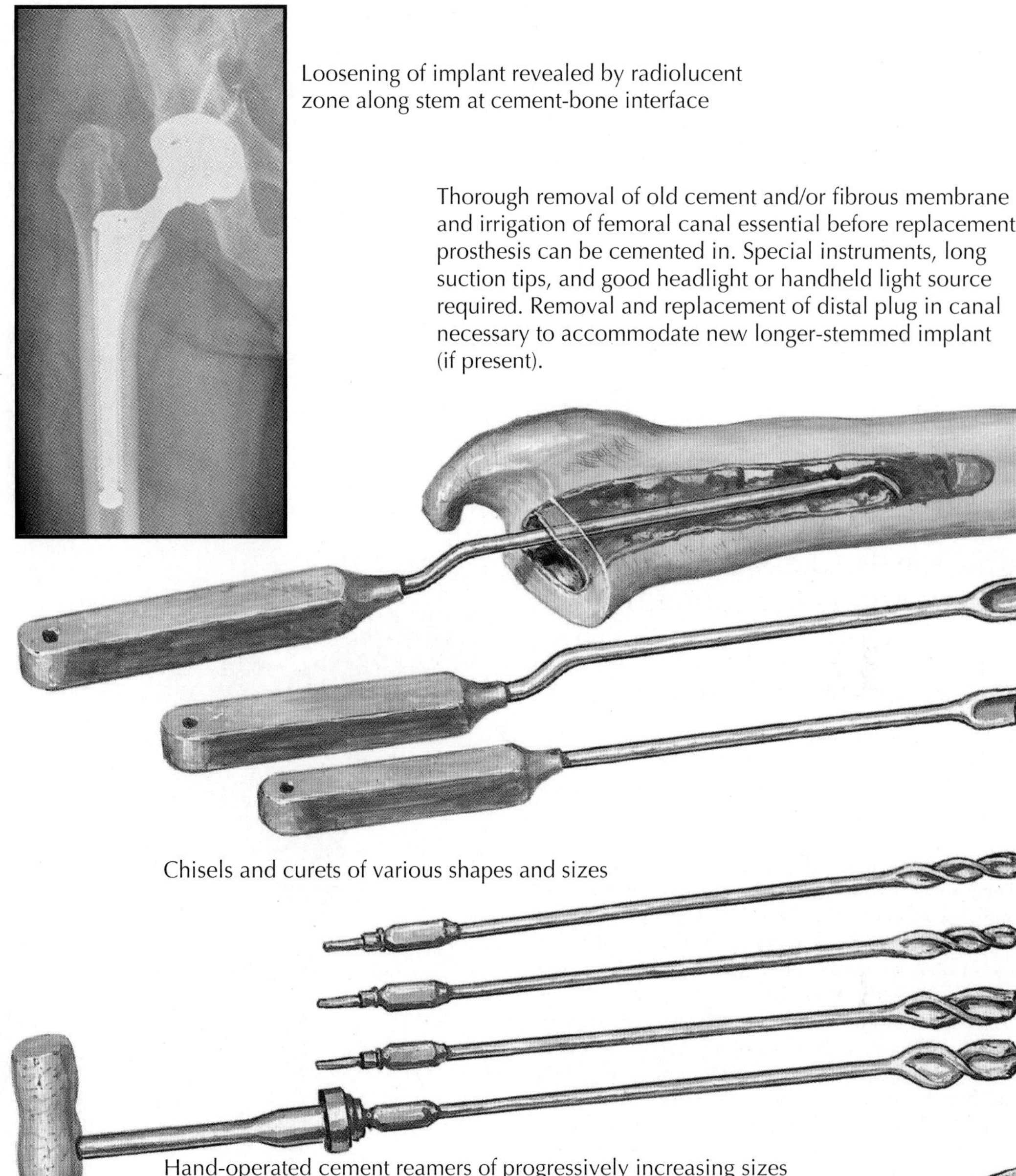
Loosening of implant revealed by radiolucent zone along stem at cement-bone interface
Thorough removal of old cement and/or fibrous membrane and irrigation of femoral canal essential before replacement prosthesis can be cemented in. Special instruments, long suction tips, and good headlight or handheld light source required. Removal and replacement of distal plug in canal necessary to accommodate new longer-stemmed implant (if present).
Chisels and curets of various shapes and sizes
Hand-operated cement reamers of progressively increasing sizes
Long-nosed forceps
F. Netter M.D.
K. Marzen

Long-handled power burr must be used with great caution to prevent penetration of cortex.

Neurologic Complications

Peripheral nerve palsy is seen in about 0.25% of cases. The femoral nerve can be damaged anteriorly by retractors, and sciatic nerve palsy may occur secondary to retractors, overlengthening of the limb, or pressure from an expanding hematoma. In hip replacement, the most common cause of sciatic nerve palsy is tension placed on the nerve by overretraction or overlengthening of the limb during surgery. This is usually manifested by extensor-evertor weakness of the foot and ankle or decreased sensation in the distribution of the more labile peroneal portion of the sciatic nerve. Although slow improvement usually occurs, complete recovery is uncommon. Rarely, acute dislocation of a total hip replacement causes sciatic nerve injury, necessitating rapid reduction and supportive care.

Total Hip Replacement: Complications (Continued)

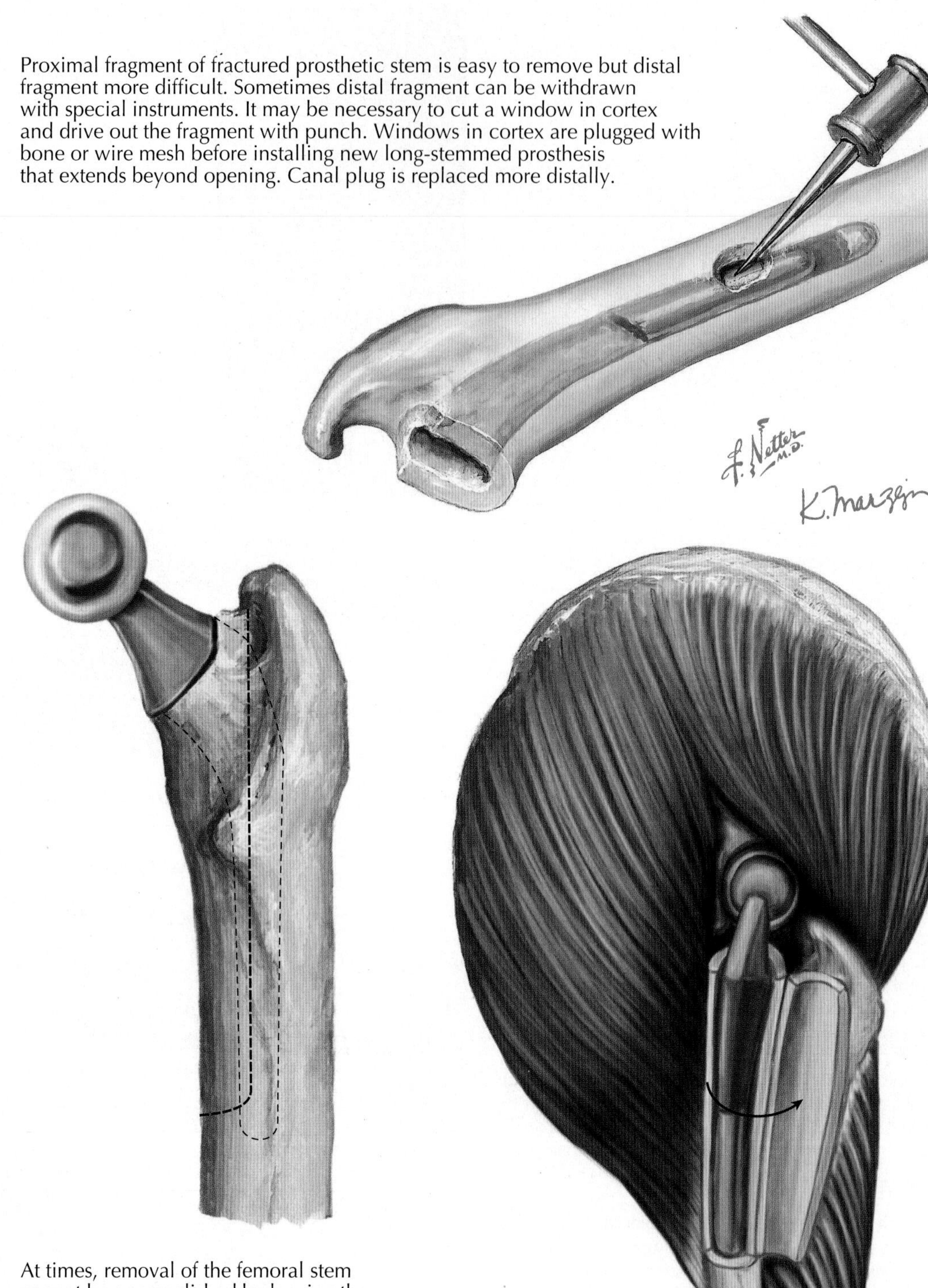

FRACTURES OF FEMUR AND FEMORAL COMPONENT
Proximal fragment of fractured prosthetic stem is easy to remove but distal fragment more difficult. Sometimes distal fragment can be withdrawn with special instruments. It may be necessary to cut a window in cortex and drive out the fragment with punch. Windows in cortex are plugged with bone or wire mesh before installing new long-stemmed prosthesis that extends beyond opening. Canal plug is replaced more distally.
At times, removal of the femoral stem cannot be accomplished by leaving the bony cylinder intact. In this scenario osteotomy of the femur is performed, making a window to facilitate removal of the component.

LOOSENING OF FEMORAL COMPONENT

Loosening of the femoral component is a late complication that usually occurs 15 to 20 years after total hip replacement (see Plate 2.51). Predisposing factors include age (<50 years), weight (>80 kg), and a high level of physical activity. Varus positioning of the femoral stem, poor cementing technique, and certain femoral stem designs are also associated with increased implant loosening. For example, the curved and diamond-shaped femoral stems are more likely to loosen, possibly because of their tendency to fragment the cement. When gaps remain between the bone and the stem of the prosthesis, because of poor cement infiltration or interposition of blood, a piston-like movement can occur and lead to progressive loosening. Porous ingrowth stems have better long-term outcomes, with some stems having a 99% 20-year survivorship when aseptic loosening is used as an end point.

Early loosening can be diagnosed by characteristic radiographic findings even before clinical symptoms appear. Evidence of loosening is a radiolucent zone at the bone-prosthesis, prosthesis-cement, or cement-bone interface. Other signs of loosening are subsidence or movement of the components. Thigh pain, the primary symptom of component loosening, is particularly evident when the patient attempts to walk. The pain, which often radiates to the knee, may begin gradually after an initial pain-free interval. Severe pain or rapidly advancing bone lysis indicates the need for revision surgery. Before a revision procedure is undertaken, however, an aspiration arthrogram and culture should be done to rule out infection, which can also cause loosening (see Plate 2.54).

Correction of a loose implant with revision surgery is more difficult than the initial total hip replacement. Careful preoperative planning is most essential. If possible, the previous incision should be used to avoid transecting scars that might compromise the vascular supply and result in skin necrosis. In select cases, a troch slide or osteotomy facilitates the revision procedure by providing the widest possible exposure. All scar tissue and pseudocapsule are excised to allow dislocation and mobilization of the proximal femur. Very loose prostheses can easily be removed. Any remaining debris must be removed carefully in a piecemeal fashion with special instruments. The distal cement plug (if present) is very difficult to remove and must often be penetrated or reamed with a high-speed power burr or hand-operated cement reamer. Long curets, cement chisels, and pituitary forceps are used for deeper access into the femoral canal. Great care must be taken to avoid perforating the femoral canal, because perforations create stress risers that can induce postoperative fractures. If perforation occurs, a femoral component with a long enough stem to reach at least two femoral cortical diameters below the defect must be used for adequate reinforcement. After the canal is thoroughly cleaned, preparation for a new porous ingrowth component is undertaken.

FRACTURE OF FEMUR

Fracture of the femur can occur around or distal to a femoral prosthesis. Even minor trauma can cause fracture if a significant stress riser is present in the femoral shaft, particularly if the bone is osteoporotic. Any bony defect

Total Hip Replacement: Complications (Continued)

can act as a concentration point for stress, including screw holes and areas of cortical penetration.

Fractures around a well-fixed component are repaired in standard fashion with open reduction and internal fixation (ORIF) with plates and screws. If the femoral component is loose, the hip is revised to a long-stemmed implant bypassing the fracture by at least two cortical diameters, and the remaining bone is fixed around the new implant with cables.

LOOSENING OF ACETABULAR COMPONENT AND FRACTURE OF ACETABULUM

The incidence of acetabular component loosening increases markedly after 12 to 15 years of function. Improper positioning and bone deficiency above the implant can also accelerate loosening. Although the average rate of polyethylene wear is very low, loosening may result from progressive osteolysis.

Pain in the inguinal region on weight bearing often heralds a loose acetabular component. Radiographs reveal a radiolucent zone around the implant. Because radiolucent zones may be evident before symptoms appear, radiographic follow-up after surgery is very important.

Revision of the loose component involves removal of the loose socket. Large defects in the medial wall of the acetabulum must be repaired with bone grafts. The new acetabular component is then impacted into place.

Segmental defects of the acetabulum are filled with acetabular trabecular metal augments that re-create a spheric acetabulum. A new trabecular metal component is then impacted into the acetabulum and secured to the augment with cement. A fracture of the acetabulum requires revision if function of the prosthesis is impaired. However, sometimes it is best to let the fracture heal first, because the new component can then be inserted more easily. Fractures of the anterior or posterior bony columns of the acetabulum may be repaired with internal fixation and the use of pelvic plates and screws.

DISLOCATION OF TOTAL HIP PROSTHESIS

Dislocation of the prosthesis can occur immediately after surgery if the patient moves the limb into a prohibited position. The patient must avoid extremes of internal rotation, flexion, and adduction for about 12 weeks until a thick capsule forms around the prosthetic joint. Treatment of an early dislocation is immediate reduction with the patient under sedation or general anesthesia. If the components are positioned properly, the patient can resume rehabilitation but must avoid the dangerous limb positions. Use of a hip-hinge abduction brace with a flexion stop is wise because it prevents unguarded movement into the proscribed positions. Recurrent dislocation should be treated according to the cause. If the position of either component is faulty, revision surgery is necessary, or if the myofascial tension is lax, advance osteotomy of the greater trochanter may be indicated when limb length is correct. If the limb is short, the neck of the femoral component may need to be lengthened.

Loosening of Acetabular Component and Dislocation of Total Hip Prosthesis

Loosening of acetabular component

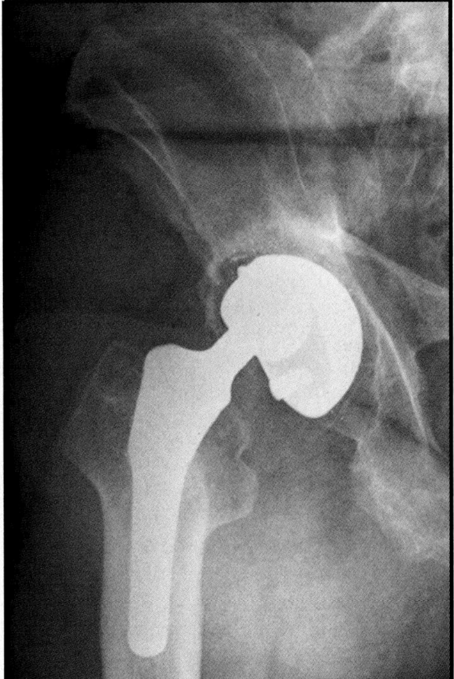

Loosening of acetabular component related to supra-acetabular bone deficiency (reconstruction with bone graft necessary).

Loosened (or fractured) cup removed. Thin bony rim of acetabulum must not be damaged. Cup may be removed piecemeal.

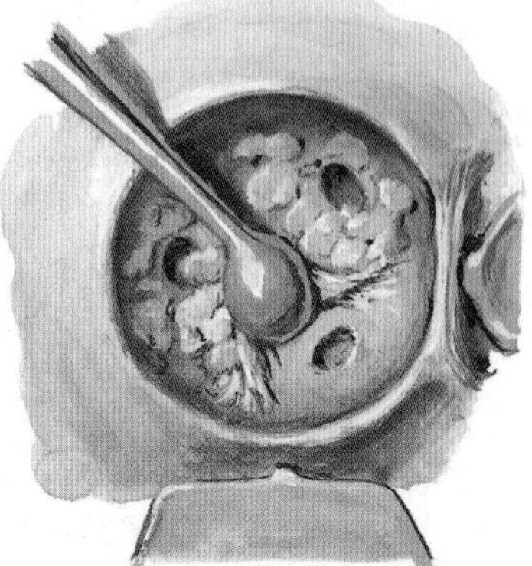

Old cement and fibrous membrane are removed, fixation holes are cleaned or rebored, and acetabulum is thoroughly irrigated.

Dislocation of total hip prosthesis

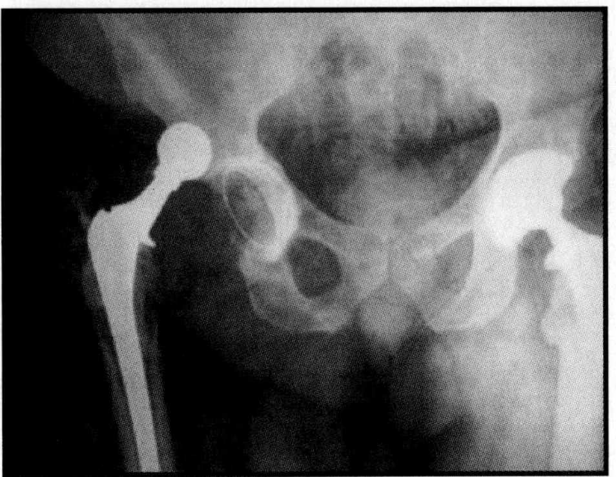

Radiograph shows dislocation of total hip prosthesis, loosening of component, and nonunion of trochanter.

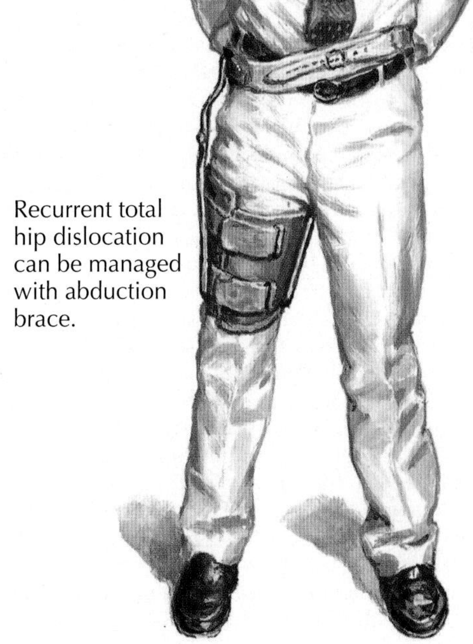

Recurrent total hip dislocation can be managed with abduction brace.

F. Netter M.D. K. Marzen

Total Hip Replacement: Infection

Suprafascial infection
Manifested by incisional pain, inflammation, and/or drainage. Usually responds well to debridement and antibiotics.

Subfascial infection

Acute subfascial infection
May be fulminant with severe systemic and febrile manifestations. More commonly mild with few or no systemic symptoms and only mild local signs. Early, deep debridement needed.

Latent infection
Pain weeks or months after surgery. Radiographs may be inconclusive. Prosthesis should be removed.

Aspiration for smear and culture.
Primary procedure for diagnosis and choice of antibiotics. Staphylococci are most common pathogens. Gram-negative infections are most difficult to treat.

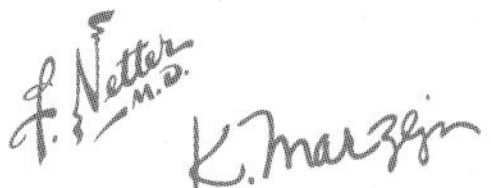

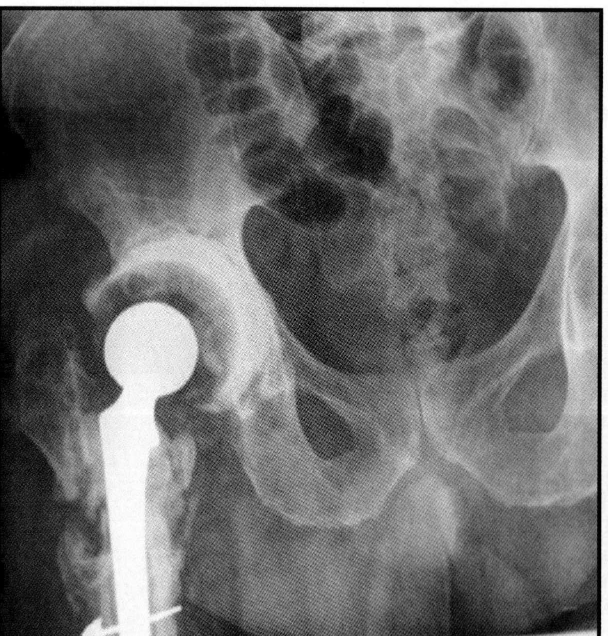

Loosening of component due to infection; note bone lysis around stem.

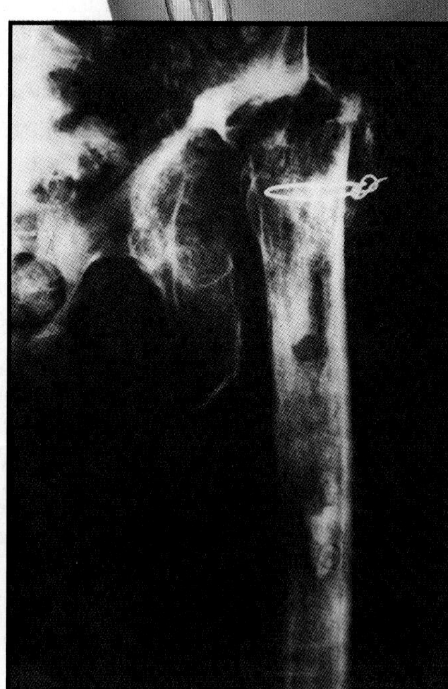

Girdlestone resection arthroplasty may be required after removal of total hip prosthesis.

Subfascial (deep) infection, whether acute or latent, is a serious complication in joint replacement surgery. It is important to identify the type of infection because prognosis and treatment differ. Also, because any implant can become a focus for infection, patients with a hip prosthesis should be given preventive antibiotics when undergoing dental, urinary, or gastrointestinal procedures.

Any unexplained wound or hip pain in the early postoperative period should arouse suspicion. Acute infections are easier to diagnose because they manifest classic systemic and local signs of sepsis. Diagnosis of latent infections is more difficult because clinical and radiographic signs are similar to those seen in aseptic loosening of the prosthesis.

Strong indications of a *suprafascial infection* are pain at the incision site, inflammation, and drainage in the first 2 weeks after surgery; fever and leukocytosis may also be present. Daily surgical wound care is therefore essential. Suprafascial infections respond well to drainage and debridement.

Symptoms of *subfascial (deep) infections* may include swelling of the thigh, increased hip pain, and elevated leukocyte count with an increased proportion of neutrophils. Accurate diagnosis depends on culture of aspirated fluid to isolate the causative organism. Blood cultures are also indicated. If the culture results are positive, surgical debridement and intravenous administration of antibiotics should be instituted immediately.

Acute subfascial infections cause a variety of signs and symptoms, depending on the organism's virulence and the patient's immunologic status. Because long-term postoperative administration of antibiotics can mask the appearance of symptoms, preventive intravenous administration of antibiotics should not be continued for more than 48 hours after surgery.

Acute deep infections must be treated aggressively with intravenous administration of antibiotics and fluid replacement, as well as immediate open debridement of the implant site. Because most nosocomial gram-positive cocci have become resistant to penicillin, early treatment with a penicillinase-resistant synthetic penicillin or cephalosporin is necessary until the drug sensitivity of the organism is determined. If the infection is controlled early enough, it may be possible to save the prosthesis. If the infection is intractable or is due to antibiotic-resistant organisms, the prosthesis must be removed. Secondary acute hematogenous infections can occur after months or years, with or without septicemia and sudden onset of hip pain.

Latent infections do not usually become evident until at least 12 weeks after surgery. They should be suspected if the patient is not recovering normally. Delayed primary infections may be due to bacterial contamination from a remote body source (mouth, urine, bowel) in the perioperative period. There may be no fever or elevated leukocyte count, although the erythrocyte sedimentation rate and C-reactive protein level are usually elevated. In a long-standing infection, radiographs may show osteopenia and a radiolucent zone around the implant. Results of bone scans are positive for both infection and a loosened implant, but the pattern of radioisotope uptake is sometimes specific enough to differentiate between the two conditions.

Treatment. Removal of the prosthesis with a temporary hip spacer is the treatment of choice. Intravenous administration of antibiotics to establish adequate bactericidal levels as confirmed by tube dilution sensitivity studies should be instituted for 4 to 6 weeks. Before revision surgery, histologic examination of local tissue is needed to ensure that the infection has been controlled.

Some organisms are so virulent and difficult to eradicate that a new implant can never be placed for fear of recurrent infection. A Girdlestone resection arthroplasty may be the only alternative procedure. Pain, severe limb shortening, and concomitant gross instability of the hip are serious disadvantages.

Bipolar Prosthesis for Hemiarthroplasty of Hip

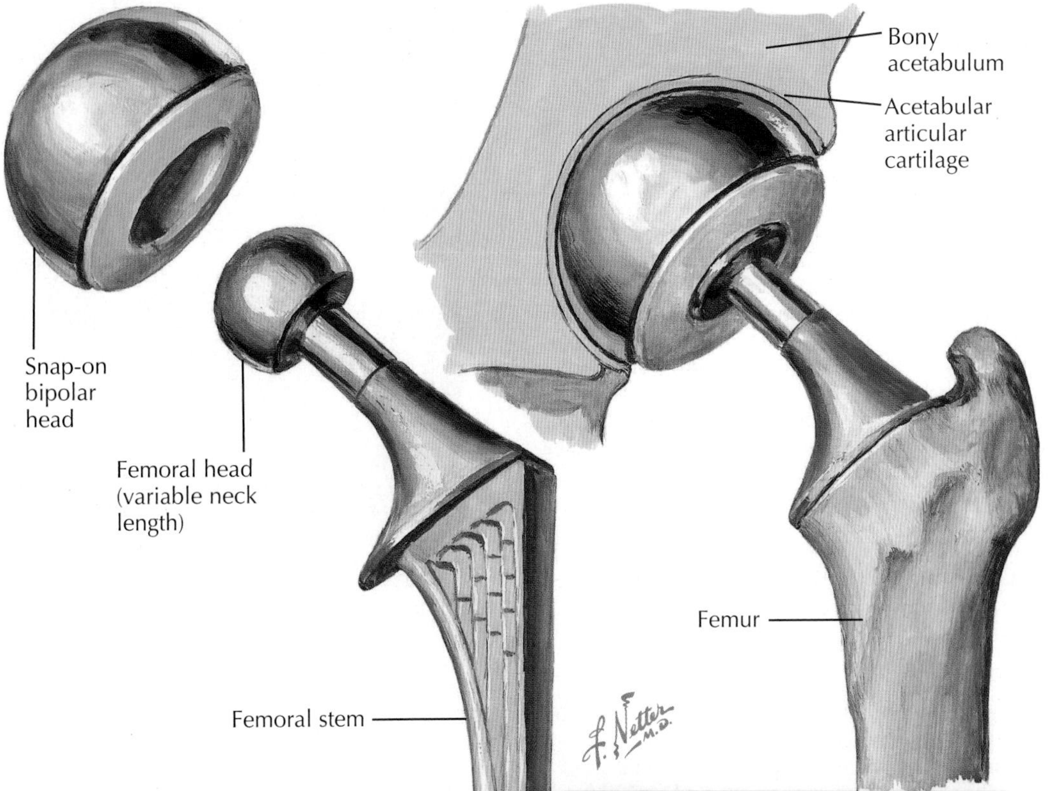

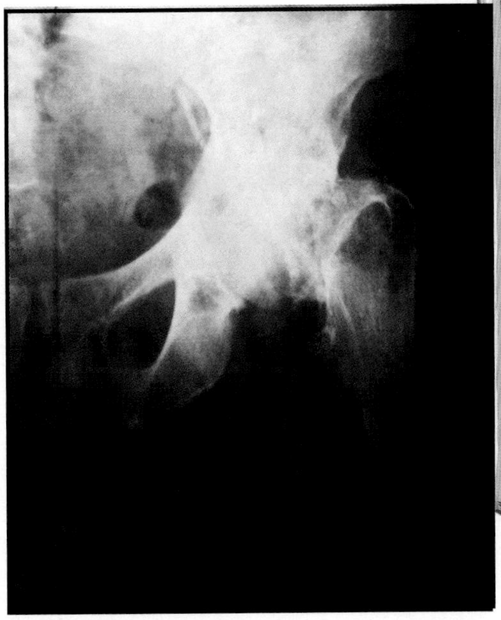

Fracture of femoral neck with articular cartilage preserved

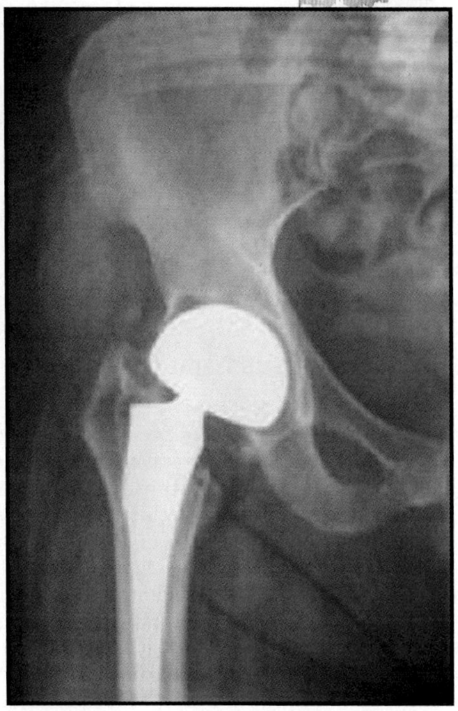

Bipolar prosthesis used to restore alignment and function

Total Hip Replacement: Hemiarthroplasty of Hip

Hemiarthroplasty, or partial reconstruction, of the hip is a less radical procedure than total hip replacement. It is performed when the acetabular cartilage is intact and the pathologic process is limited to the femoral side of the joint.

Partial hip replacement is frequently used in patients with metastatic lesions of the proximal femur, especially if there is risk of impending fracture. It is also appropriate for many patients with femoral neck fractures.

Although hemiarthroplasty is appropriate for most fractures of the femoral neck, in children and young adults every attempt must be made to save the femoral head and neck with internal fixation. This treatment may also be desirable in older patients if the fracture is only slightly displaced or impacted or if it can be stably reduced. Because the main goal of treatment in older patients is early ambulation, hemiarthroplasty may be the treatment of choice even for minimally displaced fractures, especially if the bone is markedly osteoporotic. Displaced fractures of the femoral neck should be treated primarily with hemiarthroplasty or total hip replacement because of the high incidence of complications after treatment with ORIF.

Currently accepted practice is to perform an urgent ORIF of a femoral neck fracture in young patients. In elderly patients with displaced femoral neck fractures, hip replacement is the standard of care. Currently there is debate as to whether a hemiarthroplasty or conventional total hip arthroplasty achieves better results.

In our practice, patients who are community ambulators, live independently, and do not have dementia undergo a traditional total hip arthroplasty. This avoids the potential problem of acetabular cartilage deterioration and subsequent groin pain and need for revision surgery.

In patients who suffer from impaired cognitive capabilities or those who are relatively housebound, hemiarthroplasty is performed. A hemiarthroplasty has less potential for postoperative dislocation and thus is a better option in this patient population.

HIP RESURFACING

Hip resurfacing is a surgical alternative to total hip arthroplasty. This procedure was performed in the past; however, the results were inferior to that of total hip arthroplasty. More recently, newer technology has allowed for better longevity of hip resurfacing, leading to a renewed interest in this technique.

The ideal patient for hip resurfacing is a healthy man (with no history of renal impairment) younger than the age of 55 years with good bone quality. In this cohort, resurfacing results are similar to those of total hip arthroplasty.

Resurfacing may be performed in older individuals as well as in females. However, the results of resurfacing in these patients have been inferior to the results with conventional total hip arthroplasty, and patients should be counseled about this finding. Also, females of child-bearing age should not undergo hip resurfacing. The metal ions released as the components generate wear have an unknown effect on the unborn fetus.

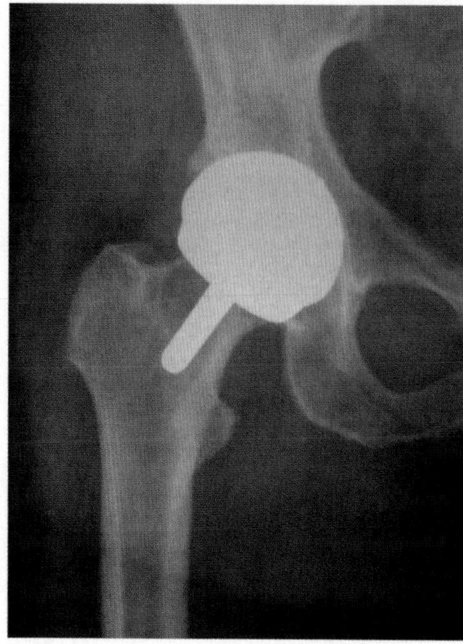
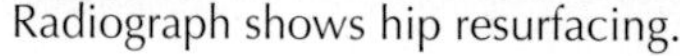
Radiograph shows hip resurfacing.

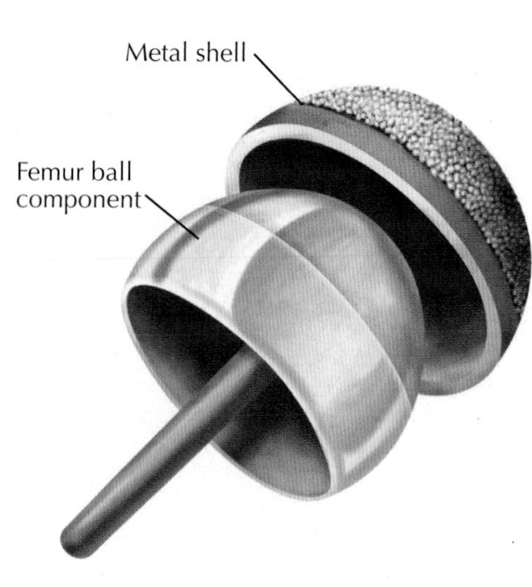

TECHNIQUE

The surgical approach is similar to that of total hip arthroplasty. A posterior or lateral approach may be used.

Once the femur is dislocated, the femoral head is sized. The acetabulum is then exposed and prepared similar to a total hip arthroplasty. The monoblock metal acetabular component is then impacted in place.

Attention is then turned back to the femur. Using a special jig, a guide pin is inserted into the femoral head. Care must be taken to place the pin in slight valgus to prevent early failure of the construct. After the pin is accurately placed, preparation of the femur proceeds. It is sequentially reamed to remove several millimeters of bone. Then several drill holes are placed in the femur, and the implant is cemented in place. Once the cement cures, the hip is reduced and checked for stability.

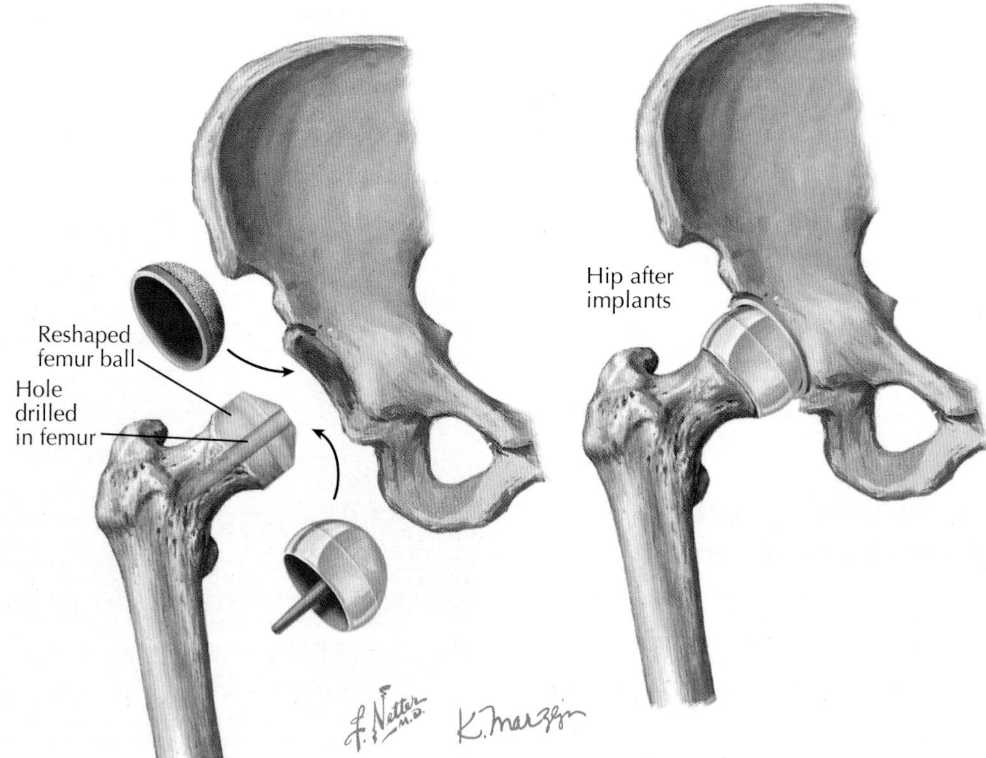

RESURFACING VERSUS TOTAL HIP ARTHROPLASTY

Hip resurfacing has several stated advantages over total hip arthroplasty. Because the femoral neck is preserved and the hip is loaded similar to a normal hip joint, some patients report a more normal-feeling hip compared with conventional total hip arthroplasty. Some surgeons will allow their patients who have hip resurfacing to resume high-impact activities (running). Also, should the femoral component fail, the conversion to a standard total hip arthroplasty is relatively straightforward; thus revision surgery years down the road may theoretically be easier. Finally, there is less risk of limb length discrepancy as well as dislocation after hip resurfacing.

There are several disadvantages to hip resurfacing. The long-term results for hip resurfacing are inferior to conventional total hip arthroplasty in all groups except males younger than the age of 55 years. In addition, there is a risk of femoral neck fracture with hip resurfacing. This risk can be minimized with proper positioning of the femoral component and the avoidance of femoral neck notching during preparation. Also, the success of resurfacing is more dependent on surgical skill (proper component positioning) than total hip arthroplasty.

Finally, hip resurfacing uses a metal-on-metal articulation, which in itself has its own inherent benefits and risks.

METAL-ON-METAL ARTICULATION

Metal-on-metal articulation in hip replacement has been in use for decades. The material has been refined over the years as technology has improved to reduce wear and allow for longer-lasting implants. Currently, a well-functioning metal-on-metal total hip arthroplasty or resurfacing can last for 15 years or longer.

However, many surgeons do have concerns with metal-on-metal articulations. As metal-on metal articulations wear, cobalt and chromium particles are generated. Elevated levels of these chemicals can be measured in the serum of patients who have received metal-on-metal articulations. The long-term effects of this are unclear. Several studies have shown a slightly increased risk of hematologic cancers in patients with metal-on-metal articulations. However, the majority of studies have shown no long-term cancer risk.

A condition unique to metal-on-metal articulation is the formation of pseudotumors or an aseptic lymphocyte-dominated vasculitis-associated lesion (ALVAL). This occurs in approximately 1% of patients. Patients present with pain after their replacement with no other cause (e.g., loosening, infection). Radiographically, rapid osteolysis may be seen. These patients may require revision because of the rapid destruction of host bone. Proper component positioning may reduce the risk of ALVAL. An acetabular component placed in excessive abduction is a risk factor for ALVAL. Avoiding this is crucial in hip resurfacing.

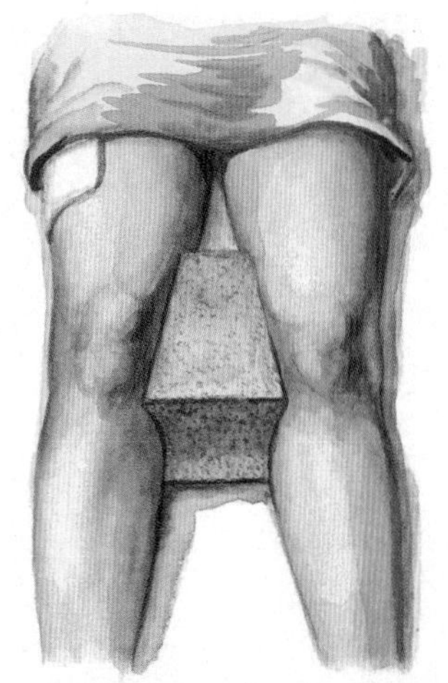

Foam wedge between thighs prevents hip adduction after surgery. Legs must never be crossed.

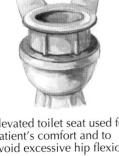

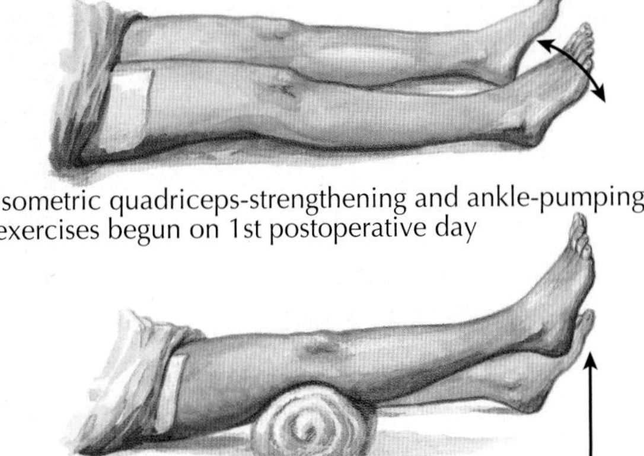

Isometric quadriceps-strengthening and ankle-pumping exercises begun on 1st postoperative day

Short-arc leg-raising exercises begun on 4th or 5th day

Elevated toilet seat used for patient's comfort and to avoid excessive hip flexion

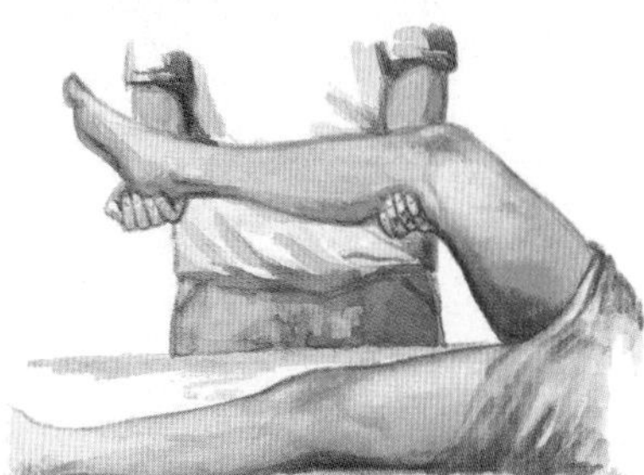

Passive, then active-assisted, exercises begun on 3rd day, with care to avoid hip adduction or flexion beyond 90 degrees

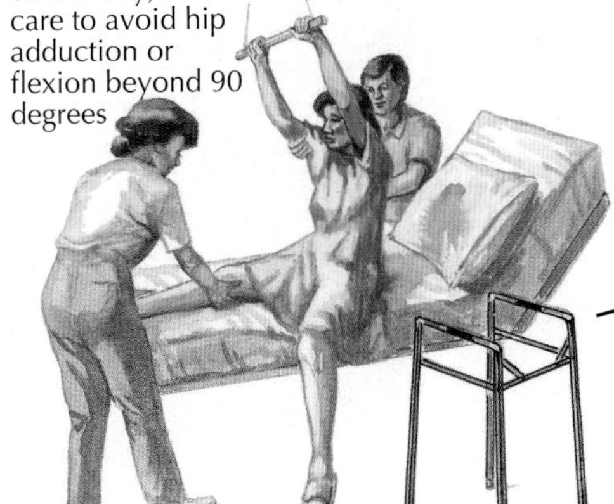

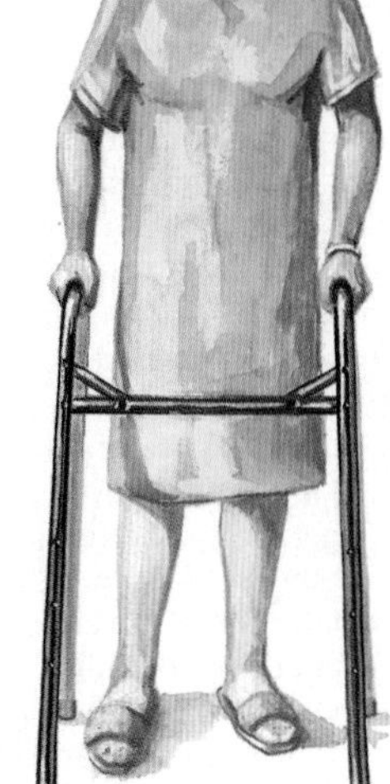

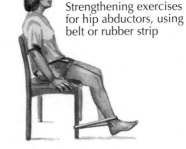

Patient first stands 10–15 minutes with walker, then walks with it; later, uses crutches, cane, and no support.

Patient assisted out of bed on 3rd or 4th day. Helped by trapeze and attendants, patient slides to edge of bed so that good leg hangs down and foot touches floor. Excessive flexion of hip avoided. Note pressure stockings.

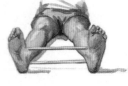

Strengthening exercises for hip abductors, using belt or rubber strip

Strengthening exercises for hip abductors using belt or elastic loop

Rehabilitation after Total Hip Replacement

On the day of surgery, the patient performs deep breathing and coughing exercises and isometric gluteus and quadriceps-setting exercises. Calf-pumping exercises are initiated to decrease the risk of thrombophlebitis. Lower limbs are maintained in position with an abduction splint. Active-assisted to mild resistive exercises are prescribed for unaffected joints and limbs. On the first postoperative day, the patient begins active-assisted range of motion of the affected hip and knee in all planes, with hip flexion limited to 80 degrees and extension limited to neutral. The patient is instructed in proper transfer techniques and is assisted in getting out of bed to stand for 15-minute periods.

On the second and third postoperative days, the patient adds short-arc quadriceps-strengthening exercises and begins progressive standing, transfers, and ambulation. Initial gait training in the parallel bars or walker assistive device provides proprioceptive feedback with partial weight bearing. During ambulation, the patient is evaluated for limb length discrepancy. The patient advances from partial weight bearing to full weight bearing as tolerated per surgeon preference and technique. The abduction wedge is removed, but it is used at night for 6 weeks after surgery.

Physical and occupation exercises continue after the third postoperative day, and then active hip flexion, extension, and abduction are added. Progressive ambulation continues until the patient achieves independent ambulation with assistive devices. Then, the patient may use supportive devices to walk without supervision. After the third postoperative day, this is often continued in a skilled rehabilitation facility until the patient is safe to be at home. Until discharge from the hospital or rehabilitation facility, the patient continues the strengthening and range-of-motion exercises and learns to negotiate steps and curbs. Hip abductor and quadriceps femoris exercises are advanced per surgeon preference to progressive resistive exercises. Instruction is given in the use of assistive devices for dressing and other activities of life. At the time of discharge, the patient is provided with written instructions to be followed at home and with adaptive equipment to compensate for the limited hip flexion (e.g., bathtub seat, elevated toilet seat, long shoehorn). When the patient is pain free, isometric exercises to increase hip muscle strength are added. The only proscribed activities are extreme hip flexion, internal rotation, adduction past neutral, and lifting weights more than 50 lb. However, applying excessive athletic stress to the prosthesis is not recommended in most cases. During the first 6 to 8 weeks after discharge, the patient normally uses a cane in the opposite hand to protect the joint. Active hip extension exercises are added after 6 to 8 weeks.

Femoroacetabular Impingement/Hip Labral Tears

The recognition and diagnosis of hip pain in the nonarthritic state has been an evolving process over the past 15 years. Patient complaints often include insidious onset of deep nonpalpable pain. This may be described as deep in the groin or, less commonly, in the buttock area. Activity-related hip pain is the norm, because this is believed to be a condition of the active population. The most common offending activities include but are not limited to running and sitting for long periods of time, with the common mechanism being hip flexion past 90 degrees with some rotation. Patients will often commonly complain of laterally based pain as well, making a true diagnosis difficult to make.

The causes of hip labral tears are believed to be a subtle abnormality of the bony anatomy of the hip joint, resulting in the so-called impingement, which leads to tearing of the labrum and possibly cartilage defects. The bony changes may exist on the femoral or acetabular in origin. Femoral (cam) impingement is the result of the loss of femoral head-neck offset, resulting in early contact of the cam with the labrum. Acetabular (pincer) impingement is the result of acetabular overcoverage. This may result from acetabular retroversion, a deep acetabular socket (coxa profunda).

A general hip examination is performed as discussed previously, with focus on hip range of motion and hip abduction strength (Trendelenburg test), as well as a gait examination. Palpation of the lateral hip should help guide the cause of pain. Palpation must take place over the greater trochanter, gluteus medius tendon, and piriformis, because they all may contribute to this syndrome. The Ober test is also performed to determine whether the iliotibial band is contracted.

Tests specific to hip impingement and labral tears include the anterior impingement test (also called the McCarthy test/FADIR [*f*lexion, *ad*duction, *i*nternal *r*otation]). This test re-creates the pinching of the anterior/anterosuperior labrum. In addition, FABER (*f*lexion, *ab*duction, *e*xternal *r*otation), a dynamic labral stress test, and a posterior impingement test may be performed. Straight-leg raising strength and iliopsoas isolation strength (hip flexion in upright seated position) should also be used to help distinguish a possible hip flexor pathologic process.

Standard radiographs include AP pelvis and shoot-through lateral views of the affected hip. These should be examined for joint space narrowing to help determine whether osteoarthritis may be the pain generator. To evaluate the hip labrum, MRI is the modality of choice. Adding an arthrogram to the study will help increase the sensitivity of the study. Also included in the arthrogram can be local anesthetic, so the injection may serve diagnostic purposes as well.

Differential diagnosis includes hip flexor strain, piriformis syndrome, hernia/sports hernia, adductor strain, osteoarthritis of the hip, avascular necrosis, lumbar radiculopathy, or trochanteric bursitis.

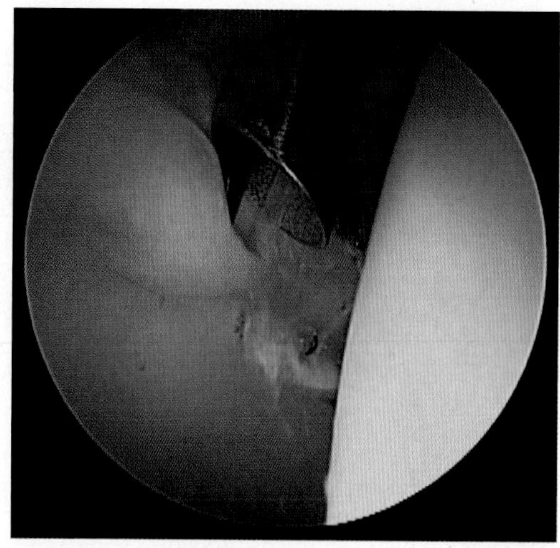

Hip lateral tears are becoming more common due to the open stance used in hitting the ball. The external rotation and extension of the hip result in increased stresses to the labrum. *From Madden C, Putukian M, Young C, McCarty E. Netter's Sports Medicine. Elsevier; 2009.*

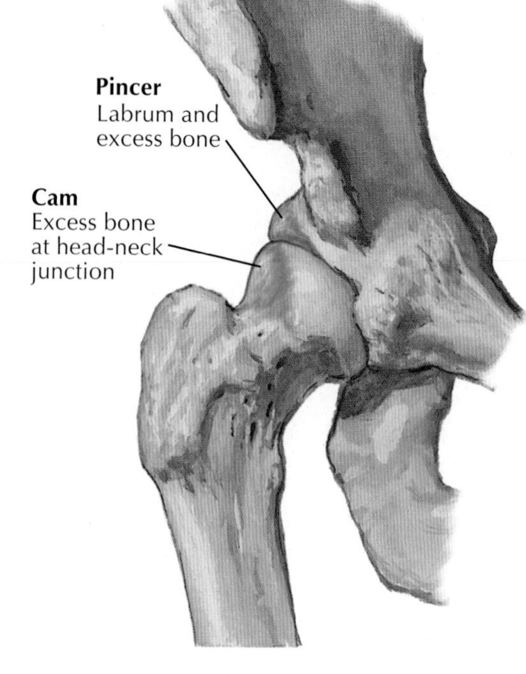

F. Netter M.D. K. Marzen

Hip Arthroscopy Portals

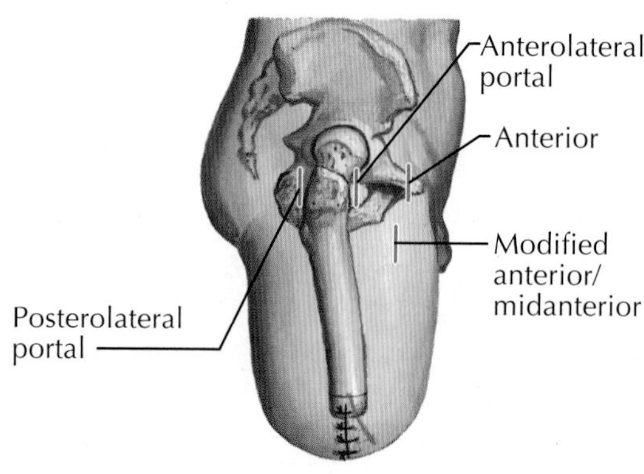

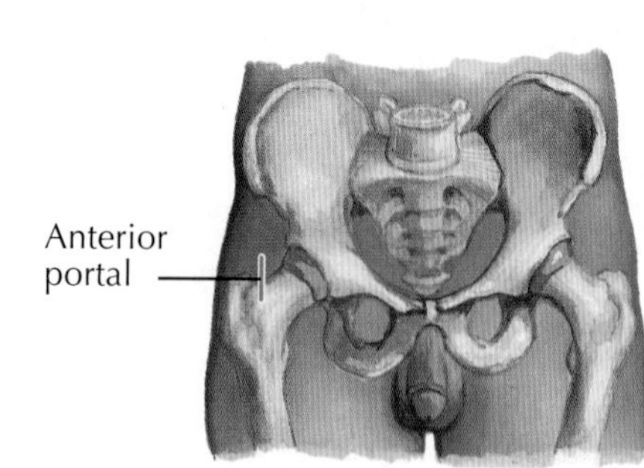

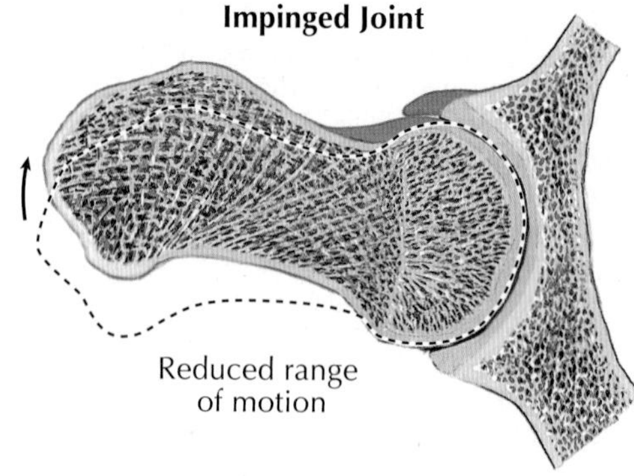

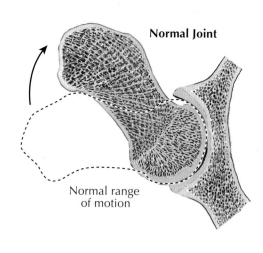

Appropriate diagnosis is essential to the treatment of hip impingement and labral tears. If a labral tear is suspected, this should be confirmed with small field-of-view MRI of the affected hip with appropriate radiographs. If a labral tear is identified without any significant hip osteoarthrosis, treatment is often surgical. The mainstay of nonoperative management is activity modification and NSAIDs. Physical therapy may be employed for muscle weakness/tendinopathy. However, pushing more motion is not recommended because labral tears are believed to be a consequence of bony impingement, and, theoretically, forcing motion means continual engagement of the offending lesion.

Once nonoperative modalities have been exhausted, or if activity modification is not an option, surgical intervention is chosen. Two options exist for the treatment of labral tears with hip impingement: open surgical dislocation or hip arthroscopy. Both treat any labral or articular cartilage pathologic processes in addition to the bony impinging lesion.

AVASCULAR NECROSIS

Avascular necrosis (AVN) of the femoral head is a debilitating disease that usually leads to osteoarthritis of the hip joint in relatively young adults (mean age at presentation, 38 years). The disease prevalence is unknown, but estimates indicate that 10,000 to 20,000 new cases are diagnosed in the United States per year, and up to 18% of total hip arthroplasties performed annually are for osteonecrosis of the femoral head.

The arterial supply to the femoral head is principally provided by three sources: an extracapsular arterial ring at the base of the femoral neck, anterior and posterior ascending branches from this ring, and arteries of the ligamentum teres. This arterial supply is well affixed to the femoral neck and is easily damaged with any femoral neck trauma.

AVN may present as nonspecific signs and symptoms. Early in the disease process, the condition is painless; however, patients ultimately present with pain, typically in the groin, and limitation of motion. Although the groin is the most common area of pain, patients may report pain in their buttock, knee, or greater trochanteric region.

AVN can be either traumatic or nontraumatic. Traumatic causes are usually very obvious to diagnose. The most common traumatic causes are hip dislocations and displaced femoral neck fractures.

The most common causes of nontraumatic AVN are high-dose corticosteroid use and excessive alcohol consumption. These factors alter lipid profiles and are thought to cause intravascular coagulation. Other causes of AVN include coagulopathies, chemotherapy, chronic liver disease, diabetes, gout, sickle cell disease, hyperlipidemia, pregnancy, radiation, systemic lupus erythematosus, and vasculitis.

Plain radiographs in the early stages may be normal or may show femoral head lucency and subchondral sclerosis.

As the disease progresses, subchondral collapse (i.e., crescent sign) and femoral head flattening become evident. Further progression of the disease results in femoral head flattening and progressive osteoarthritis.

MRI is the study of choice in patients in the early stages of AVN (before collapse) or in patients with suspected AVN but with normal radiographic findings. It can help predict the progression of disease, with smaller and more medial lesions having better outcomes.

Nonoperative treatment for symptomatic AVN is often unsuccessful. Restricted patient weight bearing with the use of a cane or crutches has not been shown to affect the natural history of the disease and is useful only in controlling symptoms. NSAIDs may be beneficial for management of the patient's pain. More recently, antiresorptive agents commonly used for the treatment of osteoporosis have shown some promise. It is thought that these drugs retard the resorptive process in AVN and therefore prevent femoral head collapse.

Surgical treatment of AVN is based on the severity of disease. Small asymptomatic lesions do not warrant surgical intervention and are closely monitored with serial examination.

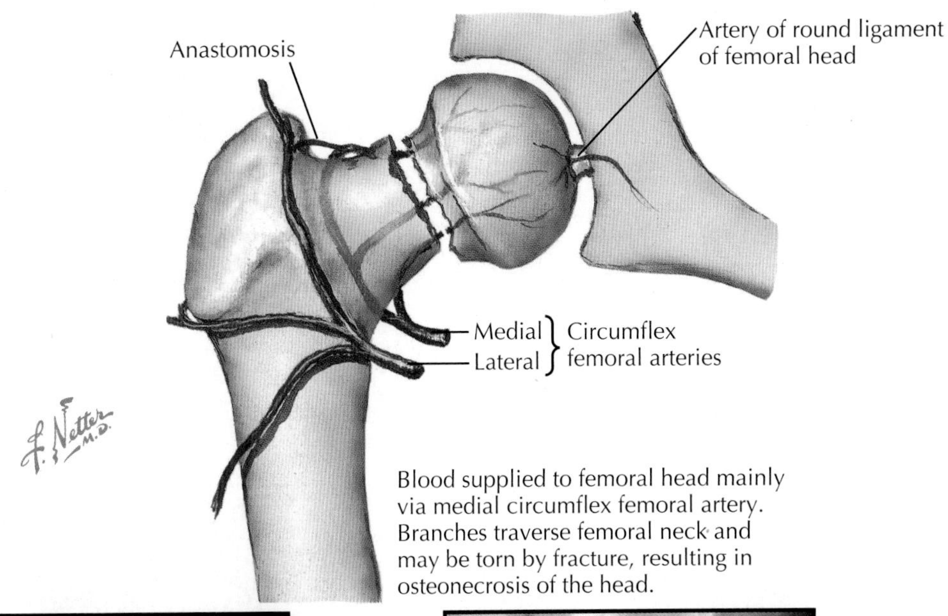

Blood supplied to femoral head mainly via medial circumflex femoral artery. Branches traverse femoral neck and may be torn by fracture, resulting in osteonecrosis of the head.

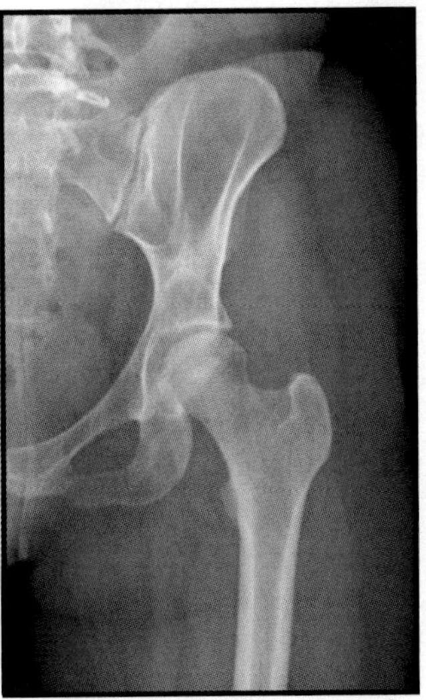

Normal hip exhibiting smooth contour and congruence

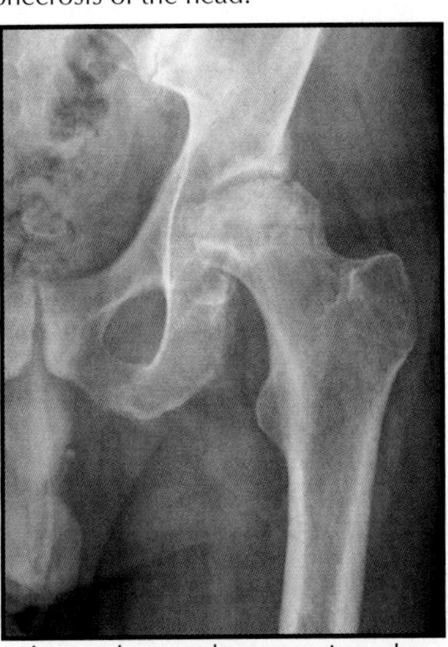

Advanced avascular necrosis and flattening of the femoral head

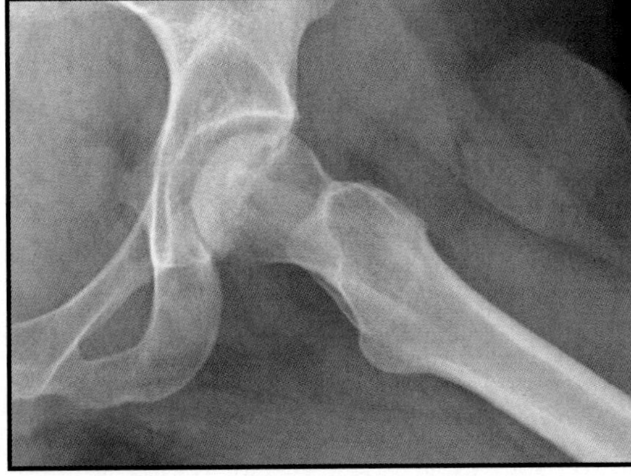

Lateral view showing aspericity and collapse

In symptomatic patients before collapse, the most commonly performed surgical intervention is core decompression. In this procedure, a hole is created through the lateral aspect of the femur, through the femoral neck, and into the lesion. This is done in an attempt to allow for a new blood supply to the devascularized region. Vascularized fibular grafting is an alternative to core decompression, although this is less commonly done.

The outcomes of these procedures are variable.

Osteotomies may be performed in attempt to move necrotic bone away from primary weight-bearing areas in the hip joint, but they have fallen out of favor because they often make subsequent arthroplasty more challenging.

Once the disease has progressed to collapse, the best surgical option is hip replacement. Total hip arthroplasty provides predictable and long-term pain relief for these patients.

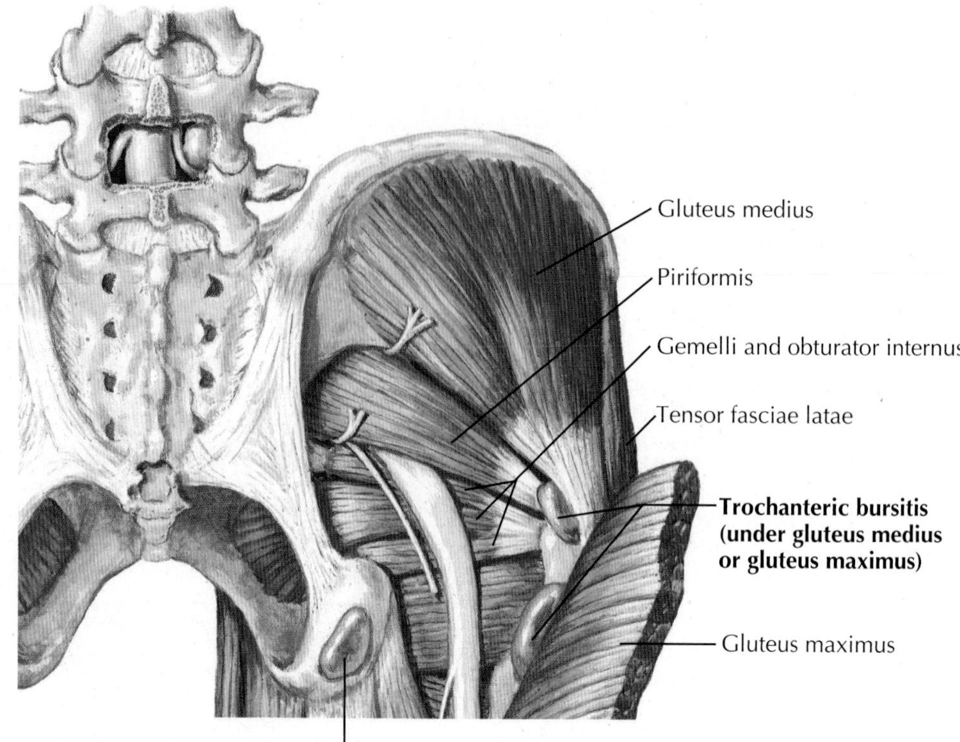

TROCHANTERIC BURSITIS

Iliopectineal bursa
Iliopsoas bursa
Ischial bursa
Trochanteric bursa

Sites for injection/ aspiration of hip joint
Site for injection/ aspiration of trochanteric bursa
Trochanteric bursa

Lateral (or trochanteric) hip pain is a very common presenting complaint. Patients often report the insidious onset of pain over the hip bone (trochanter). Occasionally, this can be caused by trauma or direct injury to the prominence. Complaints include activity-related increases in pain as well as occasionally pain at rest. Often there will be difficulty lying on the affected side for sleep. Pain is usually described as sharp and burning. It may radiate down the lateral aspect of the thigh along the course of the iliotibial band.

The true cause of greater trochanteric pain syndrome is often elusive. Onset can at times be due to a specific traumatic event. However, this is less often the situation. Trochanteric hip pain may be referred from the hip joint itself owing to osteoarthritis or a labral pathologic process. Proximal femoral anatomy (excessive proximal femoral varus) and hip abductor weakness are thought to predispose patients to trochanteric bursitis and pain.

A general hip examination is performed as discussed previously, with the focus on hip range of motion and hip abduction strength (Trendelenburg test), as well as a gait examination. Palpation of the lateral hip should help guide the cause of pain. Palpation must take place over the greater trochanter, gluteus medius tendon, and piriformis, because they all may contribute to this syndrome. The Ober test is also performed to determine whether the iliotibial band is contracted.

AP pelvis, true AP, and lateral views of the affected hip are standard. MRI of the hip is indicated with pain recalcitrant to treatment modalities when minimal osteoarthritis is seen on plain radiographs.

The differential diagnosis includes trochanteric bursitis, hip abductor tear/tendonitis, piriformis syndrome, hip osteoarthritis, and lumbar disc disease/spondylosis/sacroiliitis.

Initial treatment of trochanteric bursitis includes correcting any observable abductor weakness or iliotibial band contracture with physical therapy. NSAIDs are also used for pain relief; injection may be considered at any point. If severe pain is present on initial presentation with negative radiographs, corticosteroid injection may help alleviate the symptoms and allow the proper rehabilitation.

Persistent trochanteric tenderness often necessitates advanced imaging. MRI is used to evaluate the state of the abductor muscle complex. Partial tearing or complete rupture may be present. In this scenario, greater trochanteric pain syndrome recalcitrant to physical therapy and NSAIDs may require shock-wave therapy or injection of platelet-rich plasma into the tendinotic/partially torn area. If a labral or intraarticular pathologic process is suspected, an arthrogram may be performed at the time of the MRI with local anesthetic to determine whether the pain may be referred from the joint. Treatment at that point would be guided by results of both the arthrographic and imaging findings.

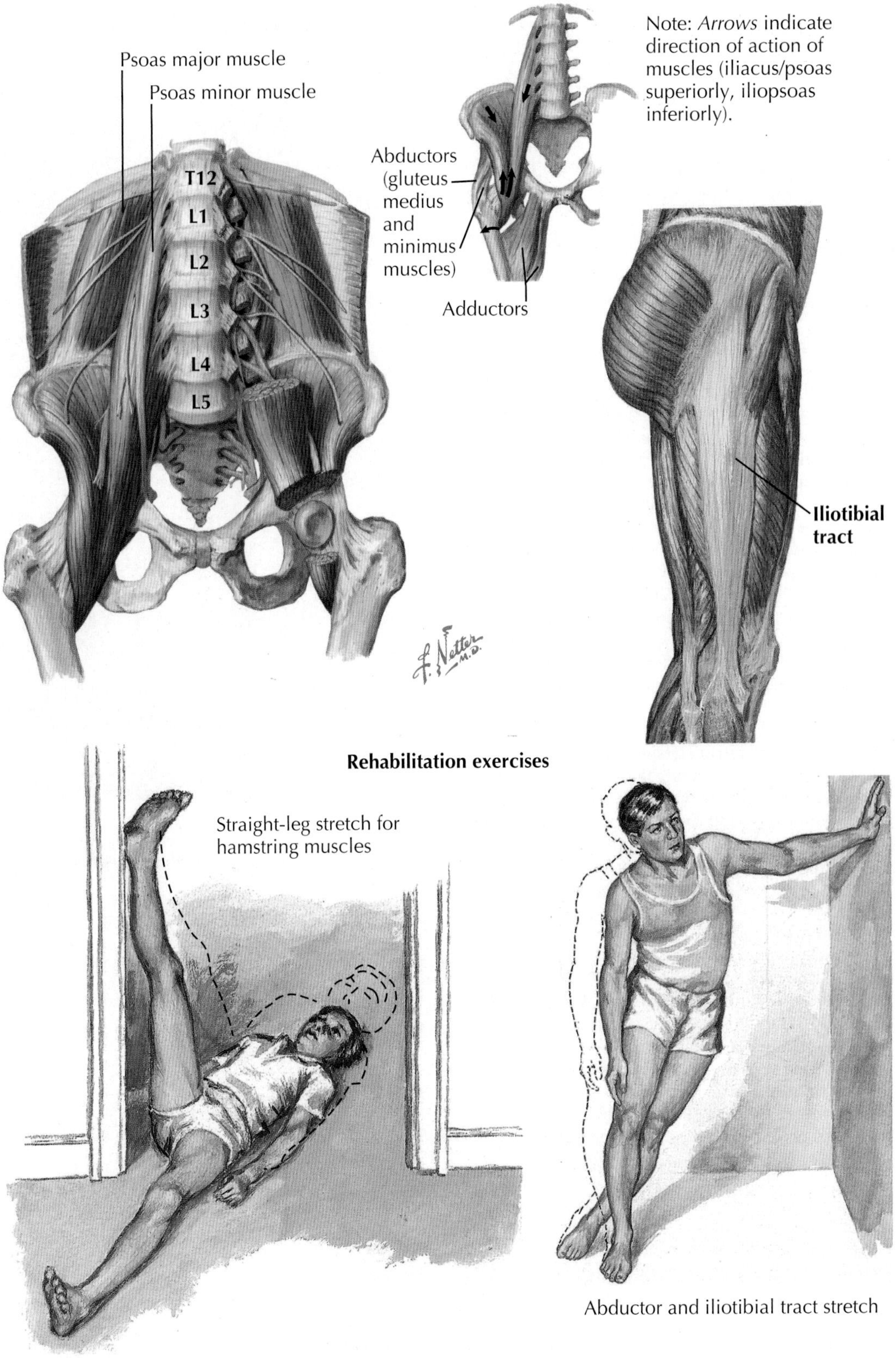

Snapping Hip (Coxa Saltans)

Patients present complaining of a painful snap or popping sensation that is exacerbated by very specific hip positions. The snapping may be either internal (iliopsoas) or external (iliotibial band). Patients with external snapping hip will often describe their hip as "dislocating." Onset is variable and most commonly associated with a change in activity or training regimen. External snapping pain will be mainly trochanteric based, whereas internal snapping causes deeper groin pain that is nonpalpable.

Differential diagnosis includes trochanteric bursitis, labral tear, or hip loose body.

A general hip examination is performed as discussed previously, with focus on hip range of motion and hip abduction strength (Trendelenburg test), as well as a gait examination. Palpation of the lateral hip should help guide the cause of pain. Palpation must take place over the greater trochanter, gluteus medius tendon, and piriformis, because they all may contribute to this syndrome. The Ober test is also performed to determine whether the iliotibial band is contracted. External snapping is often visible and audible from the other side of the examination room. Internal snapping may often be reproduced by the patient by specific movements and will be audible. On examination, this is often reproduced by taking the hip from a flexion/abduction and external rotation to extension/adduction and internal rotation or neutral.

Similar to other hip complaints, standard AP pelvis, true AP, and lateral views of the affected hip are warranted. Advanced imaging (MRI) is warranted when treatment has failed to determine an intraarticular pathologic process, as well as to examine the iliopsoas bursa. Ultrasound may also be used to diagnose the iliopsoas tendon as the snapping agent on dynamic examination.

Initial treatment for coxa saltans is physical therapy and oral antiinflammatory pain medication. For the external variety, rehabilitation is focused on core and abductor strengthening and iliotibial band stretching. Internal coxa saltans is treated with hip extension stretching and a gradual hip flexion strengthening program.

If the symptoms persist for 3 months after the initiation of therapy, injection with a corticosteroid is employed. Patients with iliotibial band snapping receive a trochanteric-based injection. Iliopsoas snapping is treated with an ultrasound-guided injection into the iliopsoas bursa. Physical therapy is then continued for another 3 months.

At this point, if symptoms still persist, surgical intervention may be considered. Hip arthroscopy is performed for each of the two types. For internal coxa saltans, a central (hip joint) examination and treatment of any labral pathologic process are undertaken. The iliopsoas tendon then can be released either from the central, peripheral compartment or directly off the lesser trochanter.

For external snapping, endoscopy or open excision of the trochanteric bursa can be performed. The area of snapping (most commonly posterior) can be identified by direct visualization and movement of the leg. The offending area of iliotibial band snapping is then excised until the snapping is no longer seen with leg movement.

Muscle Strains

Muscle strains most commonly occur at the musculotendinous junction. Most muscle strain injuries occur as the result of a forceful eccentric muscle contraction. The muscles most commonly involved are those that cross two joints (e.g., hamstrings, gastrocnemius). Another factor that makes certain muscles susceptible to strains is an increased percentage of fast twitch muscle fibers (type II).

HAMSTRING STRAIN

The hamstring musculature (biceps femoris, semitendinosus, and semimembranosus) act to extend the hip and flex the knee. The muscle group can be injured anywhere along its course from the ischium to the fibular head (biceps femoris) or medial tibia (semitendinosus, semimembranosus). Patients will often describe a pulling, tearing, or ripping sensation of the posterior thigh. The most common inciting event is a change in speed while running during athletic activity.

Examination of patients with a hamstring injury includes inspection for ecchymosis along the posterior thigh. Palpation over the point of maximal tenderness for a defect, especially proximal, should be undertaken. Resisted prone knee flexion strength at varying degrees and the ability to actively extend the hip off the examination table should be compared.

The differential diagnosis is proximal hamstring avulsion/sciatica.

Imaging for hamstring strains is often not necessary when the injury occurs in the midportion of the posterior thigh. Injuries that occur more proximal warrant plain radiographs and an MRI to evaluate for bony avulsion or soft tissue avulsion of the proximal origin.

Treatment of midsubstance or musculotendinous injury is very similar. An initial period of rest, ice, compression, and elevation to quell the acute phase of inflammation, while maintaining the length of the muscle, is initiated. Once these initial symptoms subside, isometric followed by isotonic and isokinetic exercises are progressed until a full return to activity based on symptoms is achieved. Recovery from a hamstring strain may range from 3 weeks to 6 months depending on severity. Treatment of proximal avulsions may be surgical with repair back to the ischial origin. Proceeding to surgery is guided by factors such as tendon displacement and patient expectations.

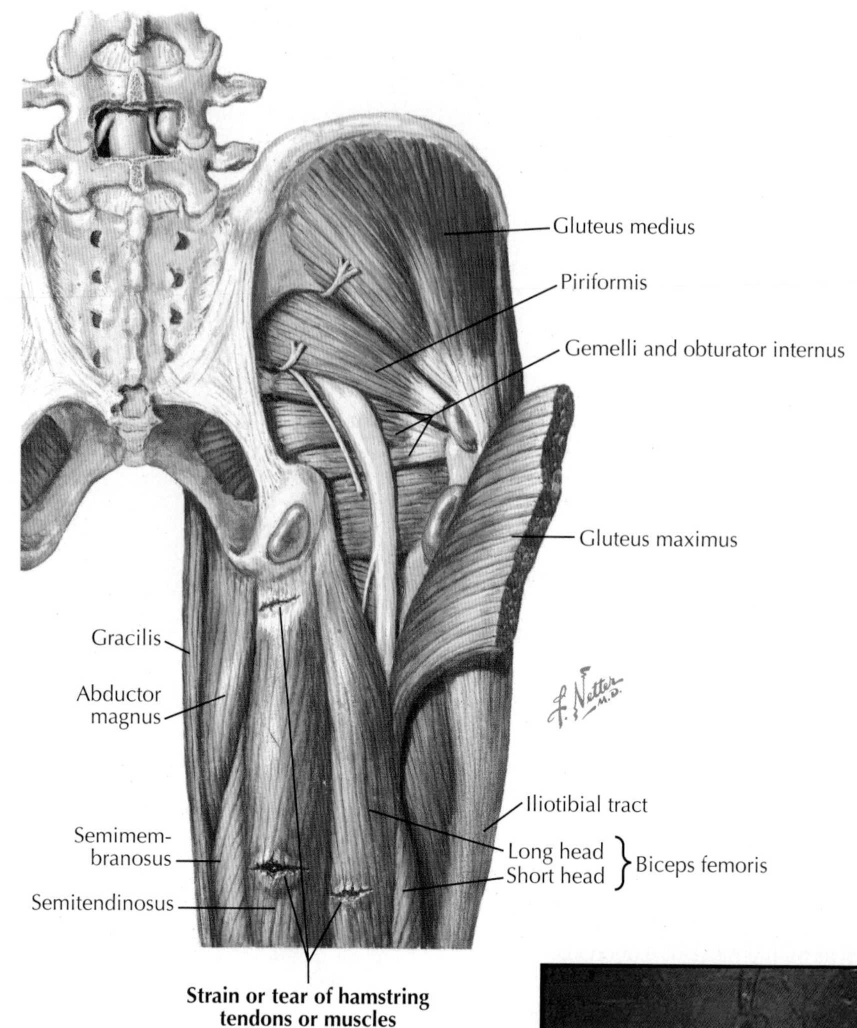

Strain or tear of hamstring tendons or muscles

MRI of proximal hamstring strain. *From Frontera W, Micheli L, Herring S, Silver J. Clinical Sports Medicine: Medical Management and Rehabilitation. Elsevier; 2006.*

ADDUCTOR STRAINS

Sudden eccentric contraction, most commonly with lateral movement and hyperabduction, is the most common mechanism of injury. Injury events range from slips on a wet floor to those sustained during a sporting activity, commonly soccer, hockey, and basketball. The adductor longus muscle is the most commonly injured muscle-tendon unit.

Examination of patients with adductor strain includes inspection for ecchymosis along the medial thigh and palpation of the adductor origin in the pubic rami. Strength comparison and causation of pain should be examined with the hips and knees fully extended and with both flexed to 45 degrees.

The differential diagnosis includes osteitis pubis (athletic pubalgia, sports hernia, hip joint irritation [labral tear]).

Plain radiographs and an MRI are used to evaluate an avulsion injury or in the case of chronic adductor issues to evaluate for partial tearing.

Groin injuries with rare exception respond to conservative management of activity modification, gradual stretching, and graded return to activities based on symptoms.

HIP FLEXOR STRAIN (RECTUS FEMORIS, ILIOPSOAS)

The rectus femoris is the most commonly injured muscle of the quadriceps muscle group. It can be injured at any point along its course. As with other strains, musculotendinous injury is most common, although proximal injuries, especially in adolescents, must be evaluated for avulsion of the anterior inferior iliac spine (origin). Eccentric contraction again is the most common mechanism, especially during sprinting. The iliopsoas is less commonly injured in isolation and may be more commonly irritated with snapping iliopsoas and iliopsoas bursitis.

Examination includes inspection for ecchymosis and palpation of the muscle belly, observing for defects. The patient's range of hip motion is tested with the Thomas test while lying supine and the Ely test lying prone, looking for hip flexion contracture and overall tightness. Strength can be tested with the straight-leg raising test (rectus femoris) and upright hip flexion (iliopsoas isolation). A strength comparison and provocation of pain with these tests help determine the cause.

Differential diagnosis is hip joint pain (labral tear, femoroacetabular impingement, osteoarthritis) or groin strain/sports hernia.

Standard radiographs of the pelvis are commonly obtained to evaluate for anterior inferior iliac spine avulsion as well as for other entities in the differential diagnosis.

The modicum of activity modification and range of motion in a pain-free range, followed by core stabilization and hip flexion strengthening, is standard for hip flexor strains.

STABLE PELVIC RING FRACTURES

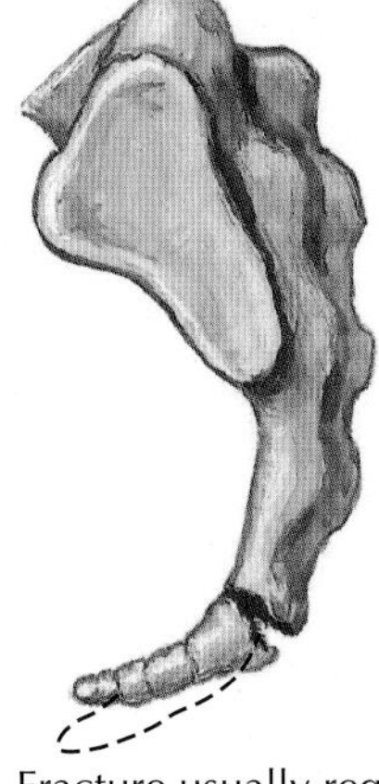

Transverse fracture of the sacrum that is minimally displaced

Fracture usually requires no treatment other than care in sitting; inflatable ring is helpful. Pain may persist for a long time.

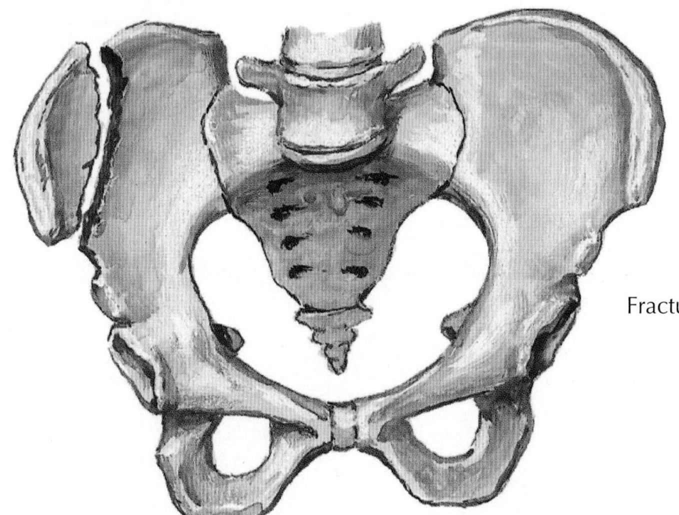

Fracture of iliac wing from direct blow

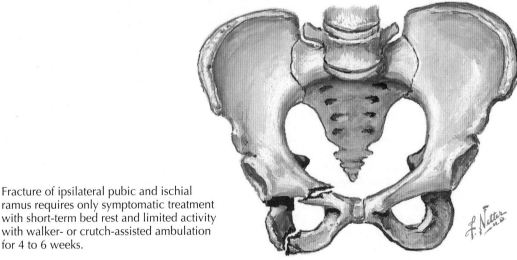

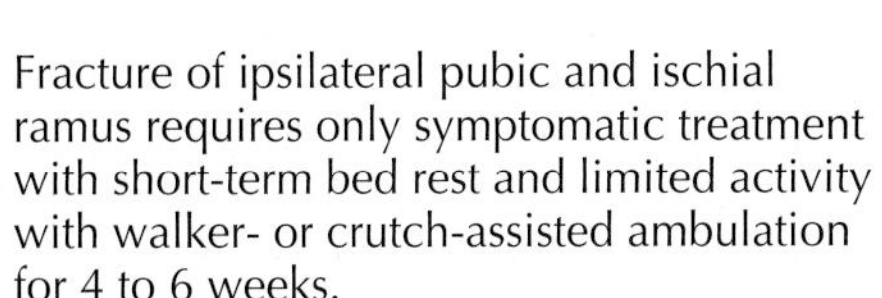

Fracture of ipsilateral pubic and ischial ramus requires only symptomatic treatment with short-term bed rest and limited activity with walker- or crutch-assisted ambulation for 4 to 6 weeks.

INJURY TO PELVIS

FRACTURE WITHOUT DISRUPTION OF PELVIC RING

Injuries to the pelvis range from minor to life threatening. In general, the severity of an injury is determined by the degree of disruption to the pelvic ring. Fortunately, many fractures about the pelvis do not affect its integrity at all.

Avulsion

In athletes, avulsions of bone from the pelvis due to strong muscle contractions are relatively common. These fractures occur at the anterior superior iliac spine as a result of the strong pull of the sartorius muscle, at the anterior inferior iliac spine from the pull of the rectus femoris muscle, and at the ischial tuberosity from the forceful contraction of the hamstring muscles. Most fractures can be treated with activity modification and medications until pain ceases. Patients may gradually resume athletic activities, usually attaining complete functional recovery within 3 months.

Fracture of Iliac Wing

An isolated fracture of the iliac wing, or Duverney fracture, is not uncommon, usually resulting from a direct compressive force to the lateral aspect of the pelvis. The strong muscle attachments on the fragment usually minimize its displacement, and, although blood loss may be substantial, shock is not common. Radiographic examination must determine whether the acetabulum is involved or whether the sacroiliac joint is disrupted. Management of the fracture involves bed rest on a firm mattress until the patient is comfortable enough to be mobilized, followed by gradual, protected weight bearing until all symptoms resolve. Occasionally, an ileus develops that is not due to abdominal visceral injury. This complication is usually relieved with nasogastric suction and intravenous administration of fluids.

Fracture of Pubic or Ischial Ramus

An isolated fracture of a single pubic or ischial ramus is a fairly uncommon injury; it usually occurs in elderly persons as a result of a fall. In this type of fracture, the pelvis remains extremely stable because the obturator foramen is a rigid, bony circle. A fracture of a pubic or ischial ramus must be differentiated from an impacted fracture of the femoral neck because treatments differ markedly. A fracture of one pubic or ischial ramus without visceral or vascular injury requires only bed rest until symptoms abate sufficiently to allow progressive mobilization with a gradual increase in weight bearing.

Fracture of Sacrum

Transverse fractures of the sacrum are usually caused by direct impact and typically have a slightly anterior displacement. Diagnosis is based on a history of injury and evidence of pain, swelling, and tenderness over the posterior aspect of the sacrum. Neurologic dysfunction may occur, evidenced by urinary retention or decrease in rectal tone. The examiner must take extreme care during the rectal examination, especially during palpation along the anterior surface of the sacrum, to avoid converting a closed sacral fracture into an open fracture through the rectum, which increases the risk of serious contamination of the retroperitoneal space. If neurologic deficit is either absent or improving, conservative treatment is indicated. If a neurologic lesion compromises bowel or bladder function, surgical decompression should be considered.

INJURY TO PELVIS (Continued)

Fracture of Coccyx

This fracture is usually caused by a direct blow to the posterior aspect of the coccyx. Symptomatic management suffices, but discomfort may persist for a long time.

FRACTURE OF ALL FOUR PUBIC RAMI

When the pelvic ring is injured at more than one site, the potential for instability increases correspondingly. Fractures of all four pubic rami disrupt the structural integrity of the anterior portion of the pelvic ring. This injury commonly results from a fall on the front of the pelvis or from lateral compressive forces on the pelvic ring. In about one-third of patients, major trauma to the lower urinary tract occurs as well. Treatment focuses on preventing any further displacement of the fracture fragments. Bed rest, with the patient in a semisitting position to relax the abdominal musculature, is followed by mobilization as soon as symptoms allow.

LATERAL COMPRESSION INJURY

Double breaks in the pelvic ring are often due to lateral compressive forces. Most of these fractures are stable because the forces cause impaction of the posterior pelvic complex, leaving the posterior ligaments intact. If the force continues or increases, the posterior sacroiliac ligaments may tear, producing an instability in the injured hemipelvis.

This injury often includes fractures of the superior and inferior pubic rami; therefore the anterior and posterior injuries are on the same side. When the patient is placed in the supine position, the displaced hemipelvis often reduces spontaneously. Radiographs may reveal only minimal displacement, but the examiner must remember that the degree of initial deformation of the hemipelvis is not known, and significant visceral injury may be present.

When a lateral compressive force is accompanied by a rotational force, the anterior fracture often occurs on the side opposite the posterior fracture; for example, an impacted fracture may occur on the left side of the sacrum, whereas fractures of the inferior and superior pubic rami occur on the right side. The hemipelvis then displaces superiorly and medially, causing the leg to appear internally rotated and shortened. The position of the hemipelvis generally remains stable, although the malrotation may compromise future function. Correcting this rotational deformity may create instability when the impacted posterior injury is reduced.

STRADDLE FRACTURE AND LATERAL COMPRESSION INJURY

Straddle fracture

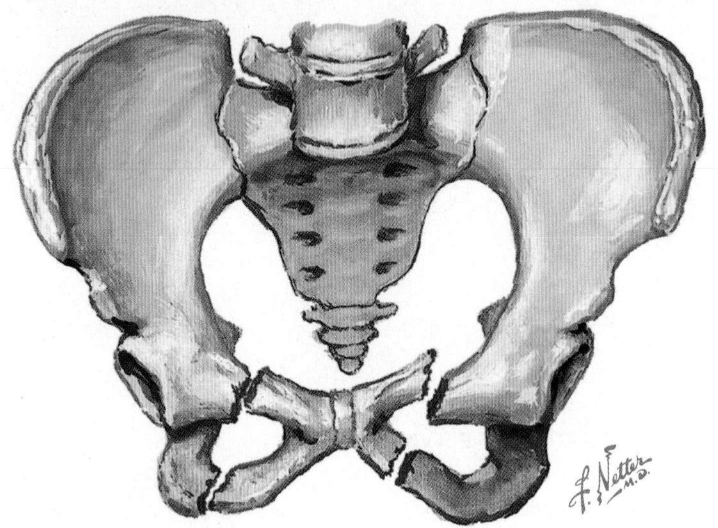

Double break in continuity of anterior pelvic ring causes instability but usually little displacement. Visceral (especially genitourinary) injury likely.

Lateral compression injury

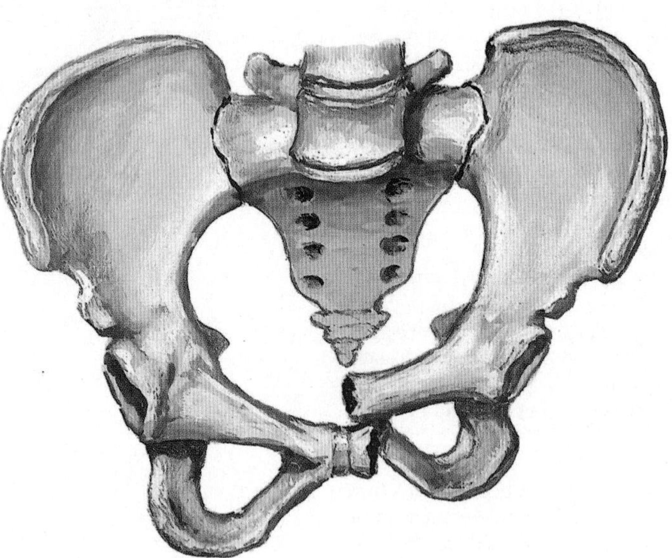

Fracture of pubic bone or pubic rami on one side, or separation of pubic symphysis with one hemipelvis driven inward to overlap other side. Widening or subluxation of ipsilateral sacroiliac joint may occur. Displacement usually minor and may self-reduce as result of tissue recoil or with manual distraction. Conservative treatment usually adequate, but visceral or vascular injury must be considered.

ANTEROPOSTERIOR COMPRESSION FRACTURE

AP compression, or open book, fractures of the pelvis are usually caused by a forceful blow from in front of the pelvis through the anterior superior iliac spines or by force applied to externally rotated femurs (see Plate 2.65). However, a blow from the rear against the posterior superior iliac spines may produce a similar injury that is characterized by disruption of the pubic symphysis and the anterior sacroiliac ligaments. Injuries range from an isolated rupture of the pubic symphysis to complete separation of the pubic symphysis accompanied by bilateral anterior subluxation of the sacroiliac joints.

Open Book Fracture

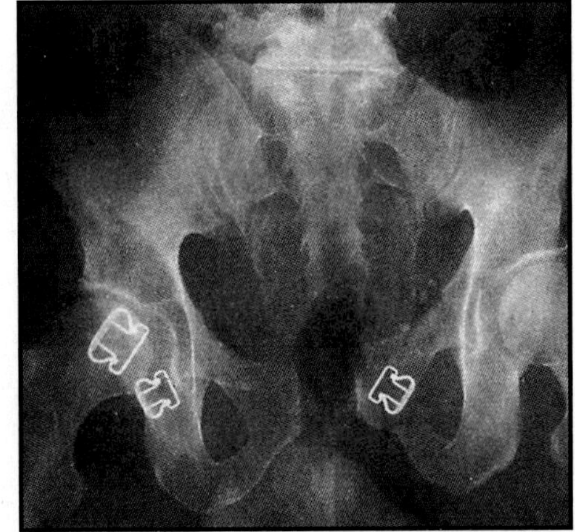

Radiograph shows open book fracture.

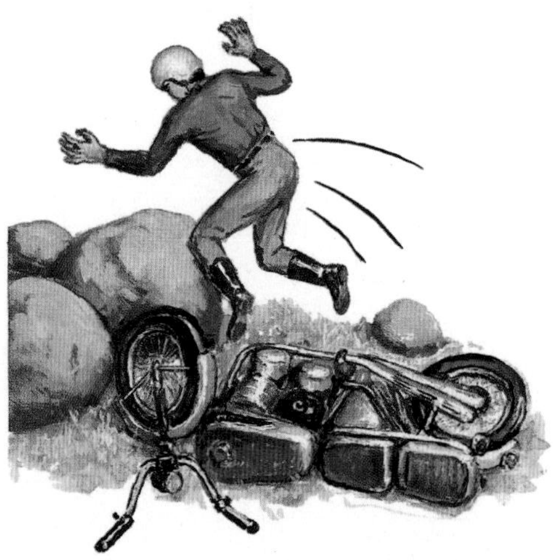

Caused by forceful impact to knee or foot transmitted to pelvis or by direct blow to pelvis

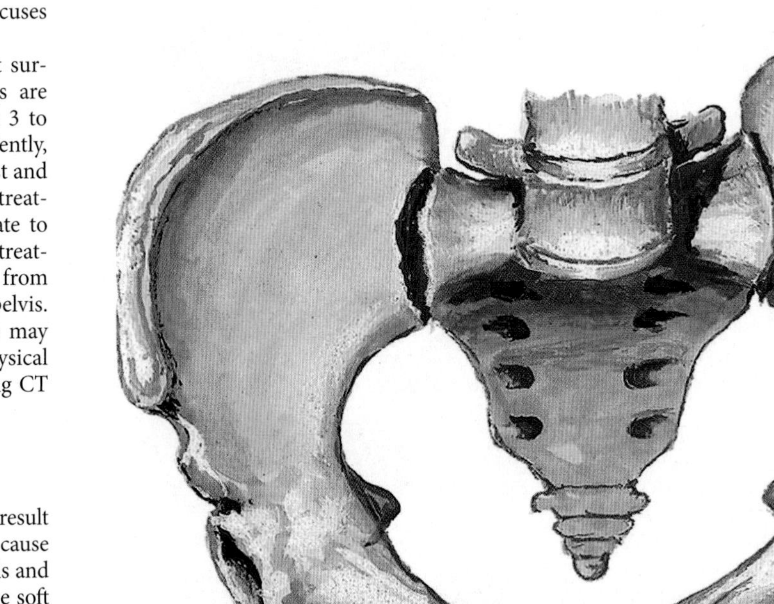

Disruption of symphysis pubis with wide anterior separation of pelvic ring. Anterior sacroiliac ligaments are torn, with slight opening of sacroiliac joints. Intact posterior sacroiliac ligaments prevent vertical migration of the pelvis.

Injury to Pelvis (Continued)

Because the sacrospinal ligaments resist external rotation of the pelvis, a separation of 2.5 cm or greater of the symphysis suggests that the sacrospinal ligaments have ruptured or have avulsed bone from the sacrum or ischial spine. Most important, the very strong posterior sacroiliac ligaments remain intact. The open book fracture is therefore relatively stable, and treatment focuses on closing the pelvic ring.

The pelvic ring can be closed with or without surgery. In nonsurgical treatment, crossover slings are used to bring the two pelvic halves together. In 3 to 4 weeks, when the soft tissues have healed sufficiently, the pelvic slings are replaced with a mini spica cast and ambulatory treatment can be initiated. If surgical treatment is chosen, ORIF is performed, using a plate to stabilize the pubic symphysis. The planning of treatment for this injury must be clearly distinguished from the treatment for a vertical shear injury of the pelvis. Because the initial radiographs of both injuries may appear similar, differentiation requires careful physical examination and supplemental imaging, including CT of the posterior pelvic complex.

VERTICAL SHEAR FRACTURE

Vertical shear, or Malgaigne, fractures of the pelvis result from severe trauma (see Plate 2.66). The force may cause unilateral or bilateral injuries to the posterior pelvis and severe and sometimes life-threatening injury to the soft tissue contents of the pelvic cavity. The injury to the anterior pelvis may include disruption of the pubic symphysis with or without fractures of two, three, or four pubic rami. The posterior injuries may be fractures of the sacrum, dislocations of the sacroiliac joint, fractures of the ilium, or fracture dislocations of the sacroiliac joint, including fractures of the sacrum or the ilium.

Avulsion fractures, particularly of the ischial spine or the transverse process of the fifth lumbar vertebra, also occur in major disruptions of the posterior pelvis. Complete instability of the affected hemipelvis indicates disruption of the sacrotuberal and sacrospinal ligaments. Because vertical shear fractures are caused by considerable force, many involve vital pelvic and abdominal tissues of the gastrointestinal, genitourinary, vascular, and nervous systems.

If the posterior hemipelvis on one side remains intact, the disrupted half can be brought to the intact side and stabilized. When both ilia are disrupted from the sacrum, stabilization is much more problematic. The aim of treatment soon after injury is to reapproximate the injured hemipelvis to the uninjured side using closed manipulation. After anesthesia or analgesia with significant muscle relaxation is obtained, the patient is positioned injured side up, with an assistant supporting the legs. The examiner pushes the displaced ilium downward and forward. If the reduction is successful, skeletal traction is often used to maintain it until significant healing of soft tissue or bone occurs.

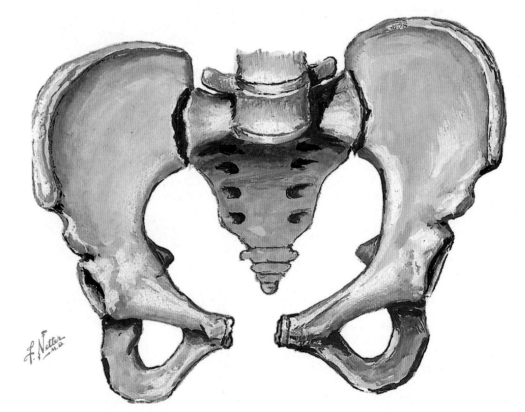

Because many Malgaigne fractures are grossly unstable, manipulative reduction is largely unsuccessful, and either external or internal fixation of the hemipelvis is needed. Fixation with an external fixation device provides relative immobilization of the hemipelvis; the stability is greater than that provided by manipulative reduction and subsequent traction. However, attempts to attain and

Injury to Pelvis (Continued)

maintain anatomic reduction with external fixators are usually unsuccessful.

ORIF of both displaced components provides the best stabilization of vertical shear fractures. Two plates may be used to secure the disruptions in the pubic symphysis and iliosacral fixation to stabilize the posterior pelvic ring.

VASCULAR AND VISCERAL TRAUMA

Vascular and visceral injuries are the chief causes of deaths associated with pelvic fractures. The likelihood of associated injury is directly related to the severity of the fracture.

Pelvic fractures normally cause bleeding from injured vessels of the pelvic marrow or from torn pelvic or lumbar arteries and veins and formation of a hematoma. The extent of the bleeding depends on the severity of the vascular and bone injuries, and the risk of death is directly linked to the severity of the hemorrhage. Patients with double breaks in the pelvic ring require transfusions twice as often as patients with single breaks or with fractures of the acetabulum. Persistent severe hemorrhage may warrant emergent investigation with transfemoral arteriography to identify bleeding sites and selective embolization using blood, gelatin, or other such substances. Arteriography may be used to identify injuries to large arteries. Pelvic binders are an important early measure to stabilize the disruption, reduce pelvic volume, and diminish blood loss.

Frequently, pelvic fractures cause injuries of the lower urinary tract. Clues to such injuries include blood at the urethral meatus or hematuria found on urinalysis. In men, rectal examination may reveal a high-riding or free-floating prostate, which usually indicates injury to the lower urinary tract. Urethrography is performed to determine whether the anterior portion of the urethra is injured. If the urethrogram appears normal, a catheter should be passed gently through the urethra into the bladder. *The catheter must not be forced.* If this procedure is accomplished, further radiographic studies can determine whether an intraperitoneal or an extraperitoneal bladder injury is present.

Most complete transections of the urethra are treated by diverting the urine stream through a suprapubic catheter placed into the bladder and, later, with repair or reconstruction of the urethra. Intraperitoneal ruptures of the bladder are repaired with suprapubic drainage to decompress the bladder. Depending on the extent of the tear, extraperitoneal ruptures may not require surgical repair; adequate drainage of the bladder is necessary to allow the laceration to heal.

Vertical Shear Fracture

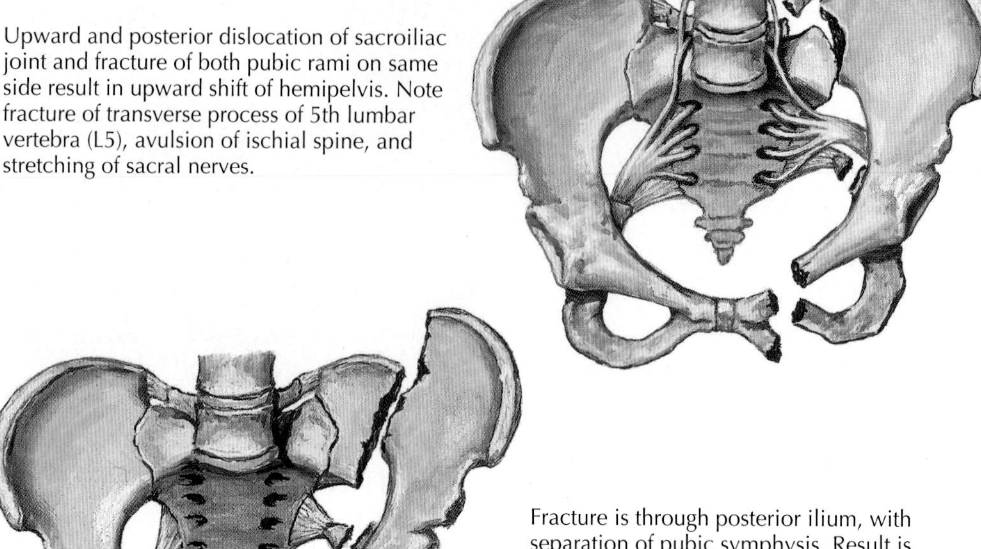

Upward and posterior dislocation of sacroiliac joint and fracture of both pubic rami on same side result in upward shift of hemipelvis. Note fracture of transverse process of 5th lumbar vertebra (L5), avulsion of ischial spine, and stretching of sacral nerves.

Fracture is through posterior ilium, with separation of pubic symphysis. Result is effectively the same as in other case shown.

Internal fixation for type of vertical shear fracture

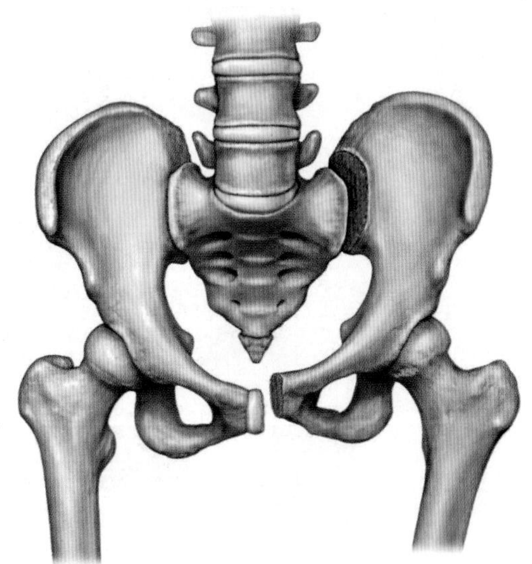

Vertical shear fracture with disruption of symphysis pubis and sacroiliac joint

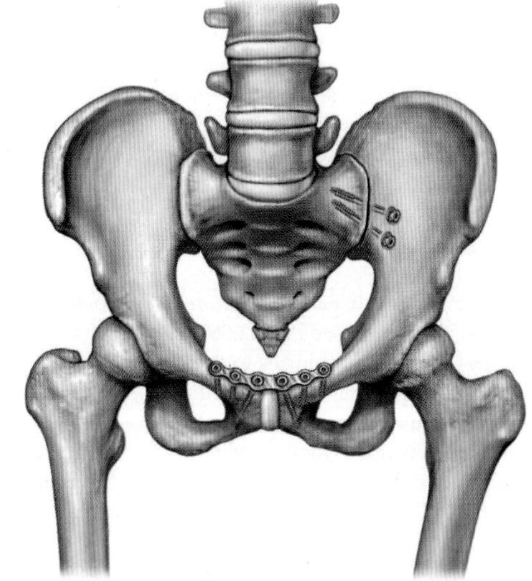

Reduction and internal fixation with percutaneous screw fixation of the sacroiliac joint and open reducti and plate fixation of the symphysis pubis disruption

The examiner must search diligently for injuries of the lower gastrointestinal tract, especially about the rectum and the anus. Blood found on rectal examination suggests that the lower gastrointestinal tract has been lacerated by bone fragments, with possible severe contamination of the extraperitoneal pelvic space. If the rectum or anus is lacerated, standard treatment includes performing a washout of the distal rectal lumen and creating a diverting colostomy to minimize pelvic contamination. In women, a careful vaginal examination is performed to detect lacerations of the vagina, which could lead to contamination and infection of the pelvis.

ACETABULAR FRACTURES

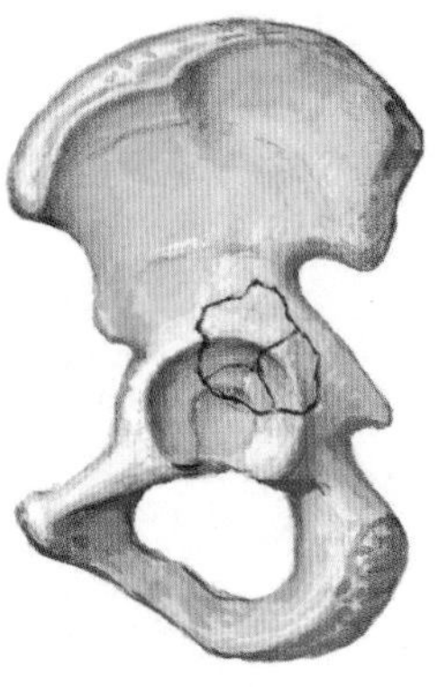
Posterior wall fracture

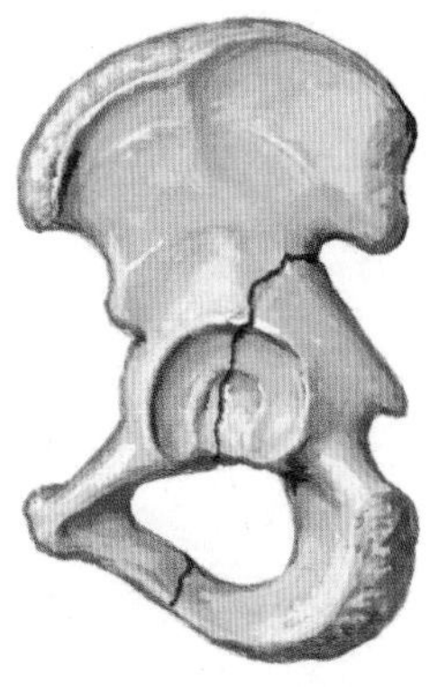
Posterior column fracture

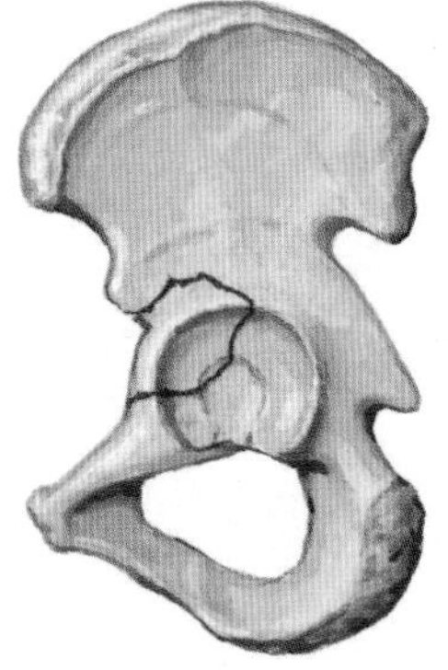
Anterior wall fracture

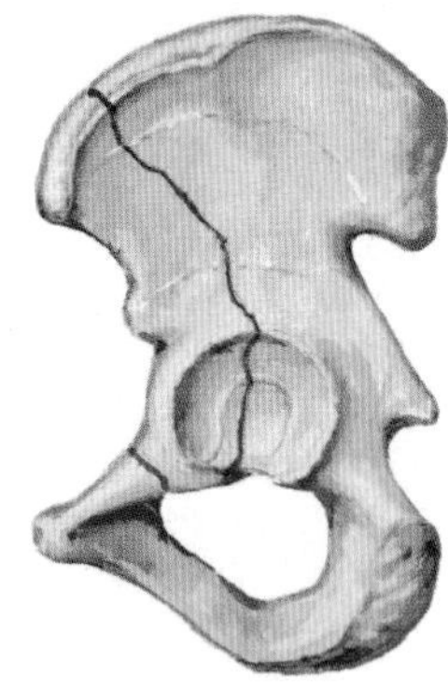
Anterior column fracture

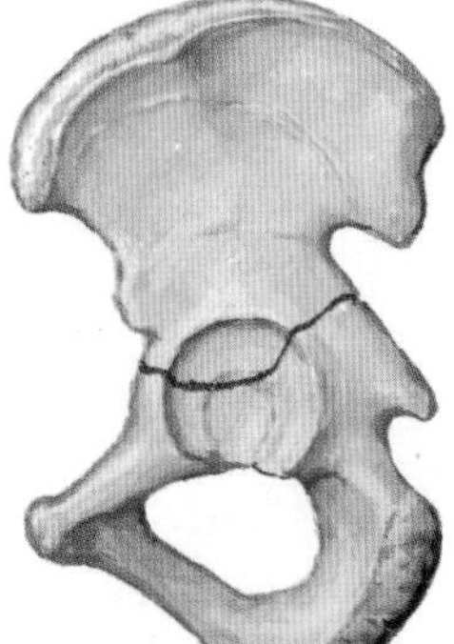
Transverse fracture

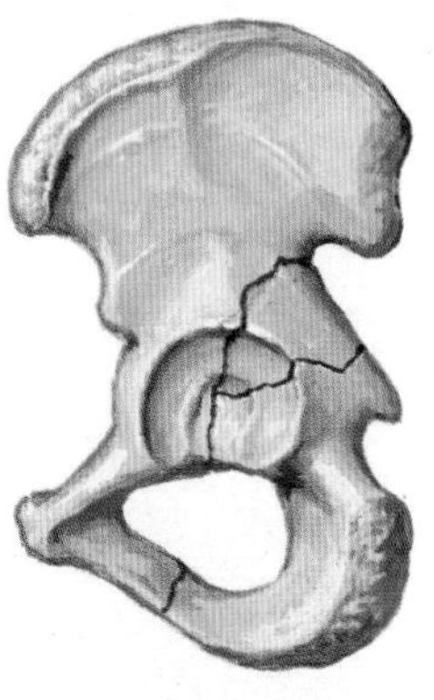
Associated posterior column and posterior wall fractures

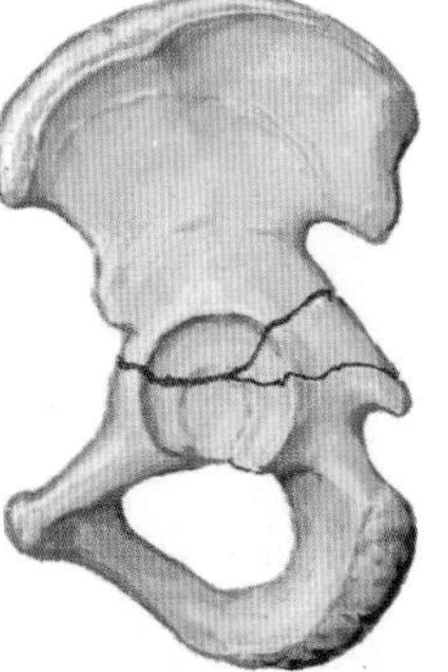
Associated transverse and posterior wall fractures

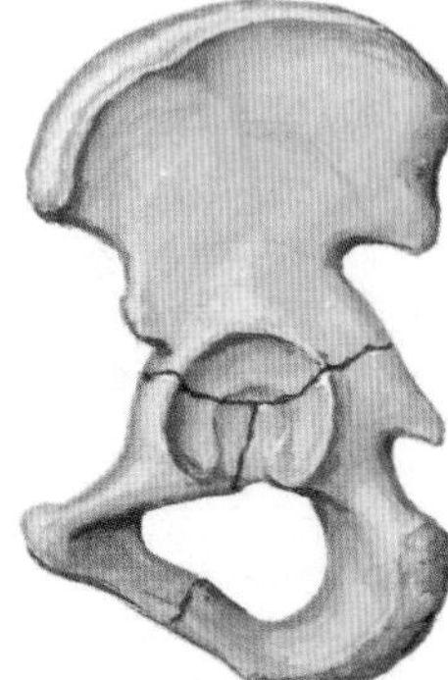
T-shaped fracture

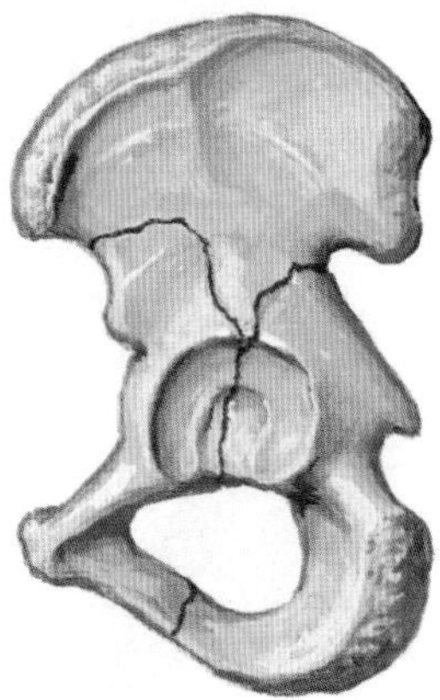
Associated anterior and posterior hemi-transverse fractures

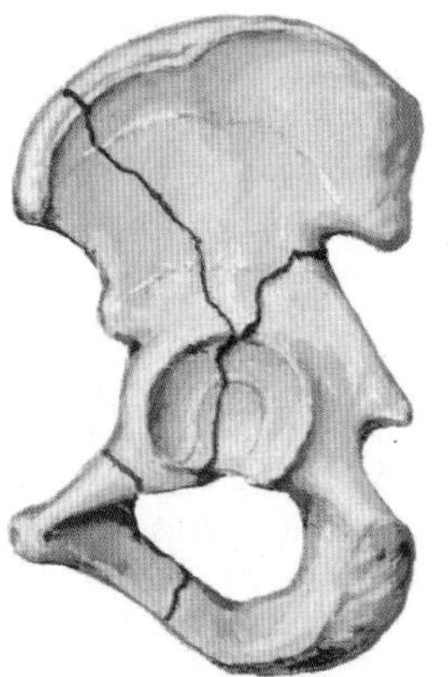
Fracture of both columns

INJURY TO HIP

FRACTURE OF ACETABULUM

The acetabulum of the pelvis makes up the socket of the hip joint. It develops at the confluence of three epiphyseal junctions between the ilium, ischium, and pubis. The growth of the acetabulum occurs with the development of this triradiate cartilage, and its shape is influenced considerably by the shape of the femoral head with which it articulates. Acetabular injuries are not as common as other injuries to the hip joint, and most result from forces generated by the femoral head against the confines of the acetabular cup. Fractures tend to occur in younger persons and involve greater violence than the typical femoral neck or intertrochanteric fracture.

Acetabular injuries range from simple avulsions of the periphery of the acetabulum to explosions of the hip socket. When the acetabulum fractures, the femoral head is usually dislocated or subluxated in relation to the part of the acetabulum that remains intact. The displacement may be anterior, central, or posterior. After reduction, an incongruence often exists between the femoral head and the acetabulum. Acetabular fractures are classified as simple and associated. Simple fracture patterns are further categorized as fractures of the anterior wall, anterior column, posterior wall, and posterior column and transverse fractures. Associated fracture patterns comprise fractures of the posterior wall and posterior column, transverse fractures with posterior wall fractures, T-shaped fractures, fractures of both columns, and fractures of the anterior wall or column with an associated posterior hemitransverse fracture.

Patients with minimally displaced fractures of the acetabulum or those who cannot, or elect not to, undergo surgical treatment are treated with nonoperative measures. Initially, the patient is placed in traction until the acute reaction of the fracture subsides. Then the hip is moved through a range of flexion, extension, abduction, and adduction, either by a physical therapist or with the use of a continuous passive motion machine. Once these movements are achieved comfortably, the patient is mobilized using crutches, with minimal weight bearing on the injured side. Radiographs are taken frequently to assess the healing of the fracture and to check for residual displacement of the femoral head.

CENTRAL FRACTURE OF ACETABULUM

Patients with severe central fracture dislocations of the acetabulum will require surgery. Those who cannot be treated with surgery can managed with more complex traction arrangements (see Plate 2.68). First, skeletal traction is applied with a pin through the distal femur or proximal tibia to establish a normal

ACETABULAR FRACTURES (CONTINUED)

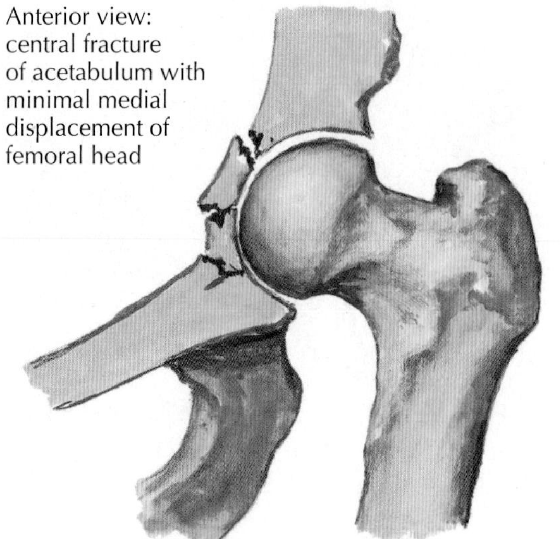

Anterior view:
central fracture
of acetabulum with
minimal medial
displacement of
femoral head

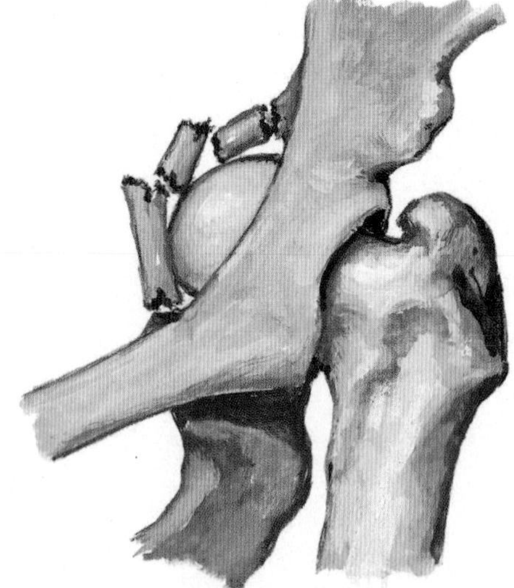

Central fracture of acetabulum with dislocation of femoral head into pelvis

INJURY TO HIP (Continued)

relationship between the superior femoral head and the dome of the acetabulum. About one-sixth of the patient's body weight is applied through the traction mechanism to restore the injured limb to its normal length. After this maneuver, a radiograph is obtained to assess the relationship of the femoral head to the intact acetabulum. If subluxation of the femoral head persists, lateral traction, applied with a sling or with a pin placed in the femur distal to the greater trochanter, is used to extricate the femoral head from the pelvis. Traction is maintained for 6 to 8 weeks. Weight bearing on the injured lower limb is limited for at least 3 to 4 months from the time of injury. Residual subluxation may occur in the same direction as the original displacement.

POSTERIOR DISLOCATION OF HIP

Posterior dislocations of the hip have become more common as the occurrence of high-energy trauma has increased (see Plate 2.69). The classic mechanism of injury is the impact of the dashboard against the flexed knee during a head-on motor vehicle collision. The dashboard collapses, striking the knee and driving the femoral head out of the acetabular socket. Generally, the resulting posterior dislocation of the hip is not an isolated injury; multiple injuries of the lower limb often occur, including fractures of the patella and femoral shaft and injuries to the posterior cruciate ligament. Aortic dissection may also be an associated injury.

Pure dislocations of the femoral head occur with the hip adducted and flexed. In this position, the force is concentrated against the soft tissues of the hip joint capsule rather than the bony architecture of the posterior acetabulum. Indentation fractures of the femoral head occasionally occur, as do abrasions of the articular cartilage. Because of its close proximity to the posterior aspect of the hip joint, the sciatic nerve (especially the peroneal division) is injured in 8% to 20% of patients with posterior dislocation or posterior fracture dislocation of the hip. Sciatic nerve injury is more common with fracture-dislocations than with pure dislocations.

When the dislocation of the hip is posterior, the major blood supply to the femoral head is injured. Avascular necrosis of the femoral head, one of the more common complications of this injury, appears to be related to the amount of time the femoral head remains dislocated from the acetabulum.

Posterior dislocation of the hip results in a classic posture: the lower limb is flexed at the hip joint, adducted, and internally rotated. Careful physical examination also reveals shortening of the limb. Many patients report a feeling of fullness in the buttocks. A neurologic evaluation of the limb must be performed, with emphasis on the musculature innervated by the peroneal division of the sciatic nerve.

Radiographs of the pelvis and hip reveal the absence of the femoral head from its normal articulation in the acetabulum. The displaced head usually appears smaller than the femoral head on the uninjured side and in a

Acetabular fracture fixation

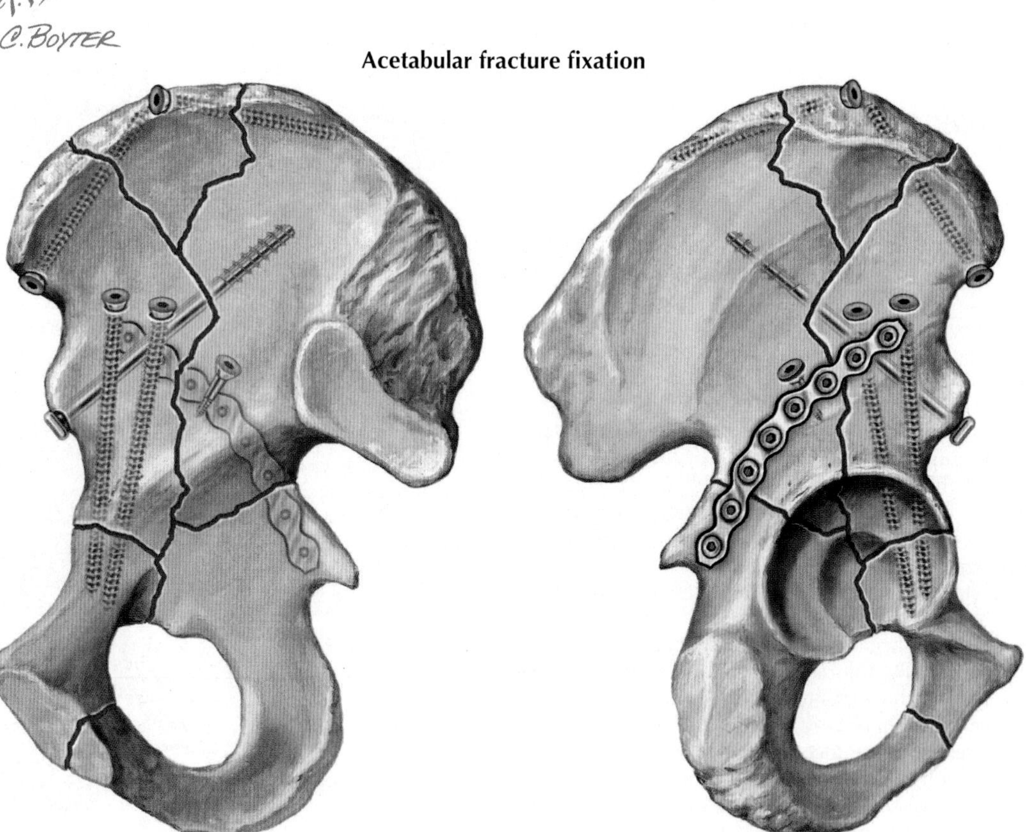

Representative fixation for both-column fracture with associated iliac wing fractures

Posterior Dislocation of Hip

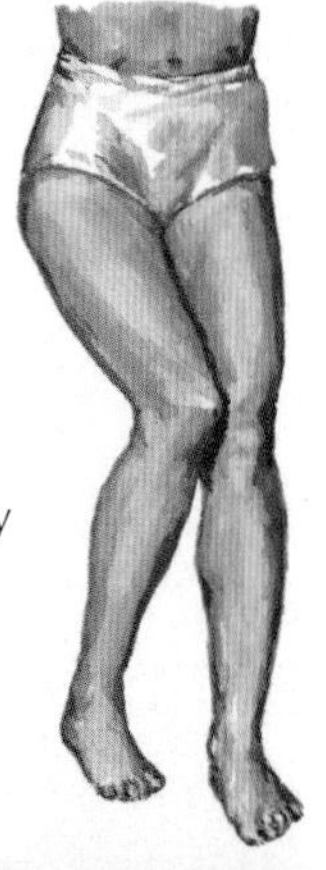

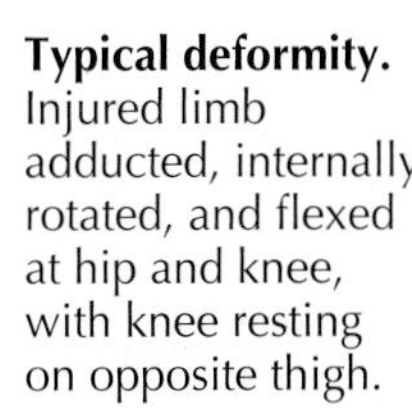

Typical deformity. Injured limb adducted, internally rotated, and flexed at hip and knee, with knee resting on opposite thigh.

Mechanism of injury often by impact with dashboard, which drives femoral head backward, out of acetabulum

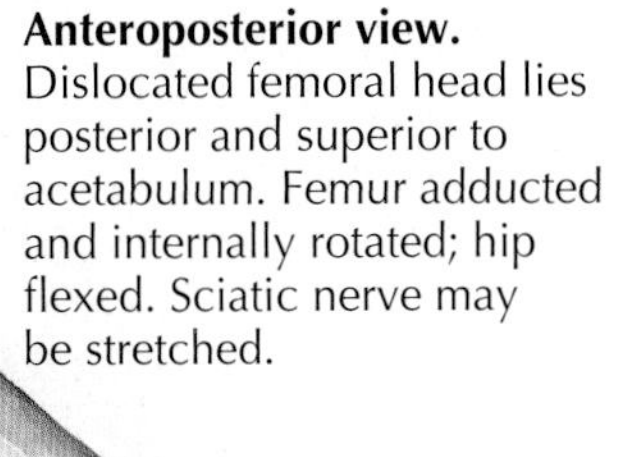

Anteroposterior view. Dislocated femoral head lies posterior and superior to acetabulum. Femur adducted and internally rotated; hip flexed. Sciatic nerve may be stretched.

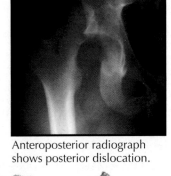

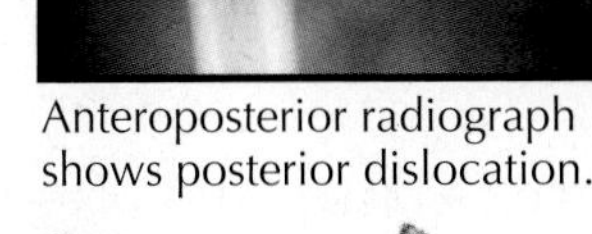

Anteroposterior radiograph shows posterior dislocation.

Allis maneuver. Patient supine on table, under anesthesia or sedation. Examiner applies firm distal traction at flexed knee to pull head into acetabulum; slight rotatory motion may also help. Assistant fixes pelvis by pressing on anterior superior iliac spines.

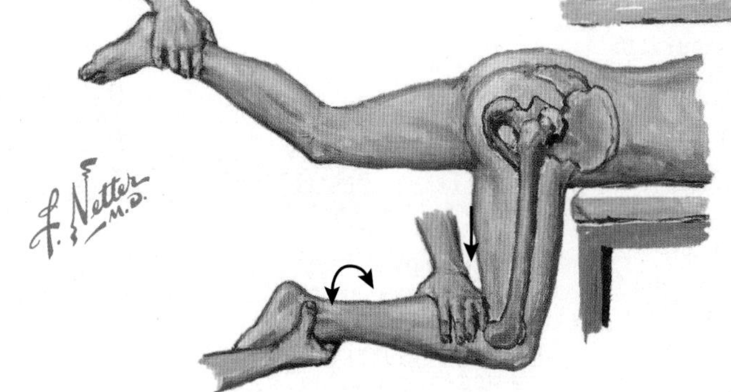

Stimson maneuver. Patient prone on table, injured limb hanging over end, its weight providing traction. Examiner applies downward pressure at calf and slight rotation at ankle. Assistant supports other limb. Anesthesia may not be necessary; sedation may suffice.

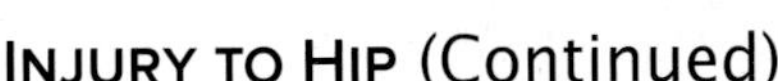

Injury to Hip (Continued)

position proximal to the acetabulum. Radiographs are important for determining both the extent of bone injury to the hip socket and any associated fractures.

In posterior dislocation of the hip with no associated sciatic nerve injury, the hip should be reduced within 12 hours of injury. Prompt reduction helps to minimize the development of avascular necrosis of the femoral head. Dislocations with associated sciatic nerve injury are acute emergencies and must be reduced to relieve extrinsic pressure on the nerve and lessen the risk of permanent sciatic nerve palsy.

In patients with multiple injuries, the most common method of closed reduction of a posterior dislocation of the hip is the Allis maneuver. The maneuver is performed with the patient supine and allows further evaluation of associated injuries to the abdomen, chest, and airway that would be difficult to perform with the patient in a lateral or prone position. With an assistant stabilizing the pelvis, the physician applies gentle traction to the lower limb in the line of the deformity. After traction has been applied, the hip is gently flexed 90 degrees while gentle internal and external rotation is applied until reduction is achieved. When it occurs, the reduction can be felt by both the physician and the assistant.

If the dislocation is an isolated injury, the Stimson gravity reduction maneuver can be used. The patient is placed prone and the injured hip flexed over the end of the examining table. An assistant stabilizes the pelvis by pressing down on the sacrum or by extending the uninjured limb. The physician flexes the involved hip and knee 90 degrees and applies gentle downward pressure behind the flexed knee. As pressure is applied, gentle internal and external rotation is added. As in the Allis maneuver, both the physician and the assistant can feel the reduction when the femoral head relocates into the acetabulum.

After reduction, it is extremely important to reassess the neurologic status of the injured limb, focusing on the function of the sciatic nerve and its peroneal division. If sciatic nerve dysfunction is now apparent, surgical exploration of the nerve should be considered. Radiographs and CT scans should be examined for evidence of joint space widening or for the presence of small bone fragments within the joint that might prevent congruence between the femoral head and the acetabulum. After successful reduction, the limb is placed in light skin traction to allow the injured hip to rest. When the local reaction to the injury subsides, the patient can be mobilized and begin gentle active range-of-motion exercises, including extension, flexion, abduction, and adduction.

Guidelines for weight bearing after this injury are not well established and remain controversial. Generally, early motion of the hip is promoted but weight bearing is delayed. If evidence of avascular necrosis develops, weight bearing is postponed even longer to prevent collapse of the femoral head. Although recurrence of posterior dislocation or subluxation of the hip is rare, posttraumatic osteoarthritic changes of the hip are not uncommon. Follow-up should continue for at least 2 years to detect any arthritic or necrotic changes.

Injury to Hip (Continued)

ANTERIOR DISLOCATION OF HIP

About 10% to 15% of traumatic dislocations of the hip are anterior dislocations, either the superior type or the more common obturator type. Anterior dislocation occurs when the hip is abducted, externally rotated, and flexed and the knee strikes a fixed object. Either the neck of the femur or the greater trochanter levers the head of the femur out of the acetabulum through a disruption of the anterior hip capsule. As the femoral head leaves the anterior aspect of the acetabulum, transchondral or indentation fractures of the femoral head can occur. Since the introduction of CT, the incidence of this type of fracture has been shown to be much greater than previously thought.

The characteristic clinical appearance is the limb flexed at the hip, abducted, and externally rotated. In assessing the neurovascular status after an obturator dislocation, the examiner must pay special attention to the presence of an injury to the obturator nerve resulting in paresis of the hip adductor musculature. Similarly, in the superior dislocation, the femoral nerve, artery, or vein can be damaged and must be assessed before reduction attempts are made. Radiographic evaluation of the injury should include AP and Judet views (oblique at 45 degrees) of the pelvis to help delineate associated injuries of the acetabulum, femoral head, and femoral neck.

The Allis maneuver is generally recommended for obturator dislocations. Strong intravenous analgesics or spinal anesthetics are given to provide adequate muscle relaxation. If closed reduction is not successful, open reduction is required. An anterior iliofemoral approach allows identification and treatment of the obstruction to the dislocation.

After reduction, new radiographs are taken to determine the extent of associated injuries to the femoral neck, acetabulum, or femoral head. Polytomography or CT may demonstrate a nondisplaced fracture of the femoral head or indentation fracture resulting from impingement of the femoral head against the acetabulum. Reassessment of the neurovascular status of the limb distal to the hip is also important. Posttraumatic osteoarthritis requiring later reconstructive surgery eventually develops in one-third of patients. Avascular necrosis may also be a residual complication. Recurrent dislocations are not common.

Postreduction care involves light traction with early active range-of-motion exercises, including extension, flexion, abduction-adduction, and rotation but avoidance of extremes of flexion, abduction, and external rotation. Just when weight bearing should begin is not clear, and the available guidelines are not consistent. Usually, as pain diminishes, the patient is allowed to begin weight bearing using crutches for support. Weight bearing is gradually increased until the support can be discarded. Follow-up should continue for at least 2 years to monitor for avascular necrosis or posttraumatic osteoarthritis.

Anterior Dislocation of Hip, Obturator Type

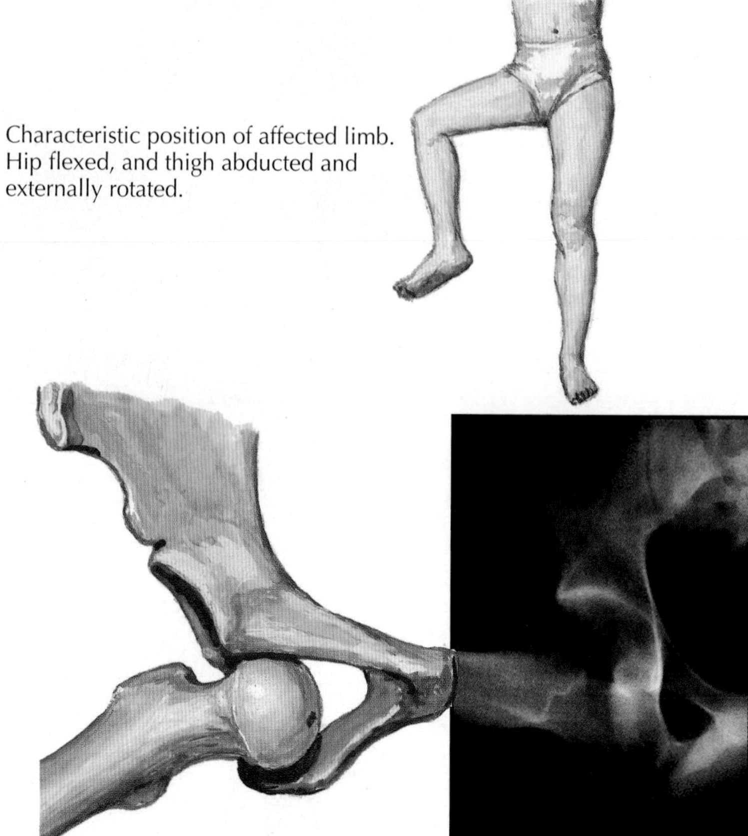

Characteristic position of affected limb. Hip flexed, and thigh abducted and externally rotated.

Anterior view. Femoral head in obturator foramen of pelvis; hip flexed and femur widely abducted and externally rotated.

Anteroposterior radiograph shows obturator-type dislocation.

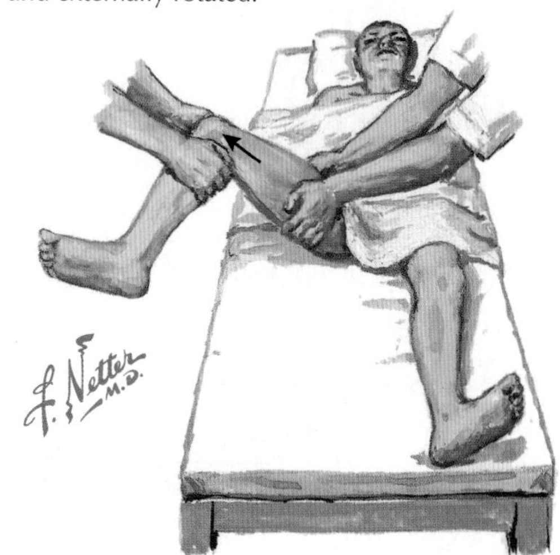

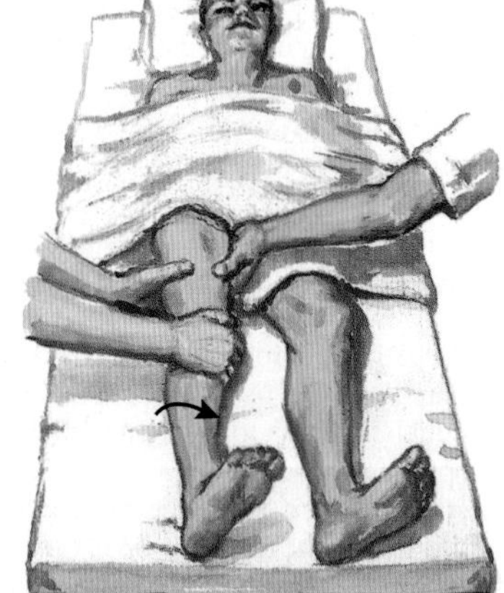

Allis maneuver. Patient supine; examiner applies manual traction in line of dislocated femoral shaft, as assistant applies lateral pressure to proximal thigh (usually performed with patient under anesthesia or sedation).

With continued traction, thigh adducted, internally rotated, and extended, thus reducing hip. No more than two attempts at reduction should be made; if they fail, open reduction is indicated.

Dislocation of Hip With Fracture of Femoral Head

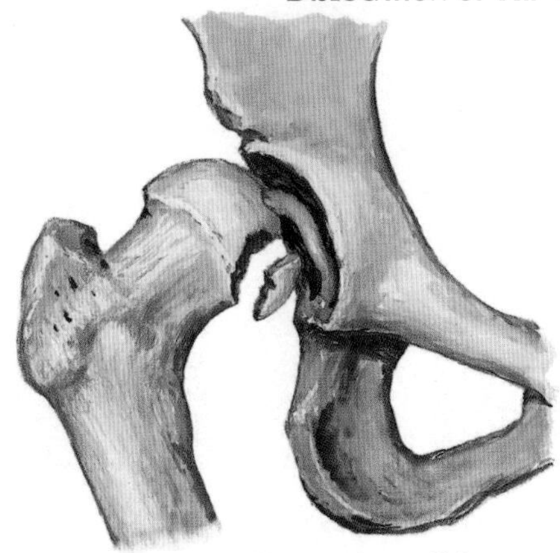

Posterior dislocation of hip with small fracture of femoral head inferior to fovea does not involve weight-bearing surface of femoral head. Such small fragments may be excised or left alone.

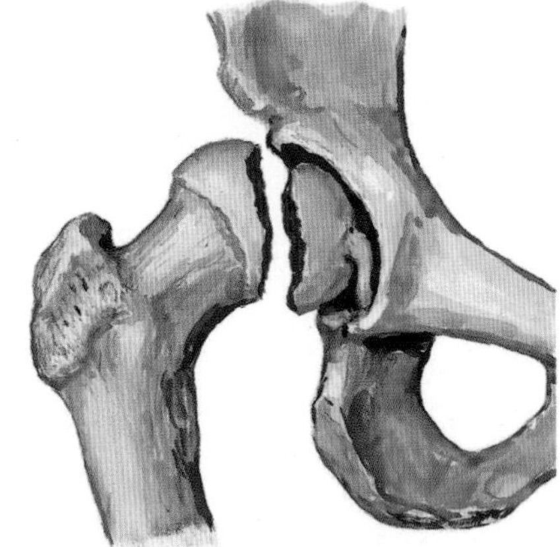

Dislocation with fracture of large fragment of femoral head extending proximal to fovea involves weight-bearing surface and may require open repair to restore articular congruity and hip joint stability.

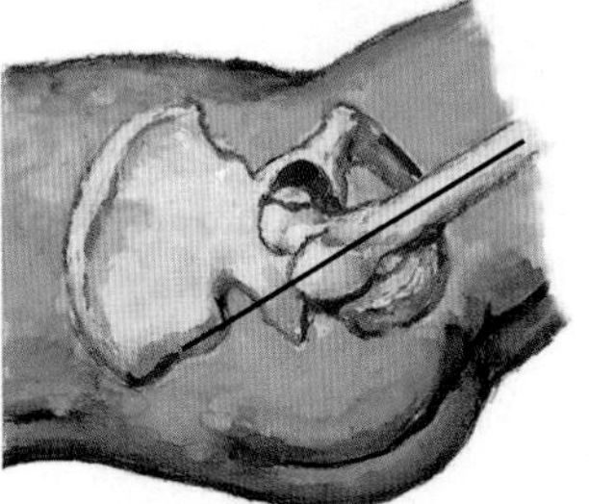

Skin and fascial incision

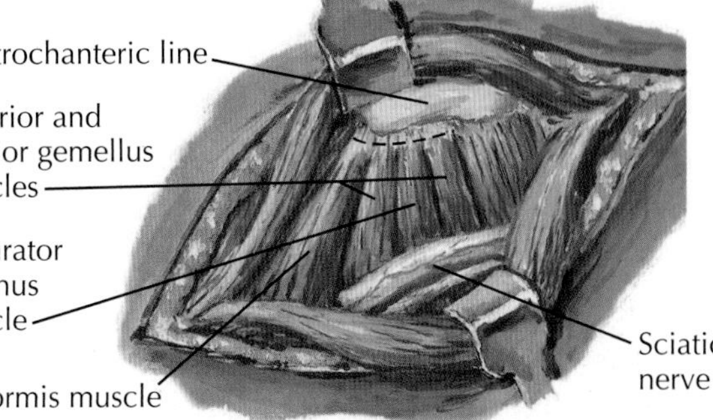

Gluteus maximus muscle is split by separation of fascicles, exposing piriformis and short external rotator muscles and sciatic nerve. Nerve must be carefully preserved.

Piriformis and short external rotator muscles are divided and reflected. Hip joint is opened, exposing femoral head and fracture fragment. If small, fragment is removed.

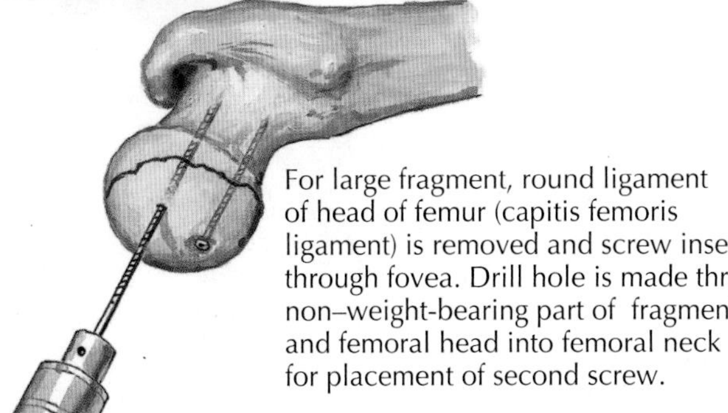

For large fragment, round ligament of head of femur (capitis femoris ligament) is removed and screw inserted through fovea. Drill hole is made through non–weight-bearing part of fragment and femoral head into femoral neck for placement of second screw.

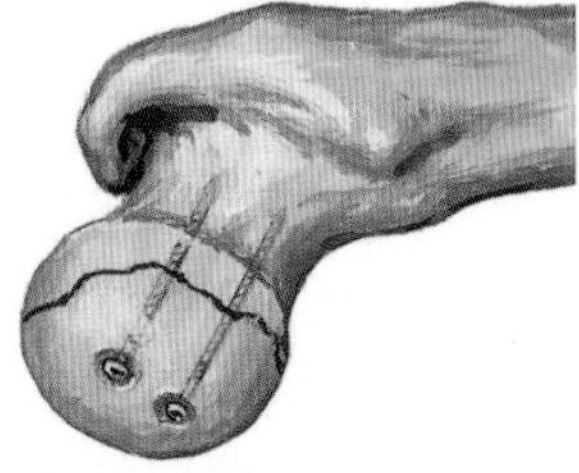

Second screw is inserted. Both screws are countersunk to prevent abrasion of acetabular cartilage.

Injury to Hip (Continued)

DISLOCATION OF HIP WITH FRACTURE OF FEMORAL HEAD

As posterior dislocations and fracture dislocations of the hip have increased in frequency, associated femoral head fractures have also become more common. These injuries are believed to occur with the hip flexed 60 degrees or less and in neutral abduction. The force of the trauma drives the femoral head against the posterosuperior portion of the acetabulum, resulting in dislocation and shear fracture of the femoral head.

Pipkin delineated four types of fracture dislocations of the hip and assigned higher numbers to the injuries with the worst prognoses. In type I injuries, fracture of the femoral head occurs inferior to the fovea of the head of the femur. Type II injuries include a fracture that is superior to the fovea. In type III injuries, a type I or type II fracture may occur in association with a femoral neck fracture, and type IV injuries involve a type I, type II, or type III injury in association with an acetabular fracture.

Because these injuries are associated with posterior hip dislocations, the neurovascular status of the limb must be determined and radiographs of the hip, including AP and Judet views, obtained before reduction is attempted. The posterior dislocation should be reduced as soon as possible to minimize avascular necrosis of the femoral head. Reduction can be performed using the maneuvers described for reduction of a simple posterior dislocation of the hip. Careful evaluation must be made of the reduction of the femoral head in the acetabulum and the reduction of the fractured portion of the femoral head to the intact head. The femoral head must be concentrically reduced in the acetabulum. The amount of step-off and gap that exists at the fracture surface must also be determined.

In type I or II injury, the fragment of the femoral head need not be removed as long as it does not impede hip motion and the hip is congruently reduced and stable. If a congruent reduction was not achieved, removal or internal fixation of the fragment to the remaining surface of the femoral head should be considered. After closed reduction, incongruence resulting in either an offset or gap greater than 2 mm should be used as the criterion for open reduction or excision of the fragment. As much as one-third of the femoral head can be removed, but many surgeons prefer internal fixation of fragments of this size.

In type III and IV injuries, the adequacy of the reductions of the femoral head fracture and dislocation is assessed first; then the reduction of the femoral neck or the acetabulum or both must be evaluated. Displaced fractures of the femoral neck may require internal fixation, and severe displacement may necessitate total hip replacement. Internal fixation of acetabular injuries should be considered if this will optimize the anatomic reconstruction of the hip joint.

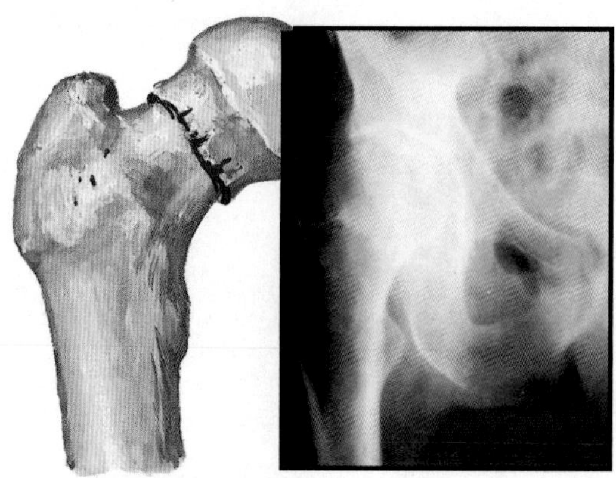

Type I. Impacted fracture.

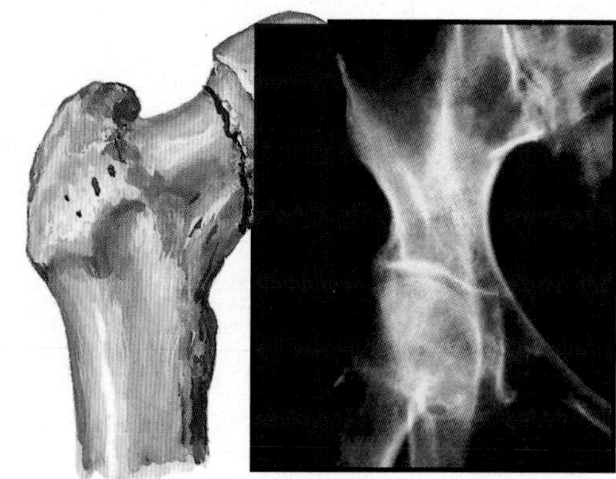

Type II. Nondisplaced fracture.

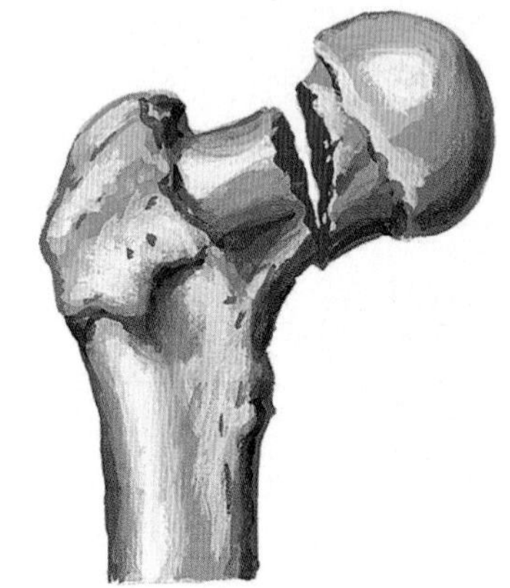

Type III. Partially displaced.

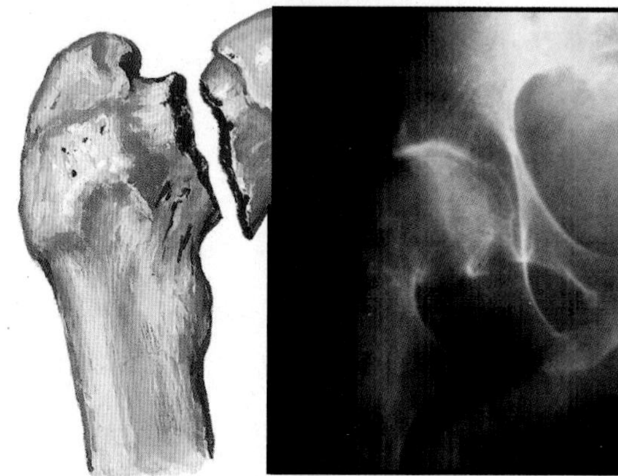

Type IV. Displaced fracture. Vertical fracture line generally suggests poorer prognosis.

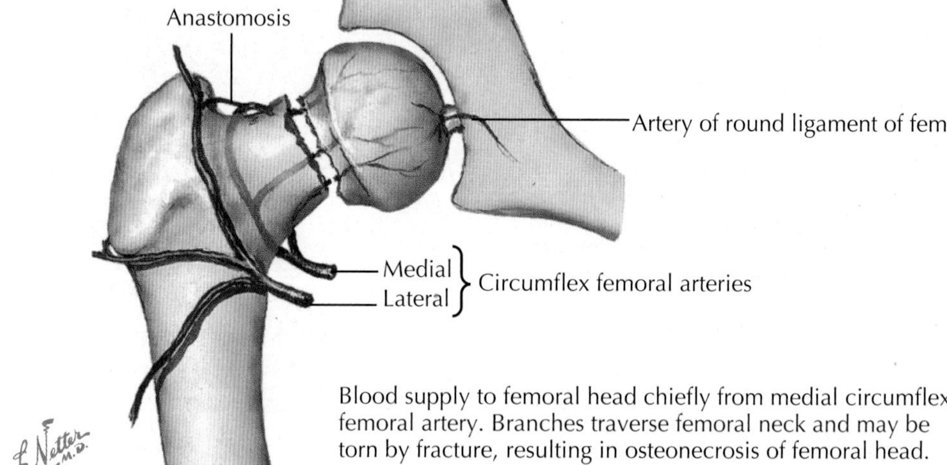

Blood supply to femoral head chiefly from medial circumflex femoral artery. Branches traverse femoral neck and may be torn by fracture, resulting in osteonecrosis of femoral head. Artery of round ligament is usually insignificant.

Intracapsular Fracture of Femoral Neck

Femoral neck fractures are very common injuries, especially in older persons. In young persons, these injuries are usually caused by severe trauma. In older patients, especially those with osteoporosis, they are associated with falls, and it is possible that the fracture occurred before the fall.

Garden has classified femoral neck fractures into four categories. In a type I fracture, the superior portion of the femoral neck is impacted into the femoral head. Type II is a complete fracture that remains nondisplaced. Type III is a fracture with partial displacement between the femoral head and neck. In a type IV fracture, the femoral head is completely displaced from the femoral neck. The Garden classification is useful because it correlates the incidence of fracture nonunion and avascular necrosis of the femoral head with fracture displacement. The incidence of these complications is very low in type I injury, whereas the type IV fracture has a 33% risk of nonunion and a 30% risk of symptomatic avascular necrosis.

Management of femoral neck fractures depends on age, bone quality, and activity level. Replacement is generally advised for older patients with poor bone quality. In patients in whom fixation is performed, accurate reduction of the fracture in both the AP and lateral planes and secure internal fixation are vital to a good outcome. Most fractures can be reduced with closed means, using a variety of reduction techniques. In the Leadbetter maneuver, reduction occurs with the hip in 90 degrees of flexion. Other techniques involve reduction with the hip in extension or in only slight flexion. There should be a low threshold for open reduction to ensure anatomic alignment of the fracture, especially in younger patients. After reduction, the femoral neck fracture is securely fixated to allow for impaction of the fracture fragments.

After surgery, the patient can begin gentle active and passive range-of-motion exercises if the fixation is secure. Active straight-leg raising is best avoided for the first 3 months. Patients who are able to cooperate with a rehabilitation program are allowed gradual weight bearing as healing of soft tissue and bone progresses. Patients who are not able to cooperate are mobilized early from bed to chair, but weight bearing on the injured limb is delayed.

Periodic follow-up is important to monitor fracture healing and to check for development of avascular necrosis of the femoral head. Initially, this tends to occur in the anterolateral segment of the femoral head, where damage to the vascular structures is greatest. If avascular necrosis is detected, intervention may be required to prevent the avascular segment from undergoing late segmental collapse, which leads to degenerative changes in the hip joint.

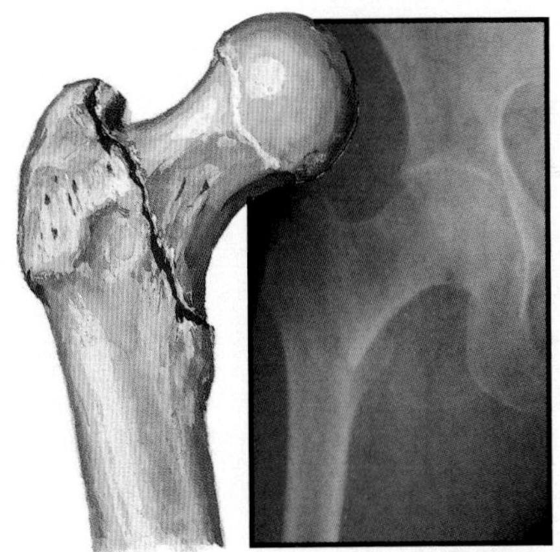

Nondisplaced fracture

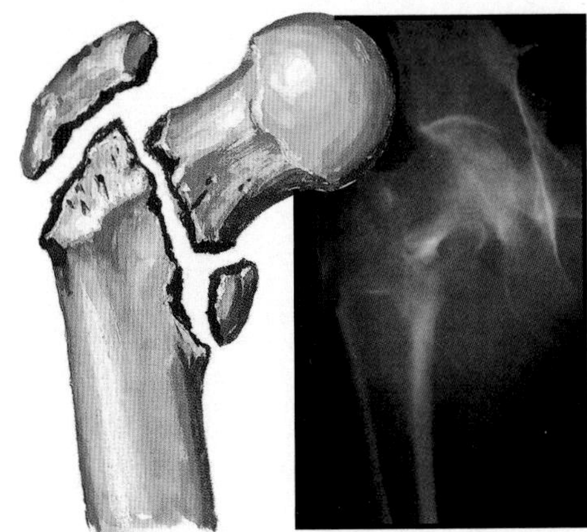

Comminuted displaced fracture

Sliding compression screw and plate. As fracture settles, screw can slide in plate, thus preventing penetration of articular surface of femoral head.

Intertrochanteric fracture reduced and fixated with sliding compression screw system. Adequate fixation of plate to distal fragment mandatory. At least four or five screws must be inserted through both lateral and medial cortices of femoral shaft.

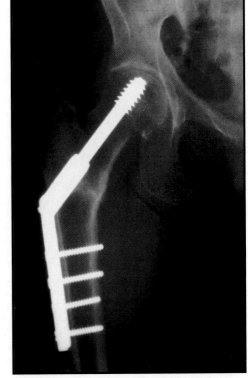

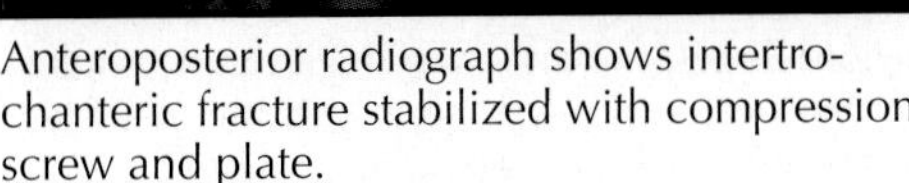

Anteroposterior radiograph shows intertrochanteric fracture stabilized with compression screw and plate.

INTERTROCHANTERIC FRACTURE OF FEMUR

Intertrochanteric fractures of the femur typically occur in the advanced elderly. These fractures occur along a line that connects the greater and lesser trochanters. Fractures can result in a simple two-part displacement or in more complex, comminuted fractures. Because the fracture surfaces created in the injury are large and filled with an abundance of cancellous bone, delayed union or nonunion is rare. Although nonoperative treatment with prolonged bed rest can be employed, the fractures are most commonly treated with ORIF.

Of the many classifications of intertrochanteric fractures, the system developed by Evans appears to be the most useful for selecting appropriate treatment. The fractures are classified into two types, stable and unstable. The system is based on whether a stable reduction of the fracture at the medial and posteromedial aspects of the fracture surface can be achieved. If stability is attained at these two sites, the fracture is likely to heal in this position with proper fixation. Evans noted that if stability could not be achieved, patients more frequently experienced loss of fixation or loss of reduction due to collapse of the fracture into a varus and externally rotated position.

Intertrochanteric fractures can be treated with screw plate implants or cephalomedullary nails. The sliding compression screw was developed to treat intertrochanteric fractures of the femur. The unstable fracture fragments telescope along the sliding portion of the device to a position of stability. The screw portion of the device is securely fixated in the femoral neck and head, and the sliding portion allows for a controlled collapse of the fracture. Recent studies have demonstrated that use of the device has reduced the incidence of complications after surgical treatment of unstable intertrochanteric fractures. However, many surgeons prefer to achieve a stable reduction of the fracture before using any device to fixate it. Stable fixation lessens the stresses applied to the sliding compression screw, which decreases the risk of implant failure. Screw plate implants are contraindicated for reverse obliquity patterns, and these are best managed with a cephalomedullary nail.

Postoperative management depends on the patient's ability to cooperate with a rehabilitation program, the quality of the bone in the proximal femur, and the adequacy of the reduction and fixation. Cooperative patients with good-quality bone and secure fracture fixation can be mobilized early with progressive weight bearing. Uncooperative patients or those unable to understand the postoperative treatment program are mobilized more slowly and cautiously. At first, these patients are simply moved from bed to chair. A similar postoperative program is recommended for patients with poor-quality bone and for those with markedly comminuted fractures and fracture instability. Comminuted intertrochanteric fractures may require bone grafting at the time of fracture fixation.

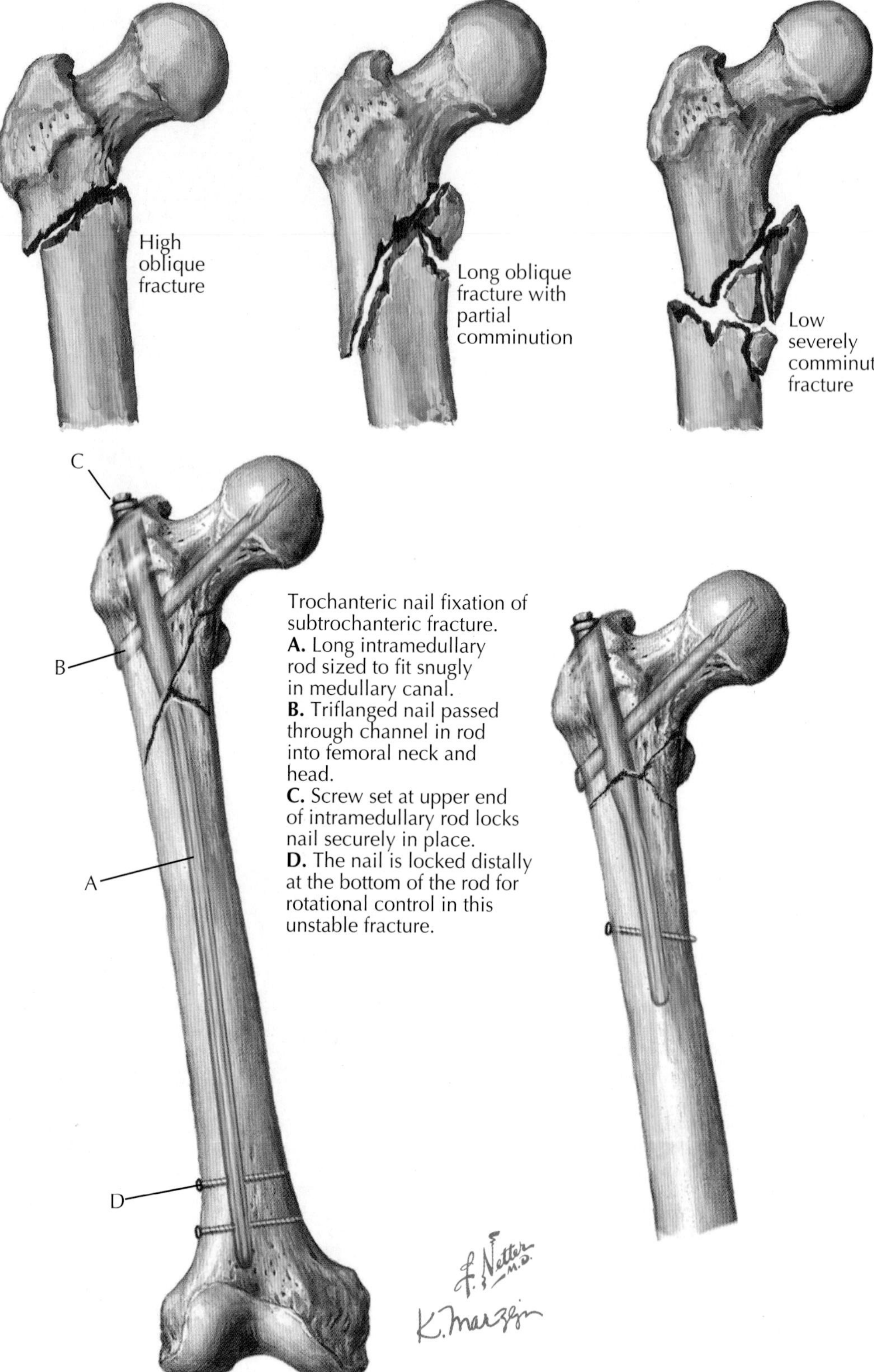
High oblique fracture
Long oblique fracture with partial comminution
Low severely comminuted fracture
C
B
A
D
Trochanteric nail fixation of subtrochanteric fracture.
A. Long intramedullary rod sized to fit snugly in medullary canal.
B. Triflanged nail passed through channel in rod into femoral neck and head.
C. Screw set at upper end of intramedullary rod locks nail securely in place.
D. The nail is locked distally at the bottom of the rod for rotational control in this unstable fracture.

SUBTROCHANTERIC FRACTURE OF FEMUR

Subtrochanteric fractures of the femur occur in two separate age groups—in young adults as a result of high-energy injuries and in very elderly persons as a result of simple falls. The fractures occur just distal to the lesser trochanter (or may involve it) and with varying degrees of comminution.

Subtrochanteric fractures are generally treated with internal fixation to allow early mobilization and rehabilitation of the patient. Closed treatment methods involving skeletal traction are rarely indicated with the advancement of modern fixation techniques.

Biomechanical analysis of the intact femur demonstrates that the highest compressive and tensile stresses on the femur are concentrated in the subtrochanteric region. Because of these very high forces, implant failure has been commonly seen with internal fixation of this type of fracture using a plate. Nonunion, malunion, and implant failure occur more often with a subtrochanteric fracture than with any other type of femoral injury. Angled plate devices, long used to treat this injury, are more likely to fail than other implant devices; the implant often breaks opposite an area of medial comminution. For this reason, proper implant selection using a cephalomedullary device is essential.

Because of problems with the use of nail plate devices, other intramedullary devices have been developed specifically for treating subtrochanteric fractures of the femur. The anterograde nail, often with a trochanteric entry point, is one of the most successful devices. The incidence of malunion and nonunion has been reduced with the use of the nail configuration, because of its intramedullary position and firm fixation in the femoral head and neck.

Postoperative management depends on the quality of fixation, the quality of bone, and the stability of fracture reduction. Patients with good bone mass, minimal comminution, and good fracture stability are mobilized early from bed to chair and then to partial weight bearing using crutches for support. In patients treated with an intramedullary device, which helps distribute the load across the fracture site, weight bearing on the injured limb progresses more rapidly than in patients treated with a plate device. Older patients with osteoporotic bone are mobilized slowly from bed to chair. Full weight bearing on the fractured limb is allowed when clinical and radiographic evaluations show adequate fracture healing.

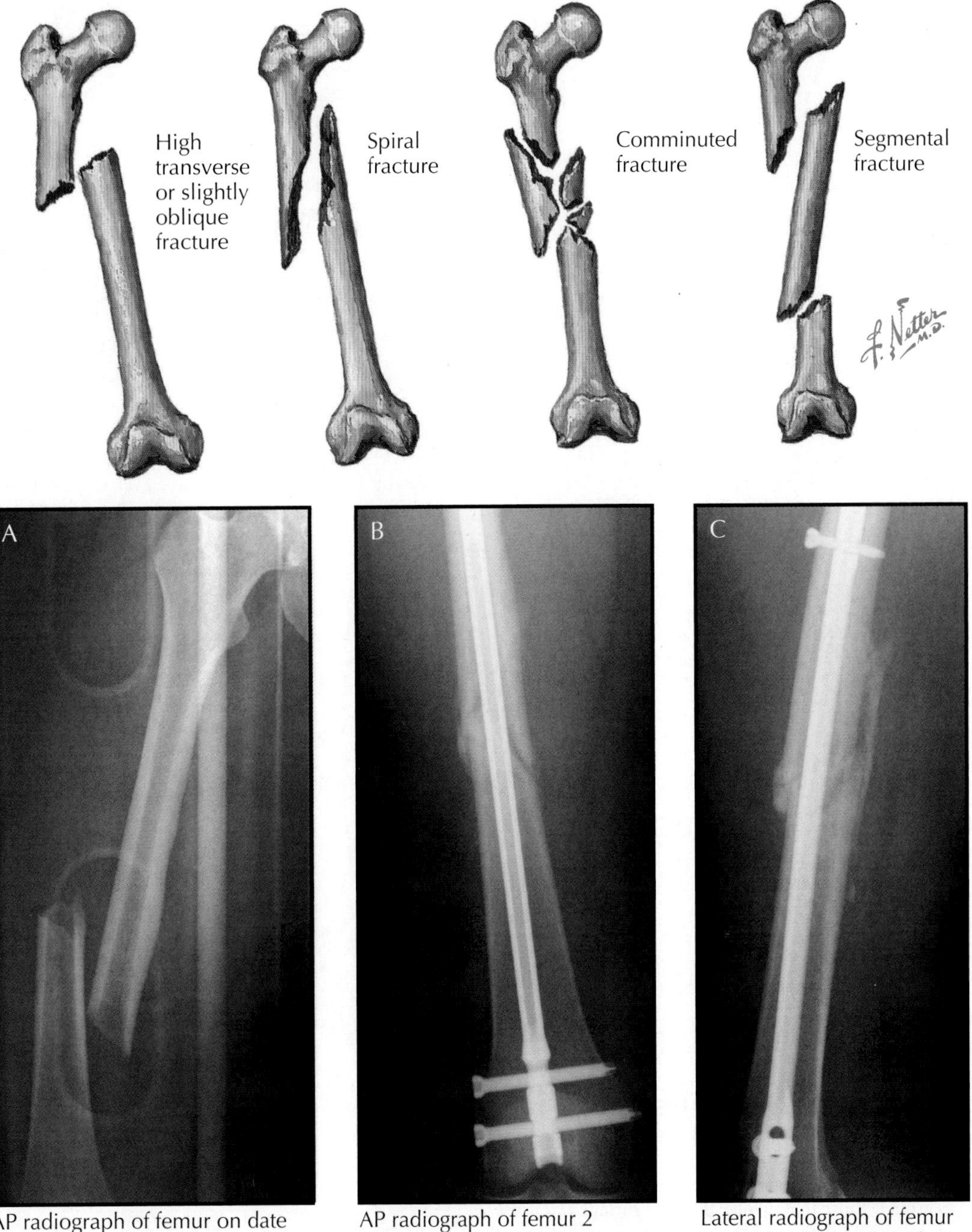

AP radiograph of femur on date of injury

AP radiograph of femur 2 months after retrograde intramedullary nailing

Lateral radiograph of femur 2 months after retrograde intramedullary nailing

A 20-year-old female was an unrestrained passenger in a motor vehicle accident. The patient sustained multiple fractures, including a closed fracture of the right femoral shaft (**A**); an open grade IIIA comminuted fracture of the junction of the middle third–distal third right tibia and fibula; a closed, comminuted fracture of the middle third of the left tibia and fibula; and comminuted fracture of the right calcaneus. On the date of injury, the patient underwent debridement of the right tibia with application of an external fixator, retrograde nailing of the right femur, and intramedullary nailing of the left tibia. Radiographs of the femur 2 months after injury (**B** and **C**) show good alignment and interval healing of the fracture.

Fracture of Shaft of Femur

Femoral shaft fractures occur in all age groups but are more common in younger than in elderly persons. Several types of fractures can result from simple trauma to high-velocity trauma. Spiral fractures are most commonly due to low-velocity torsional forces applied to the femur, whereas comminuted, segmental, and transverse fractures all result from greater forces. About 15% of femoral shaft fractures are open injuries, but associated neurovascular involvement is not common.

Skeletal traction is rarely used as a definitive treatment. Traction can be used as a temporary measure and is generally applied by placing a pin through the proximal tibia and aligning the fracture. Operative fixation is performed once the patient is resuscitated.

A major advance in the treatment of femoral fractures is the use of closed intramedullary nailing guided by a C-arm image intensifier. As the complexity of femoral fractures increased, advances in the technology of intramedullary nails also occurred. Even severely comminuted femoral fractures can now be securely fixated with standard and modified intramedullary devices. However, the major impact of intramedullary nailing has been on the treatment of femoral shaft fractures in patients with multiple injuries. Early fracture stabilization allows these patients to be upright and out of bed soon after injury, which decreases the incidence of adult respiratory distress syndrome and, possibly, of multiple organ system failure, which often accompanies multiple injuries.

When an isolated femoral shaft fracture is treated with intramedullary nailing, the patient is allowed out of bed very early. First mobilized using crutches, the patient increases weight bearing on the injured side based on the results of follow-up clinical and radiographic examinations.

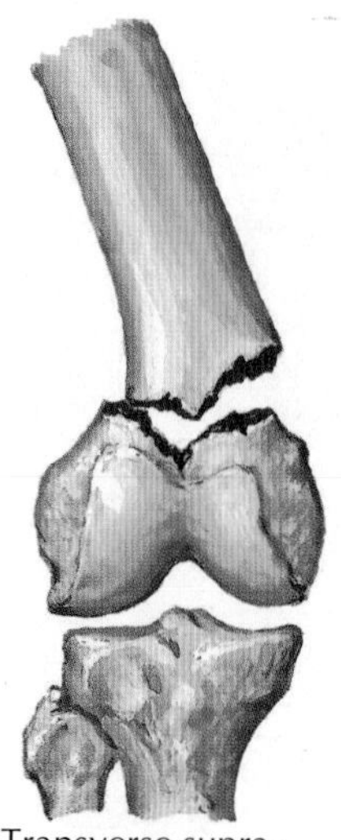

Transverse supracondylar fracture

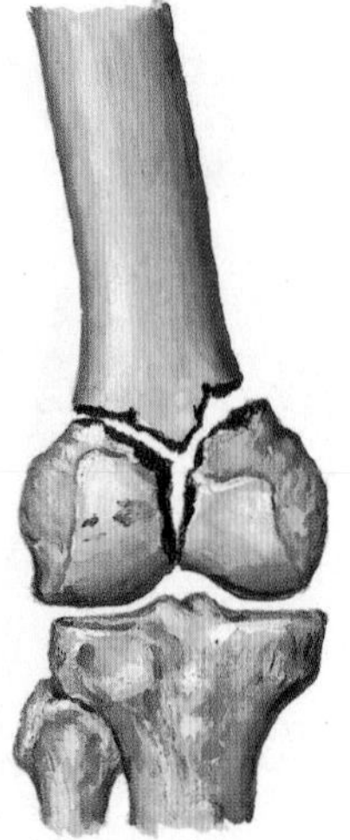

Intercondylar (T or Y) fracture

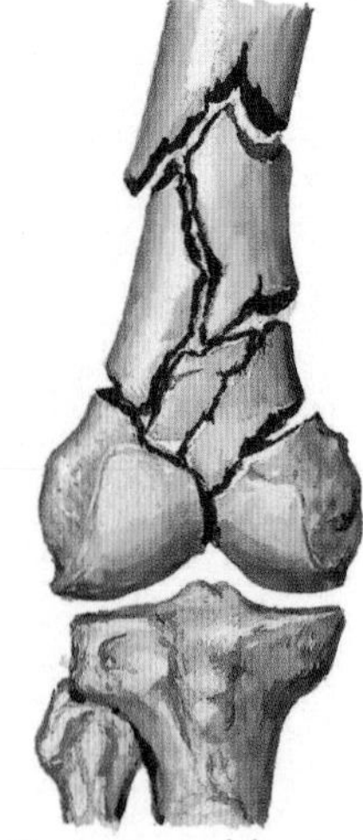

Comminuted fracture extending into shaft

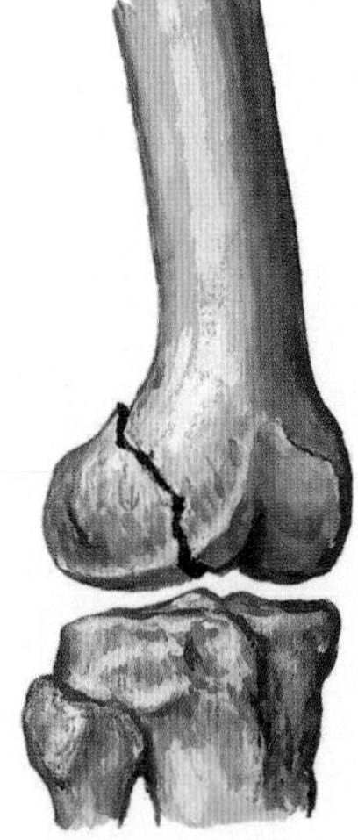

Fracture of single condyle (frontal or oblique plane)

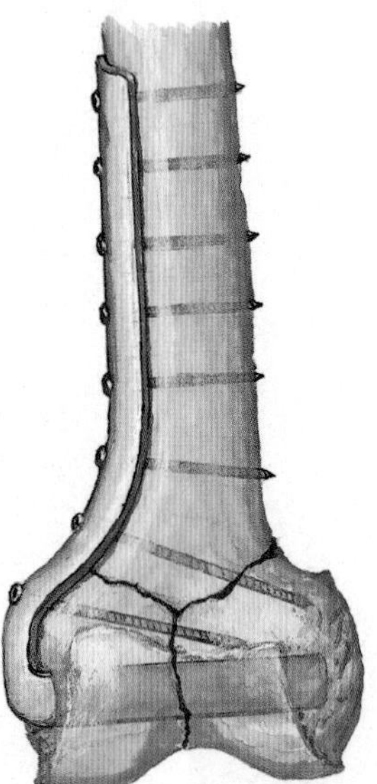

T fracture fixed with blade plate inserted into condyles and secured with screws

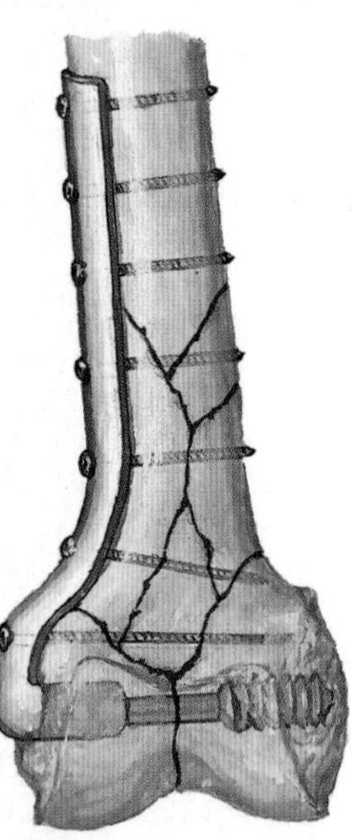

Compression screw and plate preferred for some fractures

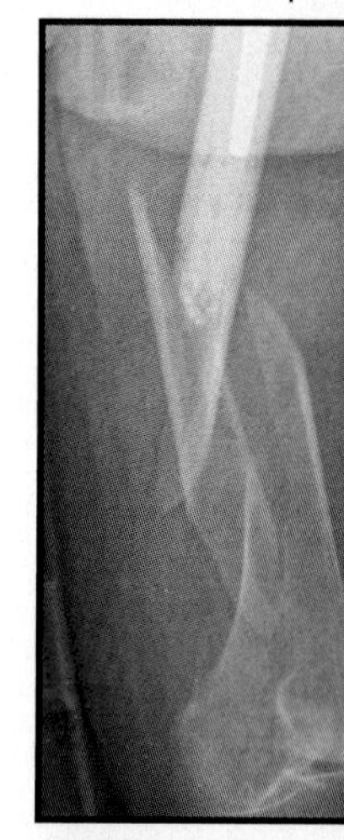

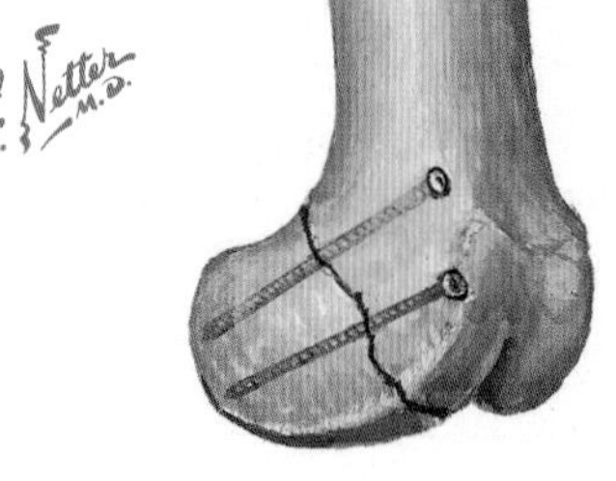

Fracture of single condyle reduced and fixed with screws

Distal femur locking plate

FRACTURE OF DISTAL FEMUR

Fractures of the distal femur are generally divided into two groups: those that involve the joint surface and those that do not. As with any intraarticular fracture, those of the distal femur can lead to significant posttraumatic osteoarthritis if the reduction and fixation of the intraarticular aspect of the fracture is not satisfactory.

The many different fracture patterns that occur in the distal femur range from the fracture type that does not involve the joint surface to the type with severe comminution of both the intraarticular and extraarticular components.

Fractures with joint involvement require treatment with ORIF, first to achieve secure fixation of the intraarticular fragments and then to join them to the intact distal femur. Intraarticular fractures are usually treated with a blade plate supracondylar screw plate or locking periarticular plate. The success of treatment with these devices depends on a meticulous surgical technique and sufficient bone quality for fixation. Retrograde intramedullary nailing may also be used for fixation of distal femur fractures.

The same problems of implant failure or fixation that occur in the treatment of subtrochanteric fractures can also complicate the treatment of the distal femur. In areas of marked metaphyseal comminution, bone grafting medially may help prevent late failure of the plate device.

Fractures of the distal femur that involve a single condyle may be stabilized securely with single lag screws or lag screws with a buttress plate. This technique allows early motion with minimal risk of displacement at the joint surface.

Extraarticular fractures of the knee at the metadiaphyseal junction or more proximal are amenable to a retrograde intramedullary nail.

Rehabilitation after ORIF is based on the security of the fixation and the quality of the bone. As clinical and radiographic examinations document healing, the patient is allowed to increase weight bearing on the injured extremity.

Amputation of Lower Limb and Hip

DISARTICULATION OF HIP

Aggressive tumors, infection, and necrosis may necessitate a disarticulation of the hip or a hindquarter amputation. With hip disarticulation, the entire femur is removed and a large posterior skin flap is preserved and brought forward. The surgeon should attempt to preserve the gluteus muscles, which can serve as a cushion for sitting and for supporting a lower limb prosthesis.

HINDQUARTER AMPUTATION

Hindquarter amputation, or hemipelvectomy, includes removal of the entire lower limb and the entire innominate bone of the pelvis. Three levels of resection have been described. The standard approach is a disarticulation through the sacroiliac joint. In a modified, or conservative, approach, the line of resection is just lateral to the sacroiliac joint, preserving a small rim of the ilium, When the tumor extends across the sacroiliac joint, an extended resection through the sacral foramina may be necessary. Regardless of the level of ilium resection posteriorly, the surgeon tries to preserve some gluteus muscles to provide coverage of the abdominal organs, which will otherwise be vulnerable to injury after resection of the ilium.

Disarticulation of hip

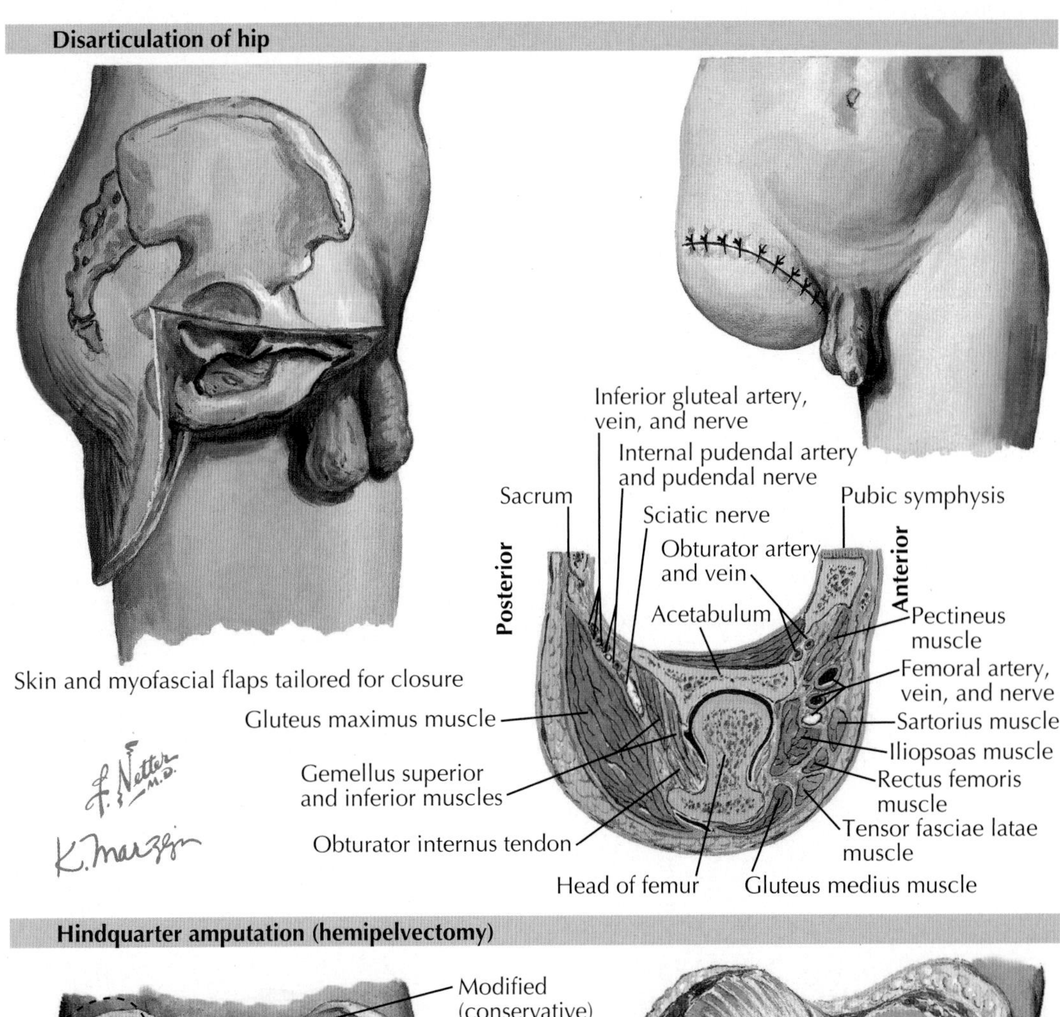

Skin and myofascial flaps tailored for closure

Hindquarter amputation (hemipelvectomy)

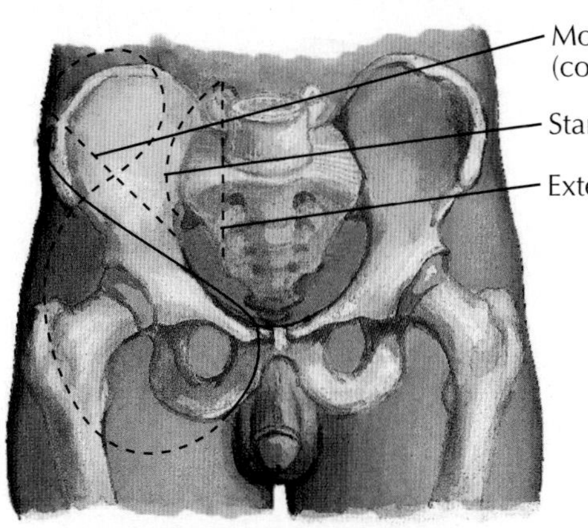

Lines of incision and resection

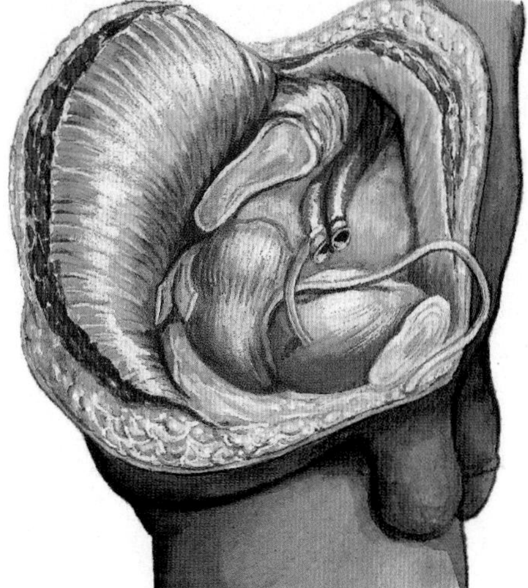

Gluteal flap formed and hindquarter removed

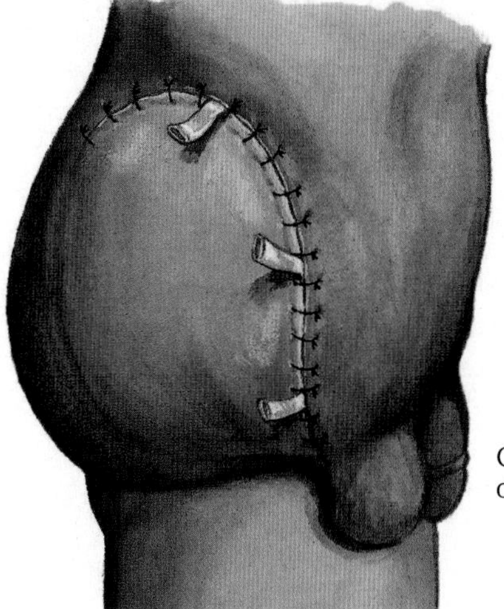

Gluteal flap closed over defect, and drain placed

KNEE

Topographic Anatomy of the Knee

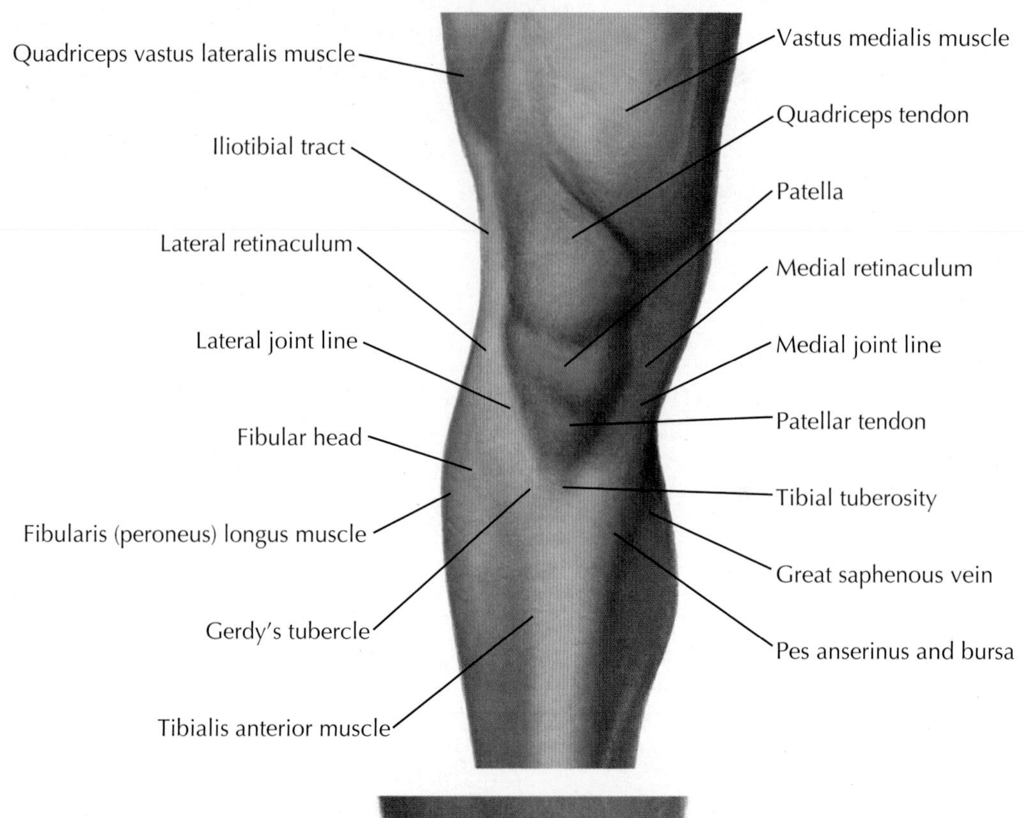

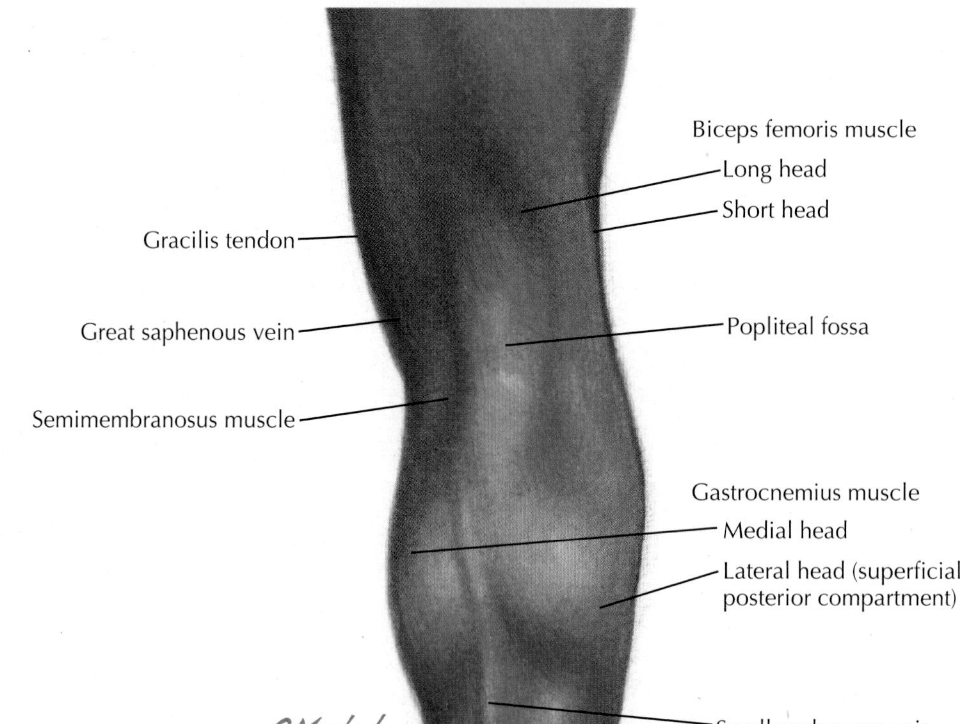

Anatomy of the Knee

KNEE JOINT

The knee primarily functions as a hinge joint permitting flexion and extension, but on closer examination its motion is revealed to be much more complex than a simple hinge. Conjunct rotation (rotation during the flexion and extension process) is also a key component of knee joint motion. Knee flexion provides looseness, which allows some voluntary rotation, whereas medial femoral rotation at terminal extension plays an important role in "locking" the knee in extension. The rotational component of motion is facilitated by larger size of the articular surface of the femoral condyles relative to that contributed by the tibial plateau. As the extended position is approached, the smaller lateral meniscus is displaced forward on the tibia and becomes firmly seated in a groove on the lateral femoral condyle, which tends to stop extension. However, the medial femoral condyle is still capable of gliding backward, thus bringing its flatter, more anterior surface into full contact with the tibia. These movements of conjunct rotation bring the cruciate ligaments into a taut, or locked, position. The collateral ligaments become maximally tensed, and a full, close-packed, and stable position of extension results. The tension of the ligaments and the close approximation of the flatter parts of the condyles make the erect position relatively easy to maintain.

The sequence of actions in flexion is reversed in extension. Flexion can be carried through about 130 degrees and is limited normally by contact between calf and thigh. Muscles from primarily the thigh but also the lower leg contribute to knee motion.

There are three articulations in the knee: the patellofemoral articulation and two tibiofemoral joints. The latter two are separated by the intraarticular cruciate ligaments and the infrapatellar synovial fold. The three joint cavities are connected by restricted openings.

The articular surfaces of the femur are its medial and lateral condyles and the patellar surface, also known as the trochlea of the knee. The condyles are shaped like thick rollers diverging inferiorly and posteriorly. Their surfaces gradually change from a flatter curvature anteriorly to a tighter curvature posteriorly and are separated from the patellar surface by a slight trochlear groove.

On the superior surface of the tibia, or the tibial plateau, there are two separate, cartilage-covered areas. The surface of the medial condyle is larger, oval, and slightly concave; that of the lateral condyle is convex

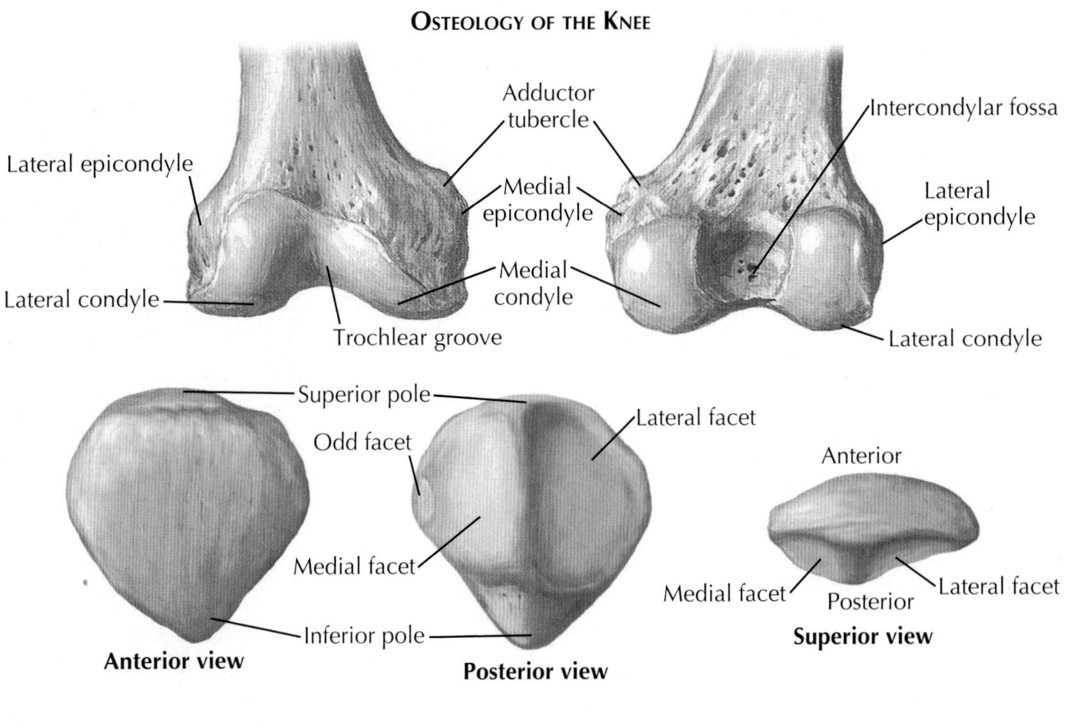

Anterior view of knee

Patellar surface
Adductor tubercle
Lateral condyle
Lateral tibial space
Lateral condyle
Medial condyle
Gerdy's tubercle (insertion of iliotibial tract)
Medial tibial space
Neck of fibula
Anterior intercondylar area
Tibial tuberosity
Oblique line
Lateral surface

Femoral mechanical axis
87°
87°
Tibial mechanical axis

—— Line of attachment of synovium (edge of articular cartilage) to distal femur
------ Line of reflection of synovial membrane

F. Netter M.D.
K. Marzen

ANATOMY OF THE KNEE (Continued)

and more circular in shape. The fossae of the articular surfaces are deepened by disc-like menisci. The composition and morphology of the menisci make them important in distribution of load about the knee during weight-bearing.

The articular capsule of the knee joint is scarcely separable from the ligaments and aponeuroses apposed to it. Posterosuperiorly, its vertical fibers arise from the femoral condyles and intercondylar fossa; inferiorly, these fibers are overlain by the oblique popliteal ligament. The capsule attaches to the tibial condyles and, incompletely, to the menisci. The external ligaments reinforcing the capsule are the fascia lata and the iliotibial tract; the medial patellar and lateral patellar retinacula; and the patellar, oblique popliteal, and arcuate popliteal ligaments. The medial (tibial) collateral ligament (MCL) also closely reinforces the capsule on the medial side.

The aponeurotic tendons of the vastus muscles attach to the sides of the patella and then expand over the front and sides of the capsule as the medial and lateral patellar retinacula. Below, they insert into the front of the tibial condyles and into their oblique lines as far to the sides as the collateral ligaments. Superficially, the fascia lata overlies and blends with the retinacula as it descends to attach to the tibial condyles and their oblique lines. Laterally, the iliotibial tract curves forward over the lateral patellar retinaculum and blends with the capsule anteriorly. Its posterior border is free, and fat tends to be interposed between it and the capsule.

The patellar ligament is the continuation of the quadriceps femoris tendon to the tuberosity of the tibia. An extremely strong and relatively flat band, it attaches above the patella and continues over its front with fibers of the tendon, ending somewhat obliquely on the tibial tuberosity. A deep infrapatellar bursa intervenes between the tendon and the bone. A large, subcutaneous infrapatellar bursa is developed in the tissue over the ligament.

The oblique popliteal ligament is one of the specializations of the tendon of the semimembranosus muscle, which reinforces the posterior surface of the articular capsule. As this tendon inserts into the groove on the posterior surface of the medial condyle of the tibia, it sends this oblique expansion lateralward and superiorly across the posterior aspect of the capsule.

Knee: Medial and Lateral Views

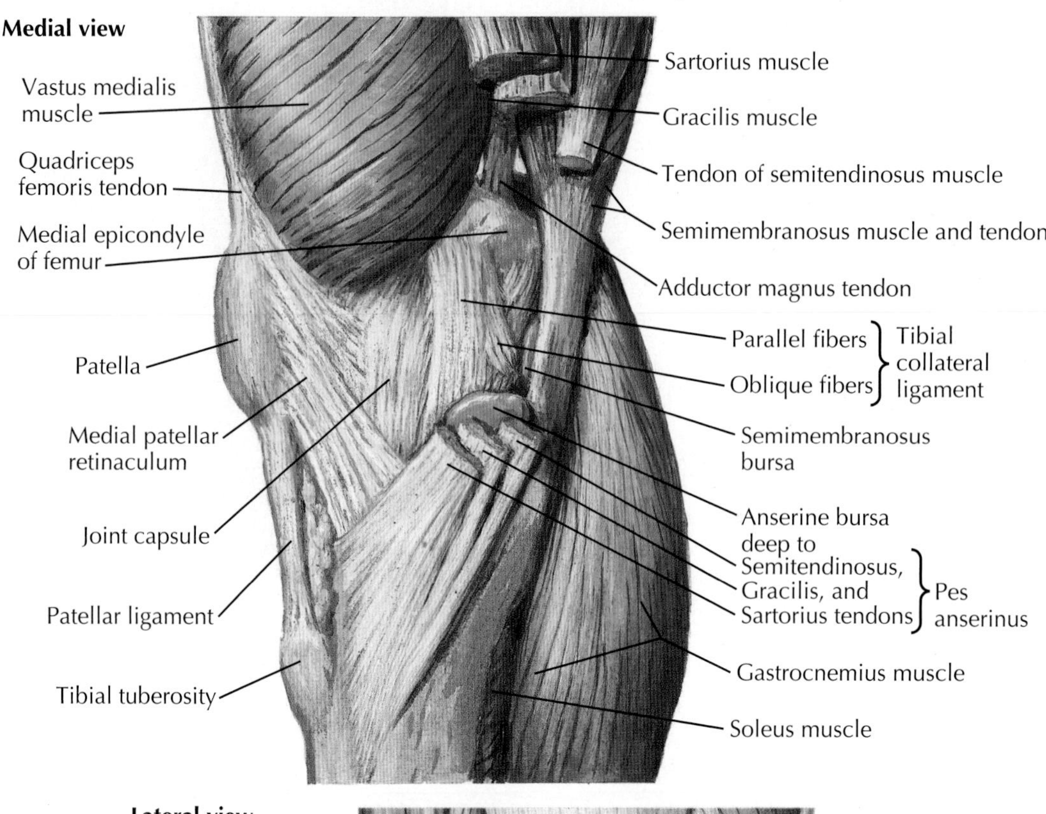

Anatomy of the Knee (Continued)

COLLATERAL LIGAMENTS

These ligaments prevent hyperextension of the joint and resist any varus and valgus forces to the knee. Both collateral ligaments are tighter in extension and progressively relaxed as the knee is brought into flexion. The inferior genicular blood vessels pass between them and the capsule of the joint, but only the lateral (fibular) collateral ligament stands clearly away from the capsule.

The MCL is a strong, flat band that extends between the medial condyles of the femur and tibia. It can be broken down into superficial and deep layers that may be separated by a thin bursa that facilitates the slight movement between these layers. The MCL is well defined anteriorly, blending with the medial patellar retinaculum. The pes anserinus tendon overlies the ligament inferiorly, the two being separated by the anserine bursa. The posterior portion of the ligament is characterized by obliquely running fibers, which converge at the joint level from above and below and give the ligament an attachment into the medial meniscus. The principal inferior attachment of the ligament is about 5 cm below the tibial articular surface immediately posterior to the insertion of the pes anserinus.

The lateral (fibular) collateral ligament is a more rounded, pencil-like cord, which is entirely separate from the capsule of the knee joint. It is attached to a tubercle on the lateral condyle of the femur superoposterior to the groove for the popliteus muscle. It ends below on the lateral surface of the head of the fibula, about 1 cm anterior to its apex. The tendon of the popliteus muscle passes deep to the ligament, and the biceps femoris tendon divides around its fibular attachment, with a small inferior subtendinous bursa intervening. Another bursa lies under the upper end of the ligament, separating it from the popliteus tendon. The synovial membrane of the joint, protruding as the subpopliteal recess, separates the popliteus tendon from the lateral meniscus.

CRUCIATE LIGAMENTS

The cruciate ligaments prevent anterior and posterior translation of the tibia relative to the femoral condyles and provide significant rotational stability to the knee joint. They are somewhat taut in all positions of flexion but become tightest in full extension and full flexion. They lie within the capsule of the knee joint, in the vertical plane between the condyles, but they are excluded from the synovial cavity by coverings of

KNEE: ANTERIOR VIEWS

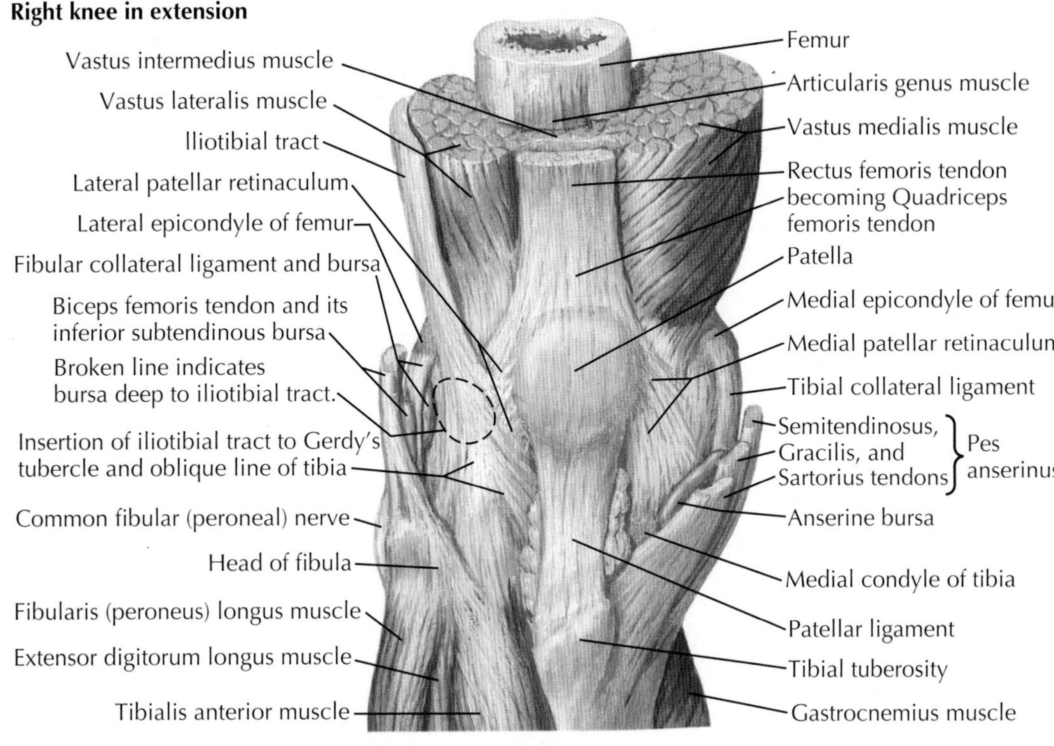

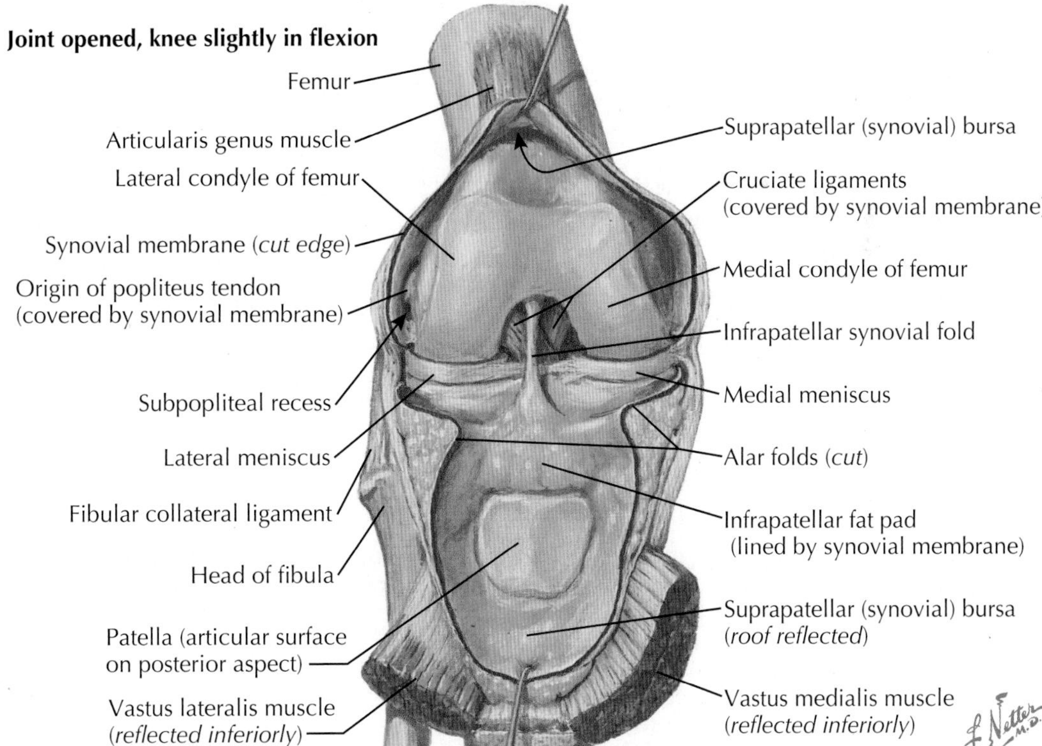

ANATOMY OF THE KNEE (Continued)

synovial membrane. Both ligaments spread linearly at their bony attachments.

The anterior cruciate ligament (ACL) arises from the rough, nonarticular area anterior to the intercondylar eminence of the tibia and extends superiorly and posteriorly to the posteromedial aspect of the lateral femoral condyle. The ACL can be divided into an anteromedial bundle and a posterolateral bundle. The anteromedial bundle is tight in flexion and provides more anterior-posterior stability; the posterolateral bundle is tight in extension and contributes more to rotational stability.

The thicker and stronger posterior cruciate ligament (PCL) passes anterosuperiorly through the knee joint on the medial side of the ACL. It extends from an extraarticular attachment over the posterior aspect of the tibial plateau to the lateral side of the medial condyle of the femur. The PCL also has two bundles: an anterolateral bundle and a posteromedial bundle. The posteromedial bundle is tight in extension, and the anterolateral band is tight in flexion.

Both cruciate ligaments receive their primary blood supply from the medial genicular artery and their innervations from branches of the tibial nerve.

MENISCI

These crescent-shaped wafers of fibrocartilage surmount the peripheral parts of the articular surfaces of the tibia. Thicker at their external margins and tapering to thin, unattached edges in the interior of the articulation, they deepen the articular fossae for the reception of the femoral condyles. They are attached to the outer borders of the condyles of the tibia and at their ends, anterior and posterior, to its intercondylar eminence.

The medial meniscus is larger and more nearly oval in outline. Broader posteriorly, it narrows anteriorly as it attaches in the intercondylar area of the tibia in front of the origin of the PCL. The lateral meniscus is more nearly circular. Although smaller than the medial meniscus, it covers a greater proportion of the tibial surface. Anteriorly, it attaches in the anterior intercondylar area, lateral and posterior to the distal aspect of the ACL. Posteriorly, it ends in the posterior intercondylar area in front of the end of the medial meniscus. The medial meniscus is also attached to the MCL, making it significantly less mobile than the lateral meniscus. The lateral meniscus is weakly attached around the margin of the lateral tibial condyle and lacks

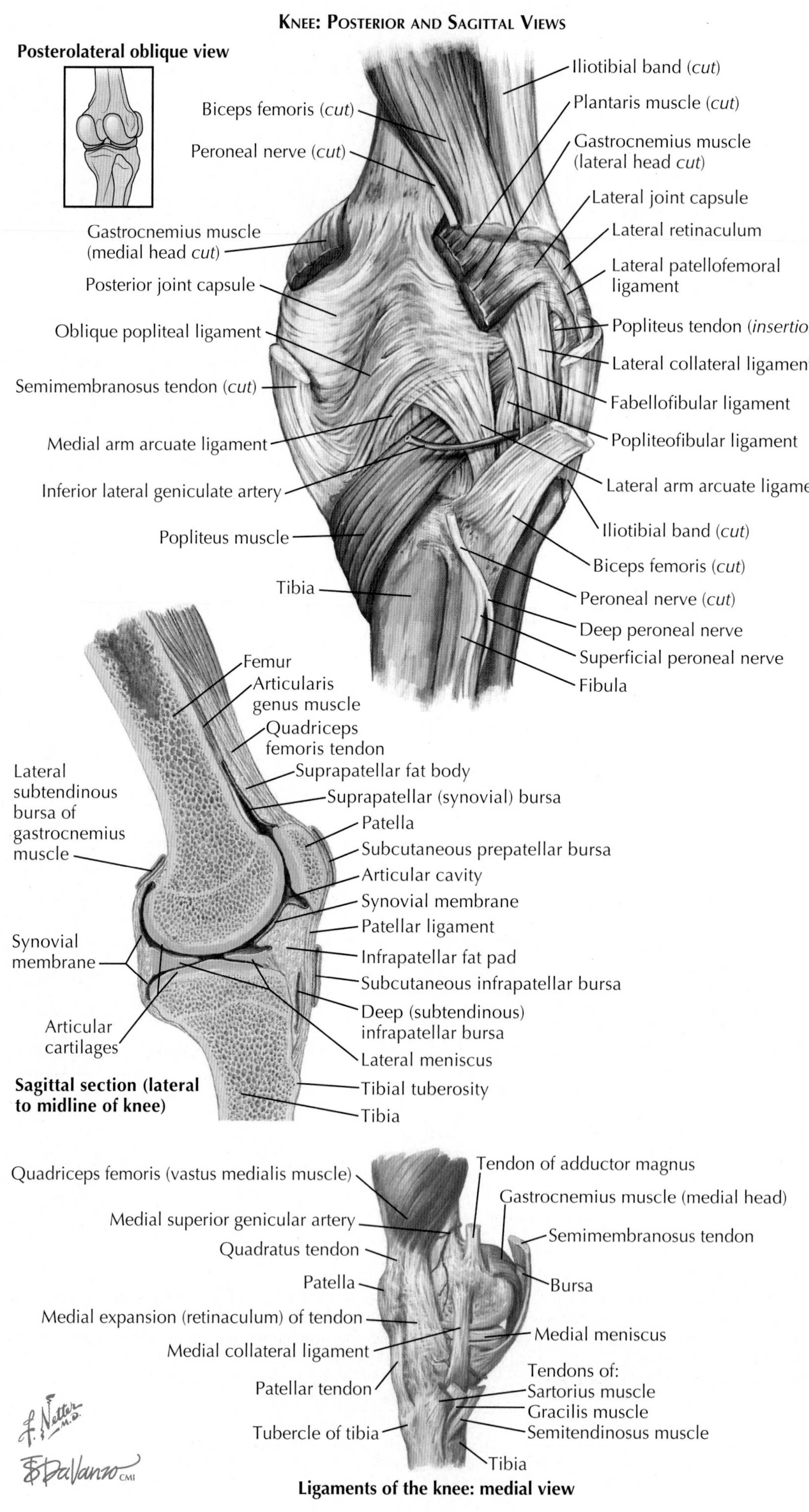

ANATOMY OF THE KNEE (Continued)

an attachment where it is crossed and notched by the popliteus tendon. At the posterior aspect of the joint, it gives origin to some of the fibers of the popliteus muscle; close to its posterior attachment to the tibia, it frequently gives off a collection of fibers, known as the posterior meniscofemoral ligament. This may join the PCL or may insert into the medial femoral condyle posterior to the attachment of the PCL. An occasional anterior meniscofemoral ligament has a similar but anterior relationship to the PCL. The transverse ligament of the knee connects the anterior convex margin of the lateral meniscus to the anterior end of the medial meniscus.

The blood supply to the medial and lateral menisci come from the superior and inferior branches of the medial and lateral geniculate arteries, respectively. There are three commonly referred to zones of the menisci based on their respective blood supply. Starting from the most vascularized peripheral (outermost) portion of the meniscus, these are the red-red, red-white, and white-white zones. These zones play a large role in therapeutic decision-making owing to the role that increased vascularity will play in the likelihood of healing, with red-red having the highest likelihood of healing a repair. Vascularity is also variable among patients of different ages, as younger patients tend to have a more robust blood supply.

SYNOVIAL MEMBRANE AND JOINT CAVITY

The articular cavity of the knee is the largest joint space of the body. It includes the space between and around the femoral and tibial condyles, extends superiorly to

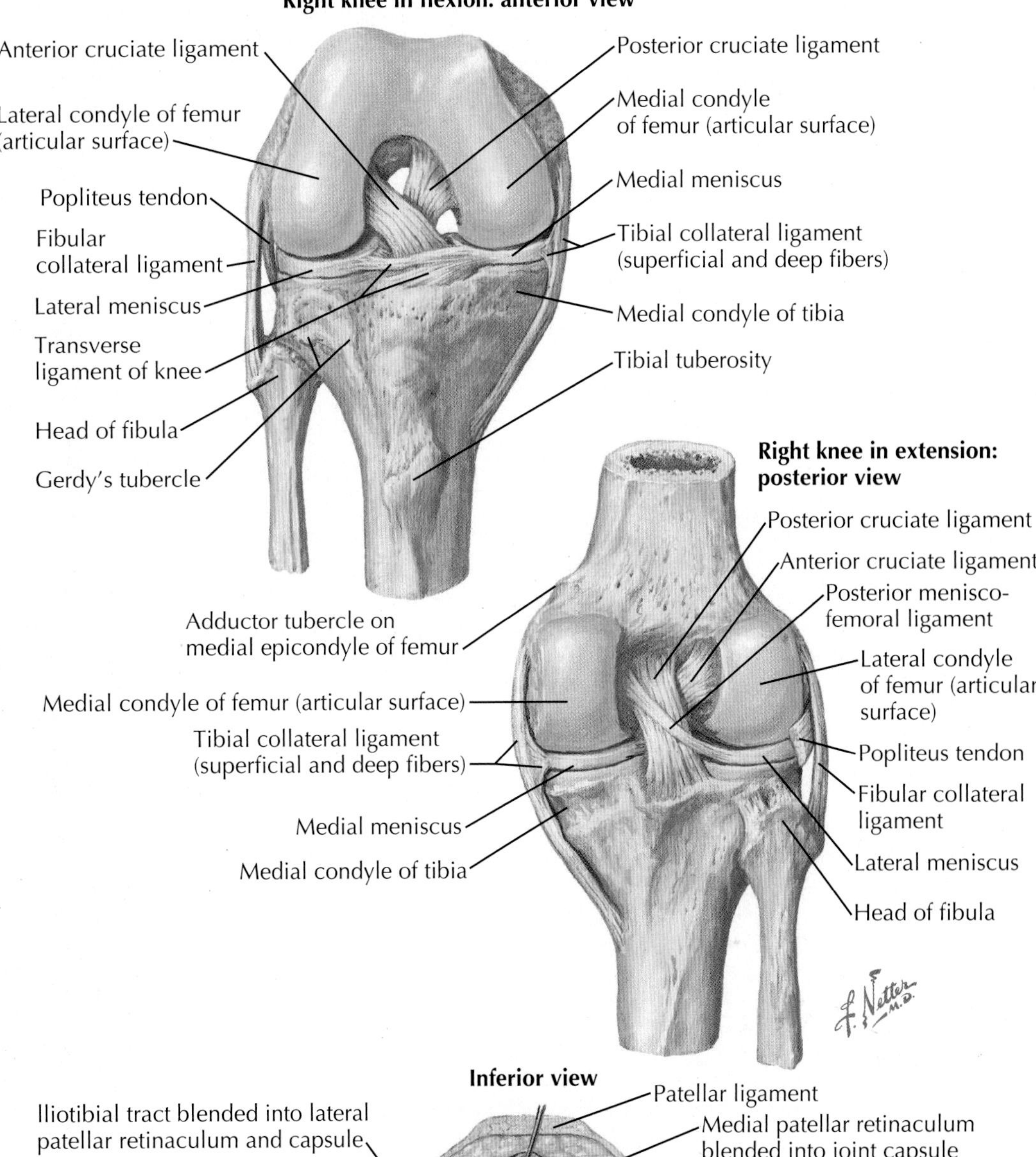

Anatomy of the Knee (Continued)

include the femoropatellar articulation, and then communicates freely with the suprapatellar bursa between the quadriceps femoris tendon and the femur. The synovial membrane lines the articular capsule and the suprapatellar bursa. Recesses of the joint cavity are also lined by synovial membrane including the subpopliteal recess. Other recesses exist behind the posterior part of each femoral condyle. At the superior aspect of the medial recess, the bursa under the medial head of the gastrocnemius muscle may open into the joint cavity.

The infrapatellar fat body or pad represents an anterior part of the median septum, which, with the cruciate ligaments, separates the two femorotibial articulations. From the medial and lateral borders of the articular surface of the patella, reduplications of synovial membrane project into the interior of the joint and form two fringe-like alar folds, which cover collections of fat. The fat pad is a normal structure, but in many cases, it may become inflamed or impinge within the patella and femoral condyle and become problematic.

BLOOD VESSELS AND NERVES

In the region of the knee there is an important genicular anastomosis. This consists of a superficial plexus superior and inferior to the patella, plus a deep plexus on the capsule of the knee joint and the adjacent bony surfaces. The anastomosis is made up of terminal interconnections of 10 vessels. Two of these descend into the joint: the descending branch of the lateral circumflex femoral artery and the descending genicular branch of the femoral artery. Five are branches of the popliteal artery at the level of the knee: the medial superior genicular, lateral superior genicular, middle genicular, medial inferior

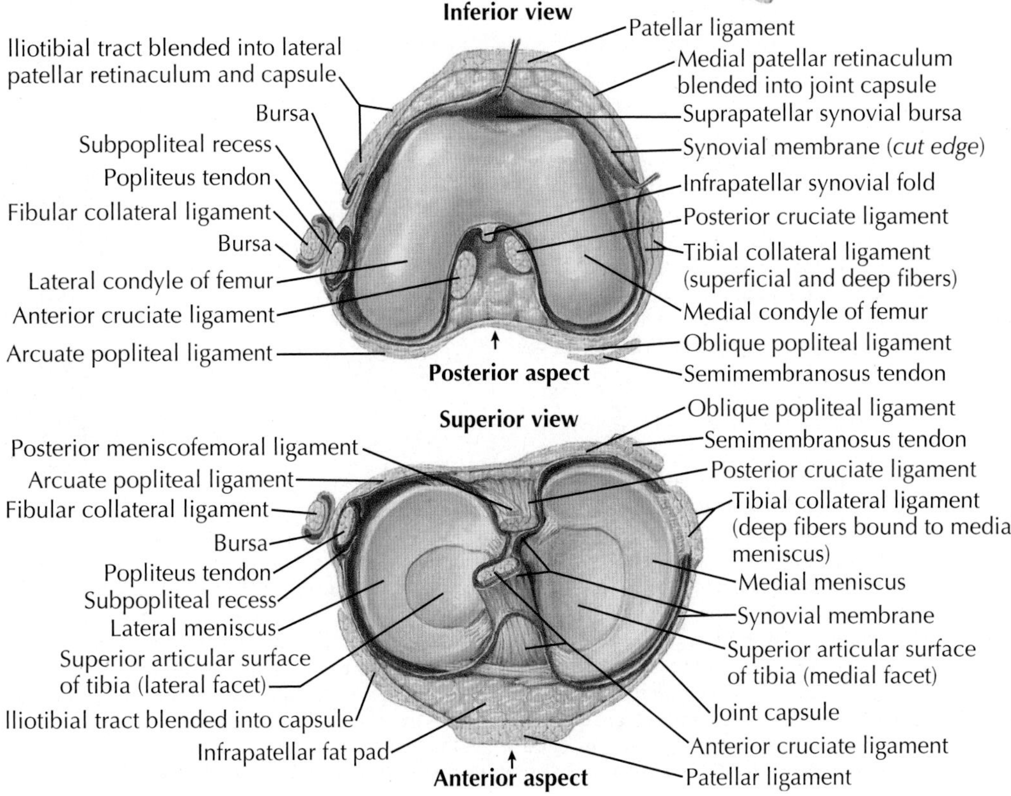

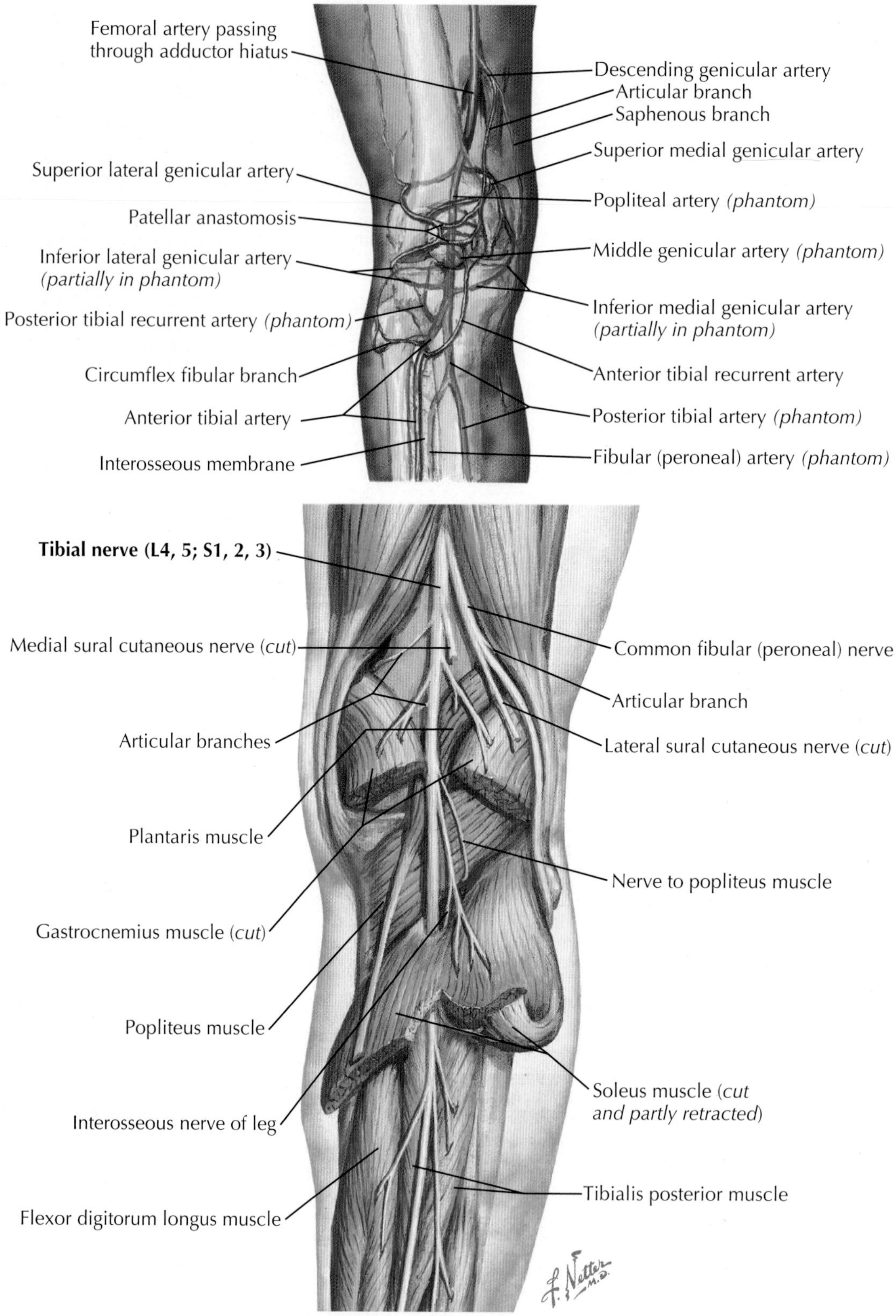

ANATOMY OF THE KNEE (Continued)

genicular, and lateral inferior genicular arteries. Three branches of leg arteries ascend to the anastomosis: the posterior tibial recurrent, circumflex fibular, and anterior tibial recurrent arteries. Veins of the same names accompany the arteries. The lymphatics of the knee joint drain to the popliteal and inguinal node groups.

The nerves of the knee joint are numerous. Articular branches of the femoral nerve reach the knee via the nerves to the vastus muscles and the saphenous nerve. The posterior division of the obturator nerve ends in the joint, and there are also articular branches of the tibial and common peroneal nerves.

PATELLA

The largest sesamoid bone is developed in the tendon of the quadriceps femoris muscle. It articulates against the anterior articular surface of the distal femur and improves the quadriceps tendon's angle of approach to the tibial tuberosity. The convex anterior surface of the patella is striated vertically by the tendon fibers. The superior border is thick, giving attachment to the tendinous fibers of the rectus femoris and vastus intermedius muscles. The lateral and medial borders, where the vastus lateralis and medialis muscles insert, are thinner. The borders converge distally to the pointed apex of the patella, which is the origin site of the patellar ligament. The articular surface is a smooth oval area, divided by a vertical ridge into two facets. The ridge occupies the groove on the patellar surface of the femur, the medial and lateral facets corresponding to articular surfaces of the distal femur. The lateral patellar facet is broader and deeper than the medial. Inferior to the faceted area is a rough nonarticular portion of the patella from which half of the patellar ligament arises.

The patella maintains a shifting contact with the femur in all positions of the knee. As the knee shifts from a fully flexed to a fully extended position, first the superior, then the middle, and last the inferior parts of the articular surface of the patella are brought into contact with the patellar surfaces of the femur. The largest amount of contact between the patella and the trochlea is at about 45 degrees of knee flexion.

Ossification of the patella develops from a single center, which appears early in the third year of life. Complete ossification occurs by age 13 years in males and at about age 10 years in females.

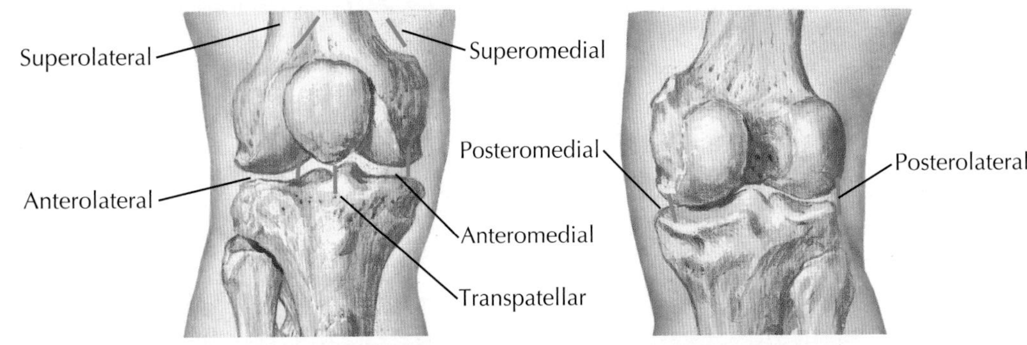

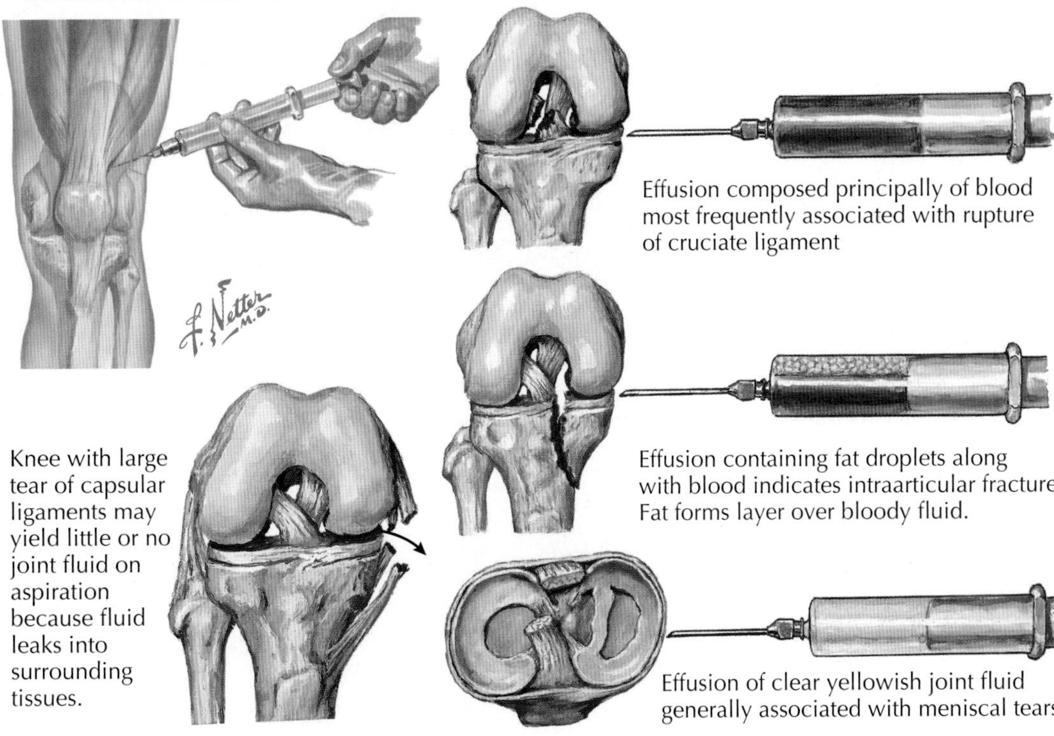

Arthrocentesis of Knee Joint

Swelling, ecchymosis, and tenderness signal a significant injury to the knee. Clinical findings may also include joint effusion, limitation of motion, and instability. Arthrocentesis is often performed to help define the nature of the intraarticular pathologic processes. A large-bore needle can be inserted into the knee via multiple approaches. If the knee is between 0 and approximately 20 degrees of flexion, an approach from just superior to the superolateral or superomedial aspect of the patella can be employed. If the knee is in approximately 90 degrees of flexion, often an anteromedial or anterolateral approach just inferior to the patella (through what would be arthroscopy portal sites) is easier to use. In both cases, care should be taken to avoid injury to the articular cartilage.

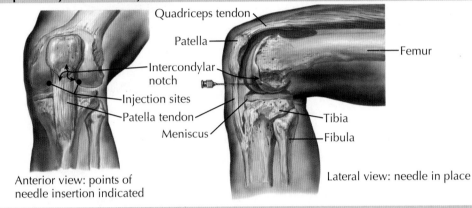

Fluid obtained from the joint is often sent for white blood cell count with differential, Gram stain, and culture and examined microscopically under polarized light to detect any crystals. Healthy joints usually yield less than 5 mL of fluid. Normal synovial fluid is clear, pale yellow, and more viscous than water. The average number of leukocytes is about 65/mm^3, and most are lymphocytes and monocytes. Acute inflammation increases the ratio of polymorphonuclear leukocytes to lymphocytes and monocytes.

Synovial effusions are categorized as group I, noninflammatory; group II, inflammatory; group III, septic; and group IV, hemorrhagic. Group I synovial fluid has high viscosity, is pale to dark yellow, and is transparent. Leukocyte count is generally less than 200/mm^3, of which about 25% are polymorphonuclear leukocytes. Glucose concentration is similar to that in serum. Group I fluid is typically found in joints with osteoarthritis.

Group II synovial fluid has low viscosity, may be yellow to light green, and is translucent. Leukocyte counts of 2000 to 75,000/mm^3 are common, and about 50% of the cells may be polymorphonuclear leukocytes. Glucose concentration is generally lower than that in serum. Group II synovial fluid is found in joints with rheumatoid arthritis.

Group III synovial fluid is obtained from a native septic joint and has a variable viscosity and color but is opaque. The leukocyte count is frequently greater than 50,000/mm^3, and polymorphonuclear leukocytes predominate (75%). The glucose level is significantly lower than that in serum.

Group IV synovial fluid is bloody, has variable viscosity, and often looks like whole blood on gross examination. A knee joint effusion consisting principally of blood (hemarthrosis) is often associated with rupture of the ACL.

An effusion containing numerous fat droplets along with blood indicates an intraarticular fracture. The volume of fat may be so great that the fat layer is visible on a lateral radiograph of the knee; after aspiration, the fat appears as a distinct layer floating on the synovial fluid and blood in the syringe. Other injuries, such as avulsion of a ligament at its insertion into bone, may produce a hemarthrosis with a few fat droplets. A large tear of the joint capsule may result in little or no detectable effusion because the blood and joint fluid leak into the periarticular tissues and they cannot be aspirated from the joint.

Meniscal Variations and Tears

DISCOID MENISCUS

The meniscus is normally a crescentic structure, although several forms of discoid lateral menisci have been described. These range from a complete disc to a very rare ring-shaped meniscus with abnormal thickness. The pathophysiology of discoid meniscus development is not completely understood. A common explanation for these variant discoid forms assumes that the normal meniscus is formed from an original discoid shape and the discoid lateral meniscus is a congenital variant in which the central portion does not degenerate with time. This theory would explain the variously shaped menisci found at surgery. However, no discoid menisci have been found in fetuses and a review of comparative anatomy shows no mammal with such a pattern of formation.

A second theory is a developmental one. Many discoid lateral menisci have abnormal attachments to the tibia. When the attachment to the posterior tibial plateau is deficient, there is a strong attachment to the medial femoral condyle by the meniscofemoral ligament (Wrisberg's ligament). This pattern of attachment may allow abnormal movement of the lateral meniscus: the posterior horn of the lateral meniscus moves into the center of the lateral compartment during full extension of the knee. With time, scarring and fibrosis of the lateral meniscus occur, with resultant thickening. These changes may account for the popping on flexion and extension that is usually noticed during childhood or early adolescence.

Treatment. Many discoid menisci are asymptomatic, and the mere presence of one is not an indication for treatment. The popping itself is not harmful unless it is accompanied by pain or swelling of the knee. Pain, swelling, and a history of trauma are relative indications for arthroscopy. Tears of the meniscus or degenerative changes on the articular surfaces may necessitate resection. Arthroscopic techniques allow for partial resection or saucerization of the discoid lateral meniscus, leaving a peripheral rim that may function properly. Resection may be difficult because of the increased thickness in such menisci. Prognosis for patients with discoid menisci is good. Discoid menisci without degenerative changes have been found in the joints of elderly persons. Therefore every attempt should be made to salvage function of the meniscus by avoiding complete excision simply to eliminate the snapping, clicking sensation.

MENISCUS TEARS

Tears of the meniscus are common findings in a patient with an acutely injured knee, especially in situations in which a traumatic twisting event has occurred. Tears may occur in either meniscus or in both menisci at the

Types of Meniscal Tears and Discoid Meniscus Variations

Types of meniscal tears

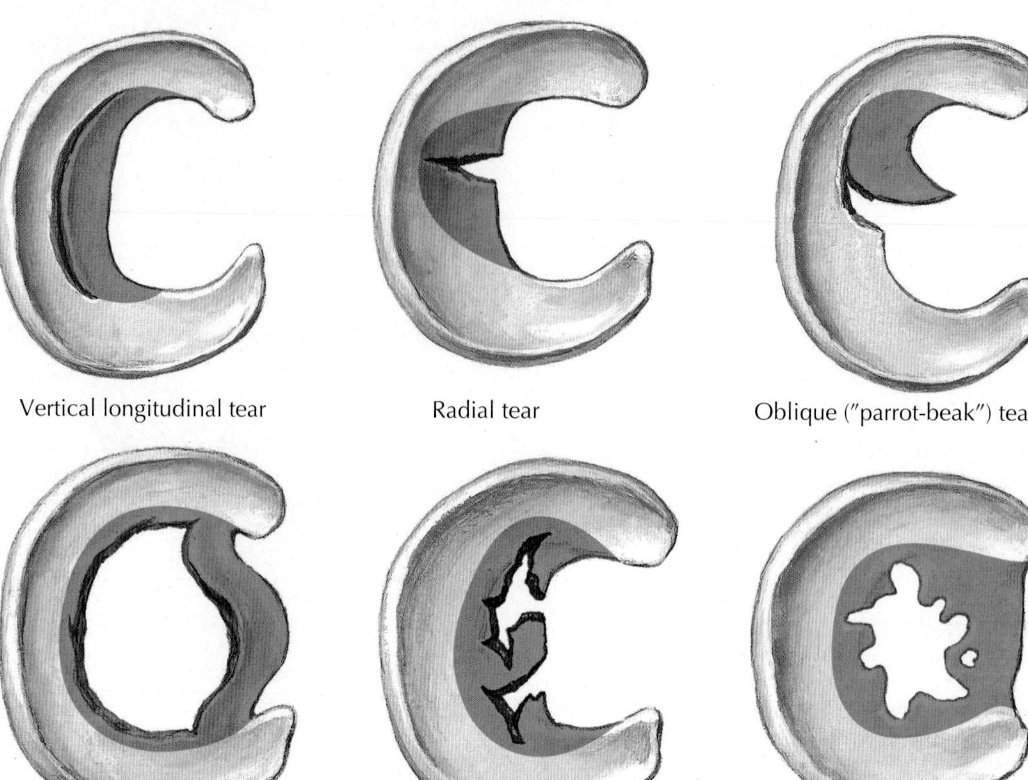

Vertical longitudinal tears involving the peripheral third are best managed by repair. Radial split tears are usually secondary to trauma, and when the split extends to the capsular rim, repair should be attempted in young people if at all possible. Oblique tears are most commonly seen and are best treated by arthroscopic partial meniscectomy (APM). Bucket-handle tears are more likely to cause locking of the knee. Horizontal (cleavage) and symptomatic degenerative tears are best treated by APM.

Discoid meniscus variations

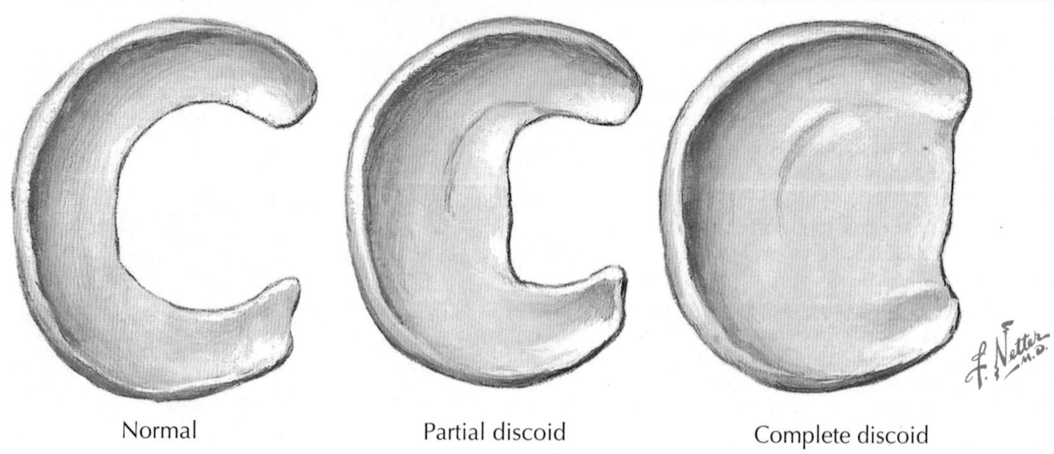

TEARS OF THE MENISCUS

Longitudinal (vertical) tear — May progress to — Bucket-handle tear

Radial tear — May progress to — Parrot-beak tear

Horizontal tear (probe in cleft) — May progress to — Flap tear

Anterior cruciate ligament
Bucket handle
Femoral condyle

Arthroscopic view of bucket-handle tear shows handle displaced into intercondylar fossa.

Arthroscopic view of parrot-beak tear with fibrillation of meniscal margin

Arthroscopic view of flap tear of lateral meniscus

Arthroscopic removal of torn meniscal fragment using motorized shaver. Scissors or scalpel may also be useful.

View 3 months later shows good fibrous healing of meniscal margin.

MENISCAL VARIATIONS AND TEARS (Continued)

same time. A meniscus tear often becomes symptomatic if its torn portion is mobile and slides into an abnormal position between the articular surfaces of the femur and tibia. Patients with a displaced meniscus tear often report pain at the joint line, recurrent knee effusions, and mechanical symptoms including locking, catching, and/or popping.

Meniscus tears can occur in a variety of types. One often symptomatic type is a bucket-handle tear, which is a longitudinal tear through the substance of the meniscus. It can resemble a bucket handle when viewed axially. The torn portion remains attached to the anterior and posterior horns of the meniscus. Another tear type is a small radial tear, which is named because the tear occurs in line with the radius of the semicircular meniscus. This tear initially often causes few symptoms, but if not treated it may progress to a deeper, more symptomatic tear type called a parrot-beak tear, which gets its name from the beak it resembles. The final tear type is a horizontal tear, which are tears in the axial plan through the substance of the meniscus. When a parrot-beak or horizontal tear occurs, an unstable flap of meniscus is often produced that can cause the aforementioned mechanical symptoms.

When an unstable portion of meniscus displaces into the intercondylar notch and becomes incarcerated, it will cause the knee to lock. Bucket-handle tears are at particularly high risk for this to occur. Manipulation of the knee may be possible and often occurs with a loud, audible, and palpable "clunk." This sound and the temporary resolution of symptoms indicate reduction of the displaced portion into its normal anatomic position.

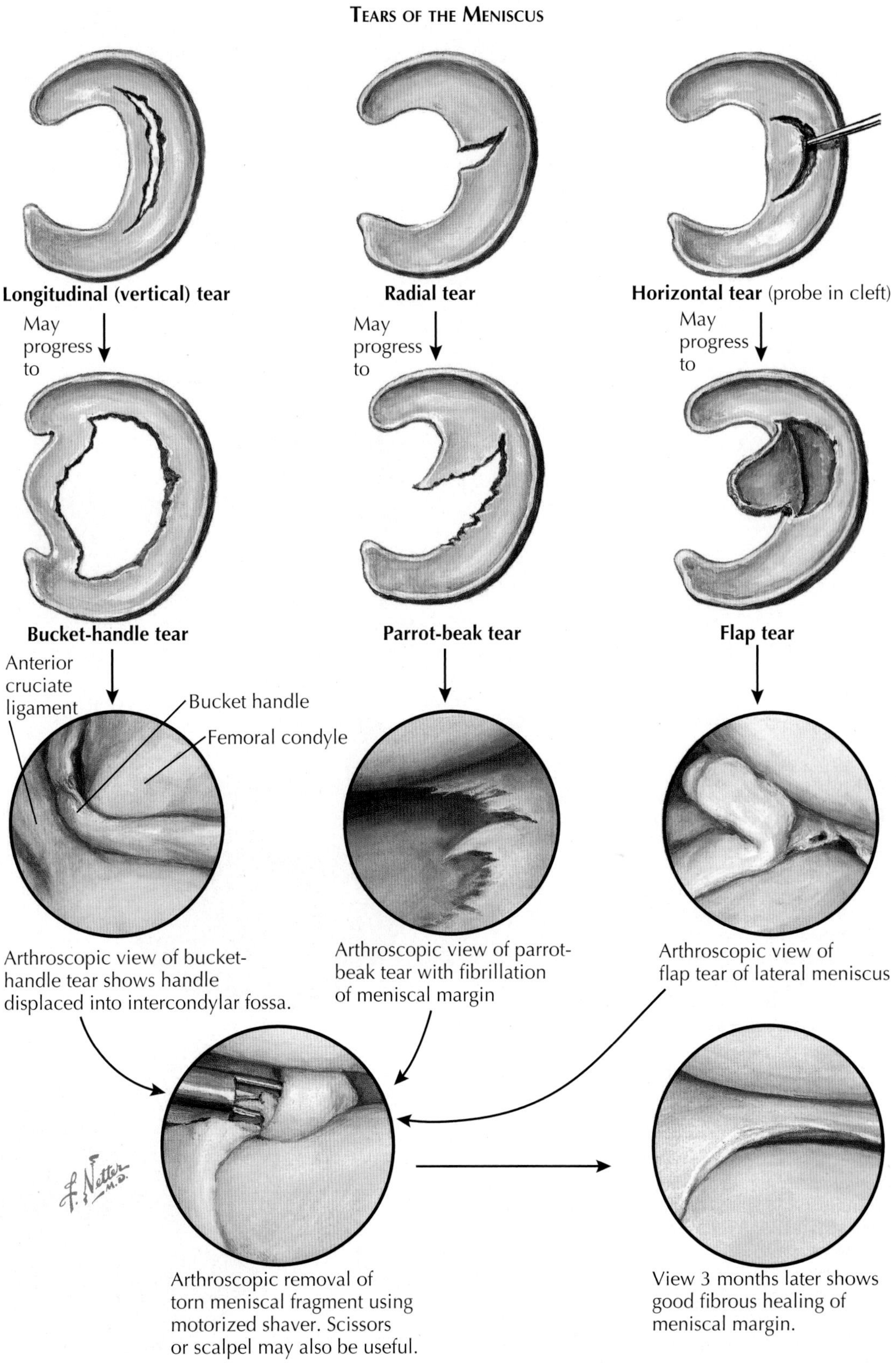

Physical Examination and Special Tests.

- *Joint line tenderness:* Tenderness along the medial or lateral joint lines is the most sensitive finding for a meniscal tear.
- *McMurray test:* The patient is supine and relaxed. The patient's knee is passively flexed to at least 90 degrees with external tibial rotation and varus stress (medial meniscus) or internal tibial rotation and valgus stress (lateral meniscus). While maintaining rotation, the patient's knee is brought into full extension. A positive test is indicated by a painful pop occurring over the medial joint line (medial meniscus) or lateral joint line (lateral meniscus).
- *Thessaly test:* The patient stands on the affected leg and flexes the knee to 20 to 30 degrees. The patient then places internal and external rotational stress through the knee. A positive test is indicated by a

MEDIAL AND LATERAL MENISCUS

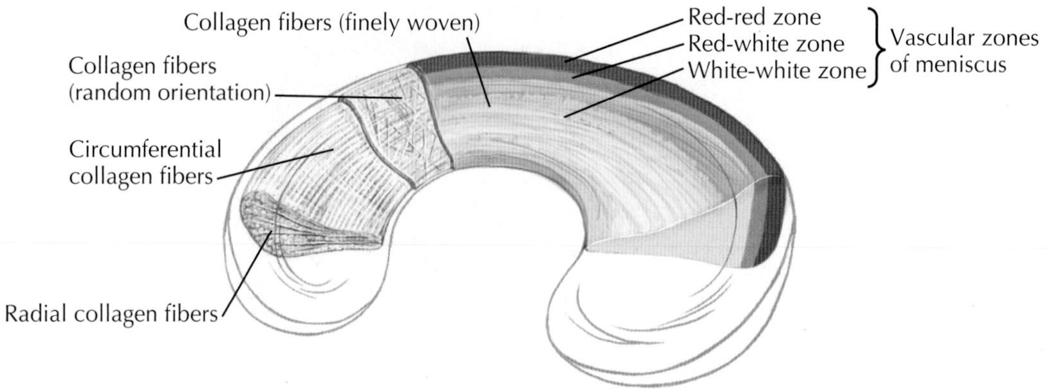

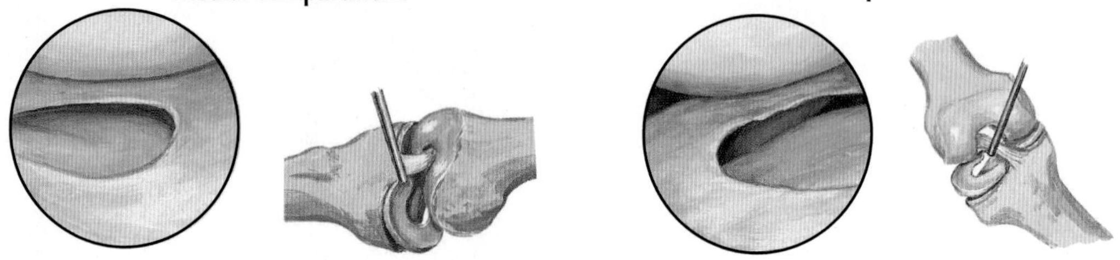

Medial meniscus visualized below femoral condyle. Meniscus rises with valgus stress, permitting inspection beneath it.

Lateral meniscus visualized. Varus stress raises meniscus from tibial condyle.

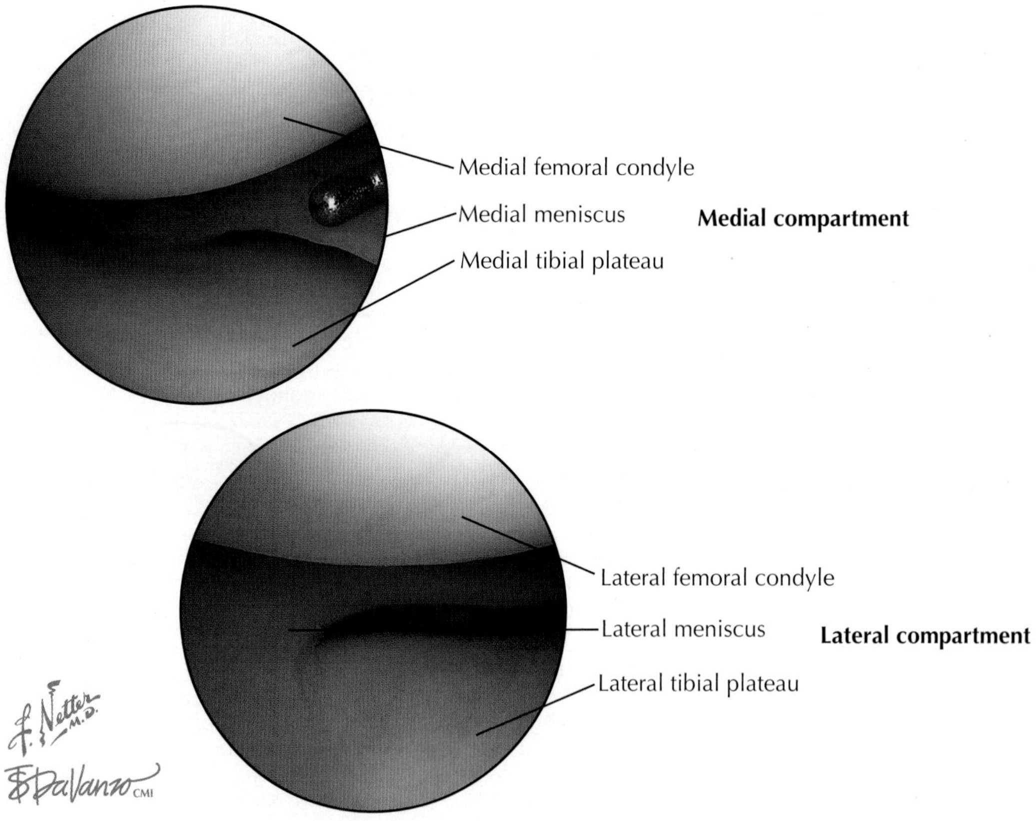

MENISCAL VARIATIONS AND TEARS (Continued)

pain and/or a painful pop over the medial joint line (medial meniscus) or lateral joint line (lateral meniscus).

McMurray and Thessaly test results may vary considerably from one examination session to the next owing to patient apprehension and chronicity of injury. A joint effusion will often be present after an acute tear.

Imaging. Radiographs are usually normal unless a meniscus tear has been present for a significant time. In that setting, they may show arthritic changes such as osteophyte formation and joint space narrowing. Magnetic resonance imaging (MRI) is the diagnostic tool of choice for identifying meniscal tears. MRI has a sensitivity as high as 95% for demonstration of medial meniscus tears but is less sensitive for detecting lateral meniscus tears.

Treatment. In young, active persons arthroscopic repair of torn menisci should always be considered. In these younger patients, the loss of a large portion of a meniscus can be devastating because meniscal deficiency can lead to earlier-onset arthritis.

At the time of the surgery, with the patient under anesthesia, a locked knee may spontaneously unlock. The knee is then examined manually to determine any ligament instability, and an arthroscopic examination is performed. To help preserve the articular cartilage, the displaced part of the meniscus can be removed during arthroscopy.

Repairs in the well-vascularized peripheral third (red-red zone) of the medial and lateral menisci have been quite successful. Multiple studies have looked at establishing which tears in the red-white and white-white zones can be repaired and whether there are biologic or pharmacologic means that may improve the potential for healing. Although these tears have less chance of healing, repair may well be indicated in younger patients. Approaches to repair include all-inside, outside-in, and inside-out techniques, with most surgeons now preferring the all-inside approach when possible.

Rehabilitation programs after arthroscopy and partial meniscectomy generally include minimal immobilization of the knee, immediate weight-bearing, and early physical therapy. Therapy consists of gait training and active and passive range-of-motion and quadriceps-strengthening exercises. Ice or heat may be applied as needed. After meniscal repair, vigorous rehabilitation and range-of-motion exercises may be delayed a few weeks.

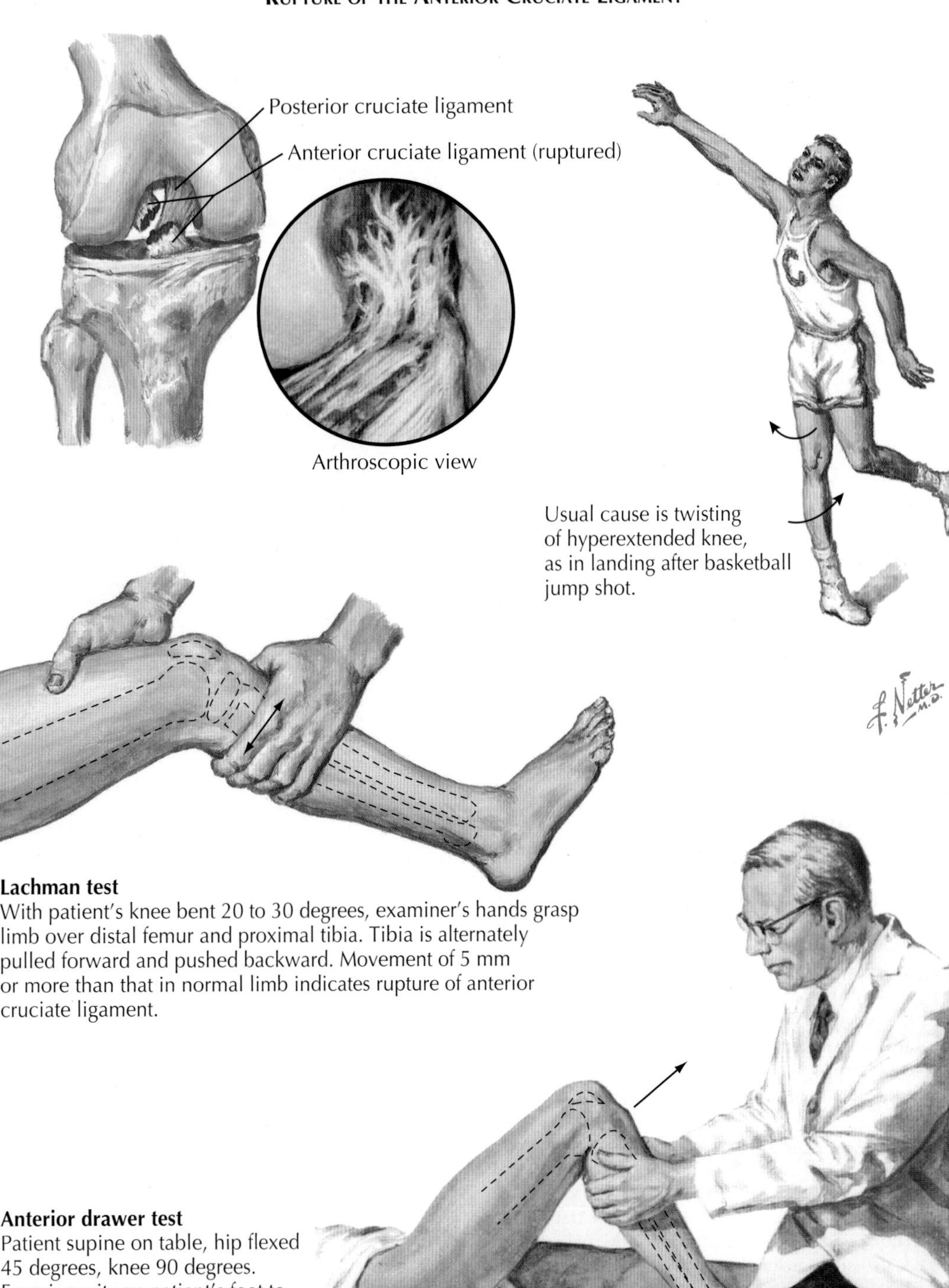

Rupture of the Anterior Cruciate Ligament
Posterior cruciate ligament
Anterior cruciate ligament (ruptured)
Arthroscopic view
Usual cause is twisting of hyperextended knee, as in landing after basketball jump shot.
Lachman test
With patient's knee bent 20 to 30 degrees, examiner's hands grasp limb over distal femur and proximal tibia. Tibia is alternately pulled forward and pushed backward. Movement of 5 mm or more than that in normal limb indicates rupture of anterior cruciate ligament.
Anterior drawer test
Patient supine on table, hip flexed 45 degrees, knee 90 degrees. Examiner sits on patient's foot to stabilize it, places hands on each side of upper calf, and firmly pulls tibia forward. Movement of 5 mm or more is positive result. Result is also compared with that for normal limb, which is tested first.

Knee Ligament Injury

Sprains of Knee Ligaments

Ligament injuries (sprains) of the knee are very common in athletes. In first-degree sprains, the ligament is stretched, with little or no tearing. These injuries produce mild point tenderness (for superficial ligaments), slight hemorrhage, and swelling. Erythema may develop over the painful area but resolves 2 to 3 weeks after injury. Joint laxity is not present, and the injury does not produce any significant long-term disability. Appropriate treatment consists of rest and muscle rehabilitation often involving physical therapy. Second-degree sprains are characterized by partial tearing of the ligament, which results in joint laxity, localized pain, tenderness, and swelling. When stress is placed on a joint during examination, the examiner should still feel a definite "end point" to the joint movement. Because the ligament is only partially injured, the joint remains stable; thus vigorous rehabilitation alone will likely be sufficient treatment. Third-degree sprains produce complete rupture of a ligament, making the joint unstable. Tenderness, instability, absence of a definite end point to stress testing, and severe ecchymosis are the hallmarks of third-degree sprains. Surgical intervention may be needed.

Sprains of the MCL are caused by a valgus force to the knee. Patients frequently report a snapping or tearing sensation and pain on the medial aspect of the knee. If only the MCL is injured, patients can usually continue to walk and may be able to continue the activity that causes the injury.

Physical examination reveals tenderness along the course of the MCL, and careful palpation can isolate the precise level of injury: at the origin of the ligament on the medial femoral condyle, at the joint line (midsubstance), or along the long distal insertion of the ligament into the medial aspect of the tibia. Patients are more comfortable if examined lying supine on the examining table with the thigh supported. The physician cradles the lower leg in both hands off to the side of the table and alternately applies varus and valgus stresses to the knee (varus and valgus stress tests). When the leg is fully extended, the ACL is the structure most responsible for mediolateral stability. However, placing the knee in 30 degrees of flexion takes the ACL "out of play" so the MCL can be tested by applying a valgus force.

Third-degree sprains of the MCL may require direct surgical repair. However, an isolated third-degree sprain may be successfully treated by controlling swelling, bracing, increasing range of motion, and rehabilitation of the quadriceps femoris and hamstring muscles through physical therapy.

Marked medial (valgus) laxity may indicate that the posteromedial corner of the knee capsule is also injured. Surgical repair is needed to prevent residual rotational instability. The MCL can also be injured as a component of a multiligamentous injury to the knee. For example, a football clipping injury may result in the

Lateral Pivot Shift Test for Anterolateral Knee Instability

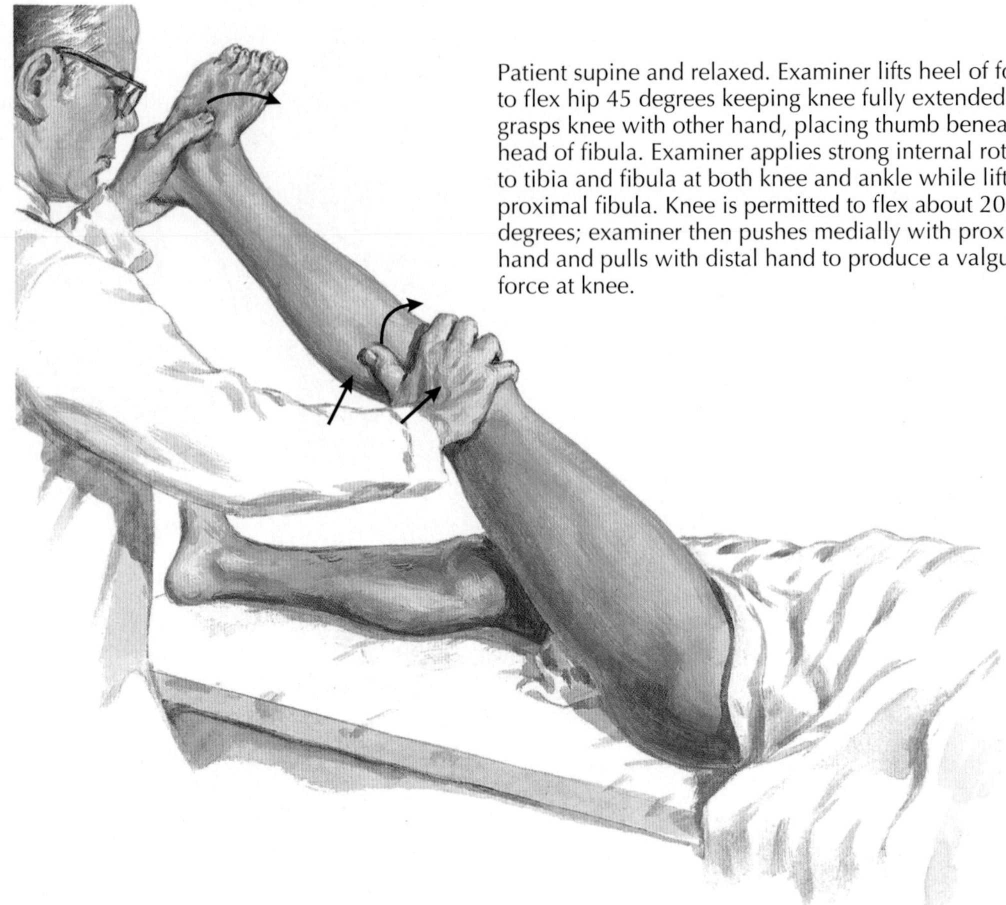

Patient supine and relaxed. Examiner lifts heel of foot to flex hip 45 degrees keeping knee fully extended, and grasps knee with other hand, placing thumb beneath head of fibula. Examiner applies strong internal rotation to tibia and fibula at both knee and ankle while lifting proximal fibula. Knee is permitted to flex about 20 degrees; examiner then pushes medially with proximal hand and pulls with distal hand to produce a valgus force at knee.

As internal rotation, valgus force, and forward displacement of lateral tibial condyle are maintained, knee is passively flexed. If anterior subluxation of tibia (anterolateral instability) is present, sudden visible, audible, and palpable reduction occurs at 20 to 40 degrees of flexion. Test is positive if anterior cruciate ligament is ruptured, especially if lateral capsular ligament also is torn.

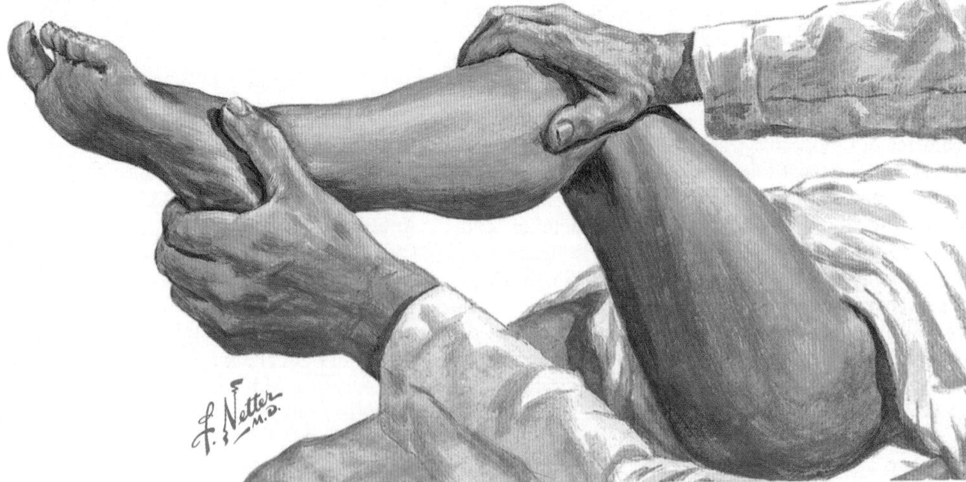

Knee Ligament Injury (Continued)

"unhappy triad" of O'Donoghue, which involves an MCL rupture, ACL rupture, and medial meniscus tear. Although this is a classically known triad, recent literature has shown that the lateral meniscus is more likely to be acutely torn at the time of ACL injury, whereas the medial meniscus is more often compromised in the chronically ACL-deficient knee. These injuries often require arthroscopically aided repair of the ligaments as necessary and repair of the injured meniscus if possible.

RUPTURE OF THE ANTERIOR CRUCIATE LIGAMENT

The ACL is the primary restraint to anterior translation of the tibia, and it also contributes to internal rotation and varus/valgus instability with the knee extension. The anatomic configuration of its two bundles (anteromedial and posterolateral) ensures functional tautness throughout the arc of motion, with the anteromedial bundle taut in flexion and the posterolateral component taut in extension. Although it may be torn by a contact injury, the ACL is most commonly injured without contact by a decelerating valgus angulation and external rotation force. In basketball, the ACL is commonly torn when a player lands from jumping with the knee in hyperextension and the tibia in internal rotation. The player hears a "pop," feels a tear and acute pain in the knee, and may not be able to continue playing. The knee may feel very unstable during weight-bearing and is often felt as a "giving way" of the knee. Patients complain that their knee slips or slides when they turn right or left with the foot planted. This sliding reflects the tibia subluxating anteriorly on the femur. Rupture of the ACL is a common cause of acute traumatic hemarthrosis.

Physical Examination and Special Tests.

- *Lachman test:* This test is simple to perform and relatively painless for the patient with an acute injury, and it is a highly sensitive physical exam for an ACL rupture. The Lachman test is performed with the knee flexed 20 degrees to reduce the stability provided by the menisci. One of the examiner's hands stabilizes the femur while the other hand grasps the proximal tibia. With the patient relaxed, the examiner attempts to slide the proximal tibia anteriorly on the femur. An intact ACL prevents the tibia from sliding forward, and if present it provides a firm end point to translation for the exam. When the ligament is injured, the tibia is moved from its normal position and can be subluxated anteriorly during the test; no firm end point can be appreciated. In the interpretation of the Lachman test, it is important to note whether the PCL is intact, as a ruptured PCL can cause the proximal tibia to sag posteriorly and produce the appearance of a false-positive Lachman.

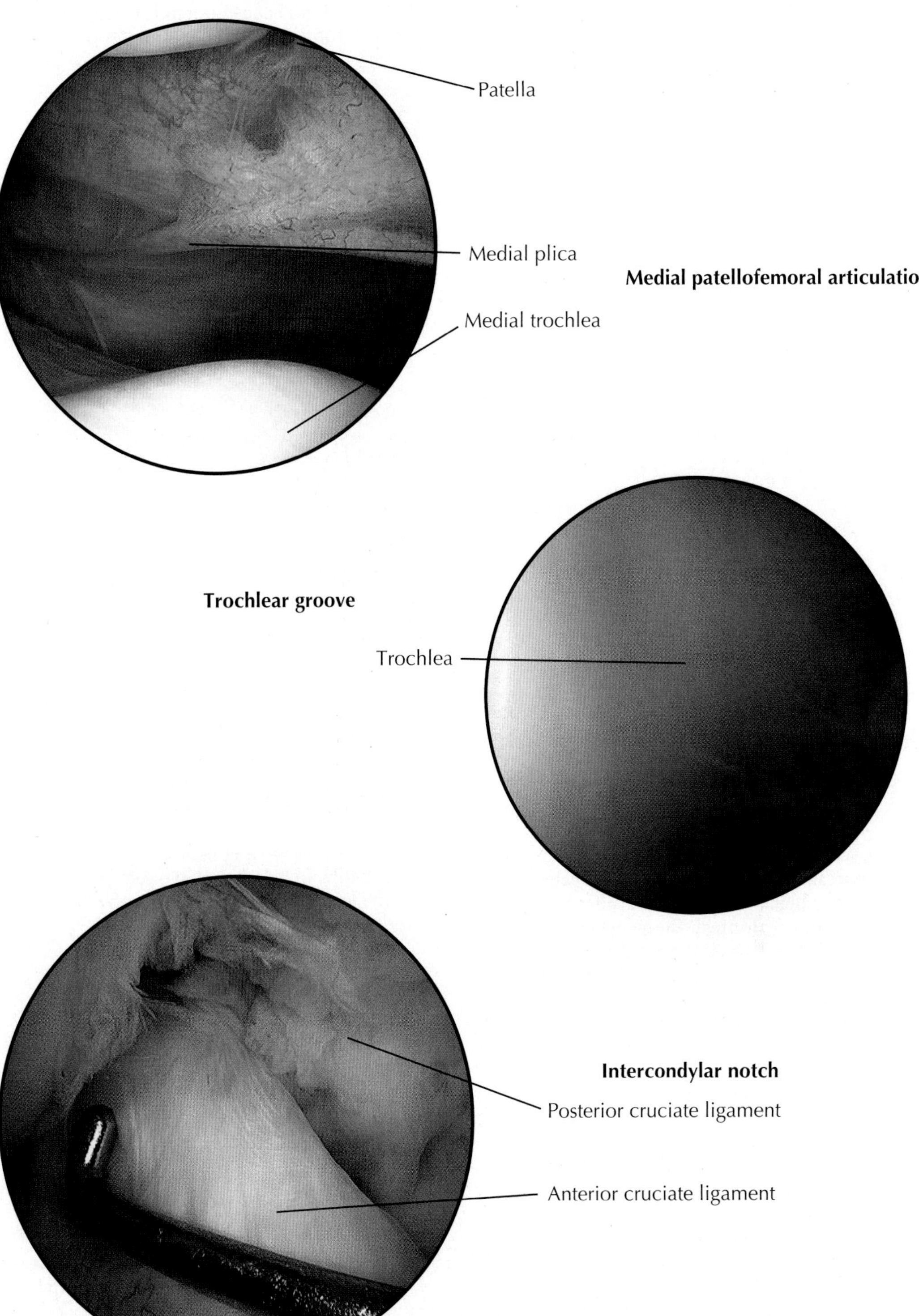

KNEE LIGAMENT INJURY (Continued)

- *Anterior drawer test:* The anterior drawer test is performed with the patient lying supine, resting comfortably with the knee flexed to 90 degrees (see Plate 3.12). The patient's foot is stabilized during the test and may be held in place by the seated examiner's thigh. The examiner grasps the patient's calf near the popliteal fossa with both hands and attempts to slide the tibia anteriorly. When the ACL is ruptured, the tibia slides anteriorly with respect to the femur; there is no firm end point to the exam in this scenario. As in the Lachman test, the injured knee must be compared with the normal one.
- *Pivot shift test:* This test identifies most cases of clinically significant knee instability, but it can be challenging to conduct in the awake acutely injured patient as it often produces a feeling of significant discomfort. Therefore the test is more effective on an anesthetized patient. The patient should be lying supine and relaxed. The examiner stands beside the injured leg, facing it. With one hand grasping the patient's foot, the examiner places the other hand on the lateral aspect of the knee, with the thumb underneath the head of the fibula. With the knee starting in full extension, a valgus force is applied at the knee while the tibia is internally rotated by the hand holding the foot. Rupture of the ACL causes anterior subluxation of the tibial plateau on the femur. As the knee is then slowly flexed, the subluxation becomes more apparent. At a point between 20 and 40 degrees of flexion, the iliotibial tract transitions from acting as an extensor (which it does when the knee is in extension) to a flexor, which causes reduction of the tibia. The reduction is palpable, visible, and frequently audible.

Imaging. On plain radiographs, a lateral capsular sign, also known as a Segond fracture, shows avulsion of the midportion of the lateral capsular ligament with a small fragment of proximal lateral tibia. This is associated with a high incidence of an ACL tear and indicates anterolateral instability.

Treatment. Not all acute injuries of the ACL require surgery. Low-demand patients who do not often engage in cutting or pivoting activities can sometimes return to activities of daily living and mild activity with solely a rehabilitation program. However, significant instability may eventually develop if injury of the ACL is neglected or treated conservatively, which puts the patient at high risk of developing degenerative meniscal tears and earlier-onset posttraumatic osteoarthritis. Patients whose knees give way during daily activities are candidates for reconstruction of the ligament. If the instability is a problem only during intense physical activity and the patient is not cutting or pivoting (such as in runners), using a brace may provide relief and allow the patient to continue to participate without surgery.

RUPTURE OF POSTERIOR CRUCIATE LIGAMENT

Usual causes include hyperextension injury, as occurs from stepping into hole, and direct blow to flexed knee.

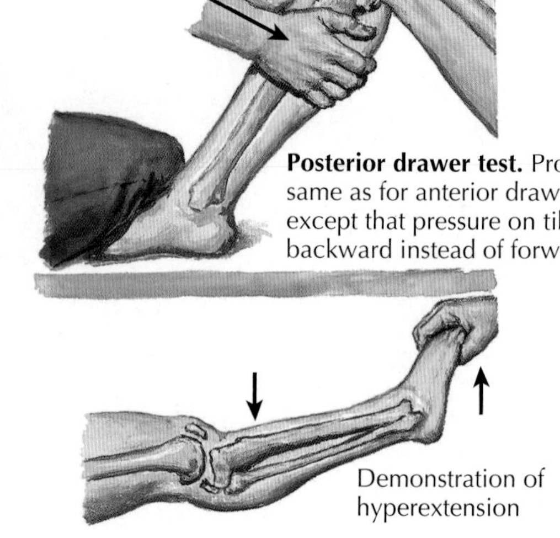

Posterior drawer test. Procedure same as for anterior drawer test, except that pressure on tibia is backward instead of forward.

Posterior sag sign. Leg drops backward.

Demonstration of hyperextension

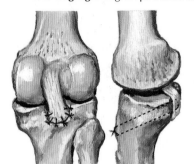

Avulsion of tibial attachment, with or without small bone fragment, may be reattached with nonabsorbable sutures to firm capsular tissue or to bone or with suture through drill holes in tibia.

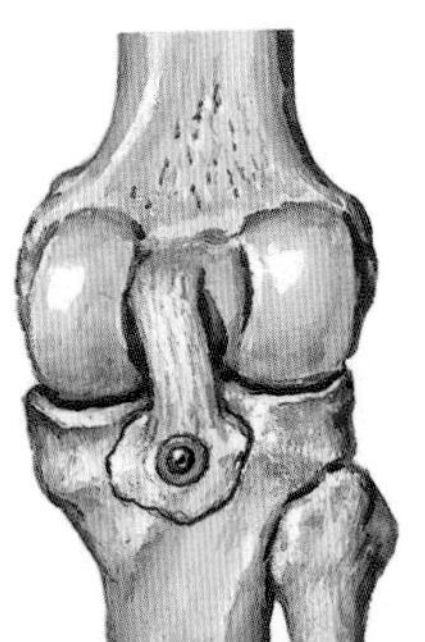

Large bone fragment avulsed from tibia may be fixed in place with screw.

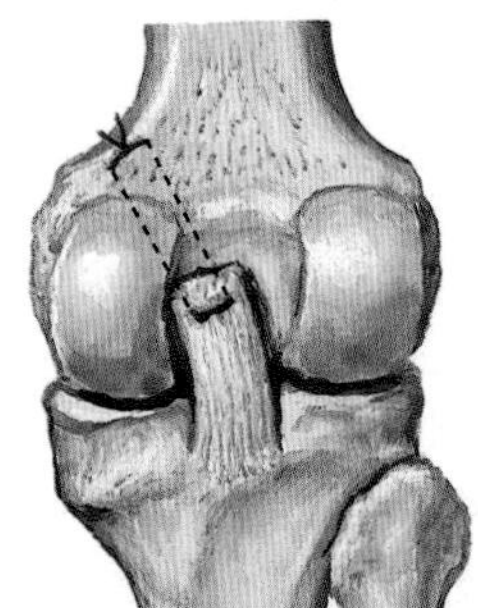

Avulsion of femoral attachment may be repaired with nonabsorbable suture through drill holes in distal femur.

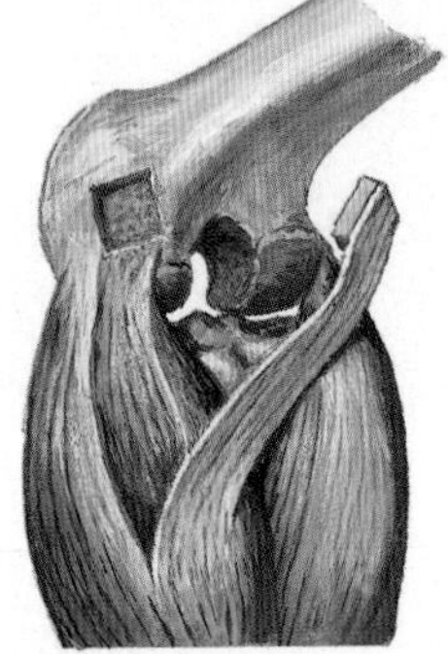

Flap formed of tendinous portion of origin of medial head of gastrocnemius muscle plus small block of bone from femoral attachment (posteromedial view).

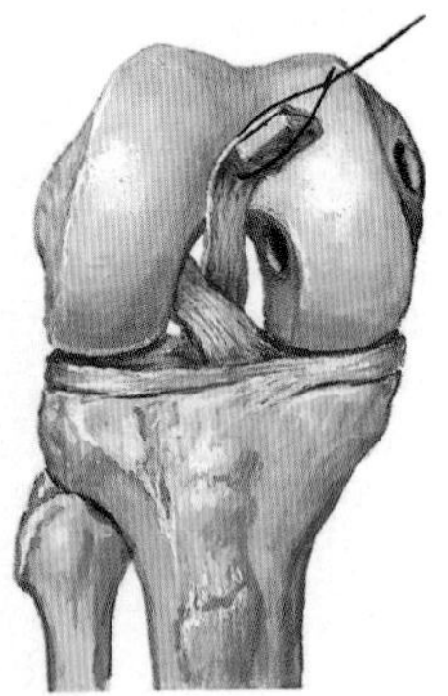

Flap passed into intercondylar notch; tunnel drilled through medial femoral condyle. Drill guide ensures accurate placement.

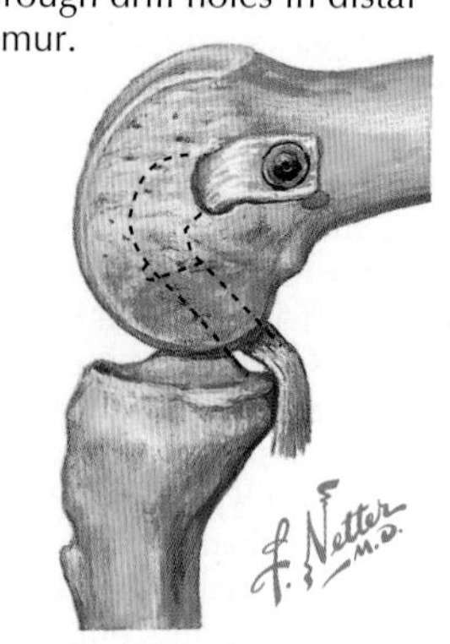

Flap with terminal bone block passed through tunnel and fixed with screw. Flap functions as substitute for posterior cruciate ligament.

KNEE LIGAMENT INJURY (Continued)

However, most patients with an acute ACL rupture require operative treatment. Young, active patients have a significantly higher chance of returning to activity if reconstruction is performed. The goals of surgery are to restore stability to the knee to permit return to activity, prolong the survival of the menisci, and delay the development of osteoarthritis.

Many techniques are used to reconstruct the ACL, with specific considerations based on each individual patient. In the skeletally mature patient, the ligament is traditionally reconstructed using an arthroscopically assisted approach. The graft choice in younger patients will usually be a hamstring or bone–patellar tendon–bone autograft, whereas older patients or those with other contraindications to hamstring harvest may use allograft tissue. In younger patients, allograft tissue yields a five times higher graft rupture rate compared with autograft, and so it is not used in that demographic. In skeletally immature patients with open growth plates, there exist multiple modifications to the traditional reconstruction methods that avoid compromising the tibial, femoral, or both open physes. Protected weight-bearing is allowed immediately, with some surgeons using braces in the early postoperative period. Early and consistent physical therapy is very important to achieve optimal results. Patients should avoid participation in high-demand sports for 6 to 12 months after surgery.

RUPTURE OF POSTERIOR CRUCIATE LIGAMENT

The most common causes of rupture of the PCL are hyperextension of the knee and a direct blow to the anterior aspect of the flexed knee (commonly a dashboard injury). Severe varus or valgus stress to the knee after injury to the collateral ligaments can cause rupture of the PCL.

Physical Examination and Special Tests. A knee lacking a functioning PCL may be hyperextended during examination. The examiner stands at the foot of the supine patient and simultaneously lifts both feet by the great toes, observing the amount of extension at each knee. A knee with rupture of a PCL exhibits noticeable hyperextension.

- *Posterior drawer test:* The posterior drawer test is performed with the patient lying supine on an examining table and the knee in 90 degrees of flexion. The patient's foot is stabilized by the examiner's thigh on the table as for the anterior drawer test. The examiner uses both hands to push the proximal tibia posteriorly to displace it relative to the distal femur. By alternately pushing and pulling the tibia, the examiner can determine whether the ACL is intact and if the proximal tibia is moving posteriorly. The examiner must recognize the starting point of the drawer test to determine accurately which of the two cruciate

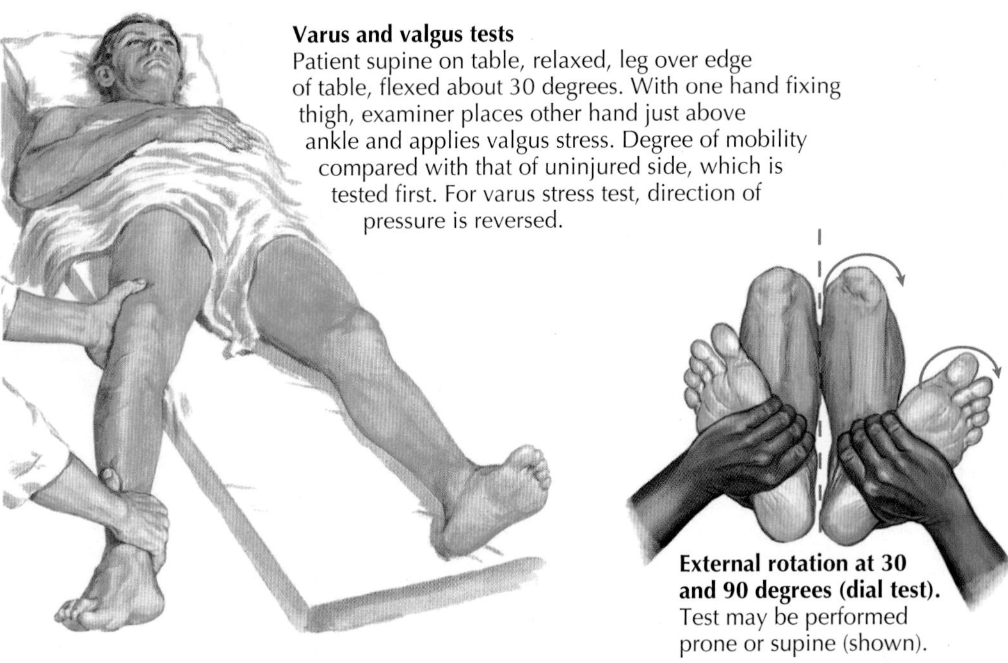

Physical Examination of the Leg and Knee
Varus and valgus tests
Patient supine on table, relaxed, leg over edge of table, flexed about 30 degrees. With one hand fixing thigh, examiner places other hand just above ankle and applies valgus stress. Degree of mobility compared with that of uninjured side, which is tested first. For varus stress test, direction of pressure is reversed.
External rotation at 30 and 90 degrees (dial test).
Test may be performed prone or supine (shown).

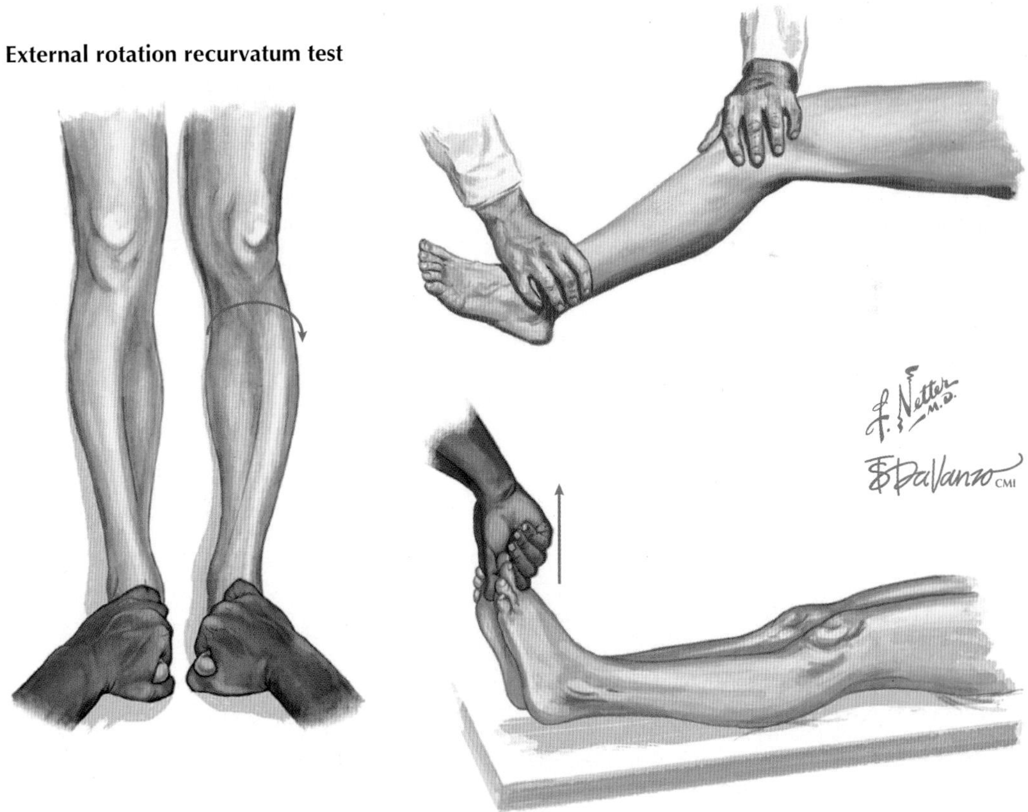

Knee Ligament Injury (Continued)

ligaments is injured; this is done by palpating the femoral condyles with the thumbs to confirm the alignment of the tibia with respect to the femur.

- *Posterior sag sign:* With the patient supine and relaxed, a pad is placed under the midthigh on the affected side; the heel is allowed to rest on the examining table, and the calf of the leg hangs unsupported. The examiner observes the knee from the patient's side. When a rupture of the PCL is present, the proximal tibia subluxates posteriorly and the anterior surface of the proximal lower leg appears to sag.

Treatment. Isolated PCL ruptures are often very amenable to nonoperative treatment with physical therapy and temporary bracing. Patients who have a high-demand level, severe instability, and failure of nonoperative management are candidates for reconstruction of the PCL. This is routinely accomplished in an arthroscopically assisted fashion. When avulsion of the bony attachment of the PCL occurs at either end, primary repair of the avulsion fragment may be performed. If the injury is purely ligamentous, reconstruction of the ligament can be conducted. Injury to the posterolateral corner of the knee capsule must also be considered and addressed when necessary at the time of surgery to avoid a poor functional result.

After surgery, the knee may be immobilized in extension for a period of 2 weeks. Vigorous physical therapy is then instituted while avoiding activities that place a load on the knee when it is flexed past 90 degrees. Achieving full extension may be very difficult and should be a goal of therapy, although manipulation under anesthesia may eventually be required.

Medial (Tibial) Collateral Ligament Injury

Injury to the MCL is often caused by a valgus force applied to the knee made more severe by external tibial rotation. This may occur from a blow to the lateral side of the joint (more common) or by a noncontact twist event (less common). The patient will initially describe pain on the medial side of the knee and, with a complete tear, complaints of the knee giving way into valgus.

Physical Examination. Injury to the MCL is noted with a positive (can be pain, more common with incomplete injuries, or laxity, as seen in complete injuries) valgus stress test with the knee in 30 degrees of flexion compared with the opposite knee. An injured MCL along with disrupted ACL or PCL will result in more gapping that occurs when the knee is tested in full extension in addition to in 30 degrees of flexion.

Imaging. Radiographs of the knee are usually unremarkable when the MCL is injured. MRI can diagnose

Sprains of Knee Ligaments

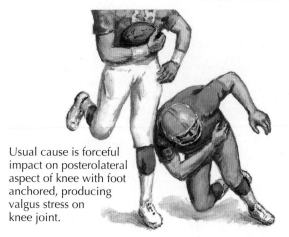

Usual cause is forceful impact on posterolateral aspect of knee with foot anchored, producing valgus stress on knee joint.

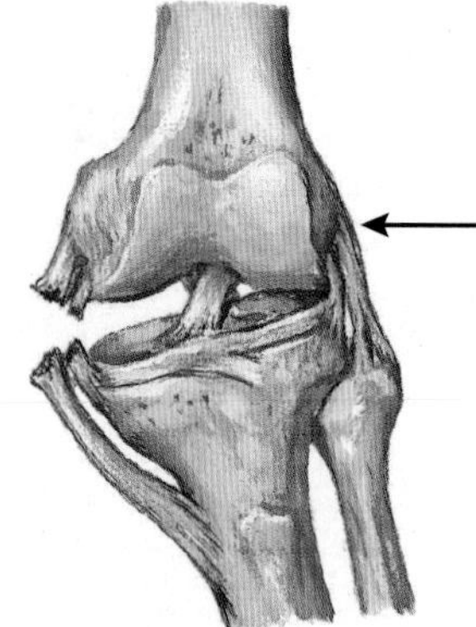

Valgus stress may rupture tibial collateral and capsular ligaments.

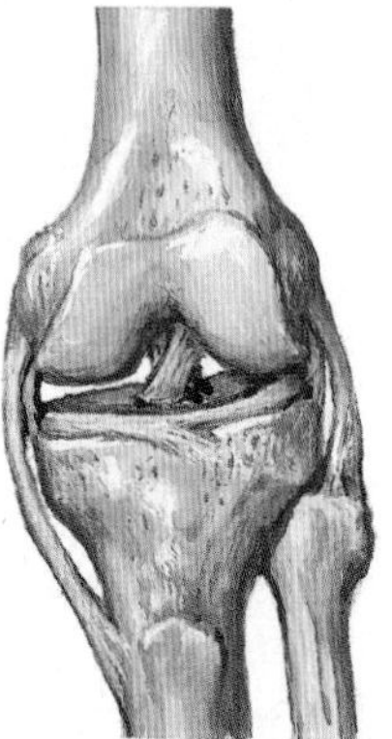

Grade 1 sprain. Localized joint pain and tenderness but no joint laxity.

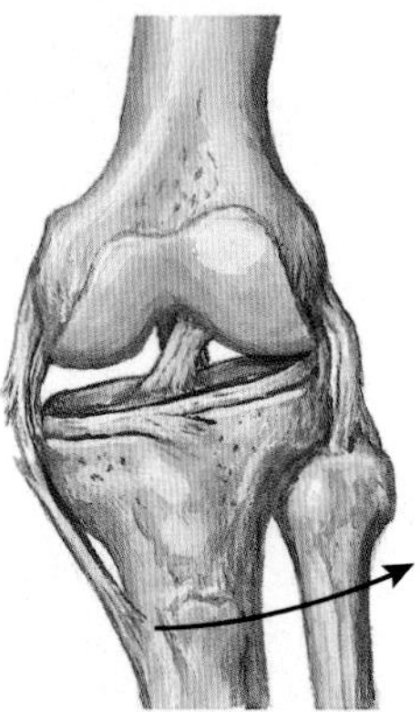

Grade 2 sprain. Detectable joint laxity plus localized pain and tenderness.

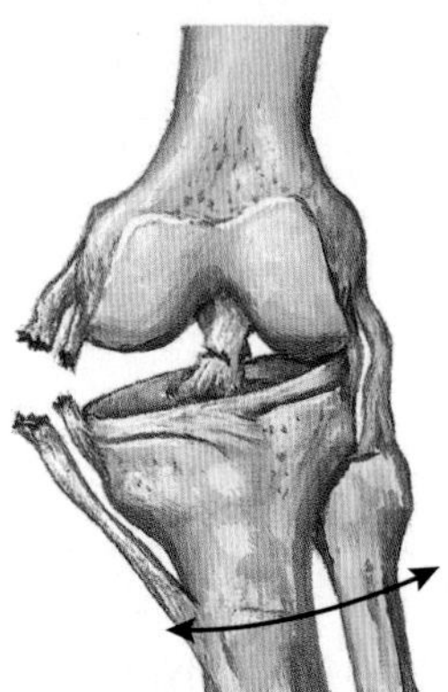

Grade 3 sprain. Complete disruption of ligaments and gross joint instability.

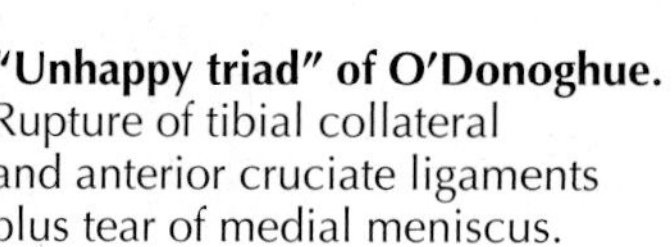

"Unhappy triad" of O'Donoghue. Rupture of tibial collateral and anterior cruciate ligaments plus tear of medial meniscus.

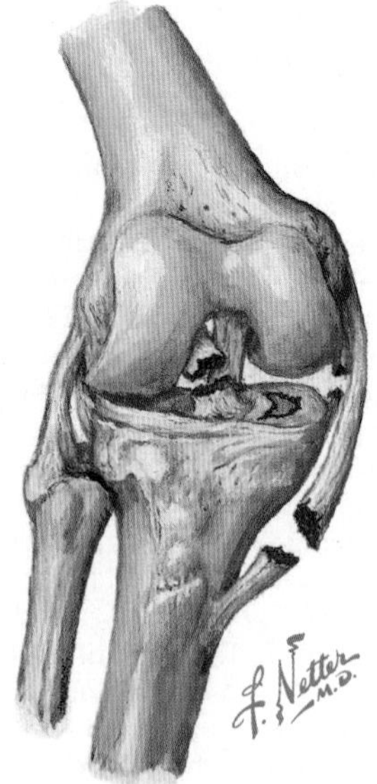

Knee Ligament Injury (Continued)

disruptions or edema in the MCL, but it is not often necessary to diagnose an MCL sprain if the history and physical exam are indicative of an incomplete MCL tear.

Treatment. Grade 1 and 2 sprains are often treated with the RICE (rest, ice, compression, elevation) protocol, along with use of crutches while weight-bearing, a brace with varus and valgus stabilizing components, and physical therapy. Unless present with other associated injuries or in a high-demand athlete, grade 3 (complete) MCL tears can also be treated with similar nonoperative measures. Surgical options include primary repair or reconstruction with autograft (semitendinosus) or allograft (can use tibialis anterior, hamstring, or Achilles tendon).

LATERAL LIGAMENT AND POSTEROLATERAL CORNER INJURIES

Injury to the lateral (fibular) collateral ligament (LCL) often occurs with a varus force or twisting moment at the knee. Injuries to this region of the knee may be associated with injuries to the popliteus tendon, iliotibial band, popliteofemoral ligament, and peroneal nerve. Posterolateral ligaments are often injured by a hyperextension mechanism, frequently with a blow to the anteromedial tibia.

Patients will complain of pain present over the lateral ligament complex. The knee may also give way when twisting, cutting, or pivoting. In chronic cases, posterolateral corner injury gives a feeling of giving way into hyperextension when standing, walking, or running backward.

Physical Examination and Special Tests. In acute cases, there may be increased gapping on a varus stress test at 30 degrees of flexion. The dial test will likely be positive in all cases of severe posterolateral ligament disruption. The dial test is conducted with the patient either prone or supine, and the examiner places an external rotation force to the knee through the ankle at 30 degrees of knee flexion. Increased external rotation of 10 to 15 degrees compared with the opposite knee indicates an injury to the posterolateral corner. If positive, the test is repeated at 90 degrees of knee flexion, and increased external rotation at this point suggests a concurrent PCL injury.

Imaging. Similar to MCL injuries, plain radiographs often do not show significant findings in LCL and PCL injuries. MRI can show ligamentous edema (suggestive of partial sprain) or tearing of both structures.

Treatment. Similar to injuries to the MCL, grade I and II sprains are treated conservatively with the RICE protocol, crutches, sometimes bracing, and physical rehabilitation. In complete tears, primary surgical repair or allograft reconstruction is usually preferable, especially if the injury involves more than just the LCL. Immobilization alone may be less successful for these injuries in patients with severe instability.

Disruption of Quadriceps Femoris Tendon or Patellar Ligament

Damage to the quadriceps mechanism generally occurs when there is active contraction of the quadriceps femoris muscle against forced flexion of the knee. Most ruptures of this extensor mechanism occur in older patients. At the time of injury, the patient experiences sudden pain, which may be associated with a tearing sensation about the knee. The tendon may be weakened by age-related degenerative changes or by pathologic changes due to psoriatic arthritis, rheumatoid arthritis, arteriosclerosis, gout, hyperparathyroidism, diabetes, chronic renal failure, or corticosteroid therapy.

Physical Examination. Palpation of the knee often reveals a hematoma, which may make examination difficult. A high-riding patella (patella alta) may indicate rupture of the patellar ligament, whereas a patella that is riding lower than normal (patella baja) suggests a rupture of the quadriceps femoris tendon. A large defect is often palpable at the site of the ruptured structure soon after injury, although if the ruptured ligament is not treated for weeks or months the sulcus may fill with scar tissue.

The most important finding during physical examination is the patient's inability to actively extend the knee fully against gravity. Also, the patient may not be able to maintain a passively extended knee against gravity. Patients with rupture of the quadriceps femoris tendon or patellar ligament without involvement of the medial or lateral retinaculum may be able to extend the injured knee actively to within 10 degrees of full extension. When there is a widely separated tear of either tendon or ligament combined with involvement of the medial and lateral retinacula, active extension is very difficult or impossible. Patients with chronic rupture of the quadriceps femoris tendon complain of giving way of the knee and marked weakness on attempting active extension. They may show an extensor lag meaning they have some active extension ability because of scarring in the injured tendon area but they cannot fully extend the knee.

Imaging. Whereas physical examination is often sufficient to diagnose disruptions of the extensor mechanism, it is recommended to obtain plain radiographs to assess for fracture and patellar positioning. MRI may be performed to assess the involved soft tissues in detail, although this is not often necessary for these patients.

Treatment. Rupture of the quadriceps femoris tendon generally occurs at its point of insertion into the superior pole of the patella, whereas rupture of the patellar ligament usually occurs at the inferior pole of the patella. In both cases, surgery is required to reestablish the continuity of the quadriceps mechanism. The tendon or ligament most often is reattached with sutures through drill holes in the patella. Then, the medial and lateral retinacula are sutured. After surgery, the knee is routinely immobilized in full extension for 6 to 8 weeks.

Patients who also have chronic metabolic disorders or receive long-term corticosteroid treatment may require a more complex repair that uses tendon, fascia, or wire to reinforce the damaged quadriceps mechanism. After postoperative immobilization, patients gradually start protected range-of-motion exercises and should use a cane or walker for some time.

Rupture of the patellar ligament may also occur at its insertion on the tibia, with or without fracture of the tibial tuberosity. In children whose growth plates have not yet closed, the ligament should be sutured, because this injury may disturb the growth of the proximal tibia. In adults, avulsion of the ligament from the tibial tuberosity is repaired by suturing the avulsed ligament though drill holes in the tibia or securing it with a metal staple or screw. A displaced fracture of the tibial tuberosity may be treated with open reduction and fixation with a metal screw. Tibial tuberosity avulsion fractures are at significant risk for developing compartment syndrome in the lower leg because the anterior tibial recurrent artery runs near the tuberosity. This structure can be easily injured concomitantly, which can lead to accumulation of blood in the anterior compartment of the lower leg and subsequently to compartment syndrome.

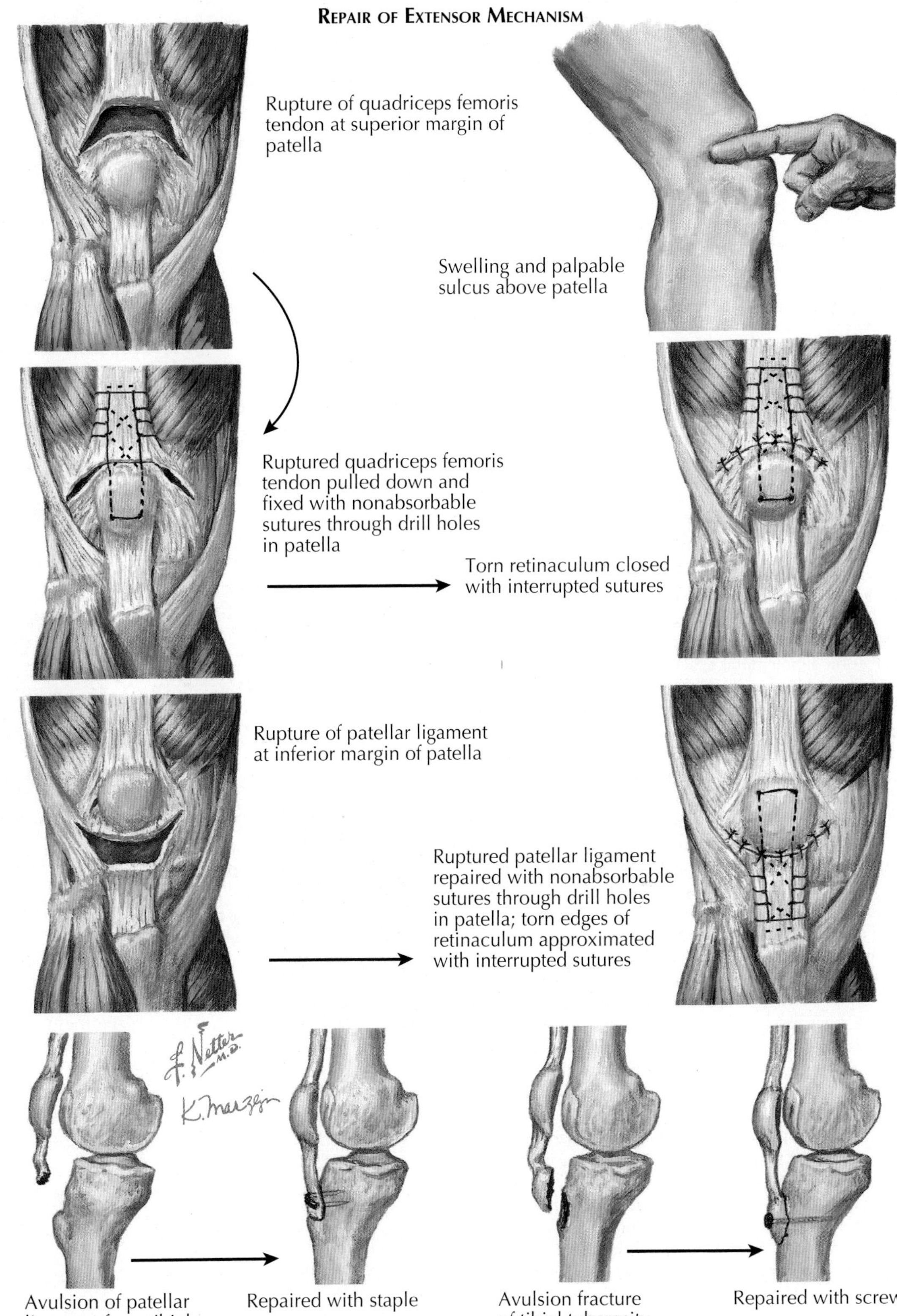
Repair of Extensor Mechanism
Rupture of quadriceps femoris tendon at superior margin of patella
Swelling and palpable sulcus above patella
Ruptured quadriceps femoris tendon pulled down and fixed with nonabsorbable sutures through drill holes in patella
Torn retinaculum closed with interrupted sutures
Rupture of patellar ligament at inferior margin of patella
Ruptured patellar ligament repaired with nonabsorbable sutures through drill holes in patella; torn edges of retinaculum approximated with interrupted sutures
F. Netter M.D.
K. Marzen
Avulsion of patellar ligament from tibial tuberosity
Repaired with staple
Avulsion fracture of tibial tuberosity
Repaired with screw

DISLOCATION OF KNEE JOINT

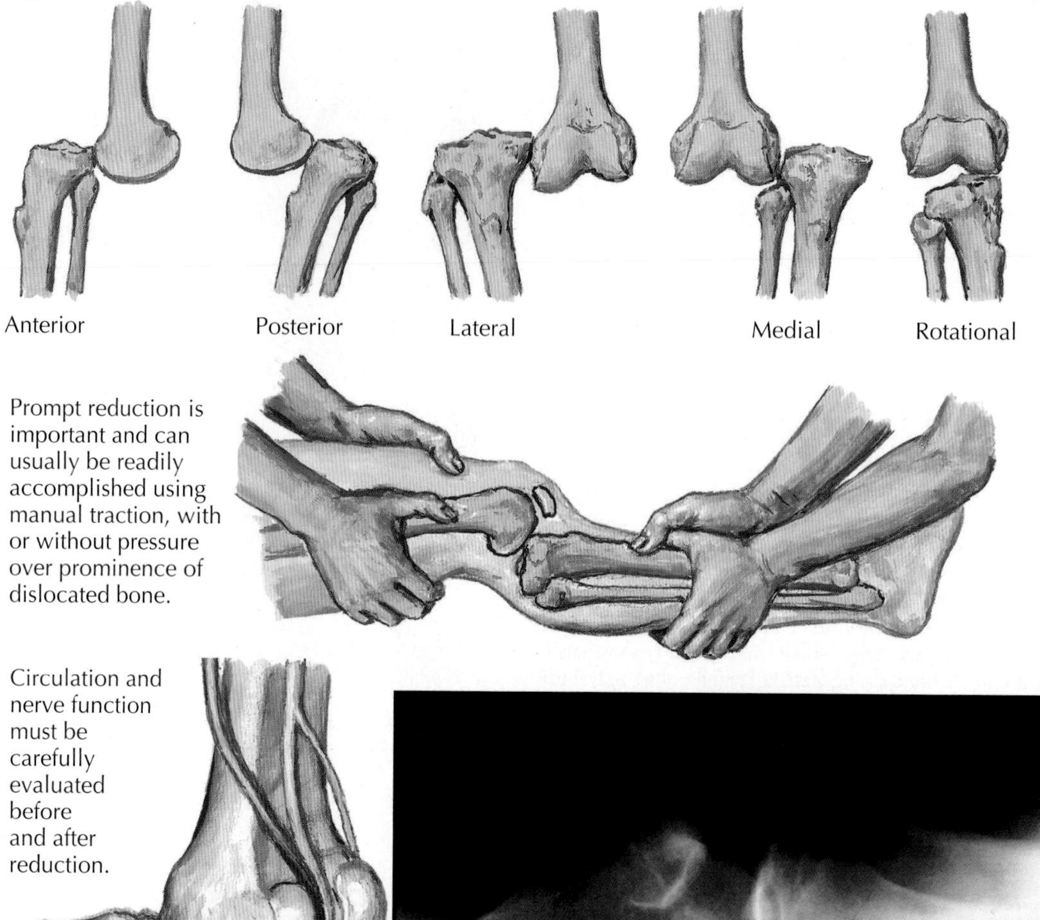

Types of dislocation
Anterior
Posterior
Lateral
Medial
Rotational
Prompt reduction is important and can usually be readily accomplished using manual traction, with or without pressure over prominence of dislocated bone.
Circulation and nerve function must be carefully evaluated before and after reduction.

Arteriogram shows occlusion of popliteal artery just proximal to joint in dislocation of knee.

Tear or thrombosis of popliteal artery is a frequent complication, requiring immediate repair or replacement. Tibial and common peroneal nerves may also be torn but usually do not require surgical repair.

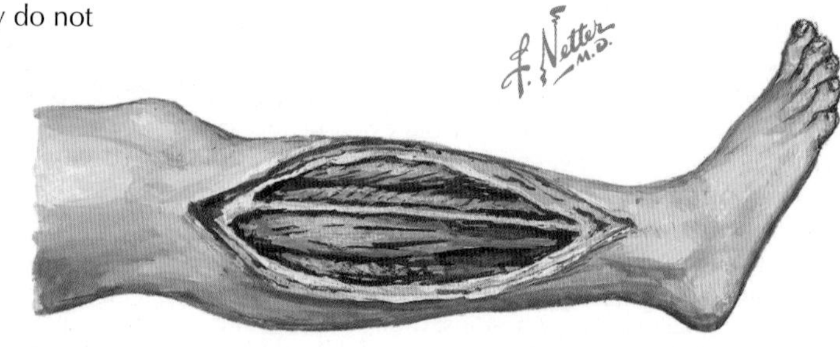

Compartment syndrome due to massive bleeding or ischemia is a common threat. Four-compartment fasciotomy must be done at the first sign of compartment syndrome.

Dislocation of the knee joint must be distinguished from dislocation of the patella. Whereas a patella dislocation involves the patellofemoral joint, a knee dislocation involves the tibiofemoral articulation. A knee dislocation is an emergency, and reduction should be achieved as soon as possible. Striking the knee against the dashboard during an automobile accident is the most common cause of injury, but athletic injuries can also be a cause. The popliteal artery and its branches are often damaged during dislocation of the knee because the trifurcation of the popliteal artery is tethered to the leg where the anterior tibial artery goes through a gap in the interosseous membrane. Therefore arterial injury must be suspected in every knee dislocation. A thorough neurovascular examination should be performed before and after reduction, and an ankle-brachial index should be obtained as well. Pulses can sometimes be present in the lower leg even in the setting of a popliteal artery injury, so suspicion should still be high for a vascular injury regardless. If there remains any question of arterial damage, arteriography or computed tomography (CT) angiography should be pursued, and, if an injury is identified, any necessary arterial repair should be done immediately.

Classification of knee dislocations is based on the position of the tibia in relation to the femur. In an anterior knee dislocation, the tibia is anterior to the femur, whereas, in a posterior dislocation, the tibia is posterior to the femur. Lateral, medial, and rotational dislocations may also occur. Associated vascular injuries are more common with anterior dislocations, whereas the peroneal nerve is more likely to be injured in posterolateral dislocations.

Diagnosis of dislocation of the knee is based on the patient's history, typical clinical findings, and radiographic findings. If the dislocation has not spontaneously reduced before the patient is examined, the diagnosis is often clear because the deformity can be very impressive. However, spontaneous reduction of knee dislocations is uncommon. When gross dislocation is not detected by physical examination or radiography but there is a history of significant knee injury, a dislocation that has spontaneously reduced may be suspected. A large effusion or hemarthrosis may not develop because large tears in the joint capsule allow the fluid to escape into the soft tissues about the knee.

The initial treatment of a knee dislocation is straightforward but must begin without delay. Reduction is performed using gentle longitudinal traction with the assistance of conscious sedation. After reduction, the neurovascular status of the limb must be carefully monitored.

Many knee dislocations are initially immobilized with splinting or a knee immobilizer, but because the reduced knee is often so unstable, it can be very difficult to maintain reduction without surgical stabilization with an external fixator. Once the patient is hemodynamically stable, it is common to obtain an MRI to assess for ligamentous and soft tissue injury. Surgical repair of torn ligaments and joint capsule is often delayed 7 to 10 days after the initial injury to allow for the soft tissues to recover.

Osteochondritis Dissecans and Osteonecrosis

OSTEOCHONDRITIS DISSECANS

Osteochondritis dissecans (OCD) is a defect in the subchondral region of the apophysis or the epiphysis of a bone, often with partial or complete separation of the bone fragment. When this occurs in the distal femur, it is a common source of loose bodies in the knee. Whereas OCD most often affects the posterolateral aspect of medial femoral condyle, it can also occur in other regions of the knee as well as the shoulder, elbow, and foot.

Etiology of OCD lesions is currently debated. Although trauma is the most likely cause of OCD, a single event is probably not responsible: this would cause a true fracture if the force is large enough. Repetitive overloading is thought to affect the local blood supply, making a region more susceptible to fragmentation and separation. Obesity increases the risk for these lesions because of increased joint loading. Normally, the knee joints are subjected to forces up to six times body weight; thus an additional 30 lb of body weight can add about 180 lb in forces to a joint. After the lesions develop, they can stay in place, or they may separate from the bone and become loose bodies in the joint. Presence of loose bodies can lead to mechanical symptoms in the joint. In treatment, restoration of the articular surface in the weight-bearing region is the most important prognostic factor.

The onset of OCD is frequently insidious, with patients reporting vague complaints, such as intermittent, poorly localized aching. Generally, the pain intensifies with exercise but may persist even at rest. The knee may feel stiff, and floating fragments of bone and cartilage can cause the knee to catch or lock. If a sufficiently large fragment becomes loose in the joint and trapped between the condyle and tibia, the patient may feel a sudden pain and the knee may "give way." These episodes may produce synovial effusions.

Physical Examination. On physical examination, forcible compression of the affected side of the joint can elicit pain and sometimes crepitus. In addition, the joint line on the affected side can be tender on palpation. Often, the physical examination is nonspecific.

Imaging. Radiographs are necessary for diagnosis, and for the knee the notch view (anteroposterior view with the knee flexed 90 degrees), tunnel view (angled posteroanterior projection with the knee flexed at 40 degrees), or lateral view all can be helpful to reveal the defect. MRI is the most helpful imaging modality to evaluate an OCD. It can define the size of the defect, indicate whether it is stable or unstable, and show better if there are any loose bodies in the joint.

Treatment. The goal of treatment is to maintain or reestablish a smooth articular surface and to remove loose fragments. Conservative measures can often be successful early. If the fragment has not separated from the femoral condyle and has an MRI appearance consistent with a stable lesion, the lesion can be considered stable and protected appropriately with activity and weight-bearing modification. Protected weight-bearing is especially important when the defect involves the

Progression of Osteochondritis Dissecans

Circles indicate arthroscopic view.

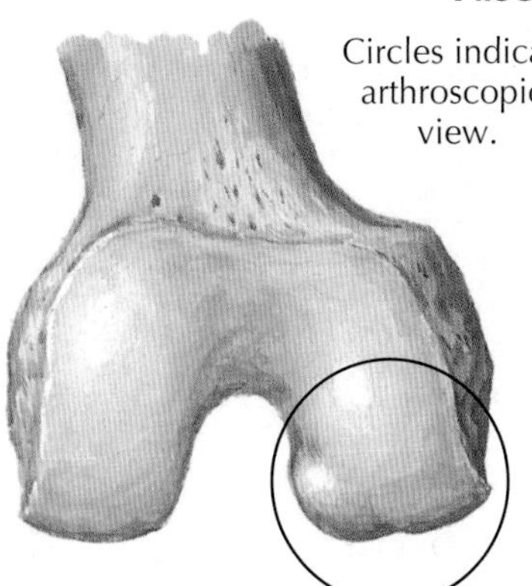

Stage 1. Bulge on medial femoral condyle due to partial separation of bone fragment. Articular cartilage intact, but defect evident on radiographs.

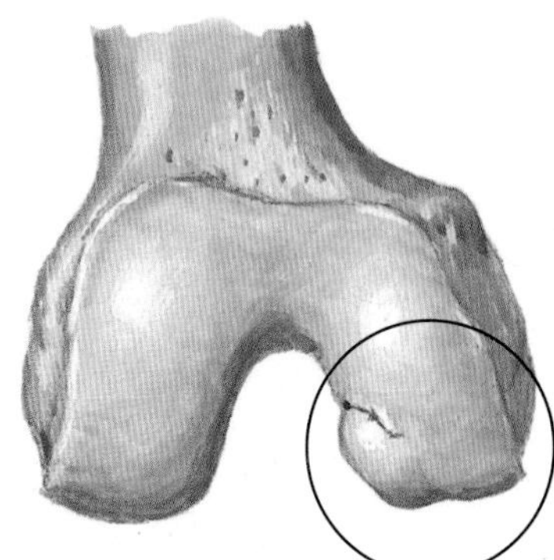

Stage 2. Partial crack.

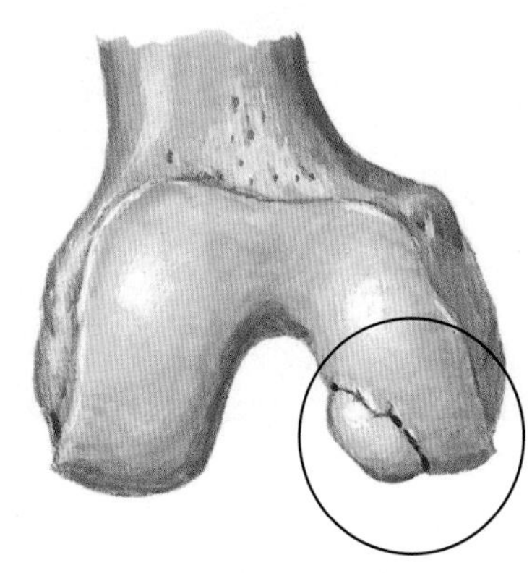

Stage 3. Fragment demarcated by separation of articular cartilage.

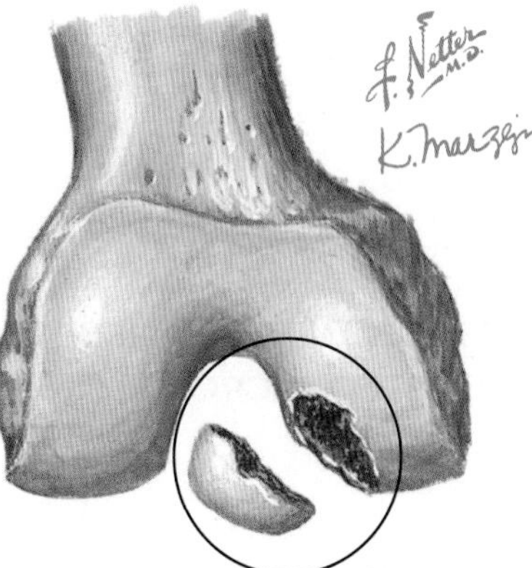

Stage 4. Fragment of cartilage and bone completely separated as loose body. This often migrates to medial or lateral.

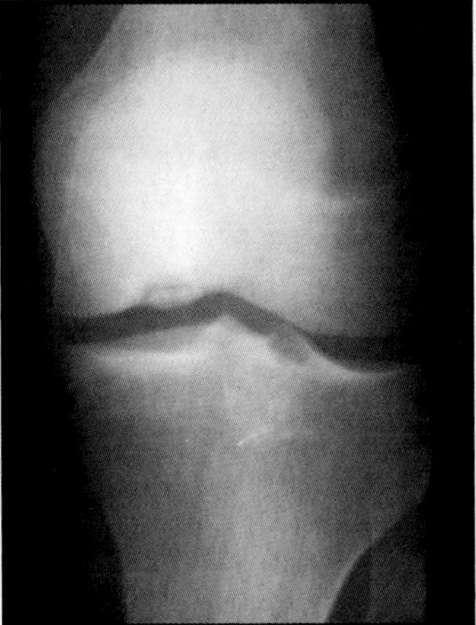

Stage 2 lesion

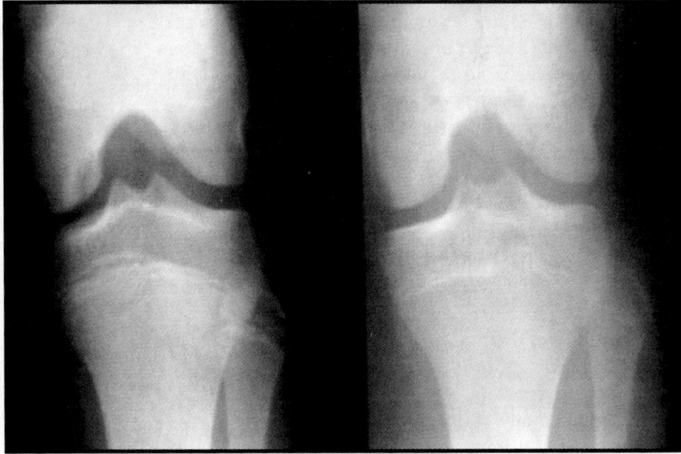

Tunnel-view radiographs of small OCD lesion involving medial femoral condyle treated with activity modification. Complete healing occurred.

Osteonecrosis

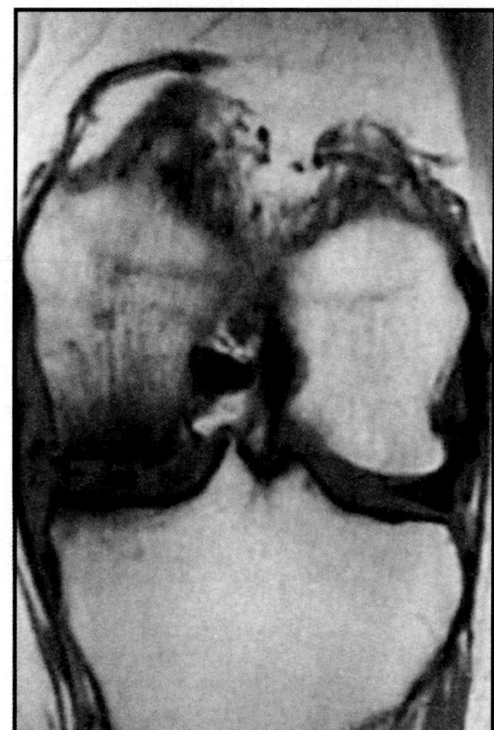

MR image of avascular necrosis (osteonecrosis) of the medial femoral condyle

Osteochondritis Dissecans and Osteonecrosis (Continued)

weight-bearing region of the femur. Immobilization is rarely needed and should be avoided whenever possible, because gentle knee motion is beneficial to the jeopardized region of the articular cartilage.

A loose or detached fragment can be removed with arthroscopy. At the same time, drilling through areas of poorly vascularized bone into regions of good vascularity may induce a vascular healing response. When the fragment represents a large part of the weight-bearing region or appears amenable to reduction, internal fixation with Kirschner wires or screws should be considered. The presence of multiple fragments lessens the chances of obtaining a congruous surface; these fragments should be removed and the base of the lesion drilled.

The prognosis for OCD of the knee depends on the age at which it occurs, the size of the defect, and the extent of the involvement of the weight-bearing regions. Defects that occur in children before the closure of the growth plate frequently heal well with conservative treatment if the fragment has not detached. In fact, many cases may go undetected; when radiographs are taken for other reasons, OCDs can sometimes even be found incidentally. However, a large defect in the weight-bearing surface of the joint in an older patient is at highest risk of developing premature osteoarthritis and a poor outcome. Lesions that occur after closure of the growth plate are less likely to heal.

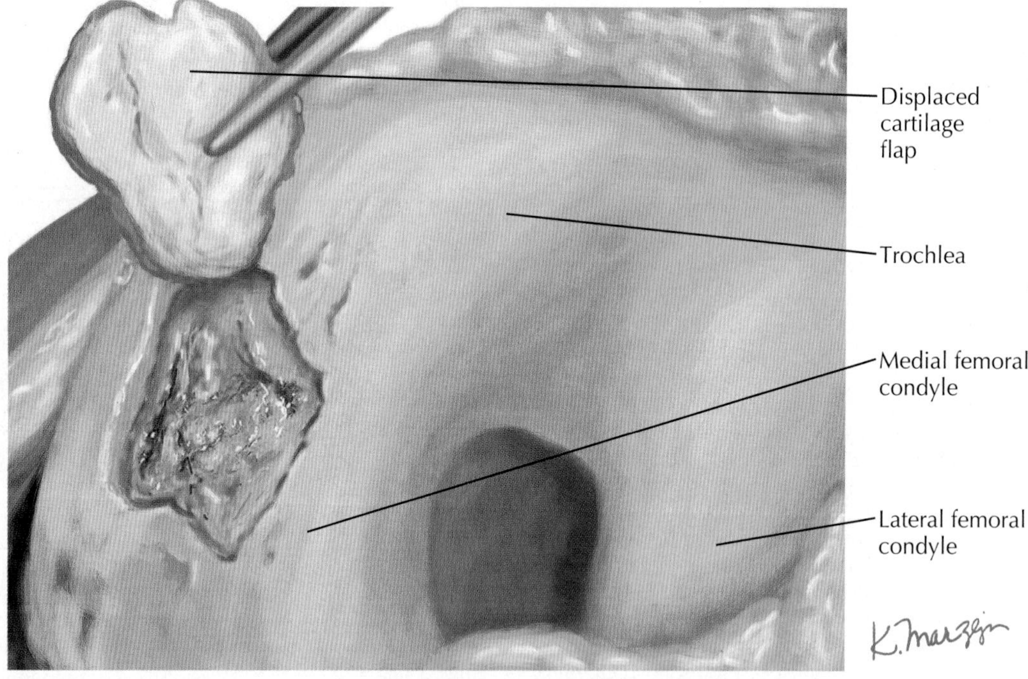

Open view of the knee showing the distal femur affected by osteonecrosis. A necrotic-appearing flap of cartilage is lifted from the diseased medial femoral condyle.

OSTEONECROSIS

Osteonecrosis is a condition where the bone dies in situ, either secondary to loss of blood supply (hence the former name of this condition, avascular necrosis) or from another etiology. This typically occurs in a female patient older than 60 years (the female-to-male ratio is 3:1) and occasionally in a younger patient with predisposing factors, such as long-term corticosteroid therapy, alcohol abuse, or sickle cell anemia. Patients with osteonecrosis can present with acute onset of pain secondary to a subchondral fracture and collapse of the articular surface, or they can present with chronic pain with a story that sounds similar to osteoarthritis. The medial femoral condyle is the most commonly involved knee structure, but osteonecrosis also may occur in the lateral femoral condyle and the tibial plateau (more often medial tibial plateau).

Imaging. Initial plain radiographs may appear normal but eventually show flattening of the articular surface, subchondral radiolucency, and sclerosis of surrounding bone. MRI can be used to depict the involved areas and may be used to detect changes not yet visible in plain radiographs.

Treatment. Smaller lesions (<5 cm^2) typically have a better clinical prognosis and may be satisfactorily treated with activity modification and use of assistive devices such as a cane. Progressive symptoms and failure of nonoperative measures may necessitate drilling of the lesion, realignment osteotomy, or total knee replacement.

Tibial spine (eminence) fracture

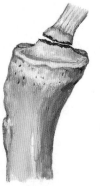

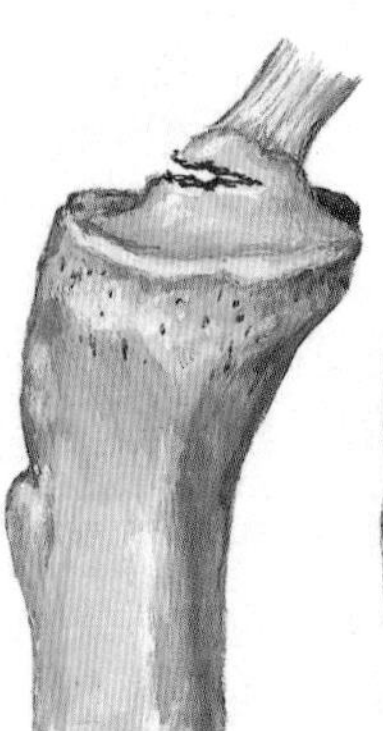

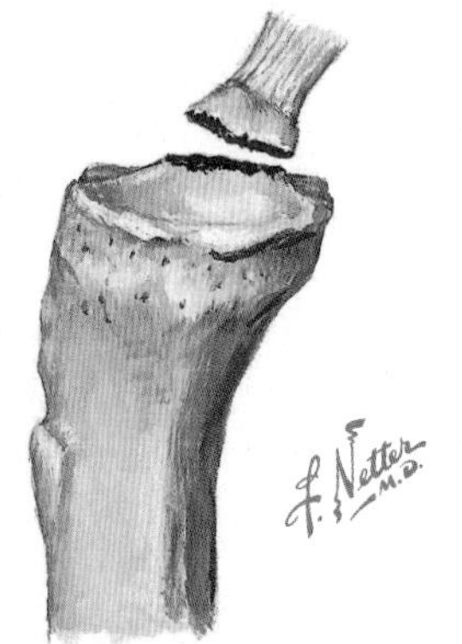

Type I. Incomplete fracture of tibia spine. **Type II.** Complete fracture, nondisplaced. **Type IIIA.** Complete fracture, displaced.

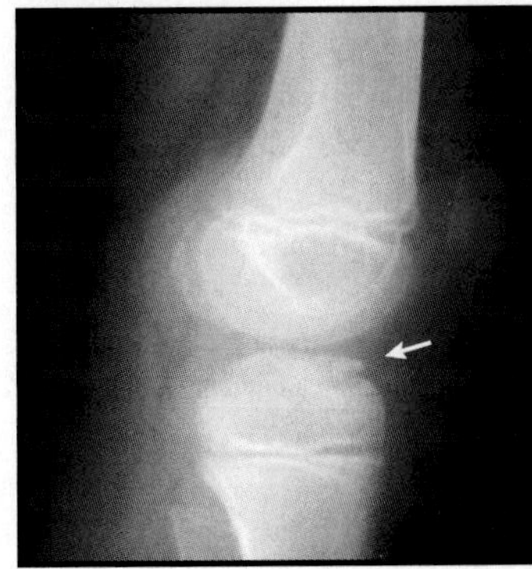

Type I tibial spine fracture

The terms *tibial spine, tibial eminence,* and *intercondylar eminence* are used interchangeably to designate the nonarticular portion of the adjacent medial and lateral tibial plateaus to which the anterior cruciate ligament is attached anteriorly. Injuries that typically cause ruptures of the anterior cruciate ligament in adults often cause a fracture of the tibial spine in children 7 to 14 years of age.

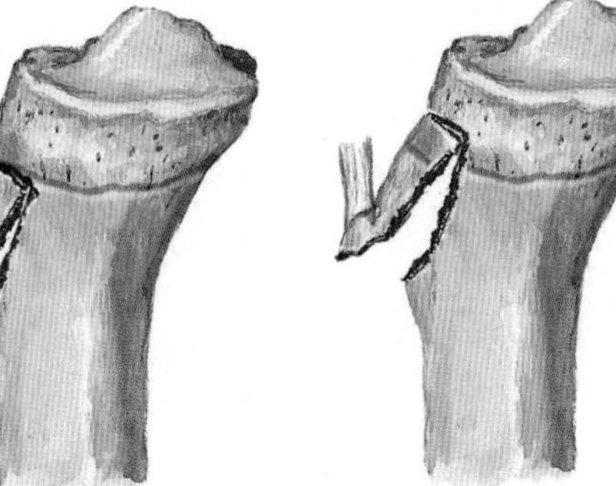

Type I Type II

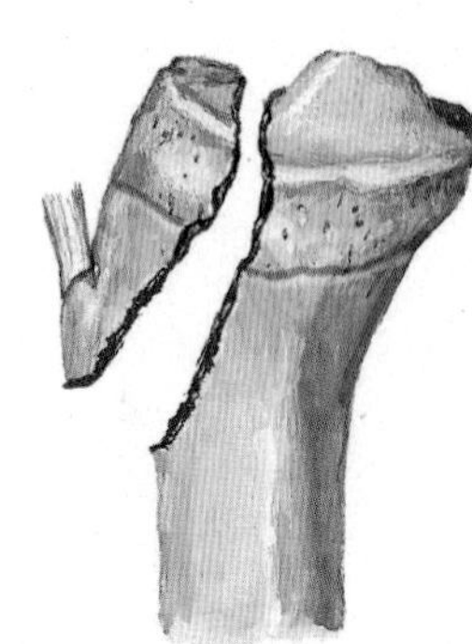

Type IIIA

Fracture of the tibial shaft

A 20-year-old female was an unrestrained passenger in a motor vehicle accident. The patient sustained multiple fractures, including a closed fracture of the right femoral shaft (**A**), an open type IIIA comminuted fracture at the junction of the middle third distal third right tibia and a closed, comminuted fracture of the middle third of the left tibia and fibula, and a comminuted fracture of the right calcaneus. On the date of injury, the patient underwent debridement of the right tibia with application of an external fixator and retrograde nailing of the right femur, and intramedullary nailing of the left tibia. Nine days after injury, intramedullary nailing of the right tibia and open reduction and plating of the right calcaneus were done.

Anteroposterior (**B**) and lateral (**C**) radiographs of the tibia 2 months after intramedullary nailing show good alignment but limited healing of the fracture, which is not unusual in open tibia fractures at this location.

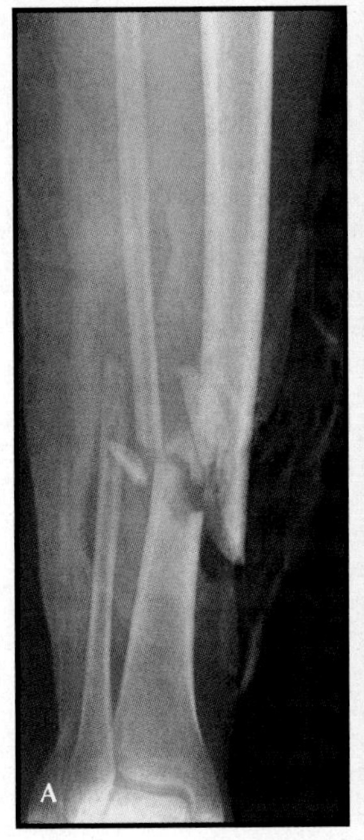

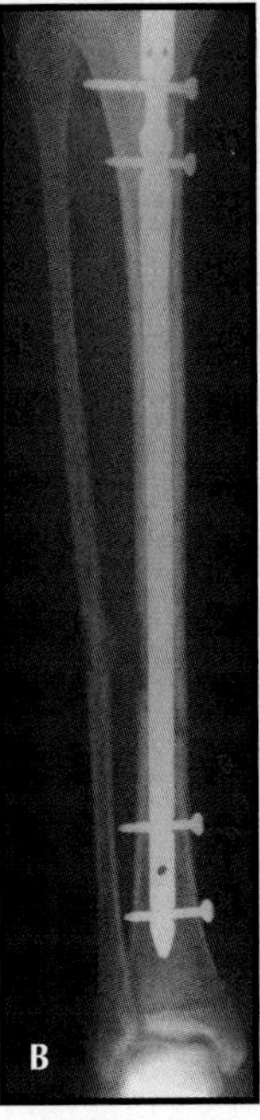

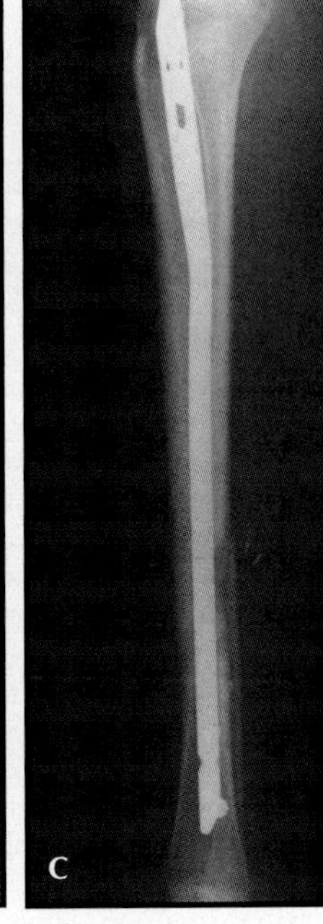

Tibial Intercondylar Eminence Fracture

Fracture of the tibial intercondylar eminence (tibial spine) indicates partial or complete detachment of the ACL from the tibia and is most commonly found in children. This fracture is usually caused by hyperextension of the knee or a sudden twisting motion. Forceful traction resulting from a direct blow to the distal femur on a flexed knee may also result in this fracture. If the fracture is displaced, the loose fragment may block motion and cause severe swelling and hemarthrosis. Type I fracture of the tibial spine is an incomplete fracture, whereas type II is complete but nondisplaced. Type III fractures are described as type IIIA (complete and displaced) and type IIIB (complete, displaced, and rotated out of position).

Type I fractures and type II fractures that reduce anatomically when the knee is in full extension may be treated by casting or rigidly bracing the knee in extension or in 20 degrees of flexion to increase relaxation of the ACL. Union usually occurs in 5 to 6 weeks, after which the patient begins active range-of-motion exercises and rehabilitation of the quadriceps femoris and hamstring muscles.

Surgery is indicated for irreducible type II fractures and all type III fractures. Because this is an intraarticular fracture, anatomic reduction is required for return of knee function. Any mechanical block to full extension is also an indication for surgery. Reduction of the fracture may be blocked if the anterior horn of either meniscus is interposed between the displaced tibial spine and its bed. During surgery, all soft tissue is removed from the fracture site and the tibial spine is replaced in its anatomic position and fixated with sutures or a screw. This can be accomplished arthroscopically or through an open arthrotomy. Because this fracture is most commonly found in the skeletally immature patient, appropriate attention must be paid to open physes during any surgical procedure. Adequate and rigid internal fixation allows the patient to regain motion quickly while the injured knee is protected in a brace. Once adequate fracture healing has occurred, postoperative rehabilitation protocols are similar to those undertaken in patients who have undergone ACL reconstruction.

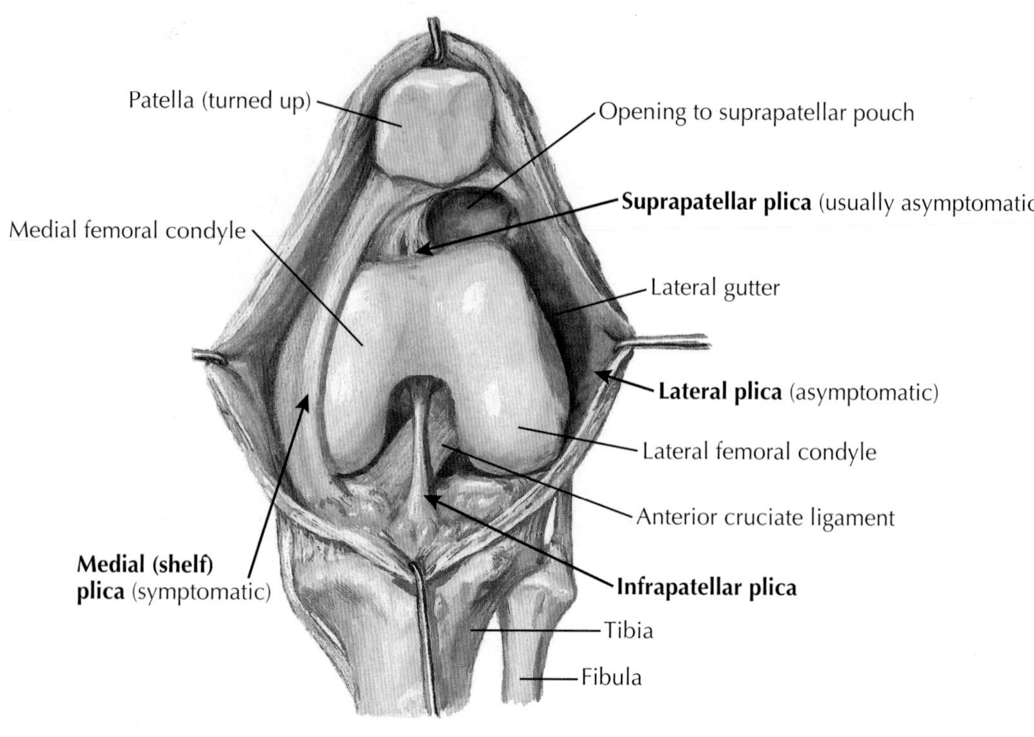

SYNOVIAL PLICA, BURSITIS, AND ILIOTIBIAL BAND FRICTION SYNDROME

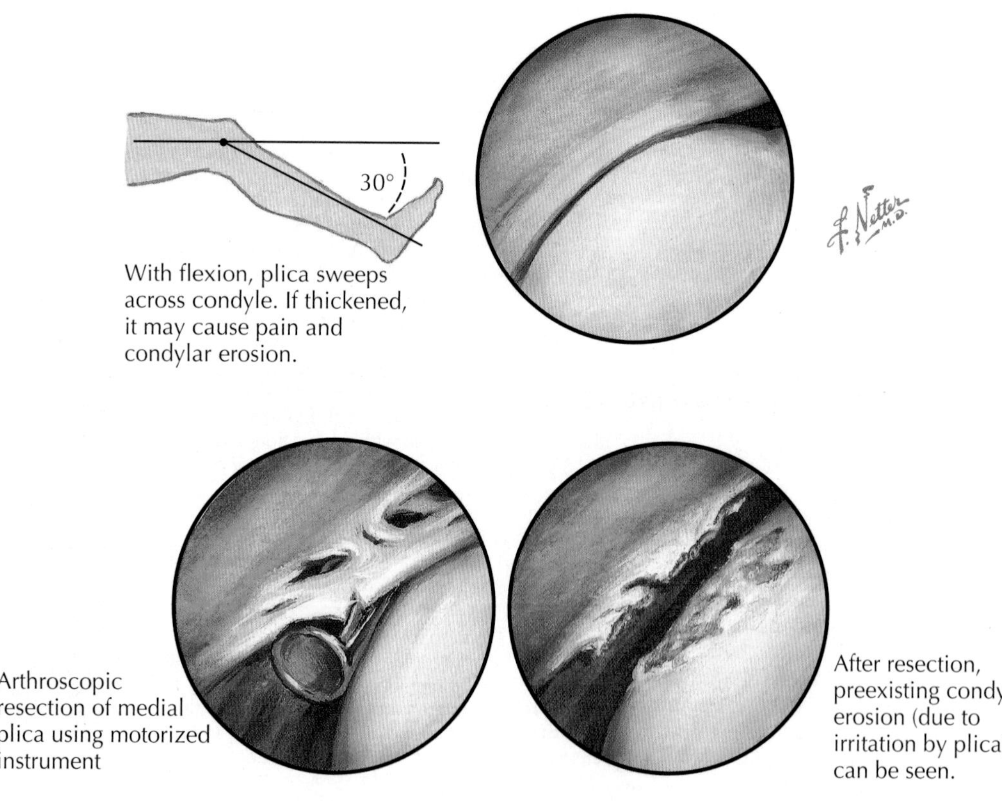

With flexion, plica sweeps across condyle. If thickened, it may cause pain and condylar erosion.

Arthroscopic resection of medial plica using motorized instrument

After resection, preexisting condylar erosion (due to irritation by plica) can be seen.

SYNOVIAL PLICA

Synovial plicae are folds of embryonic remnants of the synovial membrane. In the fetus, thin synovial membranes divide the knee joint into three compartments (medial, lateral, and patellar). In the fifth month of fetal development, these partitions usually degenerate and the knee joint becomes one space. Incomplete degeneration of one or more of the membranes can result in the formation of a plica. Most synovial folds contain a considerable amount of elastin and areolar tissue and are thus extensible and asymptomatic. Many are identified during routine arthroscopic procedures performed for other reasons.

Plicae can be found anywhere in the knee joint, but the most common location is over the medial femoral condyle. Folds in this location are called medial, or shelf, plicae. This is the area most susceptible to trauma and subsequent irritation. When the knee is extended, the patella protects the anterior aspect of the femoral condyles, but when the knee is flexed, the medial condyle is more vulnerable. Multiple traumatic events, even minor ones, that involve the condyle, repeated flexion-extension activities, or direct contusions can lead to inflammation of the plica with subsequent thickening. The thickened plica may cause local irritation and erosion of the underlying hyaline cartilage on the condyle. The symptoms of a pathologic plica may mimic those of a torn meniscus. Patients may complain of mechanical symptoms (snapping or clicking), along with pain along the medial joint line.

Physical Examination and Special Tests.

- *Plica tests:* The patient is supine and relaxed. With the tibia internally rotated, the examiner passively flexes and extends the knee from 30 to 100 degrees of flexion. Examining fingers placed along the medial patellofemoral joint may feel a click, some tenderness, or a pop of a pathologic plica.

Imaging. MRI can sometimes identify a pathologic plica, but its sensitivity is poor.

Treatment. Initially, symptomatic plicae should be managed with rest from activities that irritate the knee, use of nonsteroidal antiinflammatory drugs (NSAIDs), and application of ice. In patients whose knees do not improve with nonoperative treatment, arthroscopic excision can be effective. If plicae are an incidental finding on arthroscopy, it is up to the surgeon to determine whether excision would be beneficial based on the patient's preoperative symptoms.

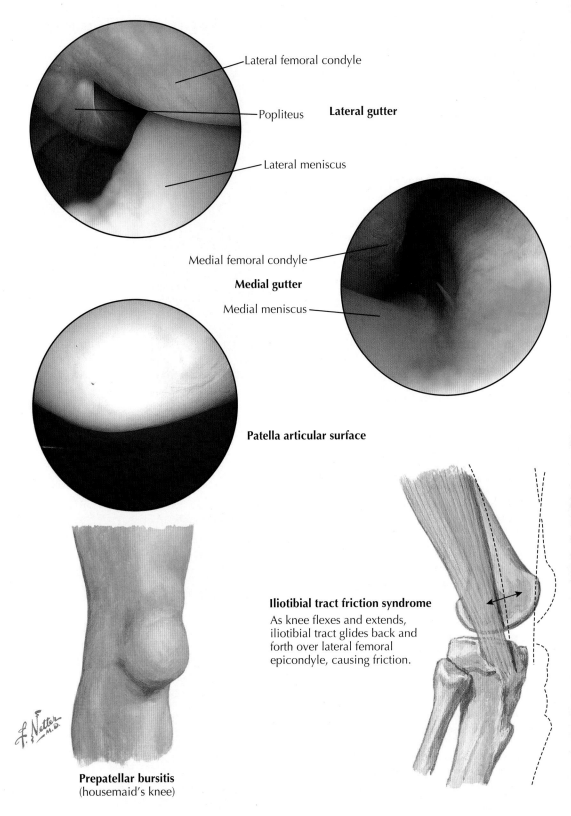

Lateral femoral condyle

Popliteus

Lateral gutter

Lateral meniscus

Medial femoral condyle

Medial gutter

Medial meniscus

Patella articular surface

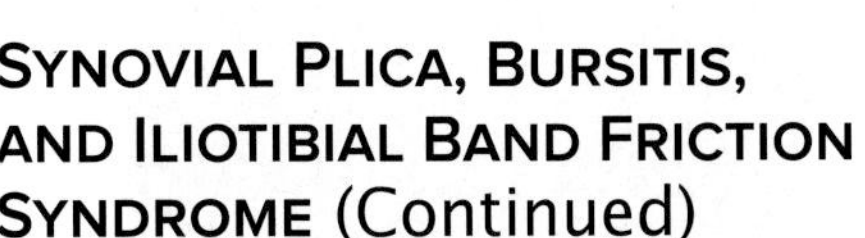

SYNOVIAL PLICA, BURSITIS, AND ILIOTIBIAL BAND FRICTION SYNDROME (Continued)

Iliotibial tract friction syndrome
As knee flexes and extends, iliotibial tract glides back and forth over lateral femoral epicondyle, causing friction.

Prepatellar bursitis
(housemaid's knee)

BURSITIS

Inflammation may occur at any of the many bursae around the knee, usually evidenced by swelling and pain. Typically, the prepatellar bursa, pes anserinus bursa, tibial collateral ligament bursa, and deep infrapatellar bursa are involved. This is usually the result of overuse but may be caused by a direct blow with bleeding into a bursa. Septic bursitis with entrance of infectious organism may also be encountered and may present as other systemic signs of infection. Careful physical examination and routine laboratory studies, such as a white blood cell count and evaluation of inflammatory markers, are both important parts of the assessment of a patient with an acute presentation of bursitis. It is also important to distinguish septic bursitis, or infection of the bursa, from septic arthritis, an infection in the knee joint itself.

Treatment. In acute cases of aseptic bursitis, improvement is commonly seen with rest, compression, ice, and padding or protection of the involved area. Short-term immobilization may also be used for a patient with an acutely inflamed knee to prevent further irritation or stress on the bursa by excessive range of motion or further trauma to the area. Aspiration of bursae should be avoided, even when suspecting septic bursitis, as bursae tend to continue to drain, and this drainage can be difficult to stop. NSAIDs are commonly used for pain relief and to reduce inflammation. In chronic cases that have failed, nonoperative treatment or in cases of acute suppurative infection, surgical bursectomy can be discussed with the patient. In the case of septic bursitis, nonoperative medical management with antibiotics (at least initially intravenous; sometimes can be transitioned to oral depending on the recommendations of infectious disease specialists) is often effective.

ILIOTIBIAL BAND FRICTION SYNDROME

This is a chronic inflammatory process involving the soft tissues adjacent to the lateral femoral epicondyle, presumably caused by chronic "friction" of iliotibial band rubbing over a bony prominence of this area. Runners are commonly affected by this overuse-type syndrome. The patient may present with lateral knee pain on activity, tightness of the iliotibial band, and occasionally popping.

Treatment. Initial treatment options include iliotibial band stretching exercises, antiinflammatory agents, and corticosteroid injection. Physical therapy protocols, particularly those including stretching regimens, are routinely used for symptomatic patients. Rarely, in refractory cases, surgery can be done to release an area of tightness or debride any focal areas of inflammation.

Pigmented Villonodular Synovitis and Meniscal Cysts

PIGMENTED VILLONODULAR SYNOVITIS

This diffuse or localized lesion develops in synovial tissue and involves the joints, bursae, and tendon sheaths. Its etiology is currently not well understood.

Diffuse Villonodular Synovitis

This condition typically occurs in adults between 20 and 40 years of age. A single joint of the lower limb, most frequently the knee, is the most common site of involvement. The synovial membrane becomes thickened and diffusely covered with long, tangled, reddish and yellow-brown villi, which may mat together to form plaques. Later, both sessile and pedunculated rubbery nodules appear. Hemosiderin-bearing stromal cells, lipid-bearing foam cells, and multinucleated giant cells are seen on microscopic examination.

Late in the disease, the pathologic changes may cause pressure indentation of bone and sometimes actual invasion of bone at the articular margins with subsequent bone destruction.

The predominant symptom is a chronic, slowly increasing swelling of the joint that is associated with mild aching. Acute episodes of pain with increased joint swelling may occur intermittently and are attributed to pinching of villi between the joint surfaces, with subsequent hemorrhage. Because the course of the disease is usually relatively benign, diagnosis and treatment are often delayed. Examination of a palpable joint often shows a diffuse, slightly warm and tender, boggy swelling. A valuable diagnostic finding is the aspiration of bloody, brown, or serosanguineous fluid from a chronically swollen, *uninjured* joint.

MRI is the most beneficial diagnostic imaging modality. Late in the disease, superficial erosions of cortical bone near the joint margin and irregular areas of bone destruction may be present.

Surgical treatment options range from arthroscopic synovectomy for more mild or inactive forms to complete open synovectomy for active diffuse forms. If the entire synovial membrane cannot be excised, localized disease can recur and radiation therapy may be indicated. If bone destruction is present, a total joint arthroplasty may be indicated depending on the degree of destruction and the patient's symptom level.

Localized Villonodular Synovitis

This more common form of synovitis occurs in small joints, bursae, and tendon sheaths. The characteristic lesion is a sessile or pedunculated, yellow to reddish brown nodule with localized villous proliferation around its base. Symptoms are mild, consisting of intermittent swelling and aching. Slight swelling and a localized nodule may be noted on examination. The tenosynovitis type, also called a xanthomatous giant cell tumor of the tendon sheath, is the most common manifestation of localized villonodular synovitis, occurring primarily in the hand or foot, where it presents as a discrete, firm, slowly enlarging nodule.

Treatment is complete excision of the nodular lesions in joints, tendon sheaths, and bursae.

Pigmented villonodular synovitis

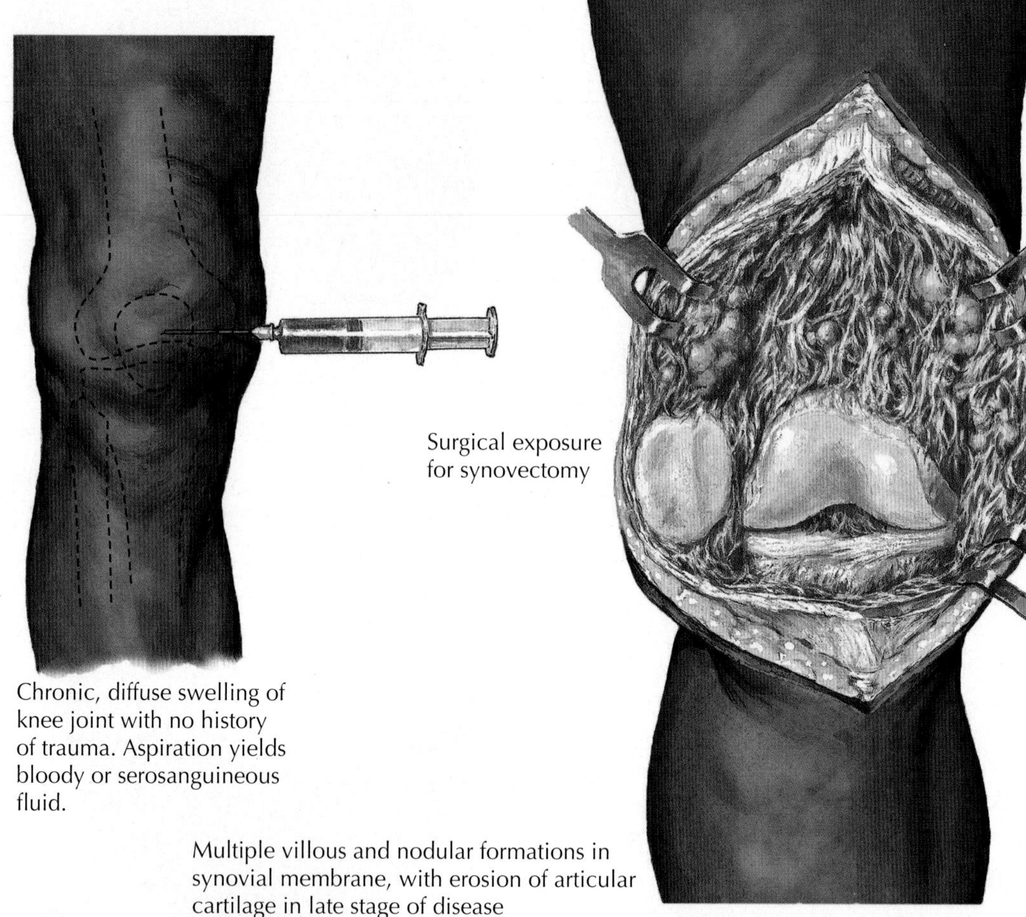

Chronic, diffuse swelling of knee joint with no history of trauma. Aspiration yields bloody or serosanguineous fluid.

Multiple villous and nodular formations in synovial membrane, with erosion of articular cartilage in late stage of disease

Meniscal cysts

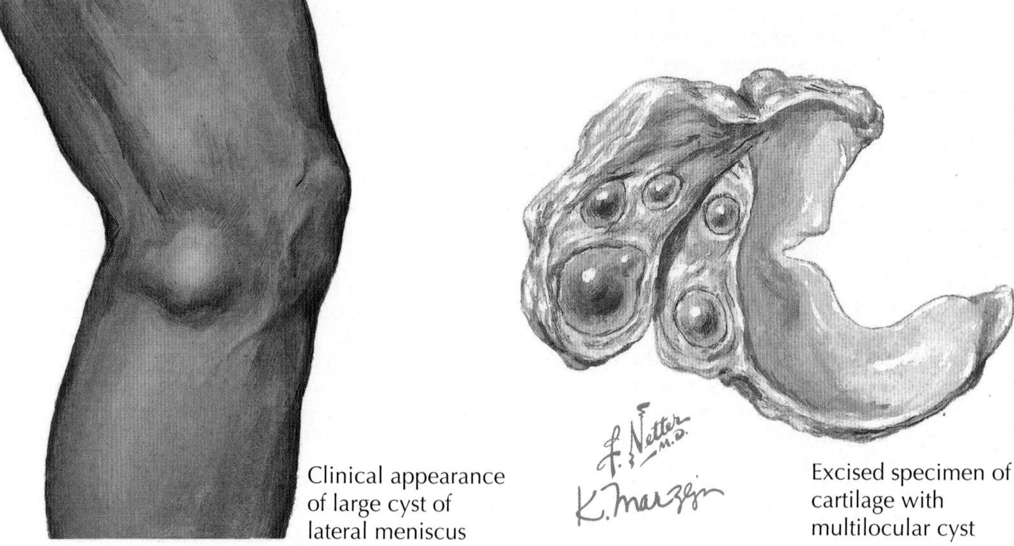

Clinical appearance of large cyst of lateral meniscus

Excised specimen of cartilage with multilocular cyst

MENISCAL CYSTS

Cysts of the meniscus of the knee are one of the most frequent causes of swelling at the lateral or medial joint line. The lateral meniscus is involved much more frequently than the medial meniscus. Although the etiology of these cysts is unknown, they may be due to trauma that causes cystic or mucoid degeneration in fibrocartilage and fibrous tissue and are often associated with tears of the meniscus. Patients vary in age from adolescence to middle age.

The cysts normally develop in the peripheral aspect of the middle third of the meniscus and in the adjacent soft tissues within the joint capsule. Usually multilocular and lined with endothelium, they contain a clear, gelatinous material.

Persistent aching in the cyst area is the main symptom. Examination reveals a tenderness to palpation of the joint line. Arthroscopic examination and decompression of the cyst and treatment of any concomitant meniscal pathology are indicated if pain and disability are significant.

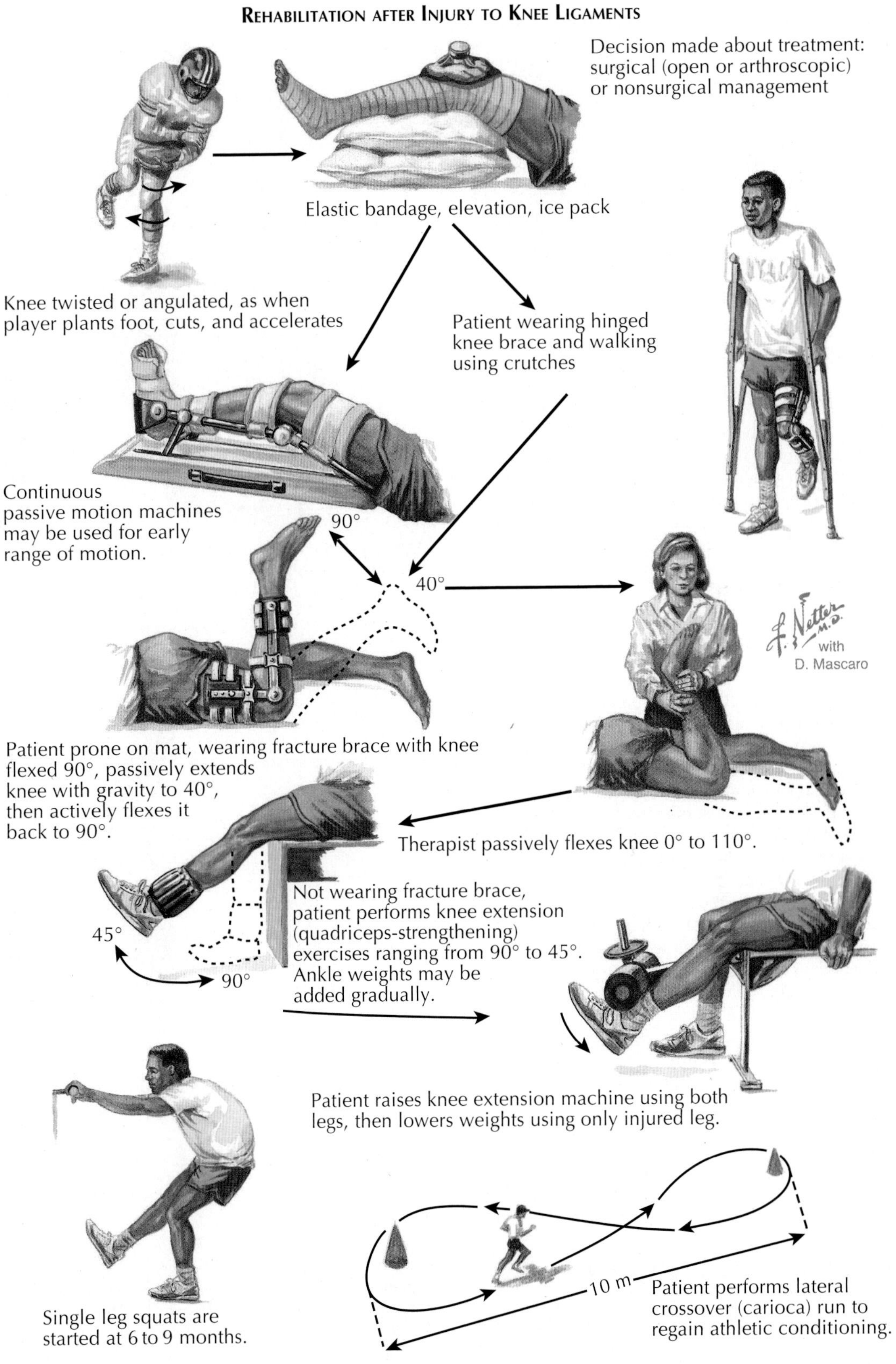

Rehabilitation After Sports Injury

The goal of nonoperative management of ligamentous injuries of the knee is to stabilize the action of the knee with the remaining uninjured, supportive structures. Rehabilitation must begin as soon as possible after injury, because disuse atrophy of the muscles occurs rapidly. Rehabilitation focuses on muscle strengthening and flexibility.

After initial injury, the knee's range of motion can sometimes be intentionally limited during exercises to 30 and 90 degrees, avoiding full extension, to decrease stress through the joint. Resistance is applied in the pain-free portion of the range of motion, with the tibia internally and externally rotated to strengthen the hamstring muscles. The exercises can be done with the patient prone or standing.

Isokinetic resistance is also initiated, starting at slow speeds and gradually increasing. Isotonic, isometric, or isokinetic extension of the knee may also be initiated. The knee should remain pain free through the entire arc of motion. End-arc discomfort may occur. Extension exercises are begun with the starting position at less than 90 degrees of flexion and termination at less than full extension. Hip flexion and abduction exercises can be isometric or isotonic. Double-foot raises (raising both heels off the floor simultaneously) in sets of 50, done with the knee slightly bent, strengthen the gastrocnemius muscles that help stabilize the knee.

Endurance training should be added to initiate cardiovascular conditioning. Use of a stationary bicycle, with the resistance set at zero, is effective and improves the range of motion in the knee. Once the knee is pain free, the resistance can be increased for further cardiovascular benefits.

Postoperative rehabilitation after surgical reconstruction of knee ligaments consists of a progressive program that is conducted in stages. Immediately after surgery, the knee can sometimes be placed in a hinged brace to allow controlled motion. For complex procedures, sometimes a continuous passive motion (CPM) machine is used to keep the knee moving constantly and facilitate recovery. Although there is no definitive evidence of the long-term improvements in outcome using CPM, the theory is that it will increase mobilization, decrease pain, reduce swelling, prevent adhesions, improve proprioceptive function, and allow for a more rapid return of joint range of motion.

The patient is then taught to use crutches to protect weight-bearing on the affected side. This protected weight-bearing is continued until the surgeon is confident that the ligaments have healed, after which the patient can progress to weight-bearing as tolerated. During the healing phase, passive range-of-motion exercises should occur, with extension being passively assisted by gravity pulling the leg toward an exercise mat and limited by the extension stop of the brace. Active flexion exercises can be started as the patient continues to recover with the patient using the hamstring muscles. Straight-leg raises, flexion-to-extension exercises within the safe range of limited motion, co-contractions, hip flexion exercises, and leg curls are also started in a progressive fashion to maintain muscle tone and strength. The amount of resistance and the number of sets or repetitions are gradually increased as tolerated.

Usually, the brace can be discontinued within 3 months after surgery, and the program for strengthening knee flexion and extension accelerated. By 6 to 7 months postoperatively, patients are often close to returning to full activity, but this may take longer if the knee required multiple ligaments to be reconstructed or repaired. Swimming and doing exercises in a pool are often encouraged after the surgical wounds have completely healed to increase strength and endurance.

Rehabilitation after Injury to Knee Ligaments
Decision made about treatment: surgical (open or arthroscopic) or nonsurgical management
Elastic bandage, elevation, ice pack
Knee twisted or angulated, as when player plants foot, cuts, and accelerates
Patient wearing hinged knee brace and walking using crutches
Continuous passive motion machines may be used for early range of motion.
90°
40°
F. Netter M.D. with D. Mascaro
Patient prone on mat, wearing fracture brace with knee flexed 90°, passively extends knee with gravity to 40°, then actively flexes it back to 90°.
Therapist passively flexes knee 0° to 110°.
45°
90°
Not wearing fracture brace, patient performs knee extension (quadriceps-strengthening) exercises ranging from 90° to 45°. Ankle weights may be added gradually.
Patient raises knee extension machine using both legs, then lowers weights using only injured leg.
Single leg squats are started at 6 to 9 months.
10 m
Patient performs lateral crossover (carioca) run to regain athletic conditioning.

Disorders of the Patella

BIPARTITE PATELLA

Congenital fragmentation of the patella is relatively common. One type, bipartite patella, occurs in 1% to 2% of the population. This anatomic variant represents a true synchondrosis (a joint whose surfaces are connected by a cartilaginous plate). Most fragmented patellae remain asymptomatic, but, occasionally, direct trauma to the patella disrupts the synchondroses, causing symptoms that mimic those of a fracture.

A true fracture is differentiated from congenital bipartite patella based on a history of significant trauma to the patella, hemarthrosis of the knee, point tenderness over the defect, and a sharply outlined fragment seen on the radiograph. If the diagnosis is still uncertain, CT or MRI can be used to differentiate an acute fracture from a congenital condition.

Asymptomatic bipartite patellae do not require any treatment. In symptomatic cases, conservative treatment, including a period of immobilization followed by stretching and strengthening exercises for the quadriceps and hamstring muscles, is usually sufficient. If the fragment remains symptomatic, it can be excised along with a lateral retinacular release.

Bipartite Patella and Baker Cyst

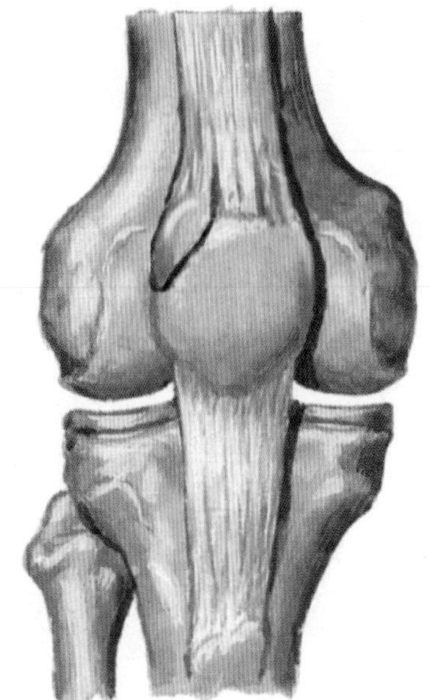

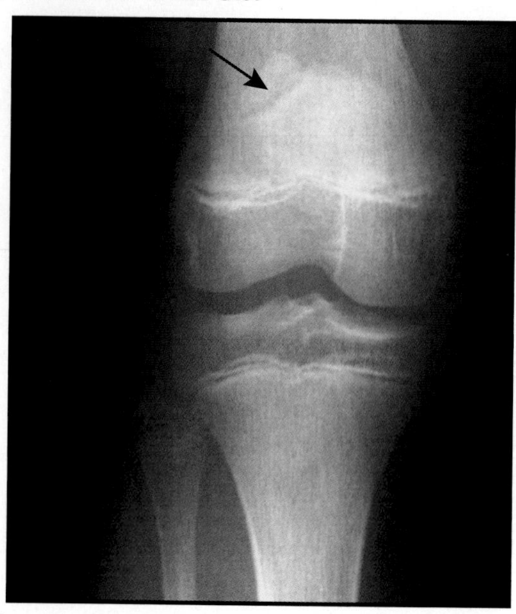

Anteroposterior radiograph of knee in a 1-year-old boy who presented with pain at superolateral aspect of patella after a fall. Radiographs show bipartite patella. Patient treated with 4 weeks of immobilization for suspected quadriceps strain/slight avulsion of bipartite fragment. Symptoms resolved and patient resumed full activity.

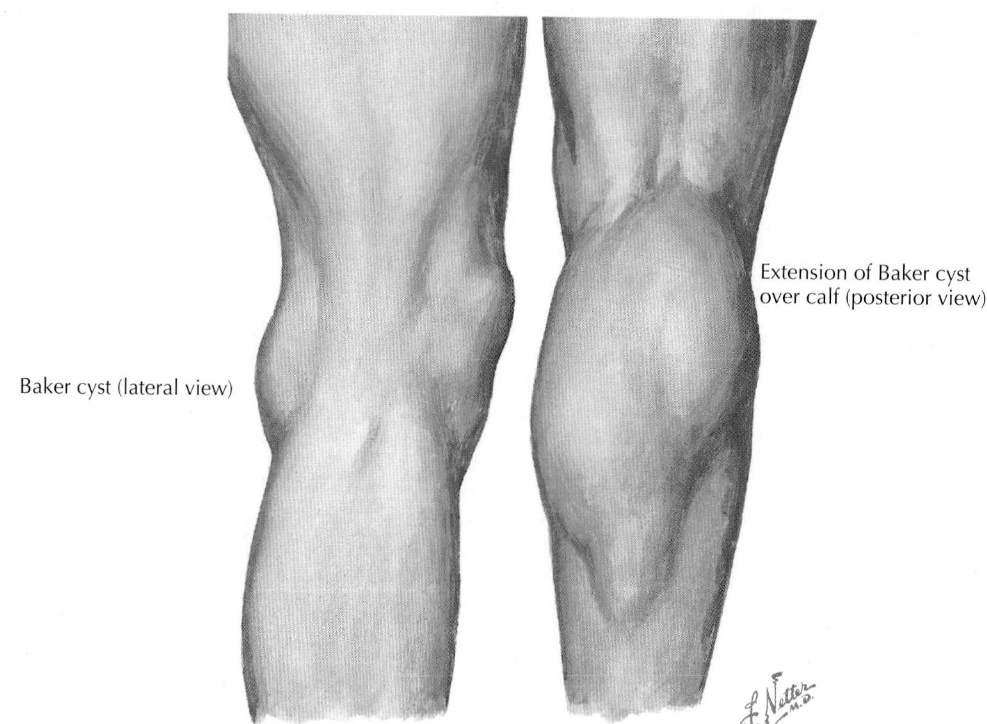

PATELLA ALTA AND INFERA

Patella alta refers to an abnormally high patella in relation to the femur. Patella alta predisposes to patellar subluxation and dislocation with resultant repetitive microtrauma and inflammation of the patellofemoral joint (patellofemoral chondrosis).

Patella infera indicates an abnormally low patella. Although it occurs most often secondary to soft tissue contracture and hypotonia of the quadriceps muscle after surgery or trauma to the knee, it may also represent a congenital variant.

Imaging. The position of the patella can best be determined on the lateral radiograph with the knee flexed 30 degrees. The Insall-Salvati ratio describes that the length of the patellar ligament is usually equal to the diagonal length of the patella. Variations of more than 20% are considered abnormal.

Treatment. Congenital patella infera is frequently asymptomatic and requires no treatment. If this condition develops after injury or surgery, it can be catastrophic. Prompt recognition of the condition is of utmost importance because treatment in the early stages can reverse it. Vigorous rehabilitation of the quadriceps muscles and mobilization of soft tissue structures around the knee should be instituted as soon as the complication is recognized.

SUBLUXATION AND DISLOCATION OF PATELLA

The patella depends on both dynamic and static stabilizers to maintain its proper position in the intercondylar groove. Although the entire quadriceps muscle contributes to the dynamic stability of the patella, the contribution of the vastus medialis muscle is critical. The distal oblique portion of this muscle resists lateral migration of the patella. The static patellar restraints, which include the bony contour of the distal femur, the joint capsule, the medial and lateral retinacula, and the medial patellofemoral ligament (MPFL), are equally important. A flat lateral femoral condyle ("tabletop" femur) allows the patella to slide laterally quite easily, whereas a deep intercondylar groove generally keeps the triangular-shaped patella well located. A large Q angle seems to increase the patient's susceptibility to subluxation or dislocation of the patella. The Q angle is formed by the intersection of two lines drawn from the anterior superior iliac spine and the tibial tuberosity through the center of the patella. This condition is also often associated with knock-knee and external tibial torsion and is most commonly symptomatic in adolescent girls and young women.

Patellar subluxation is the partial loss of contact between the articular surfaces of the patella and femur. It is most common when the ligamentous support is loose and when the vastus medialis muscles are poorly developed or atrophied. Just a weak medial quadriceps muscle permits lateral subluxation, and tightness in the lateral peripatellar tissues can pull the patella laterally.

Patellar dislocation is the complete loss of contact between the articular surfaces of the patella and femur. Congenital dislocations are rare and when present tend to be bilateral and familial. The majority of dislocations are traumatic. Underdeveloped femoral condyles, insufficient soft tissue restraints, and a weak vastus medialis muscle all predispose to patellar dislocation.

Physical Examination. Patients complain of anterior knee pain, particularly when climbing stairs, and giving way of the knee. Physical examination reveals tenderness along the medial aspect of the patella, patellofemoral crepitus, atrophy of the quadriceps femoris muscle (especially the oblique portion of the vastus medialis), and increased lateral mobility of the patella. On physical

DISORDERS OF THE PATELLA (Continued)

SUBLUXATION AND DISLOCATION OF PATELLA

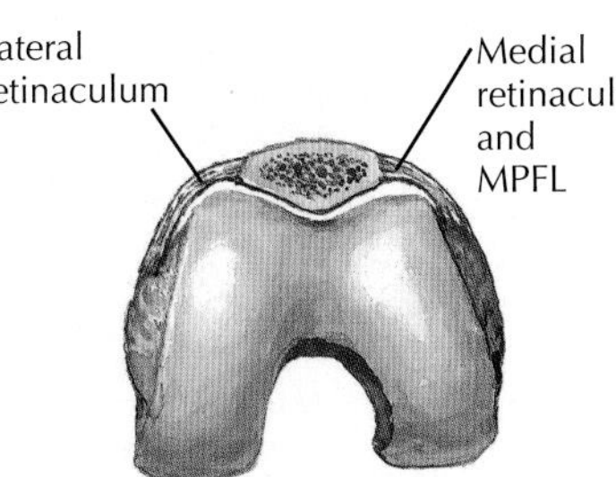

Skyline view. Normally, patella rides in groove between medial and lateral femoral condyles.

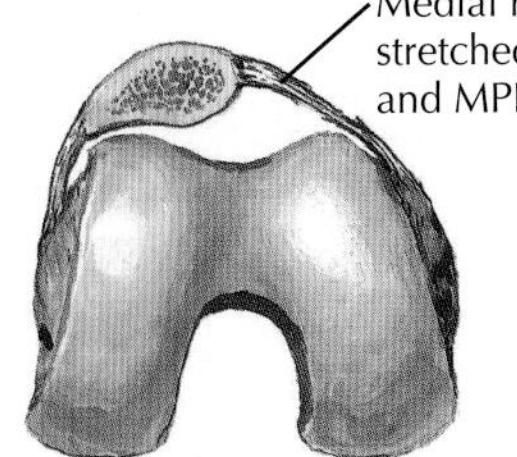

In subluxation, patella deviates laterally because of weakness of vastus medialis muscle, tightness of lateral retinaculum, and high Q angle.

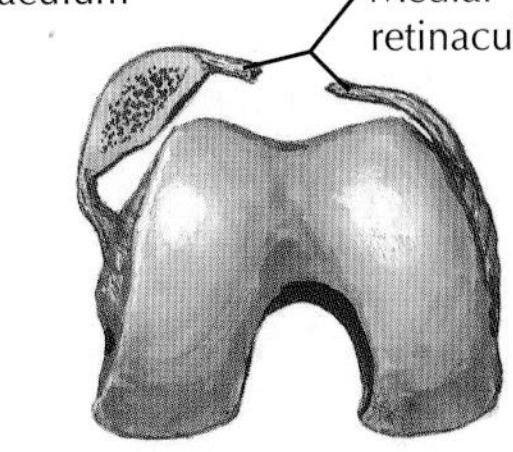

In dislocation, patella displaced completely out of intercondylar groove.

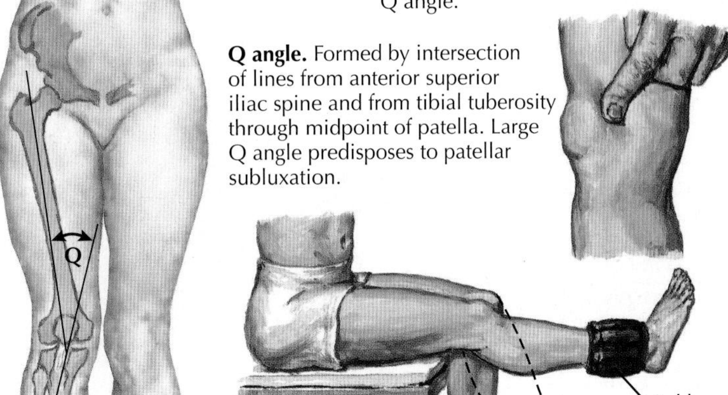

Q angle. Formed by intersection of lines from anterior superior iliac spine and from tibial tuberosity through midpoint of patella. Large Q angle predisposes to patellar subluxation.

Apprehension test. Displace patella laterally and move the knee into flexion. Unstable patella will displace laterally and pain (apprehension) is noted at approximately 20 to 40 degrees of flexion when the patella is compressed against the edge of the lateral condyle.

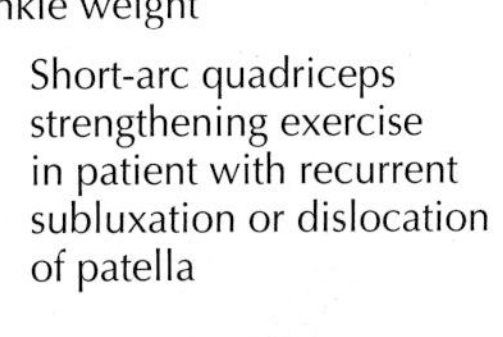

Short-arc quadriceps strengthening exercise in patient with recurrent subluxation or dislocation of patella

Surgical procedures for recurrent patellar subluxation or dislocation

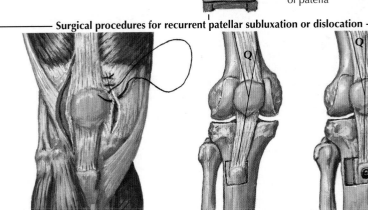

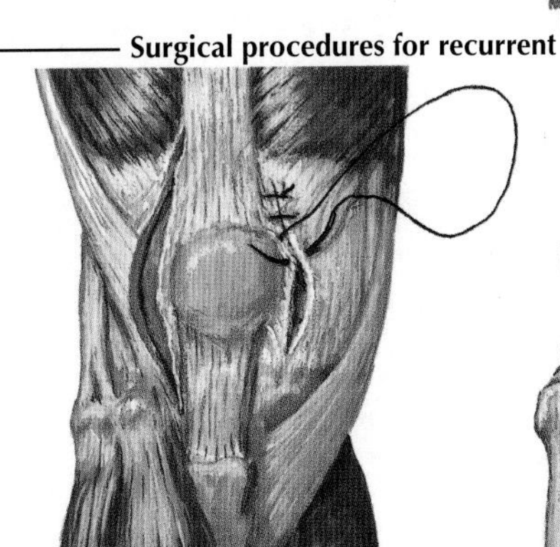

Lateral release. Lateral retinaculum incised, decreasing lateral pull on patella. Torn medial retinaculum sutured or tightened by plication.

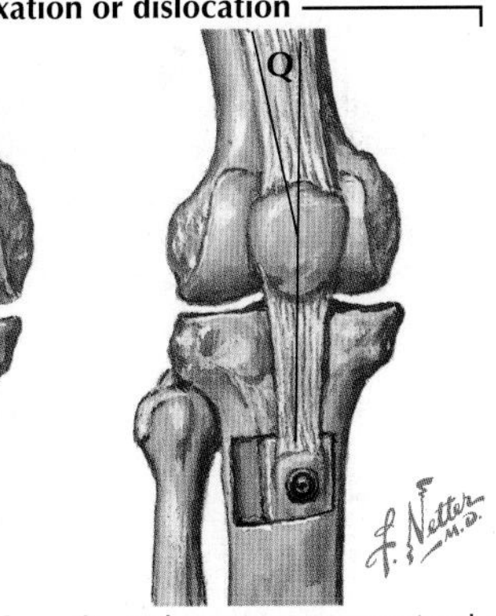

Transfer of tibial tuberosity. Tuberosity osteotomized along with attached patellar ligament. Tuberosity shifted to more medial position and fixed with screw, reducing Q angle.

examination, the patella can normally be manually displaced both medially and laterally between 25% and 50% of the width of the patella. Greater movement indicates loose patellar restraints, a finding frequently seen in adolescent females. A positive apprehension test may be elicited when the patient forcefully contracts the quadriceps femoris muscle and feels pain as the examiner attempts to displace the patella laterally. If the subluxation is not treated, the lateral retinaculum gradually becomes contracted, exacerbating the abnormal patellofemoral tracking.

Imaging. In addition to traditional anteroposterior and lateral plain radiographs, it can be beneficial to obtain an infrapatellar view with the knee flexed 30 to 45 degrees rather than the traditional "sunrise" or "skyline" view with the knee flexed beyond 90 degrees. To assess the soft tissue attachments and stabilizers and bony anatomy the surgeon may choose to obtain MRI and CT scans, respectively.

Persons at risk for patellar instability may often exhibit generalized ligamentous laxity and a poorly developed vastus medialis muscle. When these patients are sitting or standing erect in a relaxed position, the patellae often face laterally ("owl-eye" patellae). At full extension, the patella may also deviate laterally outside of the groove (J sign).

Rupture of the MPFL after lateral dislocation of the patella causes pain and tenderness along the medial retinaculum. Sometimes, the vastus medialis muscle is avulsed from the medial intermuscular septum, causing pain in the medial region of the knee. However, patellar dislocation should not be confused with a sprain of the MCL. After an acute dislocation of the patella, gentle manual lateral subluxation of the patella produces discomfort, a finding not seen with injury to the MCL.

CHONDROMALACIA PATELLAE

The term *chondromalacia* describes the softening and fissuring of the articular hyaline cartilage and frequently refers to the undersurface of the patella. Chondromalacia may result from an excessive load on the patellofemoral joint, but disuse may be a contributing factor.

In clinical practice, chondromalacia is used to describe inflammation of the articular surface of the patellofemoral joint (patellofemoral chondrosis) or degeneration of this joint (patellofemoral arthrosis). Patellofemoral chondrosis is most common in young women. Contributing factors include weakness and tightness in the quadriceps muscle, abnormalities of lower limb alignment (knock-knee, bowleg, an abnormally positioned patella), and obesity. Patellofemoral arthrosis usually occurs with aging. Patients affected by this will often report pain in the anterior knee while climbing stairs or sitting for long periods.

Physical Examination. On examination, compression of the patella may cause pain along the medial and lateral retinacula and the patellar ligament. Compression of the patella during flexion and extension of the knee usually elicits crepitation and discomfort; swelling may also be present. MRI may also reveal chondral changes along the undersurface of the patella.

Treatment. Strenuous and pain-provoking activities should be reduced until symptoms subside. Exercises to stretch and strengthen the quadriceps muscle, especially the vastus medialis muscle, should be initiated immediately. In refractory cases, patients may also benefit from arthroscopic shaving of loose articular fragments or lateral release of the patella, or both. Although removal of the degenerated tissue usually does little to alleviate the symptoms or to improve the long-term prognosis, it can decrease crepitation and synovial effusion. A lateral release may relieve excess patellofemoral contact pressure or denervate a sensitive region.

PATELLA OVERLOAD SYNDROME

Patella overload syndrome is a common and painful condition seen in rapidly growing adolescents whose bones appear to be growing faster than the attached soft tissues. This rapid growth results in tightness of the quadriceps and hamstring muscles, which can increase the compression forces between the patella and femur during knee flexion, causing irritation. Trauma can also contribute to the development of this condition, particularly if followed by immobilization or disuse. These may lead to soft tissue contracture, resulting in a tight patellofemoral joint.

Patients complain of a toothache-like pain over the anterior surface of the knee, especially along the lateral border of the patella. Conservative management with muscle and soft tissue stretching and strengthening is usually sufficient, but the patella must be protected without further irritation. If exercise causes pain, the routine must be carefully evaluated.

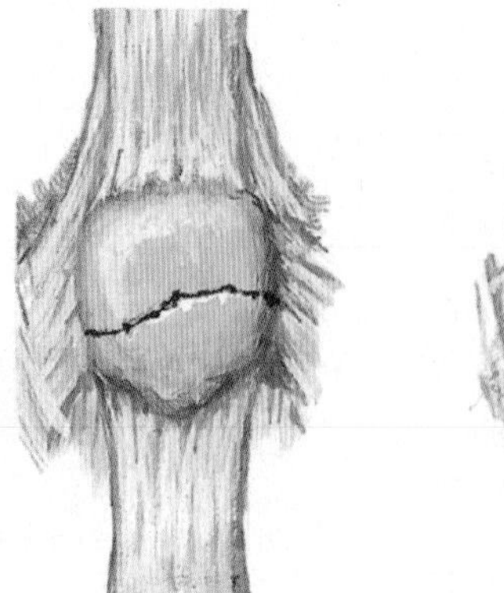

Nondisplaced transverse fracture with intact retinacula

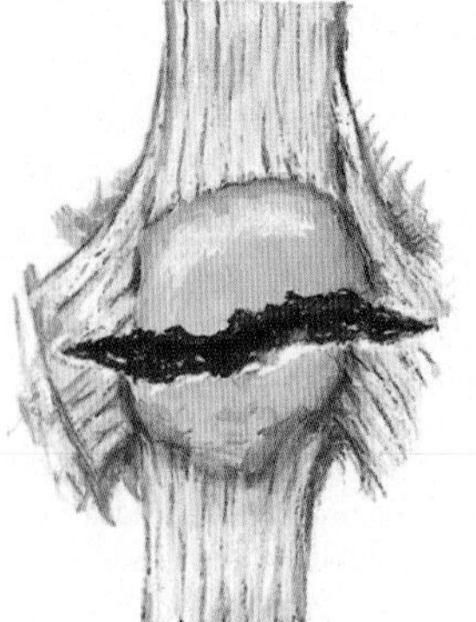

Displaced transverse fracture with tears in retinacula

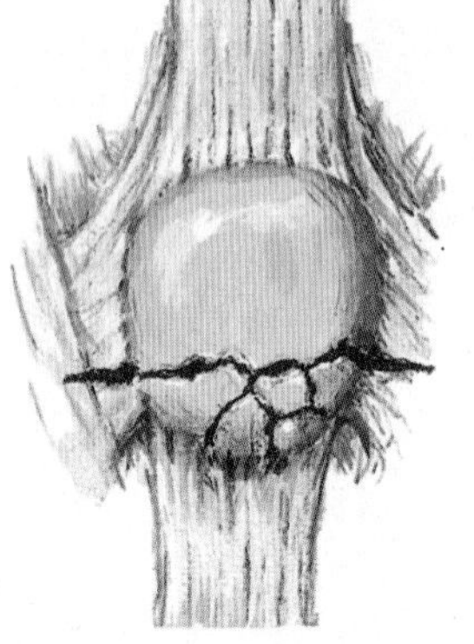

Transverse fracture with comminution of distal pole

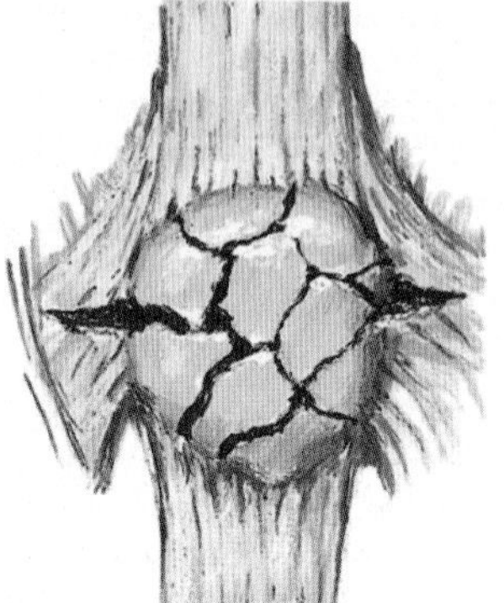

Severely comminuted fracture

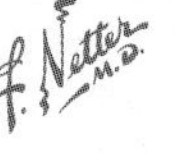

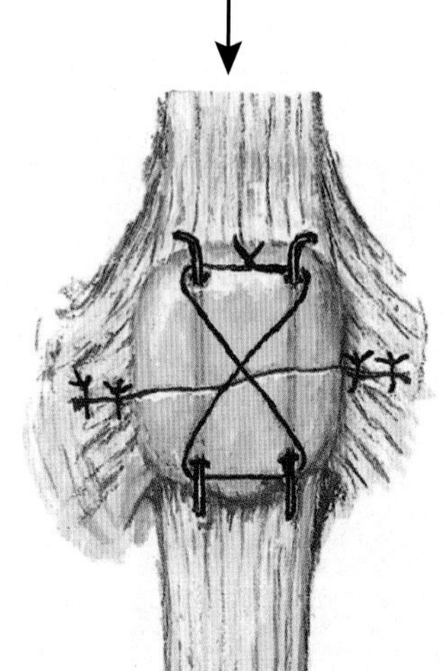

Displaced transverse or slightly comminuted fractures fixed with Steinmann pins through vertical drill holes plus figure-of-8 tension band wire and suture of retinacula.

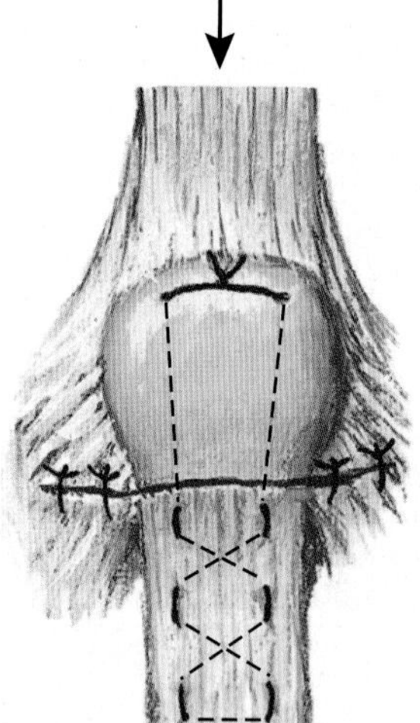

Complete excision of lower pole plus reattachment of patellar ligament to remainder of patella with wire through drill holes. Retinacula repaired.

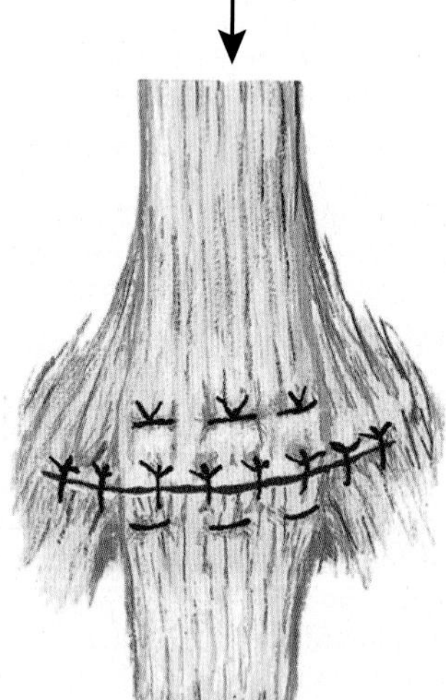

In badly comminuted fractures, patella removed, quadriceps femoris tendon sutured to patellar ligament with nonabsorbable sutures, and retinacula repaired.

Fracture of the Patella

The patella may fracture if the intrinsic strength of the patella and the extensor expansion is overcome by the pull of the quadriceps femoris muscle. Fractures are usually caused by indirect forces, particularly when the quadriceps mechanism contracts forcefully to extend a knee that is being forcibly flexed. The patient may stumble, feel the pain of a tear, hear a "pop," and fall as disruption of the patella occurs. Immediately after the patella fractures, as the quadriceps femoris muscle continues to contract and the knee continues to flex, the medial and lateral retinacula are torn. The degree of tearing dictates how much the patellar fragments separate. Indirect fractures are usually transverse, sometimes with comminution at the fracture site.

The patella, a sesamoid bone, is also vulnerable to injury from a direct blow. Striking the knee on an automobile dashboard or on the ground in a fall frequently results in comminuted, stellate fractures. These fractures often are nondisplaced, and the patient can actively extend the knee if pain is relieved. Vertical fractures of the patella occur occasionally and usually have minimal displacement.

Nondisplaced fractures of the patella are treated by immobilizing the knee in full extension with a long-leg cast, splint, or brace. Union occurs in about 6 weeks, after which active and gentle passive range-of-motion exercises should be instituted. Transverse fractures with displacement greater than a few millimeters require surgery. The fracture fragments are reapproximated to their anatomic positions. The medial and lateral retinacula are repaired when necessary, and the patellar fragments can then be held in place with a variety of fixation methods, such as the commonly used figure-of-eight tension band wire wrapped around two parallel Steinmann pins. Full knee extension should not be allowed until fracture union occurs.

If there are fractures of the proximal or distal pole of the patella with extensive comminution of the smaller fragment, partial patellectomy or fragment excision can be done. The object is to save at least one-half of the articular surface while excising the small comminuted fragments. The quadriceps femoris tendon or the patellar ligament is reattached to the remaining patella, and the medial and lateral retinacula are repaired. The knee is immobilized in full extension in a cast or splint for 6 weeks. After that, protected range of motion and weight-bearing are allowed. A patellectomy should be considered only for severely comminuted fractures without possibility of repair because removal of the patella compromises the biomechanics of the quadriceps mechanism at the knee.

Osteochondral fractures are caused by a completely different mechanism. When a lateral dislocation of the patella is forcefully reduced, a bone fragment may detach from the medial facet of the patella (occasionally from the lateral femoral condyle). Clinical findings are pain along the anteromedial aspect of the knee, marked swelling, hemarthrosis, and mechanical locking and grinding in the knee. The fracture fragments may be completely cartilaginous and difficult to see on plain radiographs but may be visualized on a skyline view of the patella. The loose body is usually removed with arthroscopy, although very large fragments may be reattached to the patella to restore articular congruency.

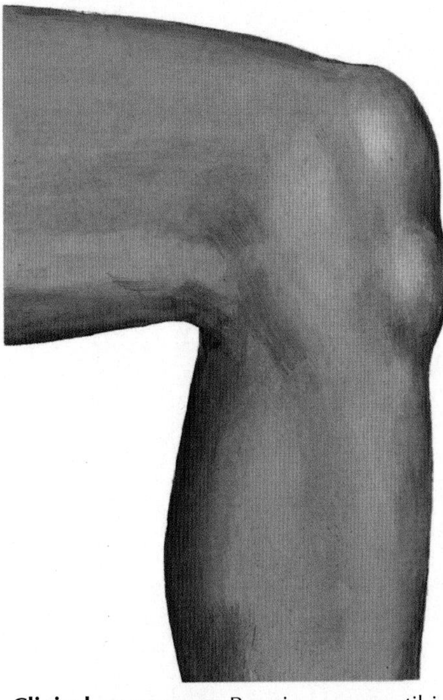

Clinical appearance. Prominence over tibial tuberosity due partly to soft tissue swelling and partly to avulsed fragments.

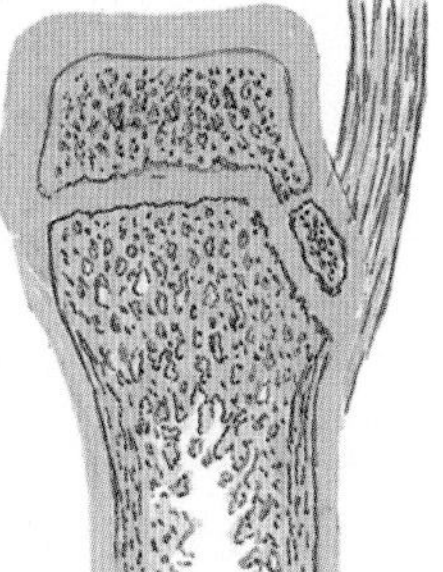

Normal insertion of patellar ligament of ossifying tibial tuberosity

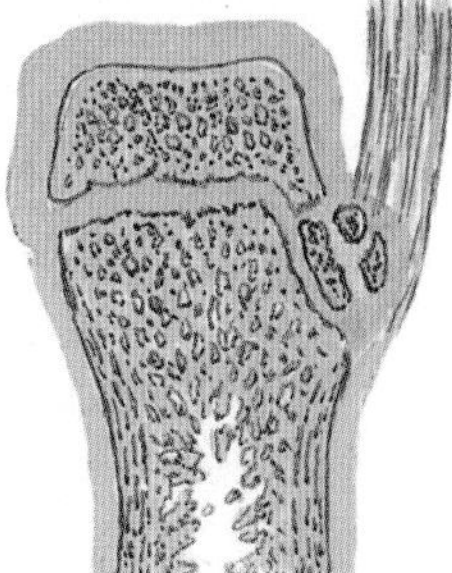

In Osgood-Schlatter disease, superficial portion of tuberosity pulled away, forming separate bone fragments.

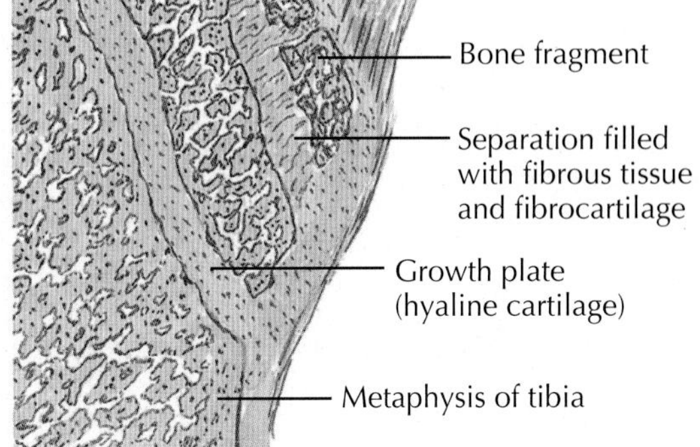

High-power magnification of involved area

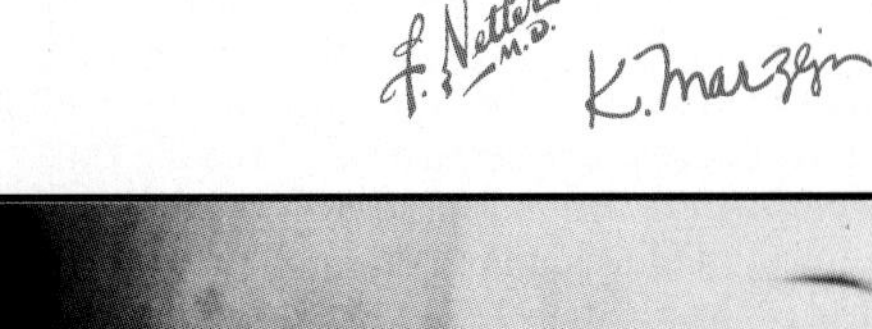

Osgood-Schlatter Lesion

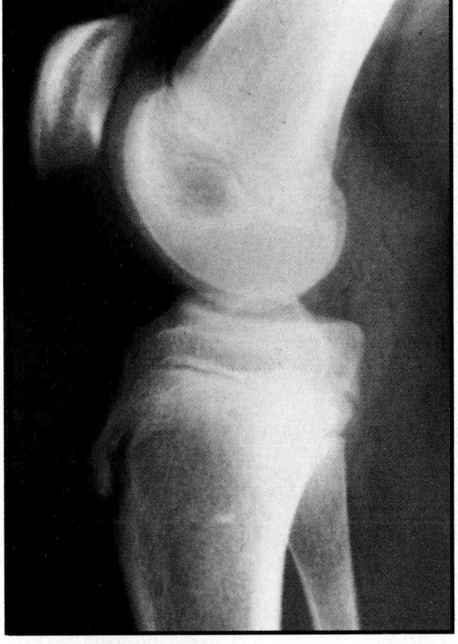

Radiograph shows separation of superficial portion of tibial tuberosity.

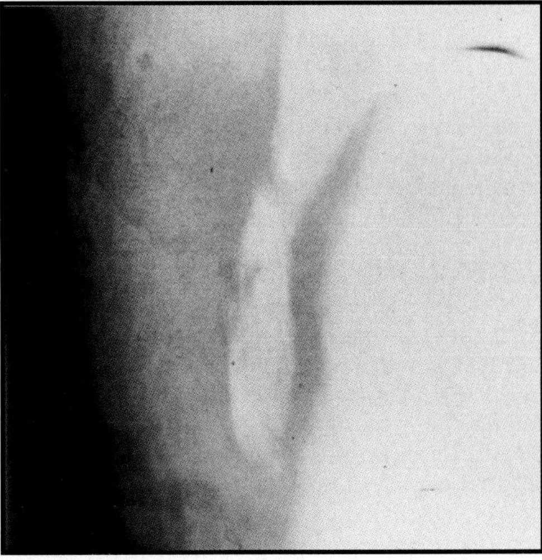

Focal radiograph shows fragment at site of insertion of patellar ligament.

Osgood-Schlatter disease occurs as a result of an overuse injury to the tibial tuberosity caused by repetitive microtrauma to the tuberosity apophysis during late childhood or early adolescence. It is a type of juvenile traction or tensile osteochondritis/apophysitis. Although it is historically more common in boys, incidence in girls has increased significantly, likely because of increased participation in competitive sports.

During fetal development, the tibial tuberosity develops as a discrete anterior extension of the epiphysis of the proximal tibia. After birth, it moves distally and develops its own growth plate, which is composed largely of fibrocartilage rather than the columnar-celled hyaline cartilage to withstand tensile stress. This fibrous composition appears to be a structural adaptation to the tension placed on the tuberosity by the patellar tendon.

By 7 to 9 years of age, the tuberosity develops its own center, or several centers, of ossification. Normally the ossification center of the tuberosity expands and eventually unites with that of the tibial epiphysis. Major or repetitive tensile stress on the tuberosity may cause the developing bone or its overlying hyaline cartilage, or both, to fail, resulting in avulsion of its superficial portion.

The avulsed fragment (or fragments) and the intact portion of the tuberosity continue to grow. The intervening area usually fills in with bone, leading to overgrowth of the tuberosity at skeletal maturity. This is manifested as a bony prominence over the anterior aspect of the proximal tibia. In some patients, the space between the fragment and the tuberosity becomes filled with fibrous material, creating a painful nonunion or even a pathologic joint.

Osgood-Schlatter disease manifests as localized swelling and tenderness over the tibial tuberosity. The pain is aggravated by direct pressure, as in kneeling, and by traction, as in running, jumping, and forced flexion. Extension of the knee against resistance may also elicit pain, but there is usually no restriction of range of motion.

The avulsion may occur while the cartilage is still in the preossification phase and thus is not radiographically evident. In this case diagnosis may be difficult. The avulsed cartilage eventually ossifies and becomes visible on radiographs as small fragments of bone that are separated from the rest of the tibial tuberosity.

The condition is self-limiting in about 90% of patients and generally resolves at skeletal maturity. Conservative treatment options to allow healing of the microscopic avulsion fractures of the apophysis include avoidance of strenuous exercise involving the knee, oral antiinflammatory medications, ice, and physical therapy focused on quadriceps/hamstring stretching and core strengthening. Surgery should be considered only in rare, resistant cases once a patient has reached skeletal maturity and after conservative treatment has failed. Surgery typically involves ossicle excision.

OSTEOARTHRITIS OF THE KNEE

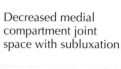

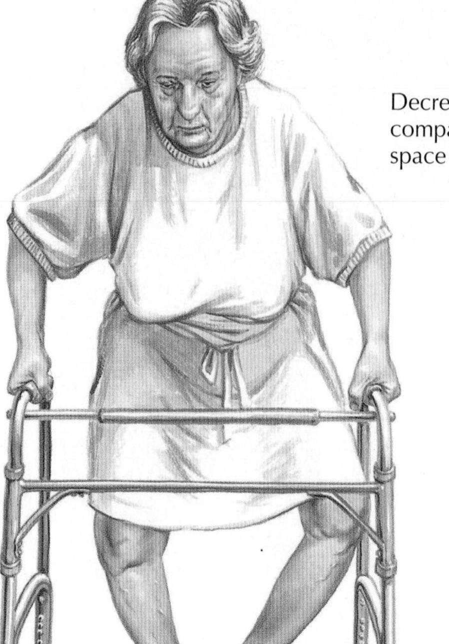

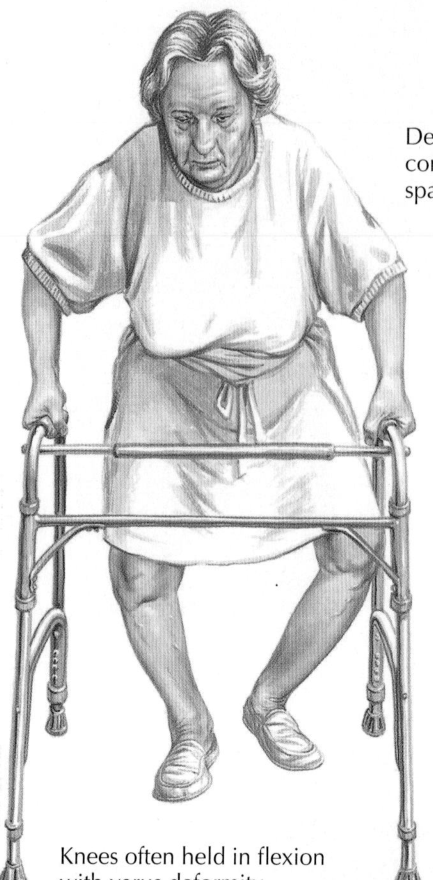

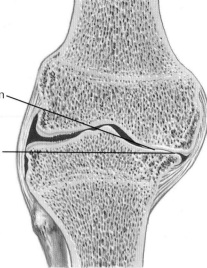

Knee with osteoarthritis exhibits varus deformity, medial subluxation, loss of articular cartilage, and osteophyte formation.

Knees often held in flexion with varus deformity

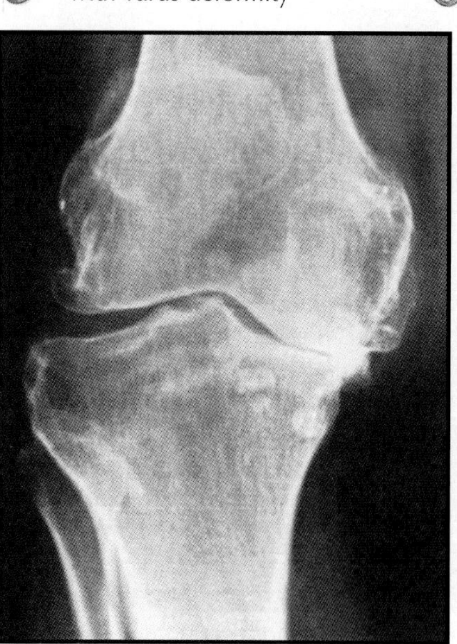

Radiograph showing varus deformity and medial subluxation of knee

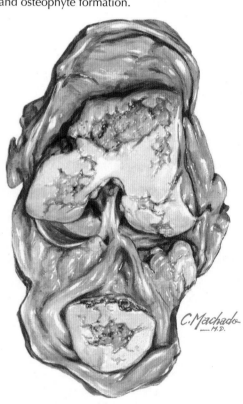

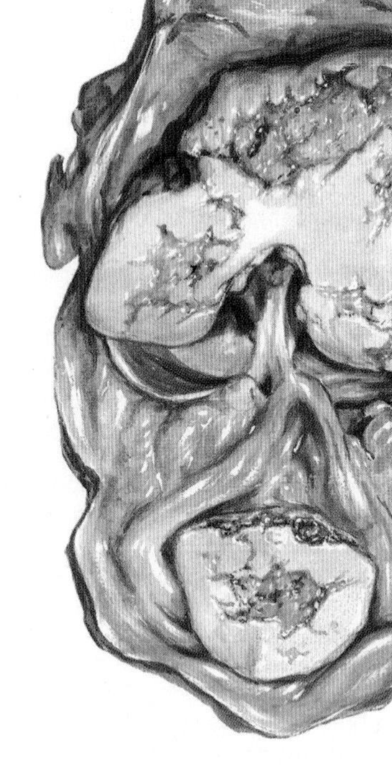

Opened knee joint showing severe erosion of articular cartilage with minimal synovial change

KNEE ARTHROPLASTY: PROSTHESES

HISTORY

Arthroplasty for the treatment of severe, painful arthritis of the knee originated in the mid-19th century when Verneuil suggested the interposition of soft tissues to replace the articular surfaces of the knee joint; materials used included pig's bladder, nylon, fascia lata, and prepatellar bursa. Resection arthroplasty was also performed. The joints developed good motion but lacked good mechanical stability. These operations were confined to patients with severe conditions, such as tuberculosis or other infectious processes that destroyed the knee.

Success with femoral mold arthroplasty of the hip prompted the development of a similar metallic device for use in the knee. In 1958 MacIntosh used an acrylic tibial plateau prosthesis, and a metal prosthesis of a similar design was developed by McKeever. Gunston applied Charnley's principle of low friction arthroplasty of the hip to develop a prosthesis for the knee joint. He used metal femoral runners that articulated with polyethylene tibial components. Each component was fixed in bone with acrylic cement. Freeman developed a single femorotibial component to replace the entire surface of each bone. The Freeman-Swanson prosthesis consisted of two components whose stability was determined by a roller-in-trough mechanism. Other designs featured fully constrained hinges that replaced the articular surfaces of the joint and did not require a balanced tension of the collateral ligaments. However, these prostheses loosened early and the rate of infection increased. Consequently, surface-replacement hinge designs were developed that allowed the knee joint to move in a normal fashion.

INDICATIONS AND CONTRAINDICATIONS

Total knee arthroplasty is routinely performed in patients with severe, incapacitating pain in the knees due to osteoarthritis, osteonecrosis, or rheumatoid arthritis, after all means of conservative management, such as administration of parenteral NSAIDs, use of a cane, intraarticular viscosupplementation or corticosteroid injections, and weight loss, have been exhausted. Arthritis due to trauma, gout, and psoriasis should also first be treated conservatively. Joint destruction secondary to pigmented villonodular synovitis may require total joint replacement after appropriate synovectomies have been performed. More recently, total knee replacement has been successfully used in patients with hemophilic arthritis.

In patients with rheumatoid arthritis, total knee replacement may be done at any age and has been successful in patients with juvenile arthritis. In these patients, growth is limited, and extra-small or custom-made prostheses may be required. In patients with osteoarthritis, total knee replacement should be confined to those older than 60 years when possible. If one or both collateral ligaments are injured, a constrained design, such as a posterior stabilized, total stabilized, or hinged-knee prosthesis should be used to provide the joint stability normally afforded by intact collateral ligaments.

In older patients with mild narrowing of the joint space and patchy articular degeneration in the femorotibial joint, severe patellofemoral arthritis may also

Total Condylar Prosthesis and Unicompartmental Prosthesis

Total condylar knee prosthesis

Femoral component

Tibial component

Anterolateral view of components in position of extension

Stem for insertion into tibia

Anterior view of components in position of extension

Femur

Tibia

Lateral sectional view of knee joint in extension with components in place

Femur

Tibia

Lateral sectional view of knee joint in extension with components in place

Lateral sectional view of knee joint in flexion with components in place

F. Netter M.D.

K. Marzen

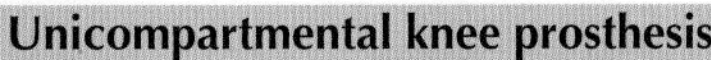

Unicompartmental knee prosthesis

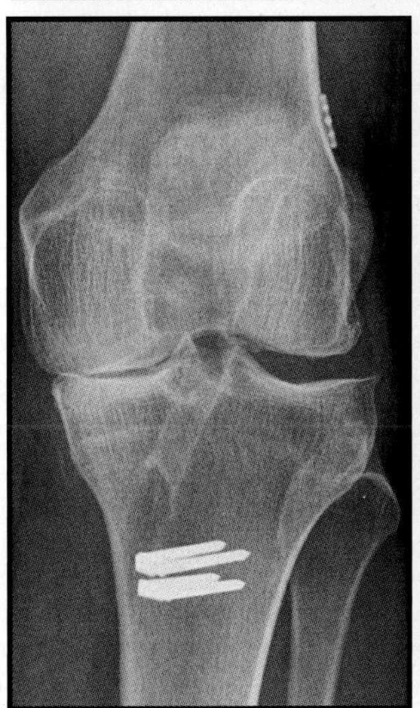

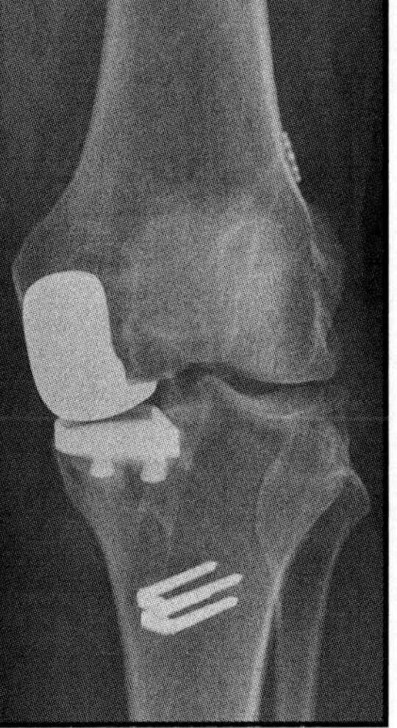

Radiographs of 41-year-old female with severe medial compartment osteoarthritis. Patient has already undergone an anterior cruciate ligament reconstruction. Preoperative view (*left*) shows marked joint space narrowing and articular deformity with preservation of the lateral compartment. The patient underwent a unicompartmental arthroplasty of the medial compartment. Postoperative view is shown (*right*).

Knee Arthroplasty: Prostheses (Continued)

be successfully treated with total joint replacement. In patients with a previous or concurrent intraarticular knee infection, arthroplasty should be delayed until the infection has been eradicated. If the infection persists and the infectious organism cannot be adequately treated, then arthrodesis, although relatively uncommon, would be an appropriate treatment. If a knee joint has been successfully fused and the patient is asymptomatic with adequate function and mobility, then knee replacement should not be performed, because there is a diminished likelihood of success and subsequent attempts at refusion of the knee may not succeed.

Other contraindications to total knee replacement include severe neuropathic joint disease, recent joint infection, painless paralytic deformities due to antecedent poliomyelitis, and cerebrovascular insufficiency. It is also recommended to delay arthroplasty as long as possible in manual laborers, athletes, or overweight persons, because the excessive mechanical stresses placed on the knee may lead to early loosening, polyethylene wear, and subsequent failure of the prosthesis, requiring early revision. Patients with posttraumatic osteoarthritis are typically young, and only in rare instances should total knee replacement be considered in this group.

TOTAL CONDYLAR PROSTHESIS

The total condylar prosthesis was developed in 1973 at the Hospital for Special Surgery. The term describes a family of prostheses with similar design characteristics that allow unconstrained movement of the knee joint.

The total condylar prosthesis requires balancing the tension of the collateral ligaments to stabilize the knee joint in flexion and extension. With appropriate design of the prosthesis and stable symmetric balancing of the collateral ligaments, the cruciate ligaments are not necessary for function of the knee joint. However, initial designs only allowed for relatively limited flexion to only 90 degrees, which left certain activities difficult for patients to accomplish. Further modifications and improvements of prosthetic design were then developed to address this issue. A total condylar design in which the PCL is retained ("cruciate retaining" prosthesis) was developed at the Brigham and Women's Hospital. This design allowed for greater flexion of the knee joint and improved the patient's ability to perform activities such as climbing stairs. Unconstrained designs have now become the implant of choice when possible in total knee arthroplasty, because they allow for the greatest amount of motion and may reduce focal contact pressures that may potentially lead to earlier implant wear and fatigue. However, it is essential in each patient to choose the implant that confers the appropriate amount of stability to the reconstructed knee.

UNICOMPARTMENTAL KNEE PROSTHESIS

For patients who have severe symptomatic arthritis involving only one compartment of the knee, there is an option to perform reconstruction of only that affected joint surface. In the more common varus deformity, an

KNEE ARTHROPLASTY: PROSTHESES (Continued)

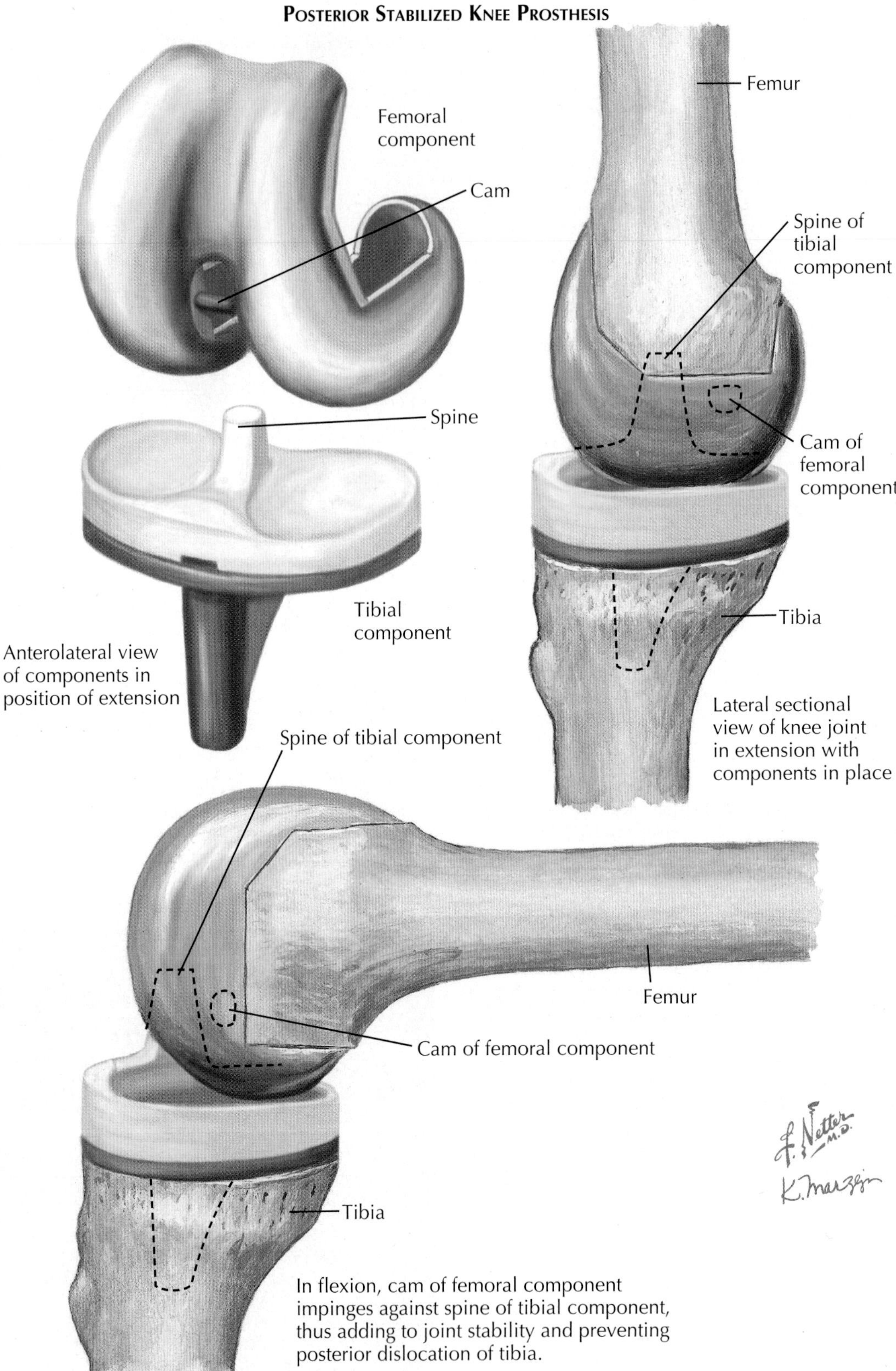

isolated medial unicompartmental knee arthroplasty can provide excellent symptomatic relief without sacrificing the remainder of the nondiseased joint surfaces and ligaments. However, successful outcomes of these procedures have been shown to be significantly determined by proper patient selection, and, if failure occurs, early revision may be required.

POSTERIOR STABILIZED CONDYLAR PROSTHESIS

The posterior stabilized condylar prosthesis, a modification of the earlier total condylar design, retains more of the function of the PCL. The articulating polyethylene component of the prosthesis has a different shape with a built-in intercondylar tibial eminence that is positioned in such a way that it engages the horizontal cam of the femoral component to mimic PCL function by preventing sagittal instability. As a result, with further flexion, the cam of the femoral component imposes a progressive rollback at the femoral condyle to prevent posterior impingement, a mechanism similar to that found in the knee with an intact PCL. Newer versions are designed to reach over 130 degrees of flexion, with a special type that allows 140 degrees of flexion available in Asia because it is compatible with the lifestyle in that region.

Potential drawbacks of the posterior stabilized prosthesis include alterations in natural gait mechanics because of the changed biomechanical environment of the knee, increased stress on the patellofemoral articulation, and transfer of the shear forces normally managed by the intact PCL to the bone-cement interface, which may result in earlier loosening and failure of the implant. However, the effects of these findings remain somewhat controversial because good long-term success of these implants has been described in the literature.

RESULTS

As new prosthetic designs and implant materials continue to be developed on a near-constant basis, it is difficult to report on long-term outcomes of the currently used devices. A 10-year follow-up study of 100 patients with the older and more traditional total condylar knee prosthesis indicated that 93% of the prostheses functioned well, did not require revision, and lasted the remainder of the patient's life. Mechanical complications were rare (2%), usually occurring in the first 2 to 3 years after surgery. Follow-up studies 2 to 8 years after replacement surgery with a posterior stabilized prosthesis reported good to excellent results in 96% of patients. It is widely considered that current implants should provide at least 10 to 15 years of good function in the average patient.

Most available prostheses include components to replace the surfaces of the patella, tibia, and femur. Although the patella should be replaced in all patients with rheumatoid arthritis, there has historically been controversy surrounding replacement of the patella in the purely osteoarthritic knee. However, studies show that results are more predictably good if the patella is resurfaced, which is most commonly done by surgeons performing total knee arthroplasties.

Total Knee Replacement Technique: Steps 1 to 5

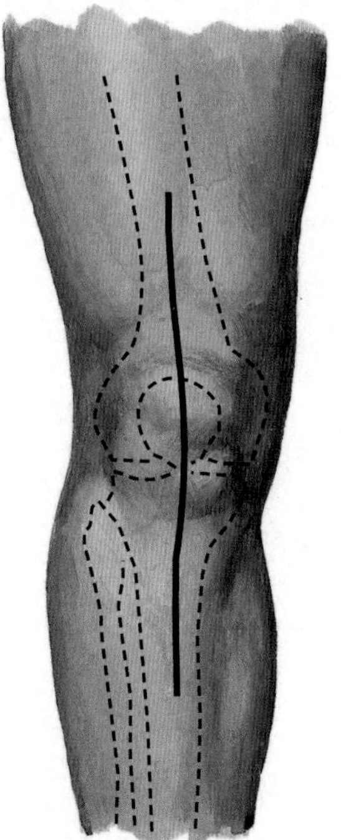

1. Longitudinal 8- to 12-inch skin incision is centered on patella.

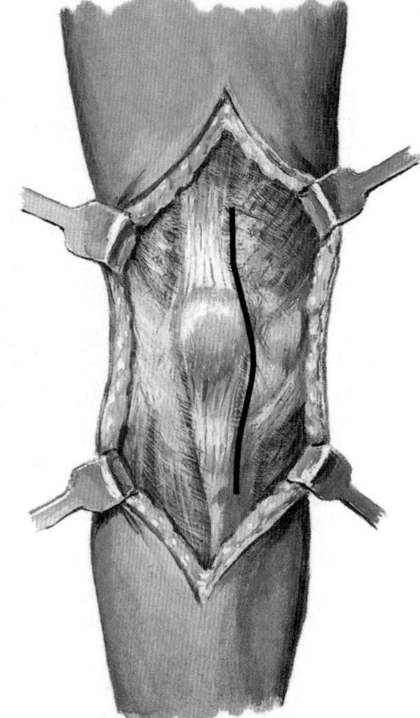

2. Capsular incision skirts medial margin of patella and courses distally through periosteum medial to tibial tuberosity.

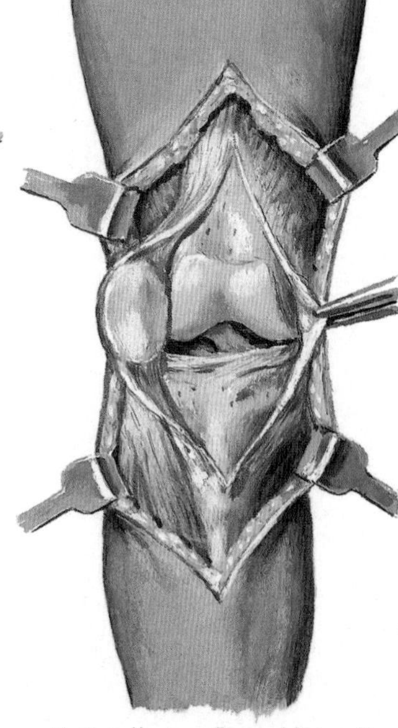

3. Patella is reflected laterally by raising patellar ligament in continuity with periosteum.

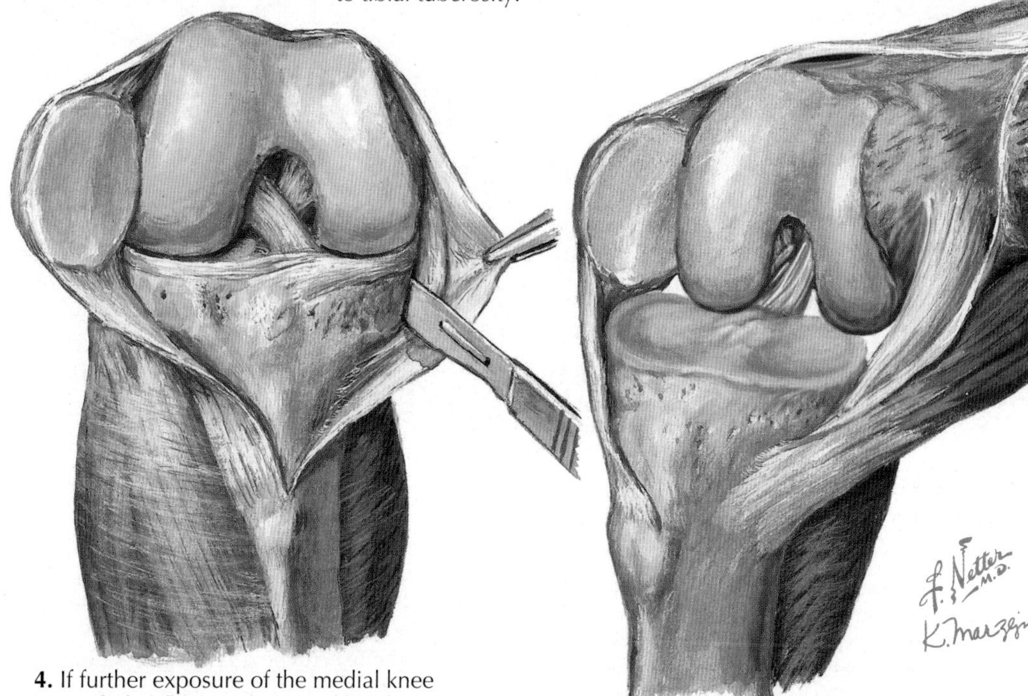

4. If further exposure of the medial knee is needed, a flap can be raised by elevating the deep medial collateral ligament and pes anserinus subperiosteally, aided by external rotation of the tibia.

5. The anterior cruciate ligament and both menisci are excised, and the tibia is subluxated anteriorly.

Total Knee Arthroplasty: Technique

EXPOSURE

Traditionally, an 8- to 12-inch longitudinal skin incision was made, centered on the anterior surface of the patella or just slightly medial to the tibial tuberosity. This incision affords the best medial and lateral exposure of the knee without placing undue tension on the skin. Currently, there is an emphasis on smaller skin incisions and minimally invasive procedures with less substantial soft tissue dissection to preserve native vascularity, making most surgeons less likely to use as large of an initial incision. After obtaining adequate visualization, the joint is then accessed by an incision proximally through the quadriceps tendon from 5 to 8 cm proximal to the superior pole of the patella and just lateral to the insertion of the vastus medialis obliquus muscle, then down around its medial margin, to a point just medial to the tibial tuberosity (medial parapatellar approach). It is essential to ensure an adequate cuff of tissue to allow proper capsular repair during closure. The medial placement helps to prevent wound dehiscence during knee flexion in the postoperative period. Other approaches, such as the midvastus and subvastus techniques, are also used to access the knee joint, although they remain less common. The periosteum directly medial to the tibial tuberosity should be left intact to help prevent avulsion of the patellar ligament from the tibial tuberosity. Every effort should be made to prevent avulsion, because reattachment of the patellar ligament is difficult and may result in limitation of knee extension.

Dissection along the anterolateral surface of the tibia and raising of the patellar ligament in continuity with the periosteum are then done to obtain lateral reflection and eversion of the patella. Any scar tissue and patellofemoral ligament attachments should be removed to facilitate eversion of the patella. The capsular incision should extend far enough proximally to allow eversion

Total Knee Replacement Technique: Steps 6 to 9

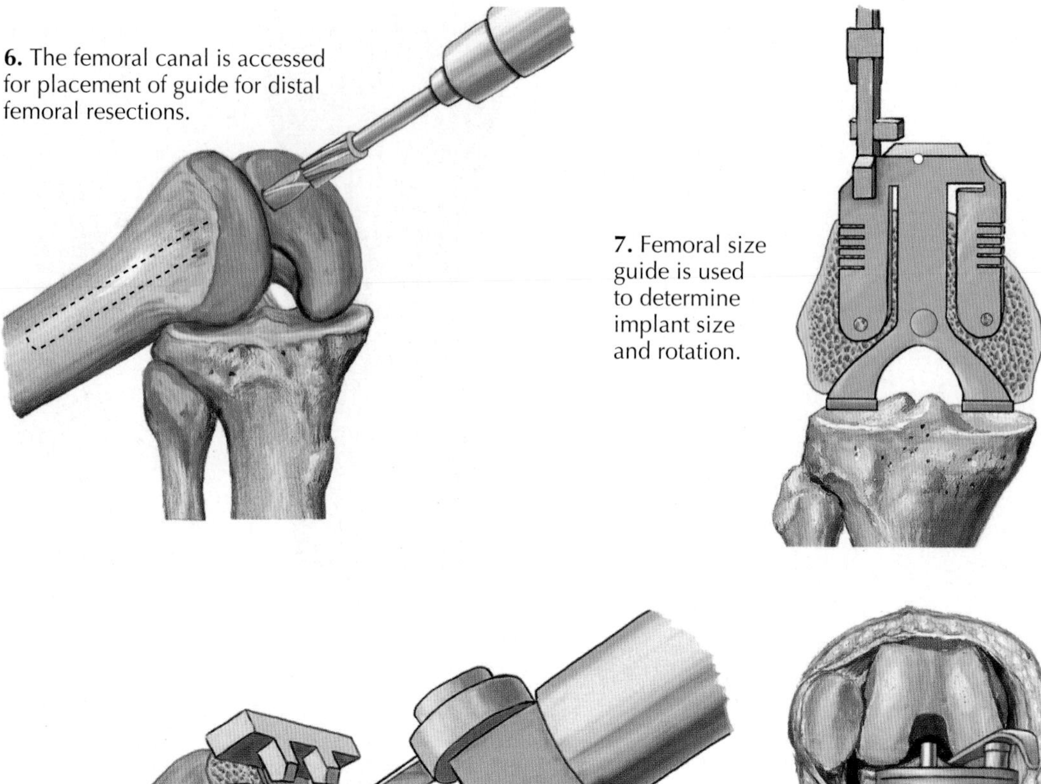

6. The femoral canal is accessed for placement of guide for distal femoral resections.

7. Femoral size guide is used to determine implant size and rotation.

8. Femoral cutting block is used for anterior, posterior, and chamfer cuts.

9. Tibial cutting block is placed using the aid of an extramedullary alignment rod (pictured; may also use an intramedullary device). The bar can be used to assess slope and alignment of the cut.

Total Knee Arthroplasty: Technique (Continued)

of the patella, but care must be taken to avoid dissecting across the quadriceps femoris tendon.

A medial flap is raised directly off the surface of the anterior tibia by detaching the insertion of the anterior horn of the medial meniscus and the soft tissue attachments and a segment of the pes anserinus tendons subperiosteally. Care is made to preserve the integrity of the MCL. Slight external rotation of the tibia may facilitate dissection of the posteromedial aspect of the bone and enables the patella to remain everted with minimal tension on the patellar ligament. Depending on surgeon preference, the fat pad may be excised at this time because it is readily visible.

Once appropriate medial and lateral exposure has been achieved, the menisci are excised to provide access to the tibial joint surface. Exposure of the tibial and femoral condyles then allows for the removal of osteophytes with either a rongeur or osteotome.

At this time, the ACL is then divided and the tibia subluxated anteriorly. This facilitates excision of the ACL and PCL (when not using a cruciate-retaining prosthesis) from their respective attachments on the femur.

BONE RESECTIONS

Now that the bone has been adequately exposed, attention is turned to the bony resection. The goal of the surgical procedure is to restore the normal mechanical axis of the knee and to provide a painless and functional articulation. Depending on the surgeon's preference and device system used, there are many options as to which surgical technique to use. There are multiple methods of achieving satisfactory balance of the soft tissue and flexion and extension gaps as well. There also exist different options for cutting guides (intramedullary vs. extramedullary) and the order in which femoral, tibial, and patellar cuts will be made. Because there

Total Knee Replacement Technique: Steps 10 to 14

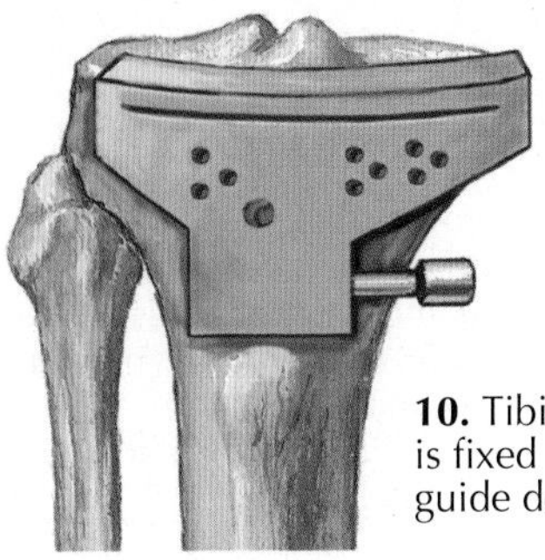

10. Tibial cutting block is fixed into place and guide device removed.

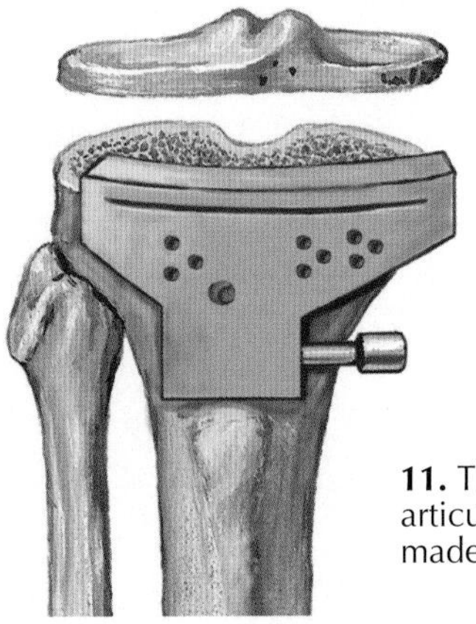

11. The proximal tibial articular surface cut is then made with oscillating saw.

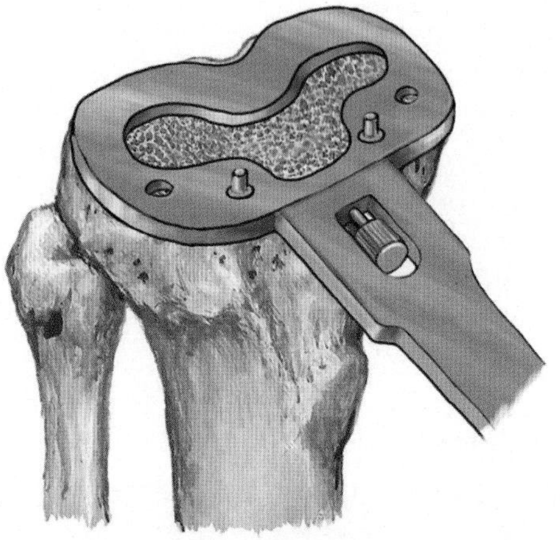

12. Trial baseplates are then used to assess the appropriate size of the implant to be used.

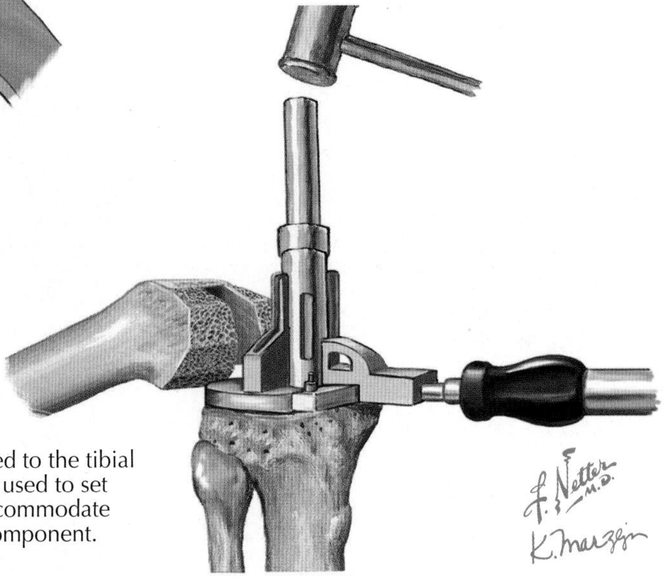

13. The trial baseplate is fixed to the tibial surface, and a keel punch is used to set rotational alignment and accommodate the stem of the final tibial component.

Total Knee Arthroplasty: Technique (Continued)

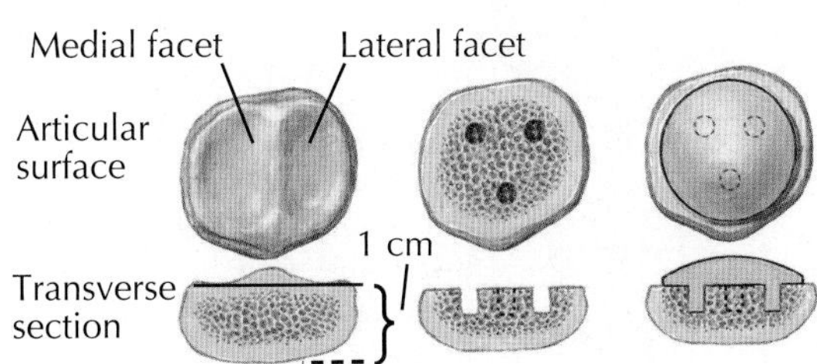

14. Articular surface of patella resected to leave flat surface. Equal amounts to be removed from medial and lateral facets, but at least 1 cm of bone must be left to ensure adequate strength. Using a patella drill template, three holes are drilled into the surface to accommodate the final patellar component, which is cemented in place.

exists no definitive consensus on these options, it is up to the surgeon to decide how to achieve the most consistent and reproducible results.

When using an intramedullary guide for distal femoral resection, the femoral canal is accessed at a point slightly anterior to the insertion of the PCL on the intercondylar notch. The cutting guide is then attached and secured in a position to obtain a resection that will equal the length of the femoral component, usually 8 to 10 cm. After this cut is made, the intramedullary guide is removed and a femoral component size guide is used to determine the appropriate implant size and subsequently determine the remaining femoral cuts. To achieve the appropriate anatomic rotation of the tibiofemoral articulation (typically 3–7 degrees of valgus), it is important to position these guides properly. There are several approaches used, including the epicondylar axis, Whiteside line, and the posterior condyles of the femur. When choosing the right size, care should be made not to allow for notching of the femur during the anterior cut and to prevent overstuffing of the joint. Notching the femoral cortex can lead to an area of stress concentration that may be susceptible to pathologic fractures of the femur if the patient falls.

After size and rotation have been determined, a femoral cutting block is secured in position and the anterior, posterior, and chamfer cuts are done. Posterior femoral osteophytes are commonly present in a severely arthritic knee, and it is essential that these be removed before positioning and fitting of the prosthesis because they can cause malposition of the component. This is regularly accomplished with an osteotome or curet. If the decision is made for a stabilized prosthesis, the necessary box cuts can be made at this time as well. A trial femoral prosthesis can then be placed.

Preparation of the tibia can also use either intramedullary or extramedullary cutting guides and jigs.

TOTAL KNEE REPLACEMENT TECHNIQUE: STEPS 15 TO 20

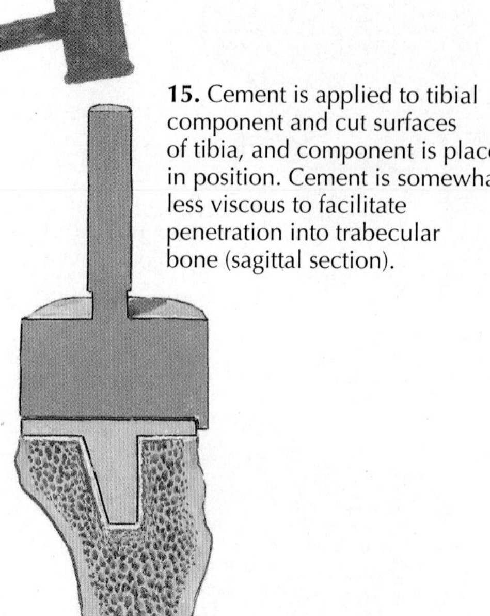

15. Cement is applied to tibial component and cut surfaces of tibia, and component is placed in position. Cement is somewhat less viscous to facilitate penetration into trabecular bone (sagittal section).

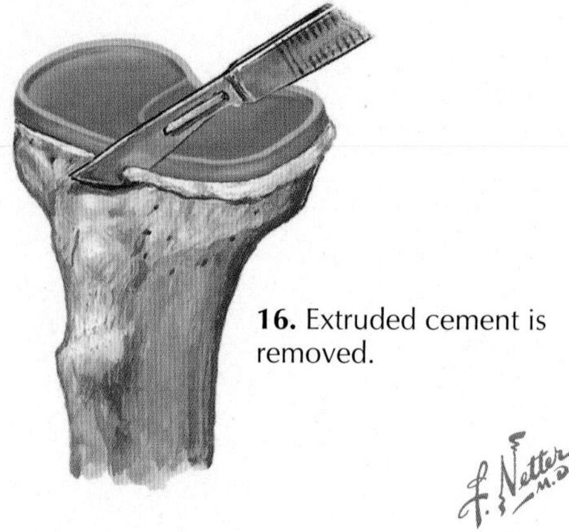

16. Extruded cement is removed.

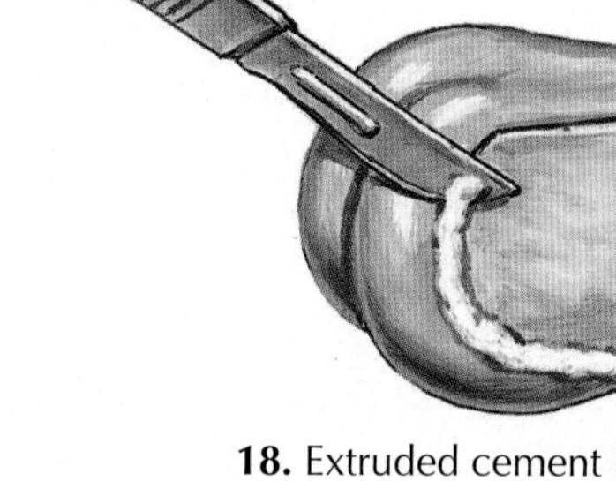

18. Extruded cement is removed.

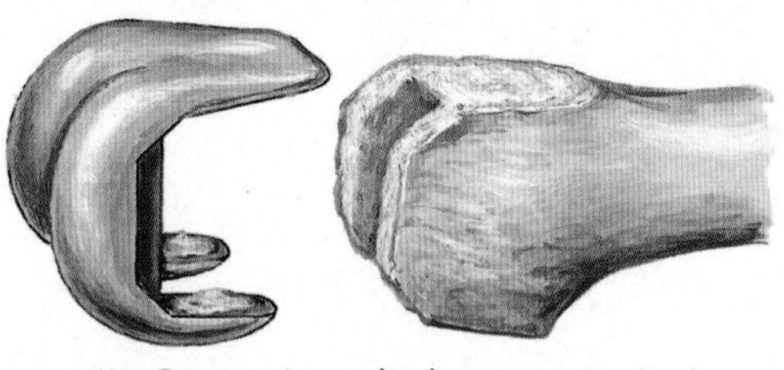

17. Cement is applied to posterior limb of femoral component and spread evenly over beveled ends of femur.

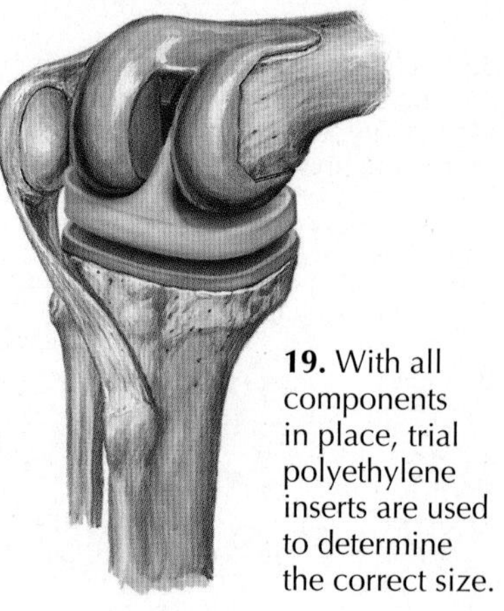

19. With all components in place, trial polyethylene inserts are used to determine the correct size.

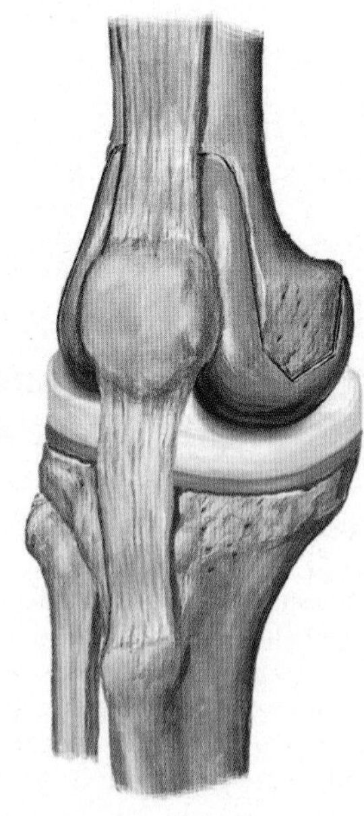

20. Once the final components are in place, the knee is placed through a range of motion and appropriate stress tests. The knee is then irrigated, hemostasis achieved, and the wound is closed.

TOTAL KNEE ARTHROPLASTY: TECHNIQUE (Continued)

When using an extramedullary guide, the bar should be centered over the tibial crest with the lateral margin of the bar at the tibial tuberosity and should distally correspond to the malleolar line or the second metatarsal. The bar is then used to determine the proper slope, and the cutting guide is positioned at the appropriate depth to make the desired tibial resection, which is most commonly done in neutral rotation. After this is completed, the guides are removed and a trial tibial baseplate can be positioned. Various sizes of polyethylene inserts can then be used to obtain the most fluid range of motion and best stability of the knee joint.

When making the cut for patellar resurfacing, there are multiple methods and guides that can be used to facilitate an adequate depth and congruous surface for the implant. Once the cut is made and the holes are drilled, a trial can be placed and patellar tracking can be assessed within the knee range of motion.

MEDIAL RELEASE FOR VARUS DEFORMITY OF KNEE

In a patient with severe varus deformity who is undergoing total knee arthroplasty, a series of interventions are necessary beyond routine soft tissue balancing to obtain proper joint alignment. These range from removal of the PCL, capsular release, resection of femoral condyle and tibial plateau osteophytes, and sequential release of the layers of the MCL. Long-term follow-up studies show that if the knee remains in a varus position the mechanical stresses placed on the tibial polyethylene component are uneven. This may lead to early wear, component loosening, and subsequent failure of the prosthesis. The release is achieved by first elevating deep the intimately related pes anserinus and deep MCL fibers subperiosteally. This is

Medial Release for Varus Deformity of Knee

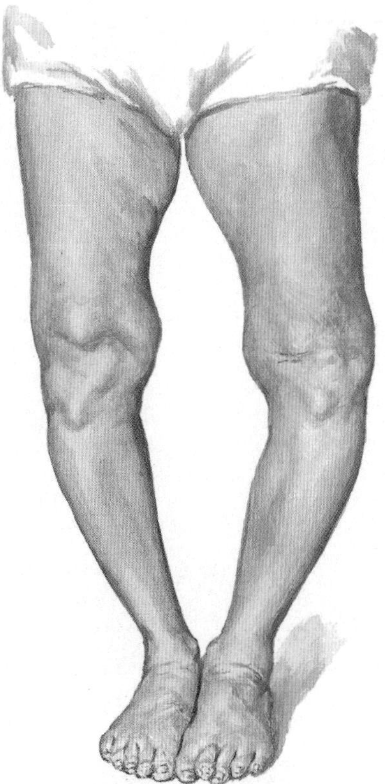

Bilateral tibia vara with severe osteoarthritis

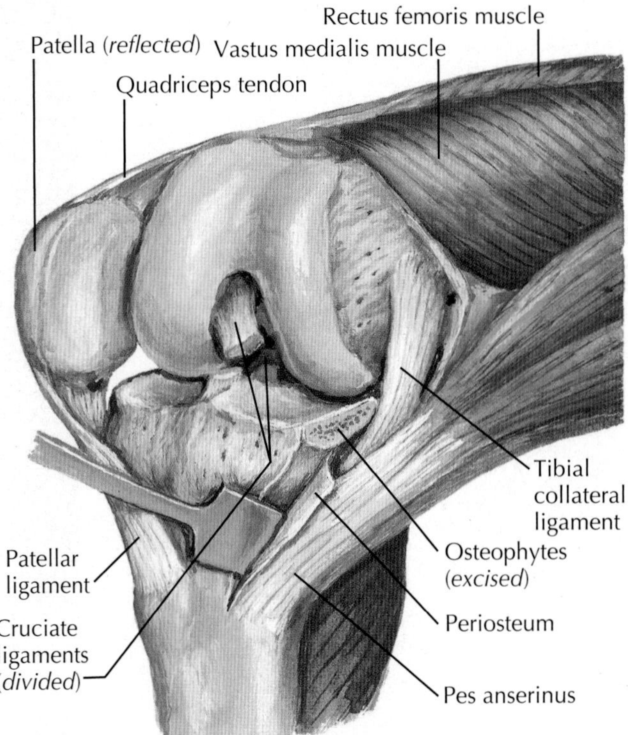

Medial release. Superficial tibial collateral ligament and pes anserinus (insertion of gracilis, sartorius, and semitendinosus muscles) stripped from upper medial tibia together with periosteal flap; osteophytes excised.

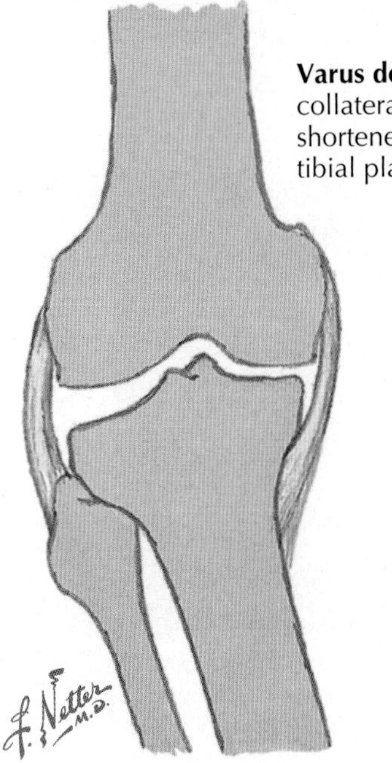

Varus deformity. Tibial collateral ligament shortened and medial tibial plateau defective.

Release of tibial collateral ligament from tibia permits balanced alignment.

Total Knee Arthroplasty: Technique (Continued)

routinely done in the initial exposure of the medial joint line. If balance is not yet achieved, release of the medial capsule and osteophyte resection is undertaken. Further release will often prove impossible without further releasing the MCL at its distal tibial attachment. During healing, the MCL reattaches itself at a more proximal level, resulting in good joint stability and obviating the need for a constrained prosthesis.

Lateral Release for Valgus Deformity of Knee

In severe valgus deformity, the lateral structures of the knee are released to return the knee joint to its normal valgus alignment near 7 degrees. The proximal attachment of the LCL and popliteus tendon is released first. The periosteum of the lateral side of the femur is then stripped proximally. If a flexion contracture is present, the insertion of the lateral head of the gastrocnemius muscle can be released. In very severe valgus deformities of more than 40 degrees, the iliotibial tract must also be released.

When the valgus deformity is combined with a flexion contracture, there is an increased risk of postoperative peroneal nerve palsy. After many years of being in a valgus and flexed position, the peroneal nerve is contracted, and correction of a severe valgus deformity stretches it to the point that the blood supply to the nerve is compromised. It is best treated by removing the bulky dressing and flexing the knee, which can be done in the recovery room. The advent of postoperative rehabilitation protocols emphasizing early motion has helped to minimize this problem. If care is taken to look for this complication, peroneal nerve function is usually restored quite rapidly. Exploration of the nerve may cause damage and is not recommended in most

Total Knee Arthroplasty: Technique (Continued)

cases. Peroneal nerve palsy occurs in less than 1% of patients with valgus knee deformities who undergo total knee replacement.

INSERTION OF COMPONENTS

Once the appropriate implants have been chosen, the trial implants are removed, the knee is copiously irrigated, and the bone surfaces are dried. It is common at this time to release the tourniquet to assess hemostasis, although this is at the preference of the surgeon. Cement (e.g., polymethyl methacrylate) is then prepared, and the femoral, tibial, and patellar components are cemented into position. It is important to remove all excess cement from the joint before closure. The polyethylene insert is then secured into position on the tibial baseplate, and the knee is again put through a range of motion. After satisfactory assessment of the components, the surgical field is then reirrigated and the joint and skin are closed. The wound is then dressed, and the patient is taken to the recovery suite.

Lateral Release for Valgus Deformity of Knee

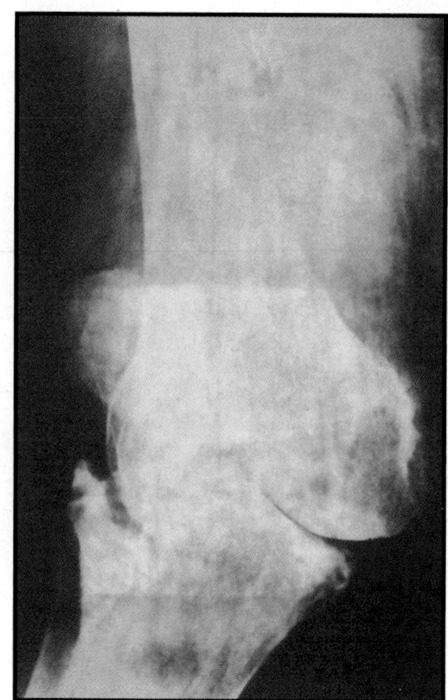

Preoperative standing radiograph shows severe valgus deformity.

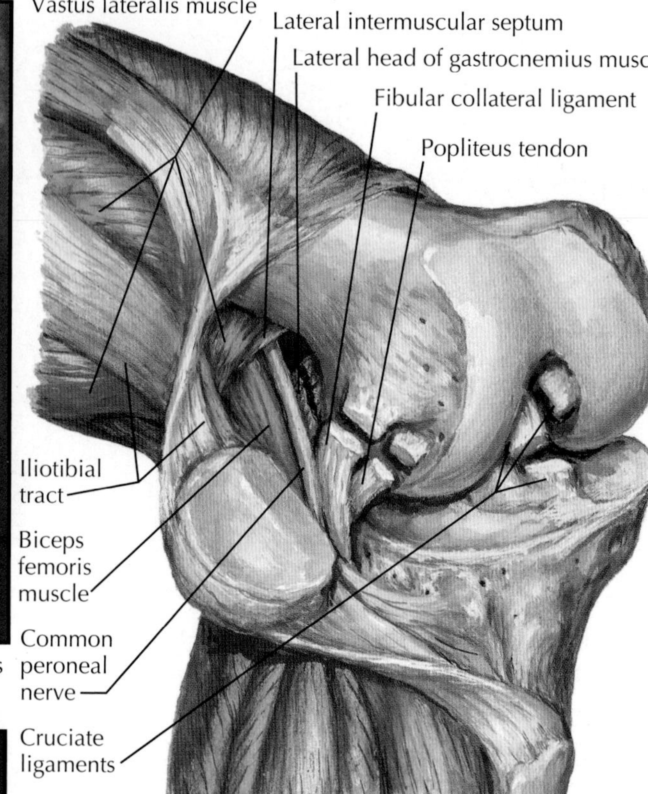

Lateral release. Patella reflected and cruciate ligaments cut. Fibular collateral ligament, lateral capsule, popliteus tendon, and part of lateral head of gastrocnemius muscle divided. If further release required, lower fibers of vastus lateralis muscle and iliotibial tract may also be severed. Common peroneal nerve carefully preserved.

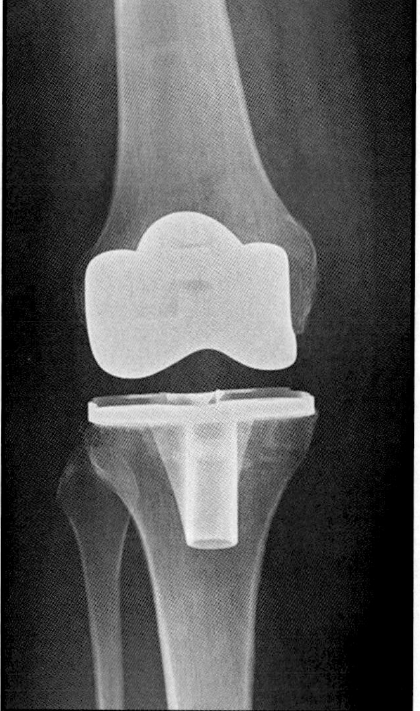

Postoperative radiograph after lateral release and total knee replacement reveals good alignment with functional stability.

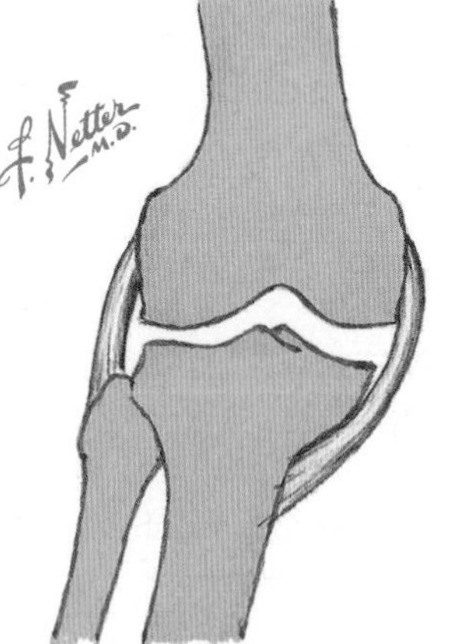

Preoperative view

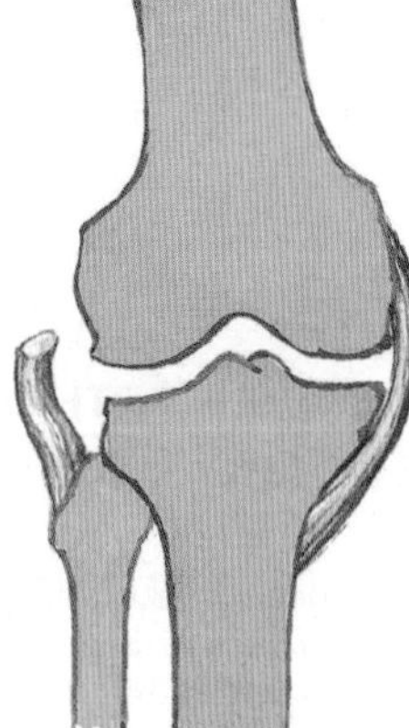

Postoperative view

Lateral release done at femoral level (in contrast to medial release, which is at tibial level). Release of lateral tension corrects valgus deformity.

POSTOPERATIVE CARE

Typically, the patient is hospitalized for 2 to 4 days. Physical therapy is provided daily and can often begin on the same day as surgery, with an emphasis on obtaining a good range of motion. It is recommended to administer 24 hours of perioperative antibiotics and provide prophylaxis against the development of deep venous thrombosis. Patients usually begin to ambulate with a walker or cane and can be discharged to the appropriate facility once they are medically stable and have a safe environment to recuperate. For as long as the prosthesis remains in place, patients must be given antibiotics before any dental procedure and urinary or gastrointestinal surgery to protect against the hematogenous seeding of bacteria, which can localize at the site of the prosthesis.

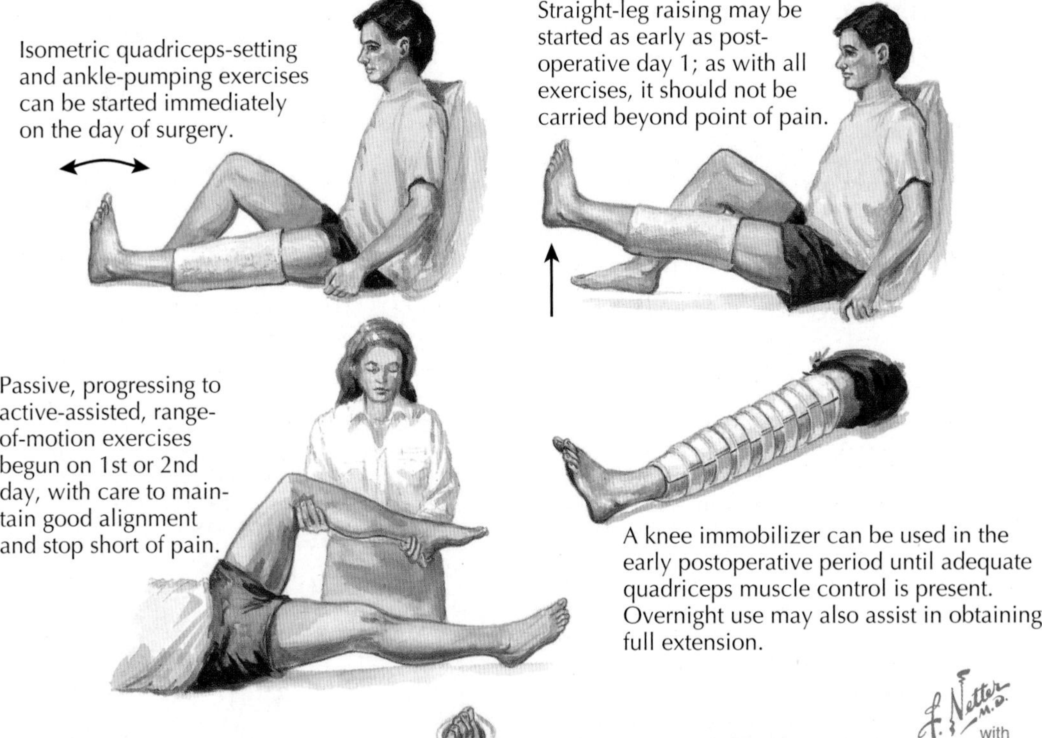

Isometric quadriceps-setting and ankle-pumping exercises can be started immediately on the day of surgery.
Straight-leg raising may be started as early as post-operative day 1; as with all exercises, it should not be carried beyond point of pain.
Passive, progressing to active-assisted, range-of-motion exercises begun on 1st or 2nd day, with care to maintain good alignment and stop short of pain.
A knee immobilizer can be used in the early postoperative period until adequate quadriceps muscle control is present. Overnight use may also assist in obtaining full extension.
F. Netter M.D.
with
D. Mascaro

Continuous passive motion machines are sometimes used in the early post-operative period. Helpful in administration of passive and active-assisted exercises; may expedite increase in range of motion and diminish postoperative pain.

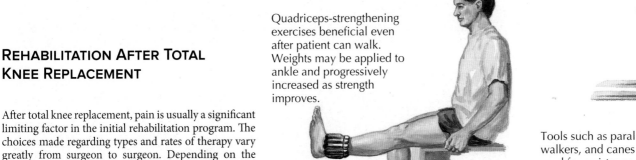

Quadriceps-strengthening exercises beneficial even after patient can walk. Weights may be applied to ankle and progressively increased as strength improves.

Tools such as parallel bars, walkers, and canes may be used for assistance in early ambulation as a patient progresses to weight-bearing without support.

Rehabilitation After Total Knee Replacement

After total knee replacement, pain is usually a significant limiting factor in the initial rehabilitation program. The choices made regarding types and rates of therapy vary greatly from surgeon to surgeon. Depending on the protocol chosen, limited exercises are typically started later the same day or on the first postoperative day. These can include calf pumping to promote circulation, gentle passive knee range of motion, assisted weight-bearing, and incentive spirometry exercises to prevent pulmonary complications. Over the following days, isometric gluteus and quadriceps-setting exercises and straight-leg raises are added. Active-assisted range-of-motion exercises are also an important part of the early therapeutic period. Some surgeons will choose to prescribe the use of a CPM machine in efforts to increase the early range of motion, reduce postoperative pain, and help avoid the need for orthopedic manipulation. Another option is the early use of a knee immobilizer, both to encourage full extension and to protect the patient while there is quadriceps weakness in the early postoperative period. However, this should be discontinued quickly to avoid the development of stiffness.

Over the next several days and weeks, both active and active-assisted range-of-motion exercises are continued to rebuild strength and gain range of motion. The patient progresses to ambulating independently with a walker, crutches, or cane if needed. Ambulation will then continue to be encouraged over greater periods of time and distances. In the early postoperative period, forcible passive exercises or manipulation is avoided.

Once adequate knee flexion has been achieved, maintenance of a normal gait pattern is essential. At this point, strengthening of the quadriceps and hamstring muscles can advance with supervision. If the patient has not achieved adequate range of motion postoperatively, the joint is manipulated under anesthesia.

The rate of progress in rehabilitation depends largely on the determination of the patient and the degree of preoperative impairment.

HIGH TIBIAL OSTEOTOMY FOR VARUS DEFORMITY OF KNEE

High tibial osteotomy is a time-proven operation performed in patients with varus deformity and medial compartment osteoarthritis. Coventry obtained excellent results by removing a wedge of bone based laterally at the level of the tibia proximal to the tibial tuberosity. In 1875 Volkmann contributed the first report of tibial osteotomy. Osteotomy has also been successfully used in revision surgery to correct a faulty primary procedure.

INDICATIONS AND CONTRAINDICATIONS

Valgus-producing osteotomy is performed in a patient with medial compartment degenerative joint disease and a varus deformity of the knee. The varus deformity should not be greater than 15 degrees, because the ligamentous laxity seen in a greater deformity would compromise the postoperative result. Osteotomy is indicated for patients younger than 60 years, although in other countries it is performed in older patients as well. (In the United States, total knee replacement is the preferred treatment in patients older than 60 years.) High tibial osteotomy may also be performed in patients with Blount disease (tibia vara), poliomyelitis, or other dysplasias of the proximal tibia.

Osteotomy is not recommended in patients with varus deformity of the knee greater than 15 degrees, valgus deformity greater than 12 degrees, instability of the collateral ligaments, associated patellofemoral arthritis, fixed flexion contracture greater than 15 degrees, and motion less than 70 degrees.

SURGICAL PLANNING AND TECHNIQUE

A preoperative standing anteroposterior radiograph is taken, and the mechanical axis is measured. Tibial osteotomy should result in an ideal alignment of 5 to 10 degrees of valgus. The amount of bone to be removed must be measured carefully. In a woman, 1 degree of correction can be obtained by a 1-mm wedge of bone; in a man, 8 degrees of correction can be obtained by removing a 10-mm wedge of bone.

Historically, a lateral incision is made at the level of the tibial tuberosity and proximal fibula; a midline incision is often the incision of choice because it may also be used if subsequent knee arthroplasty is required. The anterior muscle compartment is lifted supraperiosteally over the proximal aspect of the tibia, and the tibiofibular syndesmosis can then be identified. The fibula may be obliquely osteotomized to allow full correction. Other options for the fibula include resection of the fibular head or disarticulation of the tibia–fibula syndesmosis so that the fibula can be moved proximally after the osteotomy is closed, although these options may lead to resultant LCL laxity. Intraoperative fluoroscopy and Kirschner wires can be used as guides to plan the size of the wedge to be cut. When the base of the proposed wedge is identified, an oscillating saw and sharp osteotomes are used to remove an appropriately sized wedge of bone. The gap is then closed, the alignment checked, and fixation is applied. Prophylactic release of the anterior compartment of the leg is sometimes done at this point. The wound is then irrigated and closed in layers. A splint or cylinder cast can then be applied with three-point fixation to maintain the valgus alignment, although a bulky dressing and a knee immobilizer removed soon after surgery are often used to allow for early motion.

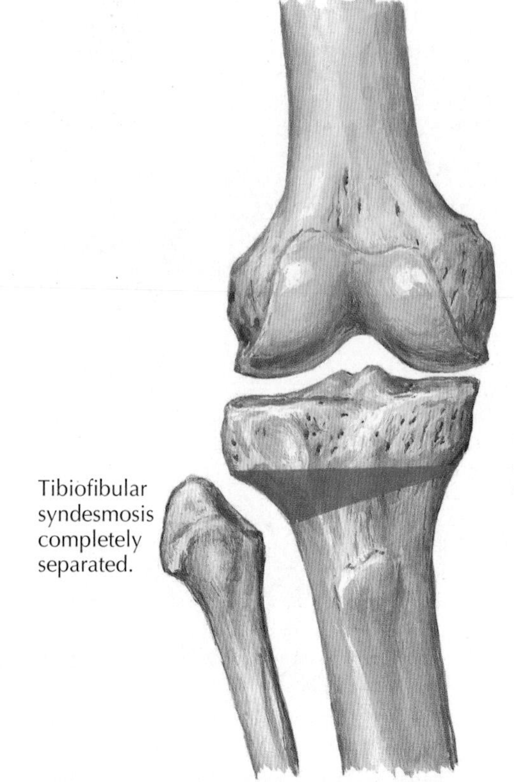

Knee with varus deformity. Blue-shaded area represents wedge of bone to be removed.

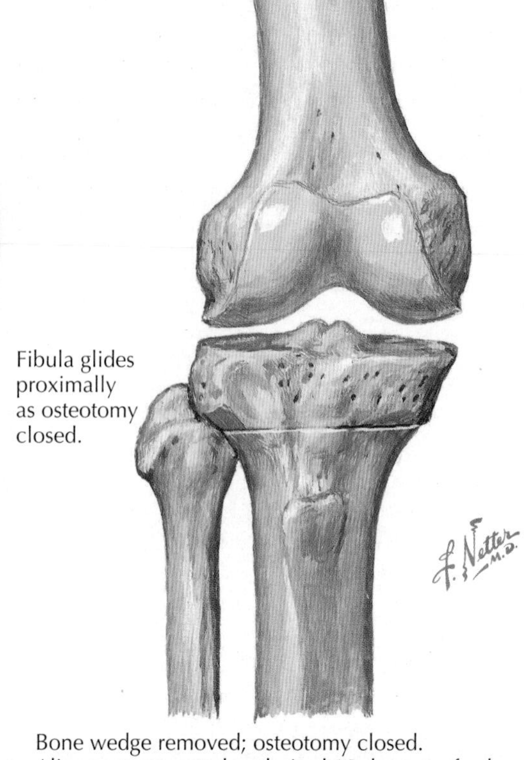

Bone wedge removed; osteotomy closed. Alignment corrected to desired 10 degrees of valgus.

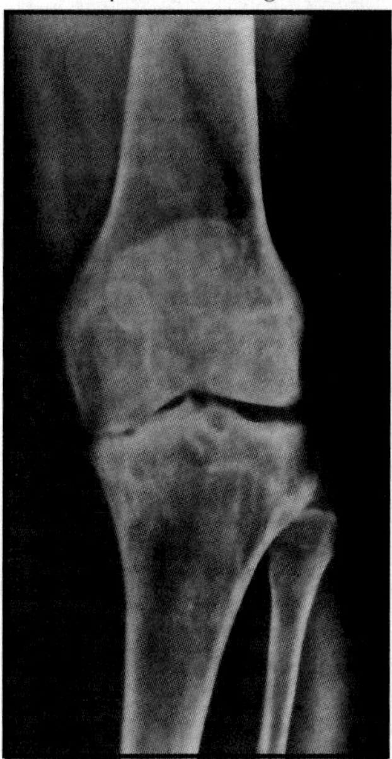

Preoperative standing radiograph reveals varus deformity.

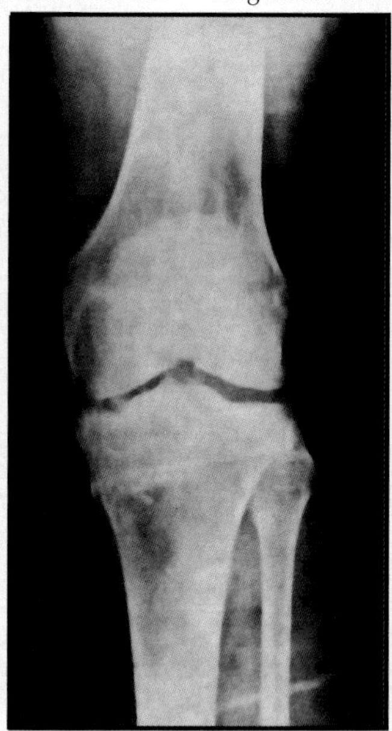

Postoperative standing radiograph shows good result: 10 degrees of valgus.

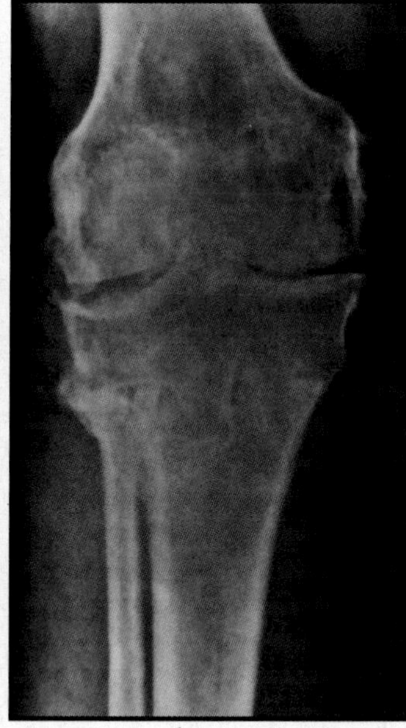

Severe joint deterioration 3 years after surgery. Total knee replacement indicated.

Postoperative care begins with gradual weight-bearing with crutches. A follow-up anteroposterior radiograph is taken after 2 weeks to make sure that the correct alignment is preserved.

RESULTS

Long-term follow-up studies have shown that the high tibial osteotomy results in a significant relief of pain for 2 to 12 years. Full range of motion is preserved, and there is no risk of complications associated with a prosthetic device. However, the same long-term studies revealed deterioration with time at the rate of 1% per year. This procedure should be regarded as one that affords temporary relief of pain until total knee replacement is required. Studies indicate that total knee replacement after osteotomy is not significantly superior to knee arthroplasty without prior osteotomy. Total knee replacement, if necessary, is usually performed about 6 years after the osteotomy. Therefore although high tibial osteotomy is the procedure of choice in younger and more active patients, in older patients the advantages and disadvantages of osteotomy versus total knee replacement should be carefully evaluated.

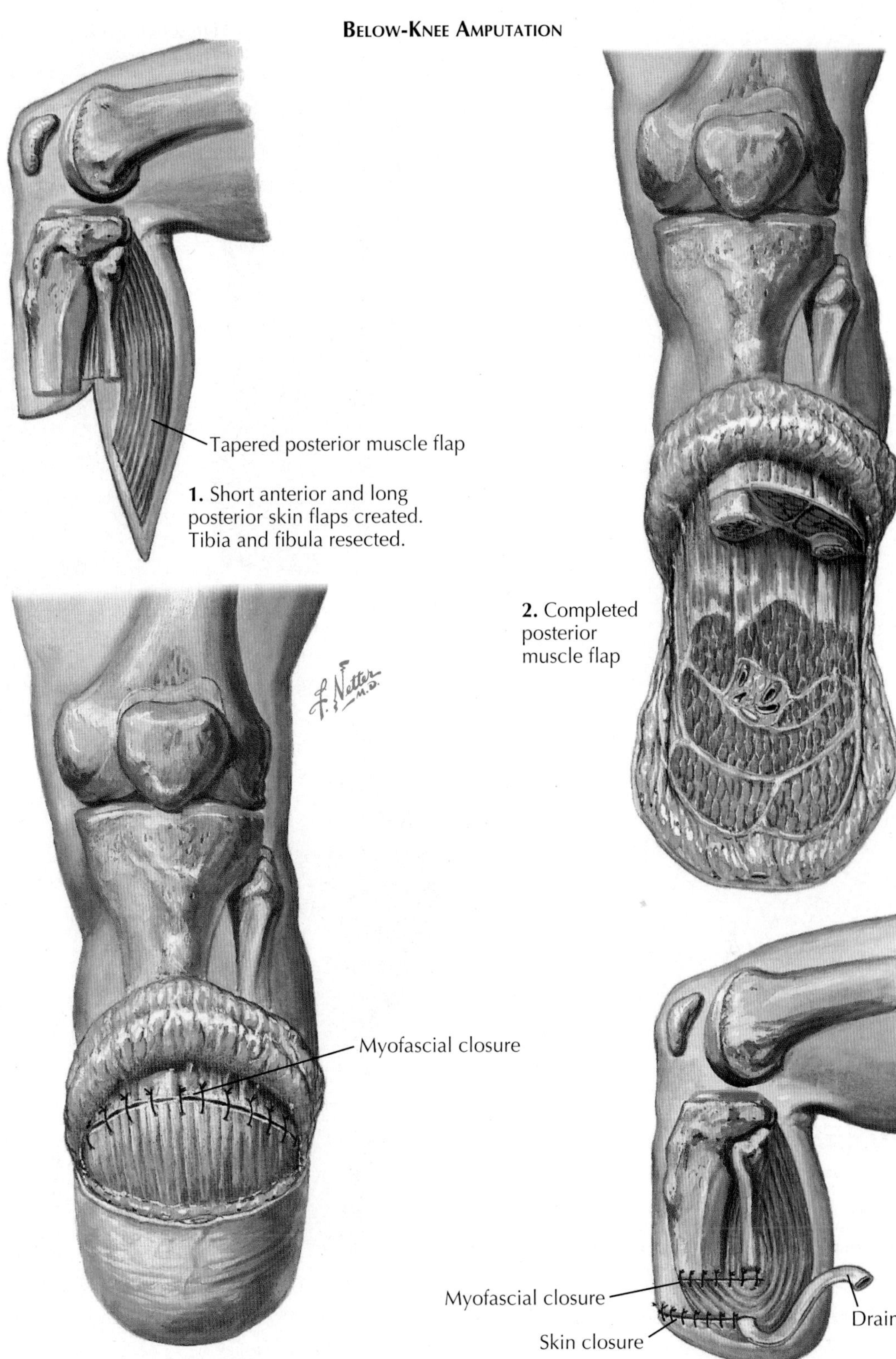

1. Short anterior and long posterior skin flaps created. Tibia and fibula resected.

2. Completed posterior muscle flap

3. Posterior muscle flap sutured to anterior fascia and periosteum

4. Completed closure

Amputation

BELOW-KNEE AMPUTATION

The most common amputation performed in patients with diabetic foot infections and gangrene of the foot resulting from peripheral vascular disease is a below-knee amputation. Both conditions can involve a significant portion of the foot, preventing successful amputation at a more distal level. Because the blood supply to the posterior muscles of the leg is usually better than that to the anterior musculature, the most common method for a below-knee amputation involves the creation of a long posterior muscle and skin flap. Usually, a below-knee amputation is performed at 10 to 15 cm below the level of the knee joint. Appropriate consideration must be made toward potential prosthetic fitting and use before making this decision. The anterior skin incision is made at this level and the tibia transected; the anterior tibial crest is carefully beveled. The fibula is usually transected about 1 cm shorter than the tibia. The posterior muscle mass is preserved 8 to 10 cm longer, along with the posterior skin and subcutaneous tissue. The posterior muscle mass is tapered with a sharp knife, and the long posterior flap is folded forward. The superficial fascia of the posterior muscle flap is sutured to the superficial fascia of the anterior compartment muscles to create a deep myofascial closure. An alternative option is to use a small-diameter drill to make multiple holes circumferentially in the tibial for myodesis using the surrounding muscle. The skin may then be either closed primarily (with or without a drain) or approximated with a vacuum dressing.

The knee joint should be preserved whenever possible. Even a below-knee amputation with a short stump of only 4 or 5 cm may permit some knee joint function, greatly facilitating the fitting of a prosthetic limb. The knee joint also allows the patient to walk more

DISARTICULATION OF KNEE AND ABOVE-KNEE AMPUTATION

Disarticulation of knee

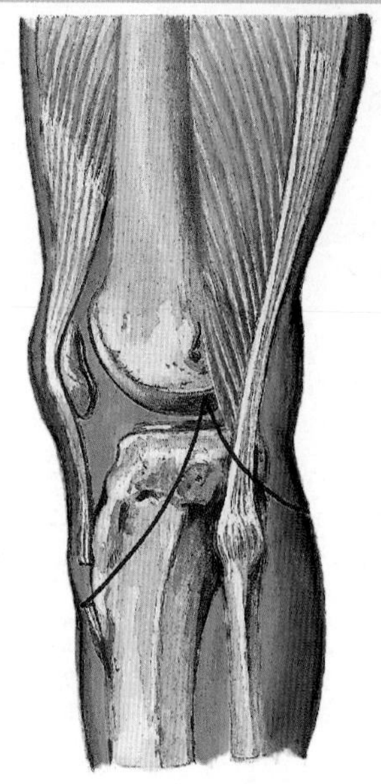

Line of incision. Patellar ligament and pes anserinus included in anterior flap.

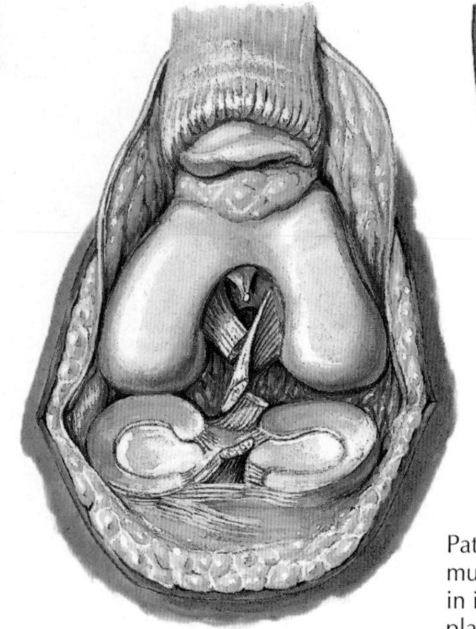

Capsular structures divided and knee disarticulated

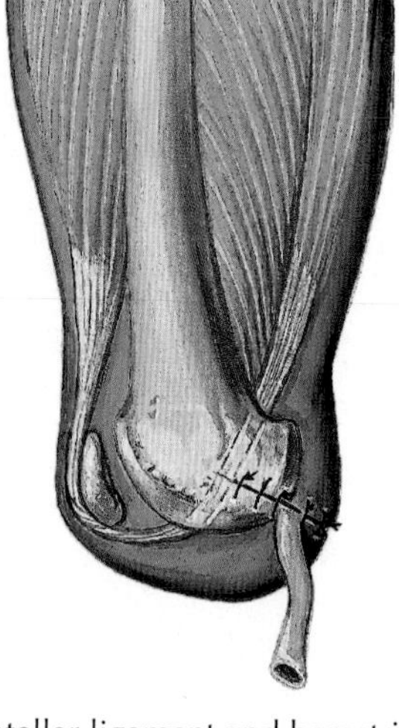

Patellar ligament and hamstring muscles sutured under tension in intercondylar notch. Drain placed and skin flap closed.

Above-knee amputation

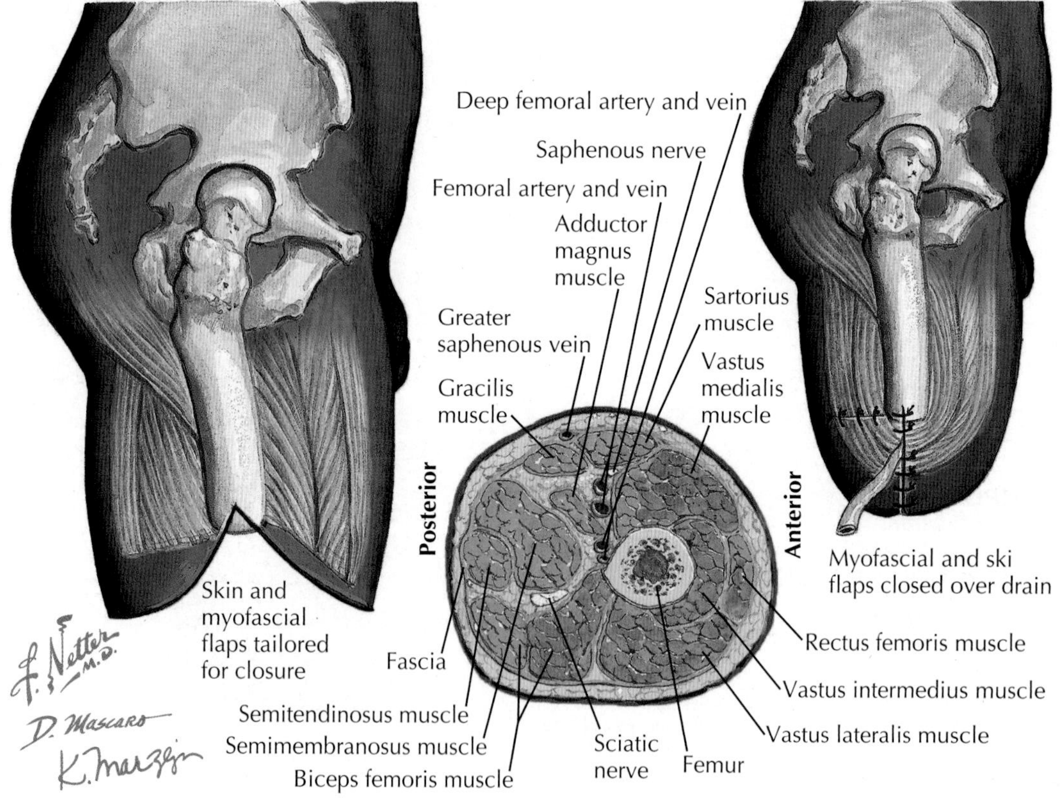

AMPUTATION (Continued)

efficiently. This efficiency is best demonstrated by measuring the oxygen demands of patients with lower limb amputations. When walking on a level surface, patients with a unilateral above-knee amputation use twice as much oxygen as patients with a unilateral below-knee amputation.

DISARTICULATION OF KNEE

This procedure may be chosen when it is not possible to preserve the limb below the level of the knee. Anterior and posterior skin flaps of equal length are fashioned, preserving the patellar ligament and patella. The patellar ligament is sutured into the stumps of the cruciate ligaments to provide a stable point of fixation for the quadriceps femoris muscle. Despite preserving a greater portion of the affected limb, outcomes of knee disarticulations are frequently inferior to above-knee amputations, especially in older patients.

ABOVE-KNEE AMPUTATION

Amputation above the knee is frequently required for severe vascular insufficiency after attempts to reconstruct the vascular tree have failed. The amputation is usually performed through the midportion of the femur. At this level, the blood supply to the muscles of the lower limb improves significantly; very often, viable muscle is encountered. Myodesis of the muscles increases the padding of the residual femur, reduces retraction of the muscles, and facilitates power in the limb by preserving the working length of the muscle unit. The skin is closed primarily, and use of a drain is recommended.

SECTION 4

LOWER LEG

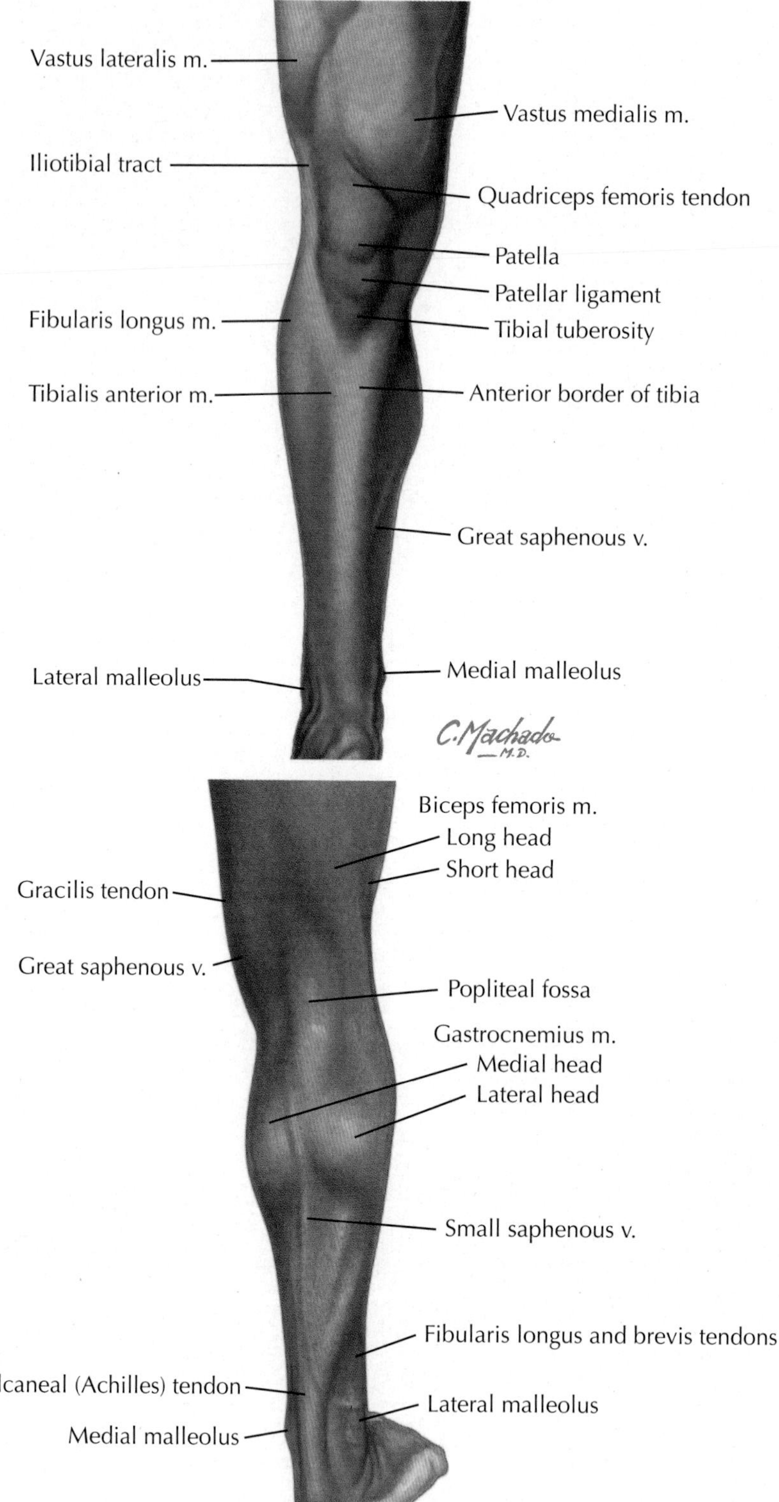

Compartments of Leg

FASCIAE AND COMPARTMENTS

The fascia lata of the thigh continues into the leg, where it is designated as the *crural fascia* (see Plate 4.2). At the knee, the fascia has many attachments—the patella, patellar ligament, tibial tuberosity, condyles of the tibia, and head of the fibula—that reinforce the medial and lateral patellar retinacula. The fascia is strengthened by expansions of the tendons of the sartorius, gracilis, semitendinosus, and biceps femoris muscles. Covering the soft parts of the leg, the crural fascia gives origin to superficial muscle fibers and blends with the periosteum of the subcutaneous surface of the tibia. Above the ankle, it blends with the periosteum of the lower part of the shaft of the fibula. Distally, it attaches to the medial and lateral malleoli and the calcaneus.

Deep extensions of the crural fascia separate certain *compartments* of the leg. The *anterior* and *posterior lateral intermuscular septa* dip deeply to attach to the anterior and posterior borders of the fibula, respectively. They define the lateral compartment of the leg, separating it from the anterior and posterior compartments. From the posterior intermuscular septum adjacent to the fibula, the *transverse intermuscular septum* (deep transverse fascia of the leg) extends medialward, ending on the tibia and in the crural fascia behind it. It separates the superficial and deep posterior compartments of the leg. This sheet is thick over the popliteus muscle and, in the lower part of the leg, lies anterior to the calcaneal tendon. At the ankle, further thickenings of the crural fascia enclose the soft parts and prevent the tendons from bowstringing. One of these is the *superior extensor retinaculum,* which spans across anteriorly from the tibia to the fibula, covers all the muscles of the anterior compartment, and restrains their tendons.

The three intermuscular septa of the leg and the interosseous membrane between the tibia and fibula and the crural fascia define the anterior, lateral, superficial posterior, and deep posterior compartments of the leg. These compartments contain groups of related muscles and vessels and nerves appropriate to them. The two posterior compartments contain preaxial muscles and are served by the tibial nerve; the anterior and lateral compartments contain postaxial muscles and are served by the common peroneal nerve (Plate 4.2).

MUSCLES OF ANTERIOR COMPARTMENT

The anterior compartment contains the tibialis anterior, extensor hallucis longus, extensor digitorum longus, and peroneus tertius muscles, which extend the toes and dorsiflex the foot. In addition, the tibialis anterior muscle inverts the sole of the foot (see Plate 4.3).

The *tibialis anterior muscle* lies against the lateral surface of the tibia. It arises from the lateral condyle of the tibia and from the upper two-thirds of its lateral surface. Fibers also take origin from the interosseous membrane, the overlying crural fascia, and the intermuscular septum between it and the extensor digitorum longus muscle. The tendon appears in the lower third of the leg and passes under the superior and inferior extensor retinacula surrounded by a synovial sheath. It inserts into the medial and inferior surface of the medial cuneiform and the base of the first metatarsal (see Plate 4.5). The tibialis anterior muscle is innervated by the deep peroneal nerve.

The *extensor hallucis longus muscle* is a thin muscle that outcrops between the tibialis anterior and extensor digitorum longus muscles in the lower half of the leg. It arises from the middle half of the anteromedial surface

Fascial Compartments of Leg

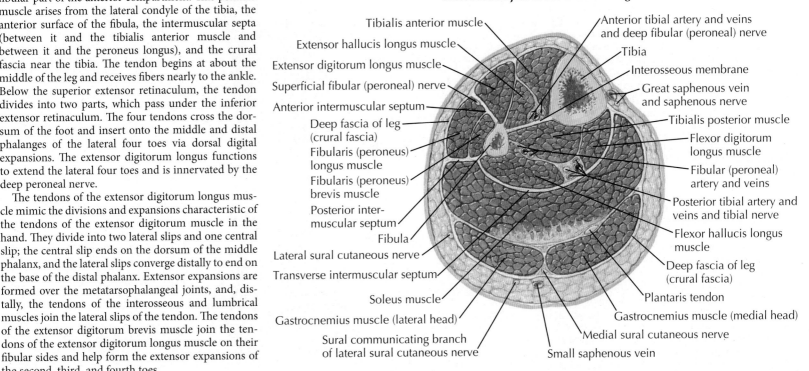

Deep fascia of leg (crural fascia)

Interosseous membrane

Anterior compartment
Extensor muscles
Tibialis anterior
Extensor digitorum longus
Extensor hallucis longus
Fibularis (peroneus) tertius
Anterior tibial artery and veins
Deep fibular (peroneal) nerve

Anterior intermuscular septum

Lateral compartment
Fibularis (peroneus) longus muscle
Fibularis (peroneus) brevis muscle
Superficial fibular (peroneal) nerve

Posterior intermuscular septum

Fibula

Deep fascia of leg (crural fascia)

Tibia

Deep posterior compartment
Deep flexor muscles
Flexor digitorum longus
Tibialis posterior
Flexor hallucis longus
Popliteus
Posterior tibial artery and veins
Tibial nerve
Fibular (peroneal) artery and veins

Transverse intermuscular septum

Superficial posterior compartment
Superficial flexor muscles
Soleus
Gastrocnemius
Plantaris (tendon)

F. Netter M.D.

Cross section just above middle of leg

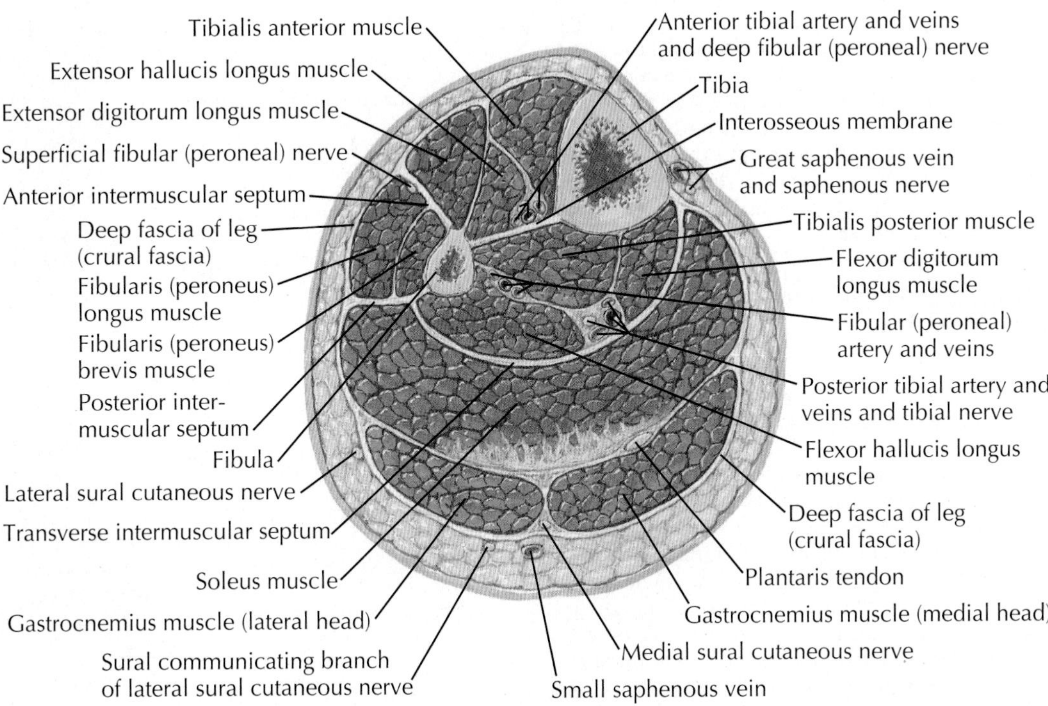

COMPARTMENTS OF LEG (Continued)

of the fibula and from the interosseous membrane for the same distance. Its tendon develops on the superficial surface, passes under the two extensor retinacula, and inserts into the dorsal base of the distal phalanx of the great toe. The extensor hallucis longus functions in extension of the great toe and dorsiflexion of the foot. It is innervated by the deep peroneal nerve (see Plate 4.3).

The *extensor digitorum longus muscle* occupies the fibular part of the anterior compartment. This pennate muscle arises from the lateral condyle of the tibia, the anterior surface of the fibula, the intermuscular septa (between it and the tibialis anterior muscle and between it and the peroneus longus), and the crural fascia near the tibia. The tendon begins at about the middle of the leg and receives fibers nearly to the ankle. Below the superior extensor retinaculum, the tendon divides into two parts, which pass under the inferior extensor retinaculum. The four tendons cross the dorsum of the foot and insert onto the middle and distal phalanges of the lateral four toes via dorsal digital expansions. The extensor digitorum longus functions to extend the lateral four toes and is innervated by the deep peroneal nerve.

The tendons of the extensor digitorum longus muscle mimic the divisions and expansions characteristic of the tendons of the extensor digitorum muscle in the hand. They divide into two lateral slips and one central slip; the central slip ends on the dorsum of the middle phalanx, and the lateral slips converge distally to end on the base of the distal phalanx. Extensor expansions are formed over the metatarsophalangeal joints, and, distally, the tendons of the interosseous and lumbrical muscles join the lateral slips of the tendon. The tendons of the extensor digitorum brevis muscle join the tendons of the extensor digitorum longus muscle on their fibular sides and help form the extensor expansions of the second, third, and fourth toes.

The *peroneus tertius muscle* is essentially a lateral slip of the extensor digitorum longus muscle; it is seldom completely separate, except at its insertion. It arises from the distal third of the anterior surface of the fibula, the adjacent interosseous membrane, and the anterior intermuscular septum. Descending under the extensor retinacula in the compartment for the extensor digitorum longus, it turns lateralward to end on the dorsum of the base of the fifth metatarsal. The peroneus tertius dorsiflexes and everts the foot. It is innervated by the deep peroneal nerve.

MUSCLES OF LATERAL COMPARTMENT

The lateral compartment contains the peroneus longus and the peroneus brevis muscles (see Plate 4.4).

The bipennate *peroneus longus muscle* arises more proximally in the leg and is more superficial. It takes its origin from the head and superior two-thirds of the lateral surface of the body of the fibula, the anterior and posterior intermuscular septa, and the crural fascia. Its tendon begins high on the superficial surface of the muscle and receives fibers (posteriorly) to almost the lateral malleolus. Behind the lateral malleolus, the tendon is posterior to the tendon of the peroneus brevis; both are enclosed within a common synovial sheath and pass deep to the superior peroneal retinaculum. The tendon of the peroneus longus muscle passes diagonally distally, inferior to the tendon of the peroneus brevis muscle, and turns medially into the foot against the anterior slope of the tuberosity of the cuboid. A sesamoid *(os peroneum)* in the tendon protects it over

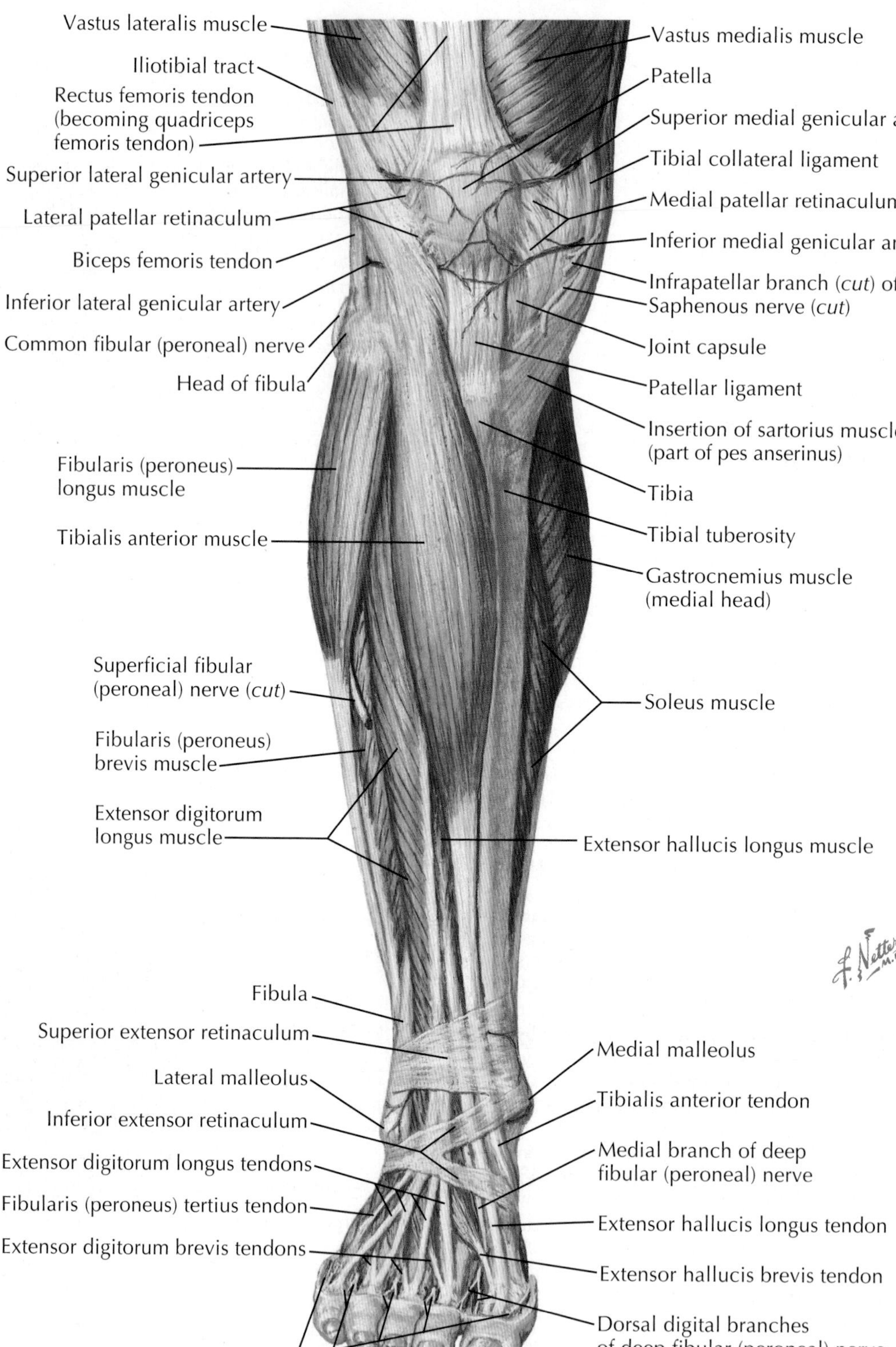

COMPARTMENTS OF LEG (Continued)

the tuberosity. Crossing the sole of the foot deep to its intrinsic muscles, the peroneus longus tendon ends on the inferolateral surface of the medial cuneiform and on the base and inferolateral surface of the first metatarsal. The peroneus longus everts, plantar flexes, and abducts the foot. It is innervated by the superficial peroneal nerve.

The *peroneus brevis muscle* lies deep to the peroneus longus muscle and is smaller and shorter. It arises from the inferior two-thirds of the lateral surface of the fibula and from the anterior and posterior intermuscular septa. Its tendon grooves the back of the lateral malleolus, lying in a common synovial sheath with the tendon of the peroneus longus. Turning anteriorly under the superior peroneal retinaculum, it passes through the inferior peroneal retinaculum to insert into the tuberosity on the base of the fifth metatarsal. The peroneus brevis muscle is an everter of the foot and is innervated by the superficial peroneal nerve.

MUSCLES OF SUPERFICIAL POSTERIOR COMPARTMENT

The gastrocnemius and soleus muscles are supplemented by the almost vestigial plantaris muscle to form a triceps surae complex in the superior posterior compartment (see Plates 4.6 and 4.7). The more superficial *gastrocnemius muscle* arises by two heads. The larger medial head takes origin from the popliteal surface of the femur immediately superior to the medial femoral condyle. The lateral head arises from the superoposterior portion of the lateral surface of the lateral femoral condyle and from the end of the supracondylar line. Bursae separate both heads from the capsule of the knee joint. The fibers of both heads converge toward the midline of the leg and unite at about its mid length into a tendinous raphe, which broadens into an aponeurosis on the anterior surface of the muscle. This aponeurosis fuses below with the tendon of the soleus muscle and, with it, forms the calcaneal tendon. The medial head is usually somewhat broader and thicker, and its muscular fibers descend a bit farther toward the heel. The gastrocnemius plantar flexes the foot, and because it crosses the knee joint it also flexes the knee. It is innervated by the tibial nerve.

The *soleus muscle* is broad and flat, lying immediately anterior to the gastrocnemius muscle but arising entirely distal to the knee. It has a triple origin from (1) the posterior surfaces of the head of the fibula and the upper third of its shaft, (2) a tendinous arch between the tibia and fibula that represents the upper part of the transverse intermuscular septum, and (3) the soleal line of the tibia and its medial border along its middle third. The muscle fibers converge into a broad aponeurosis, which fuses below with that of the gastrocnemius muscle to form the calcaneal tendon, the thickest and strongest tendon in the body. The soleus muscle plantar flexes the foot and is innervated by the tibial nerve.

The calcaneal tendon is about 15 cm long, begins at the middle of the leg, and receives muscular fibers almost to its termination. Narrowed distally, it inserts into the middle part of the posterior surface of the calcaneus; a bursa lies deep to the tendon and separates it from the upper part of the posterior surface of the bone.

The *plantaris muscle* arises from the lower lateral supracondylar line of the femur immediately above the lateral head of the gastrocnemius muscle and from the

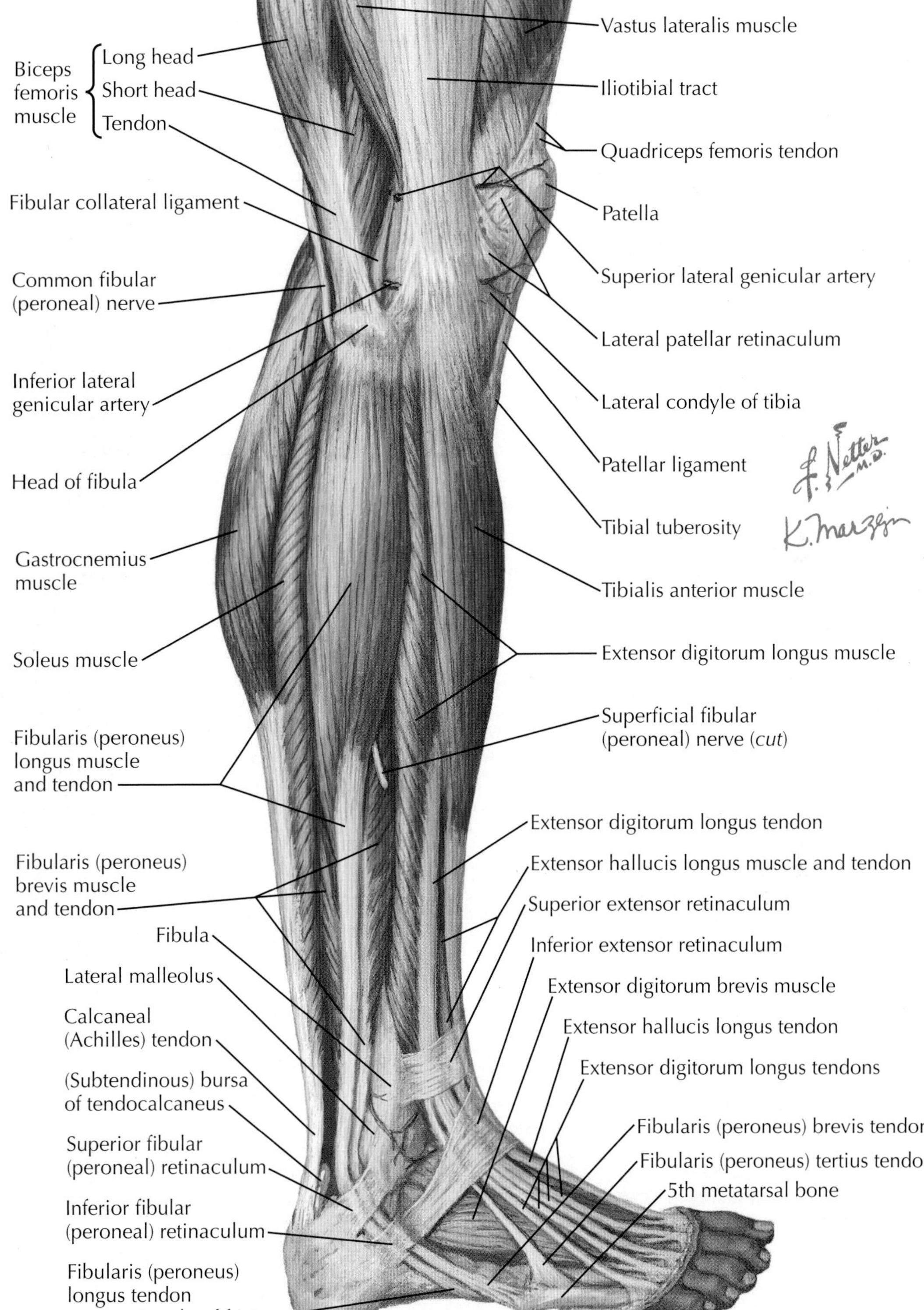

Compartments of Leg (Continued)

oblique popliteal ligament. Its short (10 cm) belly ends in a long, slender tendon that descends between the gastrocnemius and soleus muscles and then continues along the medial border of the calcaneal tendon to insert into the calcaneus. The plantaris muscle plantar flexes the foot and the knee. It is innervated by the tibial nerve.

MUSCLES OF DEEP POSTERIOR COMPARTMENT

The deep posterior compartment contains the popliteus, flexor hallucis longus, flexor digitorum longus, and tibialis posterior muscles (see Plate 4.8).

The *popliteus muscle,* a thin, flat muscle of triangular outline, occupies the floor of the inferior aspect of the popliteal fossa. It arises mainly by a stout cord from the anterior end of the groove on the lateral face of the lateral femoral condyle, close to the articular margin. The tendon passes between the lateral meniscus and the capsule of the knee joint, with the subpopliteal recess of synovial membrane lying between them. As much as one-half of its fibers may come from the arcuate popliteal ligament, with others arising in the lateral meniscus. The muscle inserts by fleshy fibers into the triangular area above the soleal line of the back of the tibia. The popliteus rotates the femur laterally on the tibia to help initiate flexion at the knee. It is innervated by the tibial nerve.

The *flexor hallucis longus muscle* lies on the fibular rather than the tibial side of the leg. It arises from the lower two-thirds of the posterior surface of the shaft of the fibula and from the intermuscular septa separating it from the tibialis posterior and peroneus brevis muscles. Its tendon grooves the posterior surface of the talus and the undersurface of the sustentaculum tali of the calcaneus. It passes forward in the sole of the foot, giving a slip to the overlying flexor digitorum longus muscle, and then passes between the two heads of the flexor hallucis brevis muscle to insert into the base of the distal phalanx of the great toe. The flexor hallucis longus flexes the great toe and provides some plantar flexion of the foot. It is innervated by the tibial nerve (see Plate 4.8).

The *flexor digitorum longus muscle* is found on the tibial side of the leg. It arises from the medial side of the posterior surface of the middle three-fifths of the tibia and from the intermuscular septum between it and the tibialis posterior muscle. Its pennate fibers converge to a tendon that lies along the medial margin of the muscle and receives fibers almost to the medial malleolus. At the ankle, the tendon of the tibialis posterior muscle is anterior to that of the flexor digitorum longus muscle. Both tendons (tibialis posterior and flexor digitorum longus) enter the foot through a groove on the back of the medial malleolus, where they are enclosed in separate synovial sheaths, that on the tendon of flexor digitorum longus muscle; the sheath of the tendon of flexor digitorum longus passes well into the foot. The tendon of the flexor digitorum longus muscle passes diagonally into the sole of the foot, crossing the deltoid ligament of the ankle joint and running superficial to the tendon of the flexor hallucis longus muscle from which it receives a slip.

In the middle of the sole, the tendon of the flexor digitorum longus muscle receives the insertion of the quadratus plantae muscle and then divides into four tendons; these insert into the bases of the distal phalanges of the second, third, fourth, and fifth toes. Like the tendons of the flexor digitorum profundus muscle in

Muscles, Arteries, and Nerves of Leg: Deep Dissection (Anterior View)

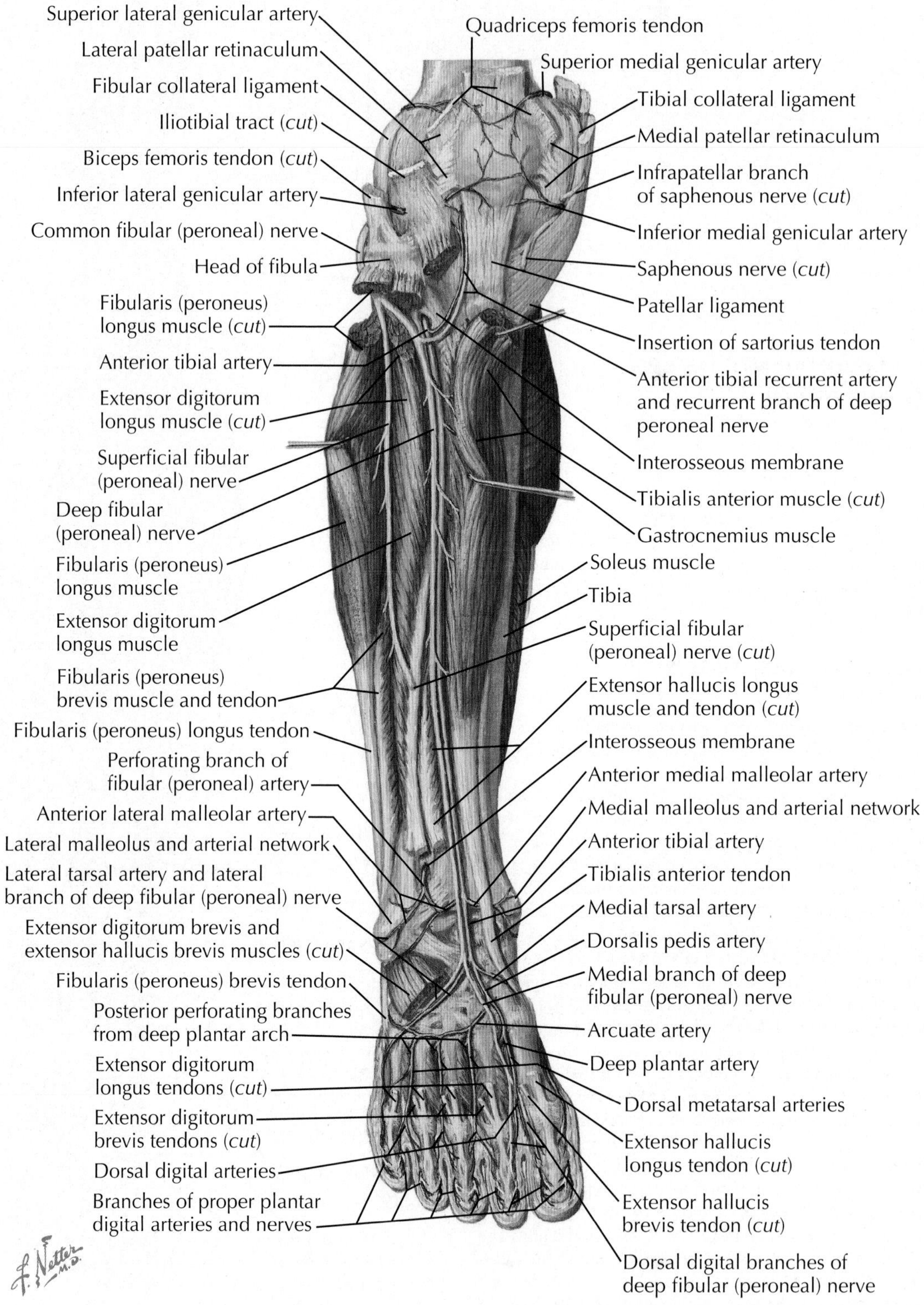

Superior lateral genicular artery
Lateral patellar retinaculum
Fibular collateral ligament
Iliotibial tract (*cut*)
Biceps femoris tendon (*cut*)
Inferior lateral genicular artery
Common fibular (peroneal) nerve
Head of fibula
Fibularis (peroneus) longus muscle (*cut*)
Anterior tibial artery
Extensor digitorum longus muscle (*cut*)
Superficial fibular (peroneal) nerve
Deep fibular (peroneal) nerve
Fibularis (peroneus) longus muscle
Extensor digitorum longus muscle
Fibularis (peroneus) brevis muscle and tendon
Fibularis (peroneus) longus tendon
Perforating branch of fibular (peroneal) artery
Anterior lateral malleolar artery
Lateral malleolus and arterial network
Lateral tarsal artery and lateral branch of deep fibular (peroneal) nerve
Extensor digitorum brevis and extensor hallucis brevis muscles (*cut*)
Fibularis (peroneus) brevis tendon
Posterior perforating branches from deep plantar arch
Extensor digitorum longus tendons (*cut*)
Extensor digitorum brevis tendons (*cut*)
Dorsal digital arteries
Branches of proper plantar digital arteries and nerves
Quadriceps femoris tendon
Superior medial genicular artery
Tibial collateral ligament
Medial patellar retinaculum
Infrapatellar branch of saphenous nerve (*cut*)
Inferior medial genicular artery
Saphenous nerve (*cut*)
Patellar ligament
Insertion of sartorius tendon
Anterior tibial recurrent artery and recurrent branch of deep peroneal nerve
Interosseous membrane
Tibialis anterior muscle (*cut*)
Gastrocnemius muscle
Soleus muscle
Tibia
Superficial fibular (peroneal) nerve (*cut*)
Extensor hallucis longus muscle and tendon (*cut*)
Interosseous membrane
Anterior medial malleolar artery
Medial malleolus and arterial network
Anterior tibial artery
Tibialis anterior tendon
Medial tarsal artery
Dorsalis pedis artery
Medial branch of deep fibular (peroneal) nerve
Arcuate artery
Deep plantar artery
Dorsal metatarsal arteries
Extensor hallucis longus tendon (*cut*)
Extensor hallucis brevis tendon (*cut*)
Dorsal digital branches of deep fibular (peroneal) nerve

F. Netter M.D.

Compartments of Leg (Continued)

the hand, the tendons of the flexor digitorum longus muscle give origin to lumbrical muscles in the foot. Also, the relationships of these tendons to those of the flexor digitorum brevis muscle and to synovial sheaths and the fibrous digital sheaths are similar to those in the hand. The flexor digitorum longus flexes the lateral four toes and provides some plantar flexion of the foot. It is innervated by the tibial nerve.

The *tibialis posterior muscle* is the most deeply situated muscle in the posterior compartment and lies between the flexor digitorum longus and flexor hallucis longus muscles. Beginning superiorly in two pointed processes, the muscle arises from the lateral part of the posterior surface of the tibia in its upper two-thirds, the upper two-thirds of the medial surface of the fibula, the intermuscular septa on either side of it, the transverse intermuscular septum of the leg, and all the interosseus membrane except the inferiormost aspect. The posterior tibialis tendon emerges from the medial side of the muscle at about the middle of the leg and continues to receive fibers almost to the medial malleolus. The tendon lies posterior to the medial malleolus and anterior to that of the flexor digitorum longus muscle, and it enters the foot under the flexor retinaculum within its own synovial sheath. It crosses the deltoid ligament of the ankle, passes under the plantar calcaneonavicular ligament, and inserts into the tuberosity of the navicular and the underside of the medial cuneiform. Expansions continue forward and lateralward to the intermediate and lateral cuneiforms and to the plantar surfaces of the bases of the second to fourth metatarsals. The tibialis posterior inverts and plantar flexes the foot and supports the medial arch of the foot. It is innervated by the tibial nerve.

MUSCLE ACTIONS

The muscles of the superficial posterior compartment all insert into the tuberosity of the calcaneus; they act together to produce plantar flexion of the foot, accompanied by some inversion. Thus they raise the heel against the weight of the body in locomotion. In standing, these muscles draw back on the leg, stabilizing the ankle joint. The gastrocnemius arises above the knee and flexes it as well. It shows intermittent activity in relaxed standing because the ankle joint is not then in its close-packed position.

In the deep posterior compartment, the popliteus muscle is a weak flexor of the knee and can rotate the leg internally. With the foot firmly on the ground, the contraction of the muscle lends to lateral rotation of the femur with retraction of the lateral meniscus and starts flexion at the knee. The other muscles of this compartment assist in plantar flexion of the foot and are invertors. The flexor hallucis longus and flexor digitorum longus muscles flex the phalanges. The flexor hallucis longus muscle shows its greatest activity at heel-off. The tibialis posterior muscle distributes body weight among the heads of the metatarsals, serving to reduce flatfoot and shifting weight toward the lateral side of the foot.

Most of the muscles of the anterior compartment of the leg dorsiflex and invert the foot at the ankle. The tibialis anterior muscle is powerful in this action. Additionally, the extensor hallucis longus muscle dorsiflexes the great toe, and the extensor digitorum longus muscle has a like action on the second to fifth toes through the insertion of its tendons into the proximal and middle phalanges of these digits. The peroneus

MUSCLES OF LEG: SUPERFICIAL DISSECTION (POSTERIOR VIEW)

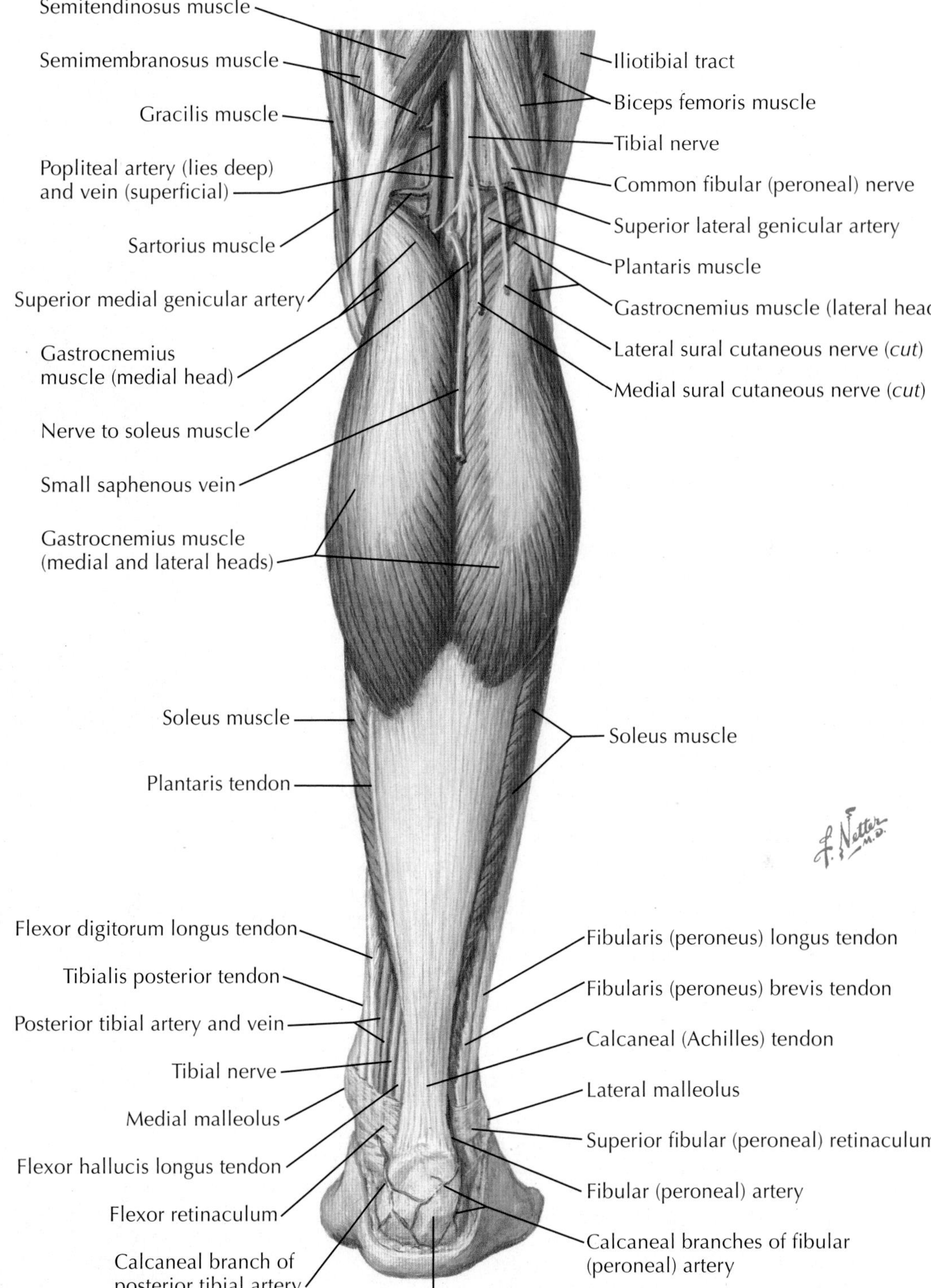

COMPARTMENTS OF LEG (Continued)

tertius muscle produces an eversion rather than an inversion effect.

The peroneus longus and peroneus brevis muscles of the lateral compartment evert and abduct the foot and assist in its plantar flexion. With respect to inversion and eversion, the insertions of the tibialis anterior and peroneus longus muscles on the same bones place the foot in a sling that is controlled immediately by the pull of these muscles.

An important fact is that a normally strong foot does not depend on muscles for ordinary static support; the muscles of the leg are generally quiescent in relaxed standing. Static support is provided by the many supporting ligaments of the joint capsules, which hold the bones in the normal arched architecture. However, in a flatfooted person or in one with other serious foot impairment, leg muscles come into play for support.

BLOOD VESSELS

Arteries

The *popliteal artery* is the direct continuation of the femoral artery at the adductor hiatus. Passing to the posterior aspect of the knee at the hiatus, the artery descends through the popliteal space with a slight mediolateral inclination between the gastrocnemius and soleus, deep to the tendinous arch of the soleus. It ends at the lower border of the popliteus muscle by dividing into the anterior tibial and posterior tibial arteries. The artery is deeper in the popliteal space than the corresponding vein and the tibial nerve, lying in the intercondylar fossa of the femur and against the posterior capsule of the knee joint. More inferiorly, it crosses the popliteus muscle. The popliteal artery gives off five genicular branches and several large sural arteries.

The *lateral superior genicular artery* passes against the plantaris muscle and above the lateral femoral condyle. Deep to the tendon of the biceps femoris muscle, it winds around the femur and supplies a superficial branch, which enters the vastus lateralis muscle and anastomoses with the descending branch of the lateral circumflex femoral artery and the lateral inferior genicular artery. It also gives rise to a deep branch supplying the knee joint and anastomosing across the front of the femur with the descending genicular and medial superior genicular arteries.

The *medial superior genicular artery* swings across the origin of the medial head of the gastrocnemius muscle anterior to the tendons of the semitendinosus and semimembranosus muscles. One branch supplies the vastus medialis muscle and anastomoses with the descending genicular (a branch of the femoral artery originating above the adductor hiatus) and medial inferior genicular arteries. A second branch supplies the knee joint and anastomoses with the lateral superior genicular artery by the anastomotic arch across the femur.

The *middle genicular artery* is a small single vessel arising from the anterior surface of the popliteal artery at the back of the knee. It pierces the oblique popliteal ligament to supply the cruciate ligaments and the synovial membrane within the joint cavity.

The *sural arteries* are usually two large muscular branches that enter the heads of the gastrocnemius muscles and send branches to the plantaris muscle and the upper part of the soleus. More proximal unnamed muscular branches supply the lower ends of

MUSCLES OF LEG: INTERMEDIATE DISSECTION (POSTERIOR VIEW)

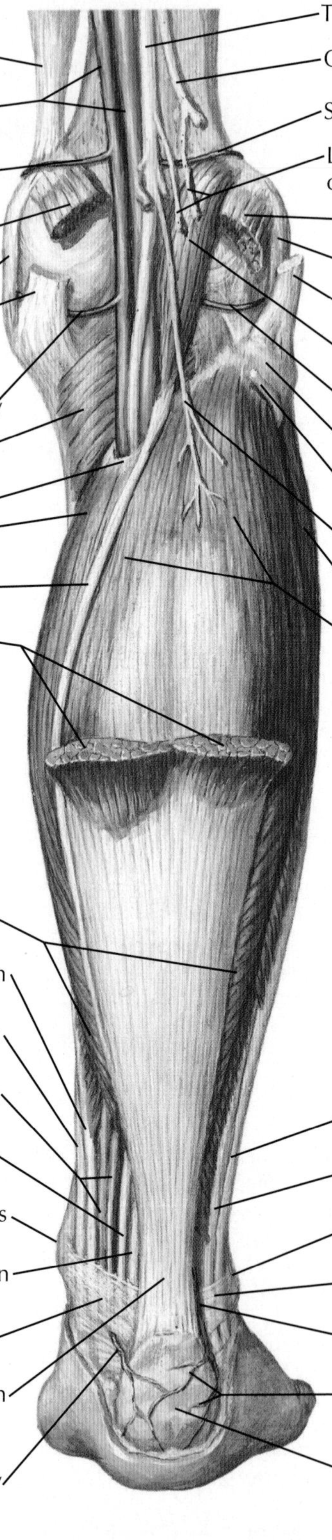

Adductor magnus tendon
Popliteal artery (deep) and vein (superficial)
Superior medial genicular artery
Gastrocnemius muscle (medial head) (*cut*)
Tibial collateral ligament
Semimembranosus tendon (*cut*)
Inferior medial genicular artery
Popliteus muscle
Tendinous arch of Soleus muscle
Plantaris tendon
Gastrocnemius muscle (*cut*)
Tibial nerve
Common fibular (peroneal) nerve (*cut*)
Superior lateral genicular artery
Lateral and medial sural cutaneous nerves (*cut*)
Gastrocnemius muscle (lateral head) (*cut*)
Fibular collateral ligament
Biceps femoris tendon (*cut*)
Plantaris muscle
Inferior lateral genicular artery
Head of fibula
Common fibular (peroneal) nerve (*cut*)
Nerve to soleus muscle
Fibularis (peroneus) longus muscle
Soleus muscle
Soleus muscle inserting into calcaneal (Achilles) tendon
Flexor digitorum longus tendon
Tibialis posterior tendon
Posterior tibial artery and vein
Tibial nerve
Medial malleolus
Flexor hallucis longus tendon
Flexor retinaculum
Calcaneal (Achilles) tendon
Calcaneal branch of posterior tibial artery
Fibularis (peroneus) longus tendon
Fibularis (peroneus) brevis tendon
Lateral malleolus
Superior fibular (peroneal) retinaculum
Fibular (peroneal) artery
Calcaneal branches of fibular (peroneal) artery
Calcaneal tuberosity
F. Netter M.D.

COMPARTMENTS OF LEG (Continued)

the hamstring muscles. A cutaneous branch descends along the middle of the back of the calf with the lesser saphenous vein.

The *lateral inferior genicular artery* crosses the upper portion of the popliteus muscle deep to the lateral head of the gastrocnemius muscle. Turning anteriorly internal to the fibular collateral ligament, it divides into branches, which anastomose with the lateral superior genicular, medial inferior genicular, anterior and posterior tibial recurrent, and circumflex fibular arteries.

The *medial inferior genicular artery* passes medialward along the upper borders of the popliteus muscle and on the medial side of the knee is deep to the tibial collateral ligament. At the anterior border of the ligament, various branches spread to anastomose with the descending genicular and medial superior genicular arteries and with the lateral inferior genicular and anterior tibial recurrent arteries.

The *anterior tibial artery* is one product of the division of the popliteal artery. It passes directly anterior above the superior end of the interosseous membrane of the leg and thereby enters the anterior compartment, lying against the medial side of the neck of the fibula. The artery descends on the interosseous membrane, first lying between the tibialis anterior and extensor digitorum longus muscles and then between the tibialis anterior and the extensor hallucis longus muscles. It is joined on its lateral side by the deep peroneal nerve. The tendon of the extensor hallucis longus muscle crosses the vessels and nerve, which then lie between the tendon of the extensor hallucis longus and extensor digitorum longus muscle at the ankle. The anterior tibial artery continues as the dorsalis pedis artery. The named branches of the anterior tibial artery are the posterior tibial recurrent, circumflex fibular, anterior tibial recurrent, anterior medial malleolar, and anterior lateral malleolar arteries and are concentrated at the knee and ankle.

The *posterior tibial recurrent artery,* sometimes a branch of the posterior tibial artery, usually arises from the anterior tibial artery in the posterior compartment of the leg. It ascends between the popliteus muscle and the back of the knee, supplies the popliteus and the tibiofibular joint, and anastomoses with the lateral inferior genicular artery. The small *circumflex fibular artery* also arises from the anterior tibial artery before that vessel leaves the posterior compartment of the leg; at times, it may be a branch of the posterior tibial artery. It passes around the neck of the fibula through the soleus muscle, supplying it, and anastomoses with the lateral inferior genicular artery. The *anterior tibial recurrent artery* arises as soon as the anterior tibial artery enters the anterior compartment of the leg. It ascends among the fibers of the tibialis anterior muscle and then branches over the front and sides of the knee joint. It anastomoses with the genicular branches of the popliteal artery and with the descending genicular and the lateral circumflex femoral branches of the femoral artery. The *anterior medial malleolar artery* takes origin at the ankle. It passes medialward, deep to the tendons of the tibialis anterior and extensor hallucis longus muscles. It supplies the skin and the ankle joint medially, anastomosing with the malleolar branches of the posterior tibial artery. The *anterior lateral malleolar artery* arises opposite the anterior medial malleolar artery and passes lateralward, deep to the tendons of the extensor digitorum longus muscle. It supplies the lateral surface of the ankle and the joint and anastomoses

Muscles, Arteries, and Nerves of Leg: Deep Dissection (Posterior View)

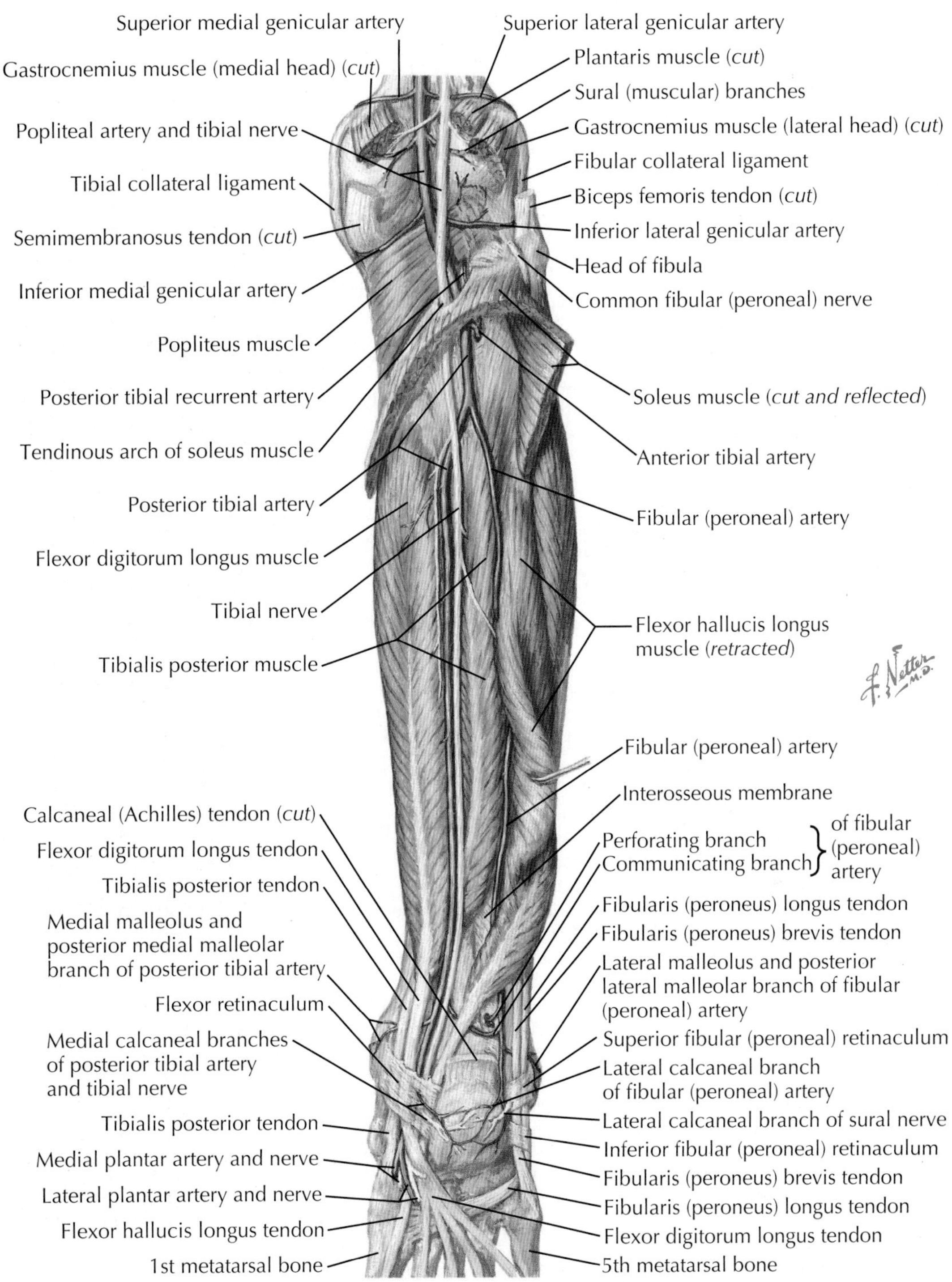

Compartments of Leg (Continued)

with the perforating branch of the peroneal artery and with ascending branches of the lateral tarsal branch of the dorsalis pedis artery.

The *posterior tibial artery* begins at the inferior border of the popliteus muscle and is the direct continuation of the popliteal artery. Accompanied by its veins and by the tibial nerve, it descends in the deep posterior compartment. At first, it inclines toward the fibula; then, after giving off the peroneal artery, it swings medially again and passes behind the medial malleolus at the ankle. It ends deep to the origin of the abductor hallucis muscle by dividing into the medial plantar and lateral plantar arteries. Apart from the peroneal artery, which is described separately, and muscular arteries throughout the leg, the branches of the posterior tibial artery are not large. A *nutrient artery* arises in the upper part of the leg to enter the tibia posteriorly. A *communicating branch* passes laterally, just above the tibiofibular syndesmosis, to join a similar branch of the peroneal artery. The *posterior medial malleolar branch* passes onto the medial malleolus and anastomoses with the anterior medial malleolar branch of the anterior tibial artery, and *medial calcaneal branches* arise just proximal to the artery's division. They reach the skin and areolar tissues of the medial side and back of the heel.

The *peroneal artery* is the largest branch of the posterior tibial artery. It supplies the muscles of the lateral side of the leg and is an important longitudinal collateral vessel through its communicating branch to the posterior tibial artery and its perforating branch to the anterior tibial artery. The peroneal artery arises 2 to 3 cm beyond the origin of the posterior tibial artery and descends near the fibula within the substance of the flexor hallucis longus muscle or between it and the tibialis posterior muscle. A *nutrient branch* enters the nutrient foramen of the fibula. The *perforating branch* passes forward at the distal border of the interosseous membrane to enter the anterior compartment of the leg. It supplies the joints at the ankle and anastomoses with the anterior lateral malleolar branch of the anterior tibial artery and with the lateral tarsal and arcuate branches of the dorsalis pedis artery. The *communicating branch* arises just below the perforating branch, runs medialward deep to the tendon of the flexor hallucis longus muscle, and joins the communicating branch of the posterior tibial artery. The *posterior lateral malleolar branch* supplies small branches to the lateral malleolus and anastomoses with the anterior lateral malleolar branch of the anterior tibial artery. It also gives off *lateral calcaneal branches.*

Veins

The veins of the leg are paired accompanying vessels of the arteries. They are supplied with numerous valves and receive many perforating communications from the superficial veins. The unions of the venae comitantes of the anterior tibial, posterior tibial, and peroneal veins are made at various levels; they form the popliteal vein. (A single popliteal vein is typically expected at about 5 cm above the knee joint.) The *popliteal vein* is typically a large single vein that ascends through the popliteal space superficial to its artery and between it and the tibial nerve. It is somewhat medial to the artery inferiorly but against its lateral side above the knee joint. Three or four bicuspid valves prevent descending flow in the vein, and one of these valves is rather consistently located just distal to the adductor hiatus. Other tributaries of the popliteal vein are genicular and muscular veins as well as the lesser saphenous vein.

Nerves of Leg: Common Peroneal Nerve

The common peroneal nerve (L4, L5, S1, S2) is the smaller, lateral terminal branch of the sciatic nerve (Plate 4.9). Its fibers are derived from the posterior divisions of the ventral rami of L4, L5, S1, and S2. From its origin, the nerve descends first along the lateral side of the popliteal fossa, overlapped by the medial margin of the biceps femoris. Then it passes between the biceps tendon and the lateral head of the gastrocnemius muscle to reach the posterior aspect of the fibular head. Finally, it winds around the posterior and lateral side of the neck of the fibula between the two heads of the peroneus longus muscle and divides into the *superficial* and *deep peroneal nerves.* At this point, the nerve is at risk for injury, as it can easily be compressed against the underlying bone.

Before dividing, the common peroneal nerve gives off three *articular branches* to the knee, which accompany the lateral superior and inferior genicular and anterior tibial recurrent arteries. It also gives off the *lateral sural cutaneous nerve,* which supplies the skin and fascia on the lateral and adjacent parts of the posterior and anterior surfaces of the upper part of the leg, and the *peroneal communicating branch,* which joins the sural branch of the tibial nerve and is distributed with it.

The *superficial peroneal nerve* descends between the extensor digitorum longus and peroneal muscles and supplies the peroneus longus and peroneus brevis muscles before piercing the deep fascia at about the junction of the middle and lower thirds of the leg. At this level, the nerve divides into medial and intermediate dorsal cutaneous nerves. The *medial dorsal cutaneous nerve* runs anterior to the ankle and onto the dorsum of the foot, supplying branches to the skin and fascia on the anterior surface of the distal third of the leg and the dorsum of the foot. Near the lower border of the inferior extensor retinaculum it splits into two *dorsal digital nerves;* one of these nerves supplies the medial and dorsal aspects of the dorsum of the foot and the great toe (except the first dorsal web space), and the other supplies the adjacent sides of the second and third toes. The *intermediate dorsal cutaneous nerve* runs along the lateral part of the dorsum of the foot, supplying the nearby skin and fascia and providing the dorsal digital nerves for the third and fourth, and fourth and fifth toes. It communicates with the lateral dorsal cutaneous nerve, the termination of the sural nerve.

The *deep peroneal nerve* passes obliquely forward and downward around the fibular neck between the peroneus longus and the extensor digitorum longus muscles to the front of the interosseous membrane. It descends lateral to the tibialis anterior muscle and is a medial relation first to the extensor digitorum longus muscle and then to the extensor hallucis longus muscle, the tendon of which crosses the nerve obliquely above the ankle. In its downward course, the nerve first lies lateral to the anterior tibial vessels, then anterior to them, and finally lateral to them again in front of the lower end of the tibia and ankle, where the nerve divides into medial and lateral terminal branches. In the leg, the nerve sends branches to the tibialis anterior, extensor digitorum longus, extensor hallucis longus, and peroneus tertius muscles; an articular branch to the ankle; and small branches to the anterior tibial vessels. The *medial terminal branch* gives rise to a *dorsal digital nerve,* which splits to supply the contiguous sides of the first and second toes, notably the first dorsal web space. It also supplies small branches to the dorsalis pedis artery and nearby metatarsophalangeal and interphalangeal joints and, occasionally, a small branch to the first dorsal interosseous muscle. The *lateral terminal branch* curves outward beneath the extensor digitorum brevis muscle, becomes slightly expanded, and gives off several slender offshoots to supply the extensor digitorum brevis muscle and its medial part (the extensor hallucis brevis muscle), the adjacent tarsal and tarsometatarsal joints, and, rarely, the second and third dorsal interosseous muscles.

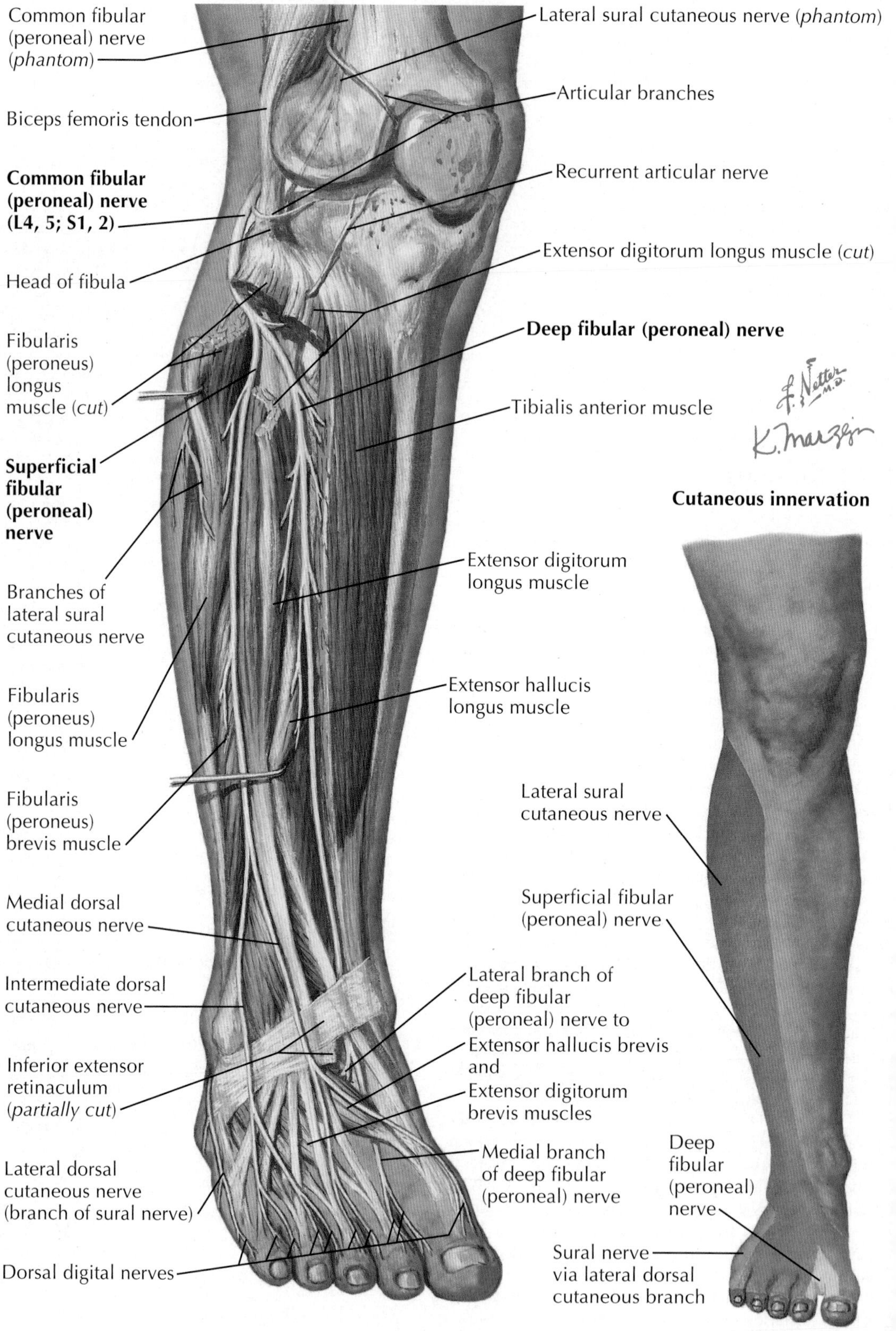

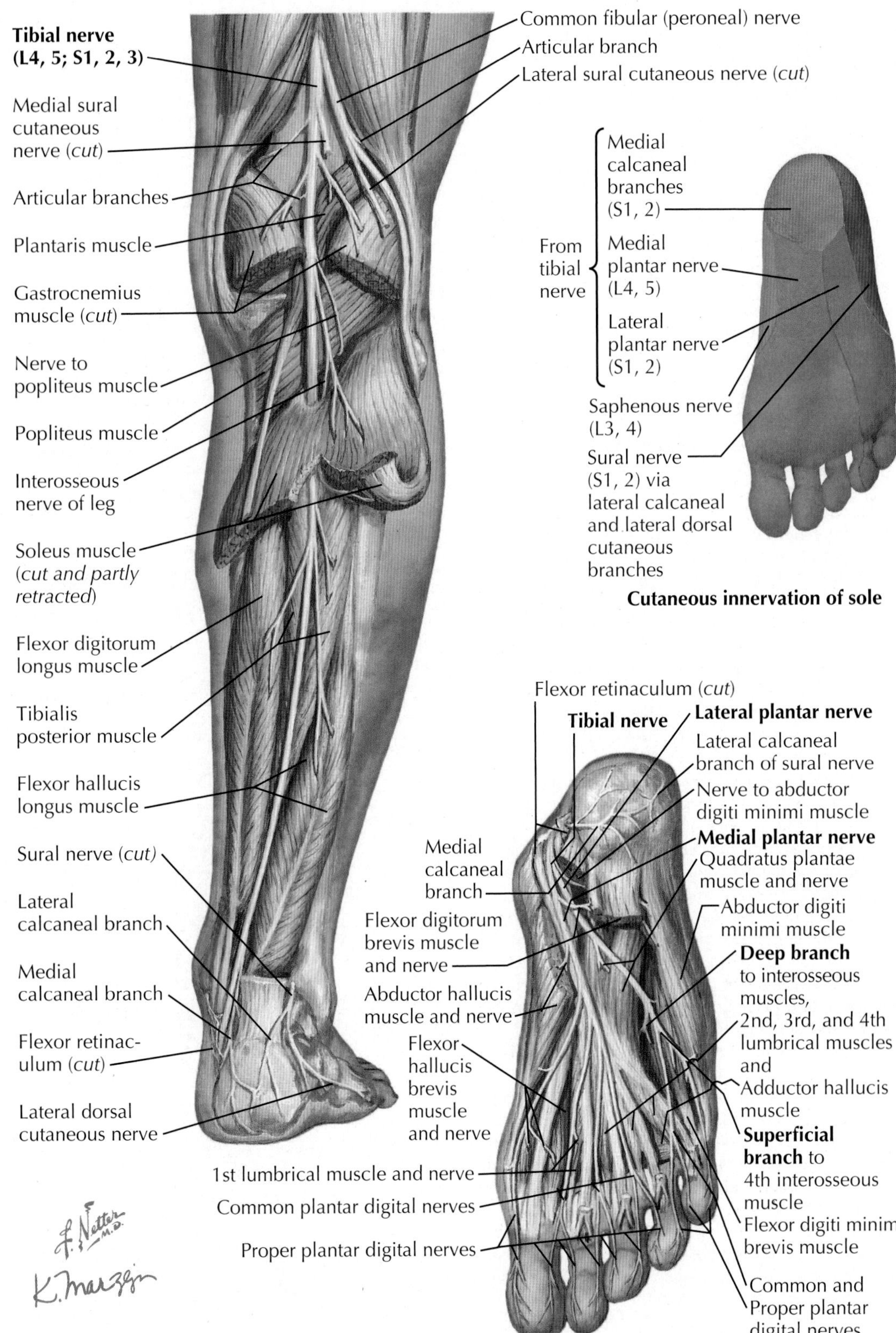

NERVES OF LEG: TIBIAL NERVE

The *tibial nerve* (L4, L5, S1, S2, S3) is the larger and medial terminal branch of the sciatic nerve (see Plate 4.10). Its fibers are derived from the anterior divisions of the ventral rami of L4 and L5 and S1, S2, and S3.

The tibial nerve continues the line of the sciatic nerve through the popliteal fossa and into the leg. At its origin, the nerve is overlapped by the adjoining margins of the semimembranosus and biceps femoris muscles. In the popliteal fossa, the tibial nerve becomes more superficial, first lying lateral to the popliteal vessels and then crossing obliquely to their medial sides before disappearing into the leg between and beneath the heads of the gastrocnemius and plantaris muscles. Passing over the popliteus muscle and under the tendinous arch of the soleus muscle on the medial side of the posterior tibial vessels, the tibial nerve next enters the space between the tibialis posterior muscle and the gastrocnemius and soleus muscles. Continuing downward, it crosses over the posterior tibial vessels to reach their lateral sides, so as to lie between the contiguous margins of the flexor digitorum longus and flexor hallucis longus muscles. In the distal third of the leg, the nerve is covered only by skin and fascia as it descends toward the ankle region, where it curves anteroinferiorly into the sole of the foot behind the medial malleolus, deep to the flexor retinaculum and between the tendons of the flexor hallucis longus and the flexor digitorum longus muscles. The nerve ends at this level by dividing into the *medial* and *lateral plantar nerves.*

The tibial nerve consists of muscular, articular, sural, calcaneal, and medial and lateral plantar main branches; it also gives off smaller osseous (medullary) and vascular twigs.

The *muscular branches* supply both heads of the gastrocnemius muscle and the plantaris, popliteus, soleus, tibialis posterior, flexor digitorum longus, and flexor hallucis longus muscles. Branches to the gastrocnemius, plantaris, and popliteus muscles and a few that enter the posterior surface of the soleus muscle arise in the popliteal fossa. The branch to the popliteus muscle descends over the posterior surface of the muscle, hooks around its inferior border, and ascends to enter its anterior surface. Branches to the deep surface of the soleus and to the tibialis posterior, flexor digitorum longus, and flexor hallucis longus muscles are given off in the upper third of the leg. Vasomotor branches to the popliteal vessels arise from the main tibial nerve or from its branches in the popliteal fossa.

The *articular branches* help supply the knee, ankle, and superior and inferior tibiofibular joints and may arise in common with small branches supplying adjacent muscles, bones, and vessels.

TIBIA AND FIBULA

Bones of right leg

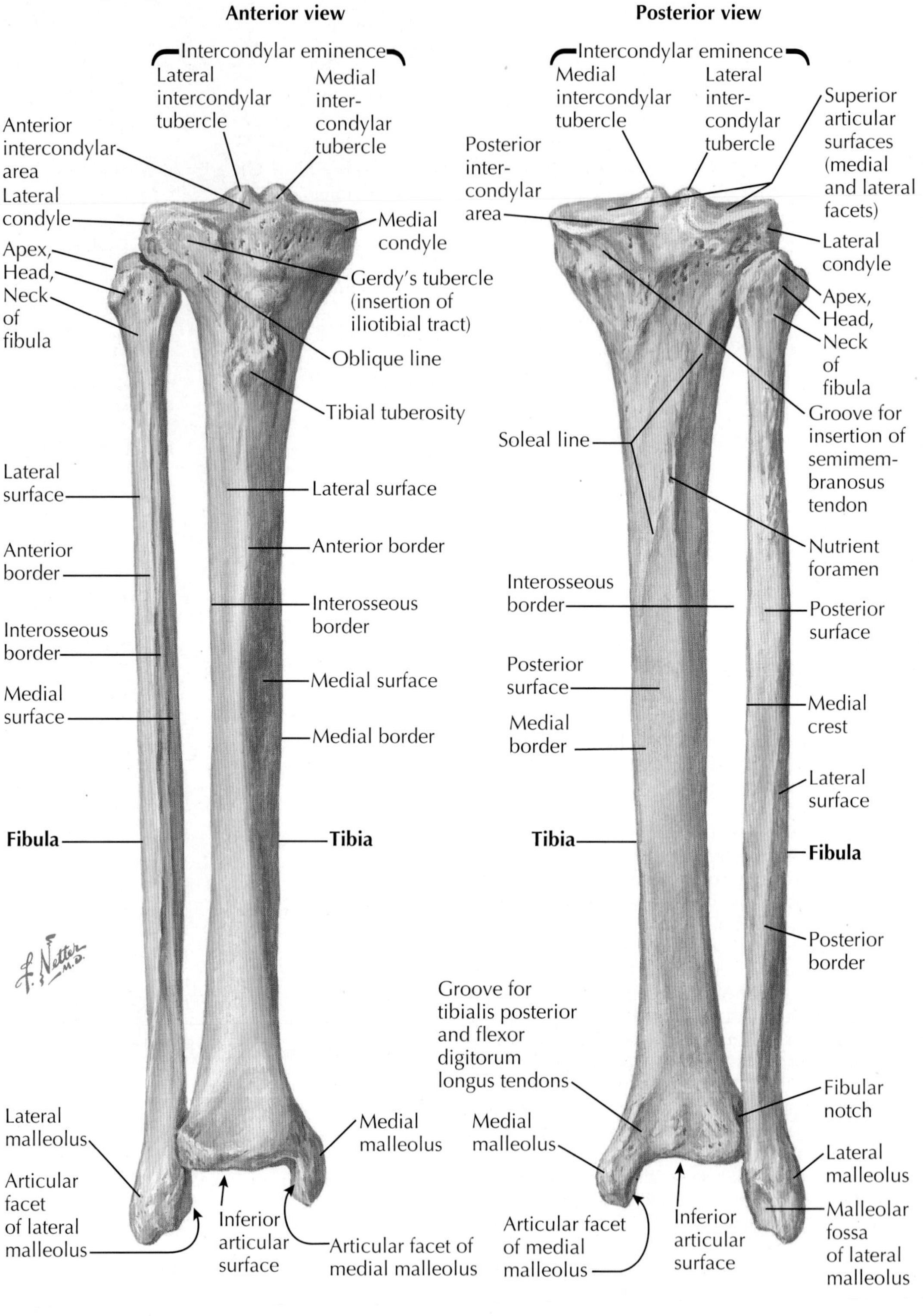

BONES OF LEG

TIBIA

The tibia is the weight-bearing bone of the leg, with the fibula serving for muscular attachments and completing the ankle joint on the lateral side (see Plate 4.12). The tibia is a long bone with expanded extremities, especially superiorly where it is widened to receive the condyles of the femur. Here, there are medial and lateral buttresses, which form the medial and lateral condyles. The *superior articular surface* has two facets. The medial facet is oval and slightly concave. The lateral facet is nearly round. It is concave from side to side but convex from front to back. The central parts of these facets receive the condyles of the femur; the rims give attachment to the menisci of the knee joint.

An *intercondylar eminence* is elevated between the two articular facets and is marked by a medial and a lateral intercondylar tubercle (tibial spine). The anterior intercondylar area in front of the eminence provides attachment for the anterior ends of the medial and lateral menisci and for the anterior cruciate ligament. The posterior intercondylar area exhibits a broad groove that lodges the posterior cruciate ligament; in front of this, the area gives attachment to the two menisci. Anteriorly, the two condyles pass over into a triangular area marked by vascular foramina and sloping to the tibial tuberosity below. The triangle is bounded by the *oblique lines.*

The *tibial tuberosity (tibial tubercle)* has a smooth upper portion for the attachment of the patellar ligament; its roughened lower portion is only separated from skin by a subcutaneous infrapatellar bursa. The rough medial surface of the medial condyle gives attachment to the fascia lata; posteriorly, the medial condyle shows a transverse groove for the insertion of the tendon of the semimembranosus muscle. On its posteroinferior surface the *lateral condyle* has a nearly circular facet that articulates with the head of the fibula. Anterior to this facet, an oblique line and Gerdy's tubercle provide attachment for the iliotibial tract.

The *shaft* of the tibia is triangular in cross section; it is wider proximally and distally and tapers to its narrowest at the junction of the middle and distal thirds. It has medial, lateral, and posterior surfaces and anterior, medial, and interosseous borders. The anterior border, slightly sinuous, begins at the lateral margin of the tuberosity above and ends on the medial malleolus below. It is subcutaneous and prominent and is sharpest in its middle third. The medial border, sharper in its lower half, extends from the posterior aspect of the medial condyle to the posterior border of the medial malleolus. The interosseous border is on the fibular side of the bone and is sharp throughout its length. Just above the ankle, the interosseous border bifurcates and encloses a triangular area for the attachment of the ligamentous tissue representing the tibiofibular syndesmosis. The medial surface of the shaft of the bone is smooth; it provides for the insertion of certain thigh muscles, such as the pes anserinus muscle, in its upper third. The rest of its surface is subcutaneous. The lateral surface of the shaft is hollowed in its upper two-thirds for the origin of the tibialis anterior muscle. Its lower third is smooth; it spirals anteriorly and is covered by tendons of the muscles of the anterior compartment of the leg.

The *soleal line* is a prominent marking of the posterior surface. It begins behind the facet for the head of the fibula and runs obliquely downward to the medial border of the bone at the junction of the upper and middle thirds of the shaft. The triangular area above the soleal line gives insertion for the popliteus muscle. The soleal line gives origin for the soleus muscle. The nutrient foramen of the tibia is below this line. Also below the soleal line arise the flexor digitorum longus and tibialis posterior muscles, separated by a vertical ridge of bone that sometimes is distinct.

The *inferior extremity* of the tibia projects medialward and downward as the *medial malleolus;* this forms a subcutaneous prominence at the ankle. The malleolus is grooved posteriorly for the tendons of the tibialis posterior and flexor digitorum longus muscles and tibial nerve; there may be a groove more laterally for the tendon of the flexor hallucis longus muscle. The lateral surface of the inferior extremity forms a triangular *fibular notch,* roughened by the ligamentous tissue uniting

TIBIA AND FIBULA (CONTINUED)

BONES OF LEG (Continued)

the bones. The borders of the notch are sharp for the attachments of the anterior tibiofibular and posterior tibiofibular ligaments. The distal end forms a quadrilateral *inferior articular surface* for articulation with the body of the talus. This surface is wider anteriorly than posteriorly and concave anteroposteriorly. It is continuous with the *malleolar articular surface* on the internal aspect of the medial malleolus. The malleolar articular surface lies almost at right angles to the inferior articular surface of the shaft and extends about 1.5 cm beyond it. From the lower edge of the medial malleolus, the deltoid ligament passes to the bones of the foot.

The tibia is *ossified* from three centers, one for the body and one for each extremity. They appear in the seventh week of intrauterine life for the body; in the upper epiphysis, shortly before birth; and in the lower end, between ages 1 and 2 years. The lower epiphysis joins the body of the bone first at roughly age 16 years in males and age 14 years in females. The upper epiphysis joins later at approximately age 17 years in males and 15 years in females.

FIBULA

The fibula lies parallel to the tibia and is long and slender (see Plate 4.11). It is not weight-bearing but gives attachment to muscles and aids in forming the ankle joint. It has a slender body and two somewhat expanded extremities.

The *head* of the fibula is knob-like and bears on its slanted superior aspect the almost circular articular surface of the head. The apex of the head projects upward at the posterolateral limit of the articulation; it gives attachment to the fibular collateral ligament of the knee joint and, on its lateral aspect, to the tendon of the biceps femoris muscle. Upper fibers of the tibialis anterior and soleus muscles also arise from the head of the fibula. Like the tibia, the shaft of the fibula has anterior, interosseous, and posterior borders and medial, lateral, and posterior surfaces. The neck of the fibula is grooved by the common peroneal nerve.

The sharp *anterior border* begins just below the head. Distally, immediately above the lateral malleolus, it divides to enclose a triangular subcutaneous surface. This border gives rise to the anterior intermuscular septum. The *interosseous border* is close to the anterior border. It begins in front of the head above, lies anteromedially along the shaft, and divides below into the borders of the tibiofibular syndesmosis. The interosseous border of the fibula is joined in the lower third of the shaft by the *medial crest.* The nutrient foramen of the fibula is located posterior to the distal end of the medial crest. A relatively indistinct posterior border gives attachment to the posterior intermuscular septum. The surfaces of the fibula give origin to the muscles of the adjacent compartments of the leg (see Plates 4.2 and 4.11).

The *lateral malleolus* is the pointed distal extremity of the fibula. Its tip descends about 1.5 cm below the tip of the medial malleolus of the tibia. Its lateral surface, convex and subcutaneous, is continuous with the subcutaneous area of the shaft. The medial surface of the malleolus consists of the triangular malleolar articular surface and the fossa of the lateral malleolus. The *malleolar articular surface,* angulated outward below, makes contact with the lateral side of the talus. The *fossa of the lateral malleolus* provides the area of attachment of the transverse tibiofibular and posterior talofibular ligaments. The borders of the malleolus give attachment to ligaments of the ankle joint, and the posterior border is grooved for the tendons of the peroneus longus and peroneus brevis muscles.

The fibula has *three centers of ossification.* One in the center for the shaft appears in its middle during the eighth week of uterine life; the ends of the bone are still cartilaginous at birth. Ossification in the lower extremity begins at about the end of the first year; in the upper extremity, it begins in the fourth year in the male and early in the third year in the female. Fusion of the lower epiphysis of the fibula with the shaft takes place first at roughly age 14 years in females and at age 16 years in males. Fusion of the proximal fibular epiphysis takes place later roughly at ages 17 to 18 years in males and at age 15 to 16 years in females,

Anterior view with ligament attachments

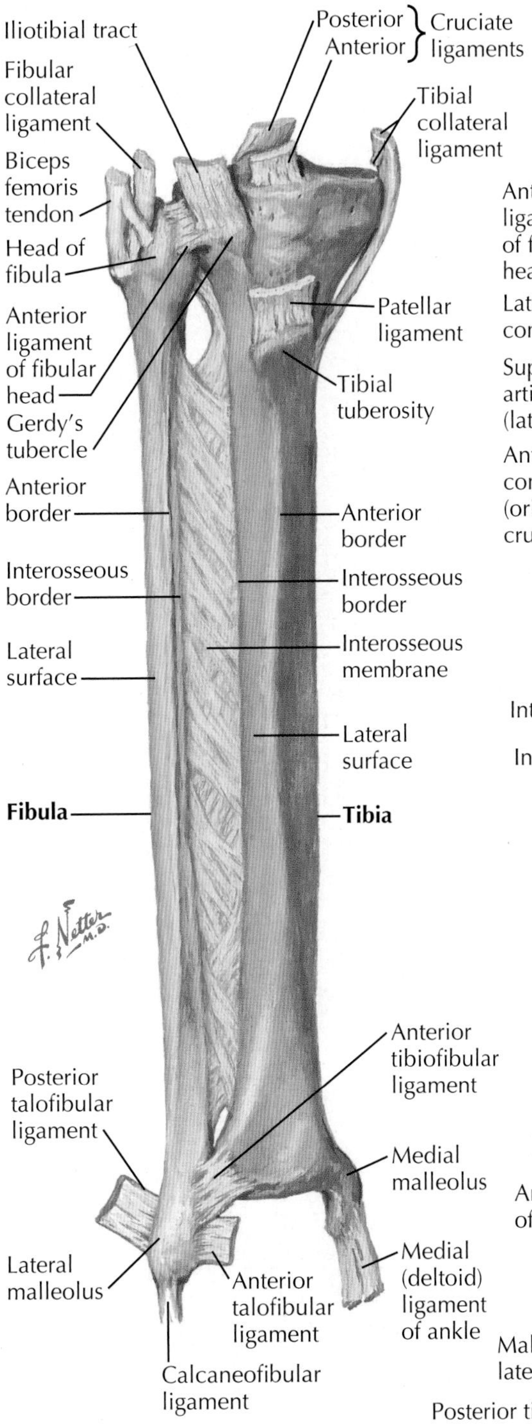

Iliotibial tract
Fibular collateral ligament
Biceps femoris tendon
Head of fibula
Anterior ligament of fibular head
Gerdy's tubercle
Anterior border
Interosseous border
Lateral surface
Fibula
Posterior talofibular ligament
Lateral malleolus
Calcaneofibular ligament
Anterior talofibular ligament
Posterior / Anterior } Cruciate ligaments
Tibial collateral ligament
Patellar ligament
Tibial tuberosity
Anterior border
Interosseous border
Interosseous membrane
Lateral surface
Tibia
Anterior tibiofibular ligament
Medial malleolus
Medial (deltoid) ligament of ankle

Superior view

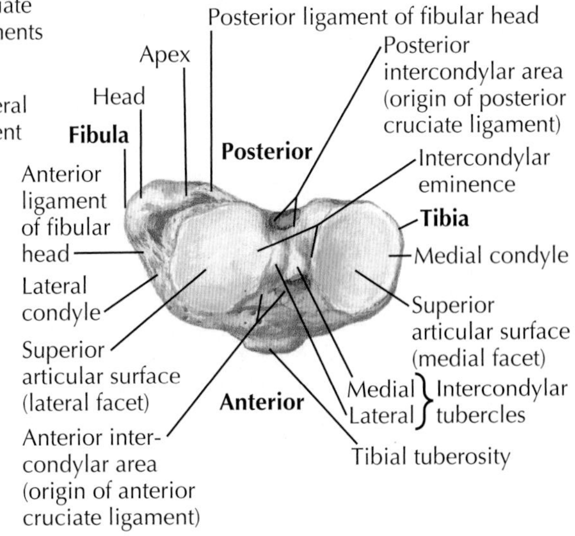

Posterior ligament of fibular head
Apex
Head
Fibula
Anterior ligament of fibular head
Lateral condyle
Superior articular surface (lateral facet)
Anterior intercondylar area (origin of anterior cruciate ligament)
Posterior
Anterior
Posterior intercondylar area (origin of posterior cruciate ligament)
Intercondylar eminence
Tibia
Medial condyle
Superior articular surface (medial facet)
Medial / Lateral } Intercondylar tubercles
Tibial tuberosity

Cross section

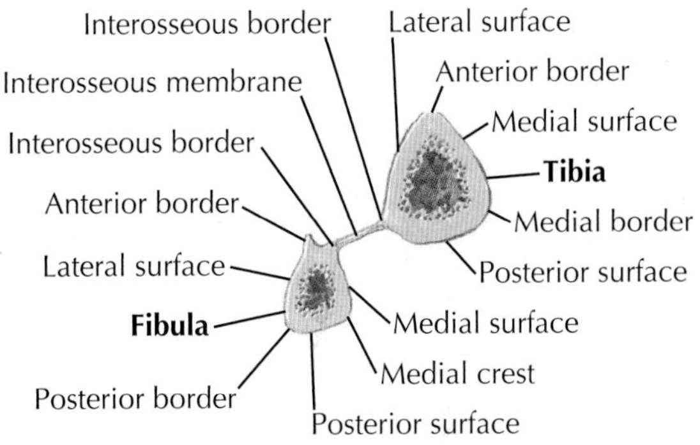

Interosseous border
Lateral surface
Interosseous membrane
Anterior border
Medial surface
Interosseous border
Tibia
Anterior border
Medial border
Lateral surface
Posterior surface
Fibula
Medial surface
Medial crest
Posterior border
Posterior surface

Inferior view

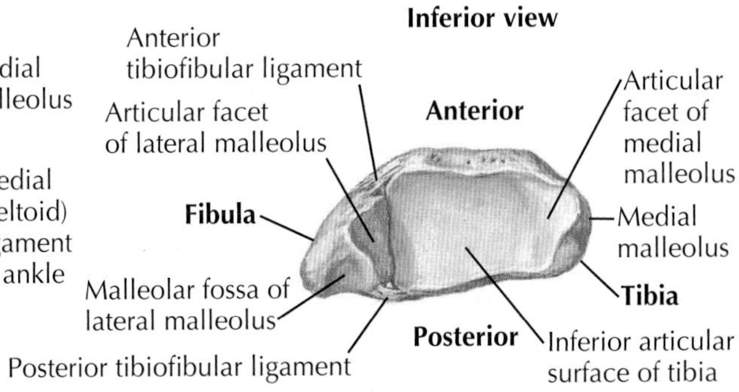

Anterior tibiofibular ligament
Articular facet of lateral malleolus
Anterior
Articular facet of medial malleolus
Fibula
Medial malleolus
Tibia
Malleolar fossa of lateral malleolus
Posterior
Posterior tibiofibular ligament
Inferior articular surface of tibia

F. Netter M.D.

Bones of Leg (Continued)

although individual differences are common. The fibula may be taken as a vascularized bone graft, but care must be taken to leave the proximal 4 cm and distal 6 cm at minimum.

JOINTS BETWEEN TIBIA AND FIBULA

The functional union of the tibia and the fibula is in three parts: the tibiofibular articulation proximally, the interosseous membrane, and the distal tibiofibular syndesmosis (see Plate 4.12).

The *tibiofibular articulation* is a plane joint between the circular facet on the head of the fibula and a matching surface on the underside of the lateral condyle of the tibia. The articular capsule, attached at the margins of the tibial and fibular facets, is strengthened by accessory ligaments. The *anterior ligament of the head of the fibula* consists of fibrous bands that pass obliquely from the front of the head of the fibula to the front of the lateral condyle of the tibia. The *posterior ligament of the head of the fibula* is a single broad band running obliquely between the head and the back of the lateral tibial condyle. It is crossed by the tendon of the popliteus muscle, and the subpopliteal recess of the knee joint cavity is sometimes in communication with the cavity of this joint. The articulation between the tibia and fibula transmits roughly one-sixth of the axial load and helps resist torsional stresses and lateral bending forces in the lower extremity. Subluxation at the proximal articulation may be seen most commonly in preadolescent females and usually resolves with skeletal maturation.

The tibiofibular articulation receives arteries from the lateral inferior genicular and anterior tibial recurrent arteries, and its lymphatics drain to the popliteal lymph nodes. Nerves to the joint come from the common peroneal nerve, the nerve to the popliteus muscle, and the recurrent articular nerve. Movement is slight at this joint, but it imparts a certain flexibility in the relations of the two bones during ankle movement and in response to the action of the muscles attached to the fibula.

The *interosseous membrane* of the leg extends between the interosseous borders of the two bones. It consists largely of fibers that pass from the tibia lateralward and downward to the fibula with some fibers traveling in the opposite direction as well. The upper margin does not reach the tibiofibular articulation, and the anterior tibial vessels pass across the upper edge of the membrane to the anterior compartment of the leg. The membrane is continuous below with the interosseous ligament of the tibiofibular syndesmosis and is perforated by several vessels, especially the perforating branch of the peroneal artery. It separates the anterior and posterior compartments of the leg and gives origin to muscles of both groups.

The *tibiofibular syndesmosis* is a fibrous joint in which the rough convex surface of the medial aspect of the lower end of the fibula is attached through the interosseous ligament to the corresponding rough, concave surface on the lateral side of the tibia. The *interosseous ligament,* continuous with the interosseous membrane above, consists of short, strong, fibrous bands uniting the two bones. The *anterior inferior tibiofibular ligament* and the *posterior inferior tibiofibular ligament* pass, respectively, from the borders of the fibular notch of the tibia to the anterior and posterior surfaces of the lateral malleolus of the fibula. Each is inclined downward and laterally. The *inferior transverse tibiofibular ligament* is largely deep to the posterior tibiofibular ligament. It arises from nearly the whole inferior border of the tibia posteriorly and attaches to the upper portion of the malleolar fossa of the fibula. This is a thick and strong ligament, and it projects below the bony margin to form part of the articulating fossa for the talus. A recess of the articular cavity of the ankle joint and its enclosing synovial membrane extend upward between the tibia and fibula to the lower end of the interosseous ligament.

The blood supply of the tibiofibular syndesmosis is principally from the perforating branch of the peroneal artery and the malleolar arteries; its nerve supply is from the deep peroneal and tibial nerves. This articulation forms the firm union of the tibia and fibula required in the box-like mortise of the ankle. Its fibrous tissue and ligaments allow a slight yielding of the bones for the accommodation of the talus in the movements of the ankle.

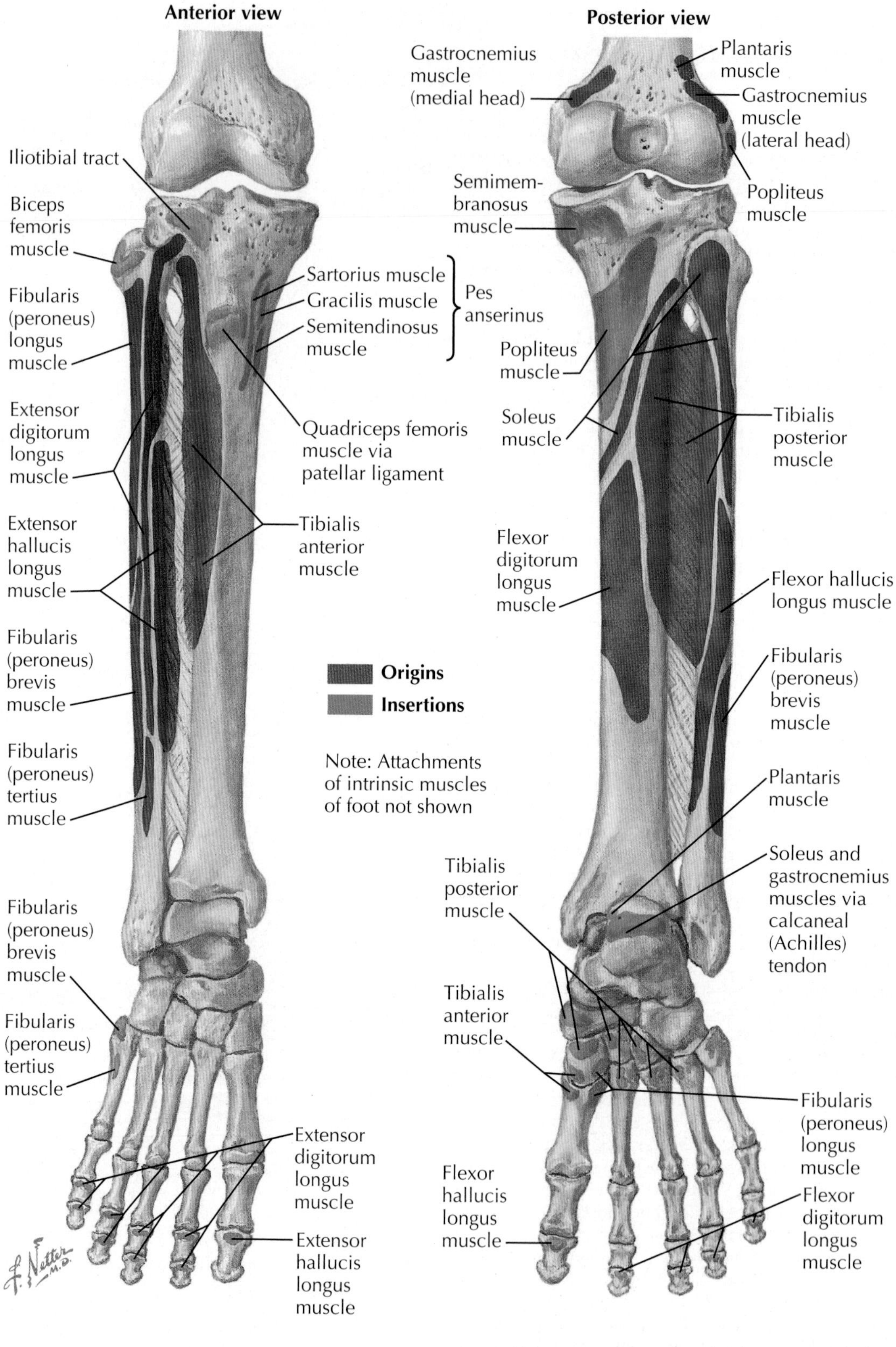

Fracture of Proximal Tibia Involving Articular Surface

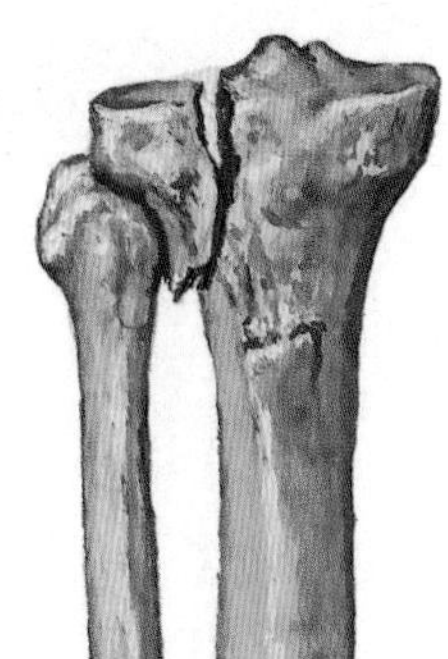

Split fracture of lateral tibial plateau

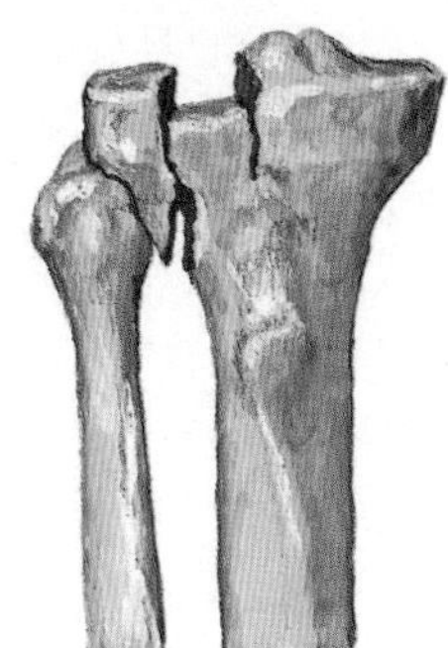

Split fracture of lateral condyle plus depression of tibial plateau

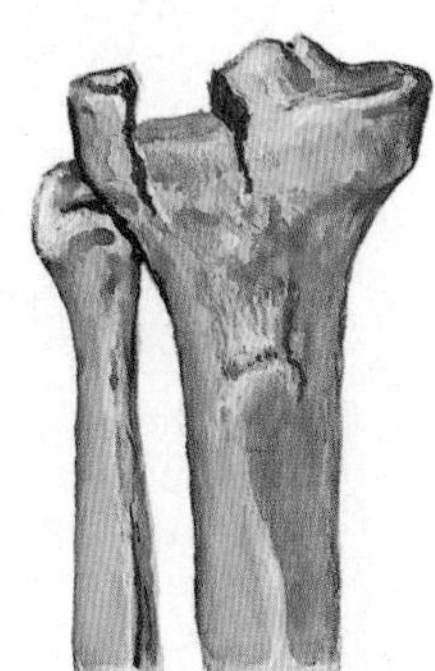

Depression of lateral tibial plateau without split fracture

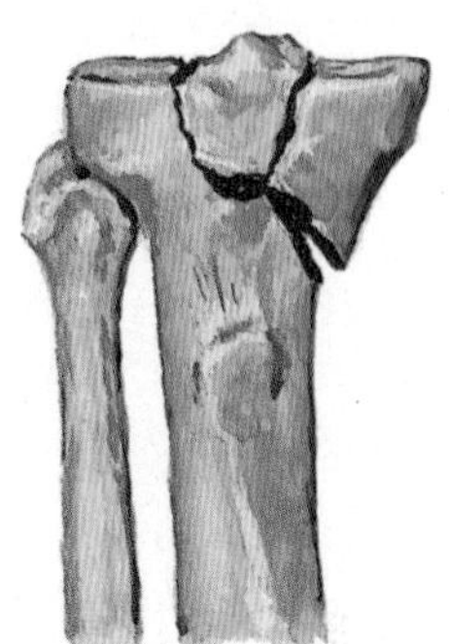

Comminuted split fracture of medial tibial plateau and tibial spine

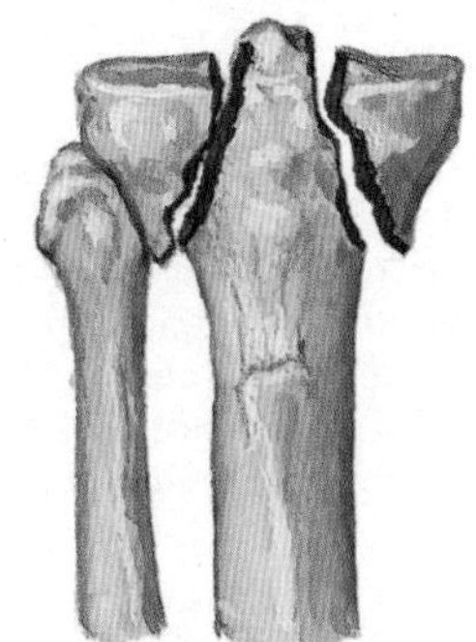

Bicondylar fracture involving both tibial plateaus with widening

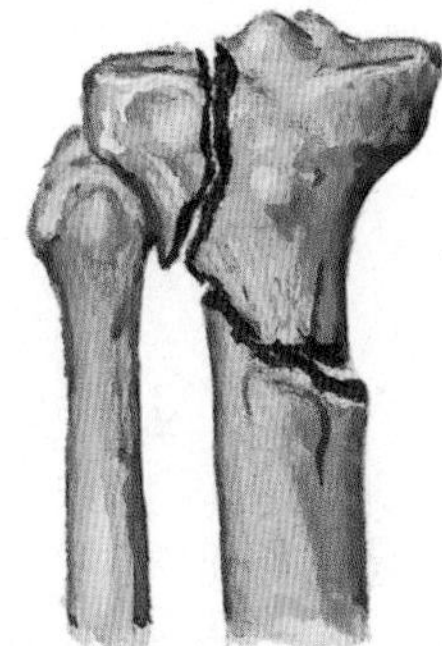

Fracture of lateral tibial plateau with separation of metaphyseal-diaphyseal junction

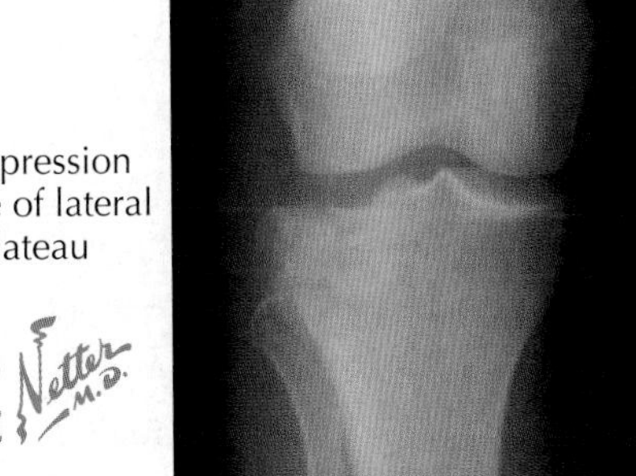

Split depression fracture of lateral tibial plateau

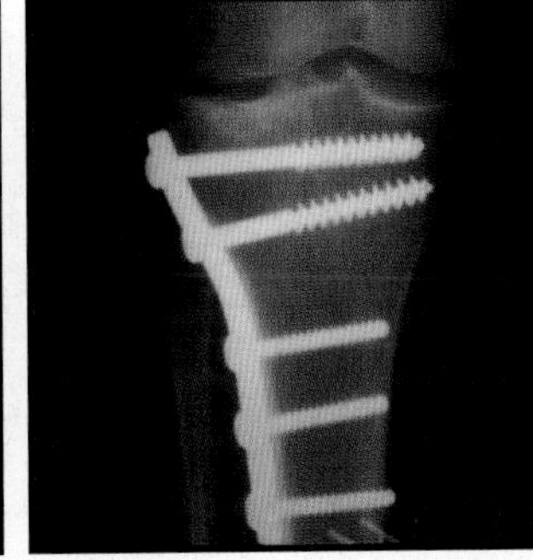

Repair by elevation of depressed segment plus bone graft and buttress plate

Fractures of the proximal tibia involving the articular surface at the knee are referred to as fractures of the tibial plateau. Tibial plateau fractures result from a combination of varus/valgus stress and axial loading. The medial tibial plateau is stronger, and as such the lateral tibial plateau (condyle) is more frequently fractured; isolated fractures of the medial tibial plateau and fractures of both tibial condyles occur less frequently and result from higher energy mechanisms and thus typically have more associated injuries. Fractures of both the tibial plateau and the shaft of the proximal tibia are rare injuries. Fractures of the lateral tibial plateau generally involve either cleavage of the plateau from the remaining portion of the articular surface (split fractures) in younger patients with harder bone and a depression or cleavage of the plateau with an associated depression of part of the plateau (split depression). Both types of fracture often require anatomic reduction of the fracture fragment to the intact portion of the articular surface.

The evaluation of tibial plateau fractures must contain a thorough examination for associated injuries both locally and in other areas. The soft tissue must be carefully evaluated to determine whether the fracture is open, and ambiguous cases may require a saline load test of the knee for confirmation. Open fractures should be treated accordingly. Because of the axial loading mechanism, the joints above and below should be carefully evaluated (as well as the full length of the tibia, femur, and fibula) and the lumbar spine assessed. Ligamentous and meniscal injuries are common, especially in younger patients and those with higher energy mechanisms. A thorough neurologic examination of the leg should be performed with special attention to the peroneal nerve, which is most commonly injured with medial-sided injuries. A vascular examination is also essential because the popliteal artery is tethered posteriorly in the knee; intimal arterial injuries may lead to thrombus and ischemia. It is imperative to assess the compartments of the leg for compartment syndrome, and observation may be required for higher energy injuries. Adequate radiographs are necessary to evaluate the articular surface, and traction views and computed tomographic scans are frequently beneficial.

Tibial plateau fractures may be classified using the AO/OTA classification system or the Schatzker classification. In the Schatzker system there are six types of fracture, with types 1 to 3 considered as having lower energy patterns:

- Type 1—lateral split
- Type 2—lateral split-depression
- Type 3—lateral depression
- Type 4—medial fracture
- Type 5—bicondylar fracture
- Type 6—fracture with complete separation of metaphysic and diaphysis

Multiple techniques and implants are available to fix tibial plateau fractures. In split fractures in which adequate closed reduction can be achieved, stabilization can be accomplished with percutaneous screws. In depressed fractures, the depressed portion must be elevated to its proper position. When this articular fragment is elevated, a defect remains in the underlying cancellous bone that must be filled with bone graft or substitute to support the fragment in its anatomic position and prevent its collapse. Fixation often involves use of plate and screw constructs to maintain the reduction of the tibial plateau. If fixation is needed on both the medial and lateral sides, two incision techniques are used to maintain soft tissue viability.

As with many joint injuries, the joint surface must be restored, the fracture firmly stabilized, and joint motion resumed as early as possible. Plate 4.14 shows complicated fractures of the proximal tibia, which require complex methods of fixation to maintain reduction and allow early joint motion.

After surgery, the patient begins early active range-of-motion exercises, but weight-bearing is delayed. When clinical and radiographic examinations demonstrate that healing is progressing normally, weight-bearing can begin (usually within 10–12 weeks). If the internal fixation is not secure or the patient's bone quality is poor, internal fixation is often supplemented with a cast or functional brace, which allows early motion while providing support during healing.

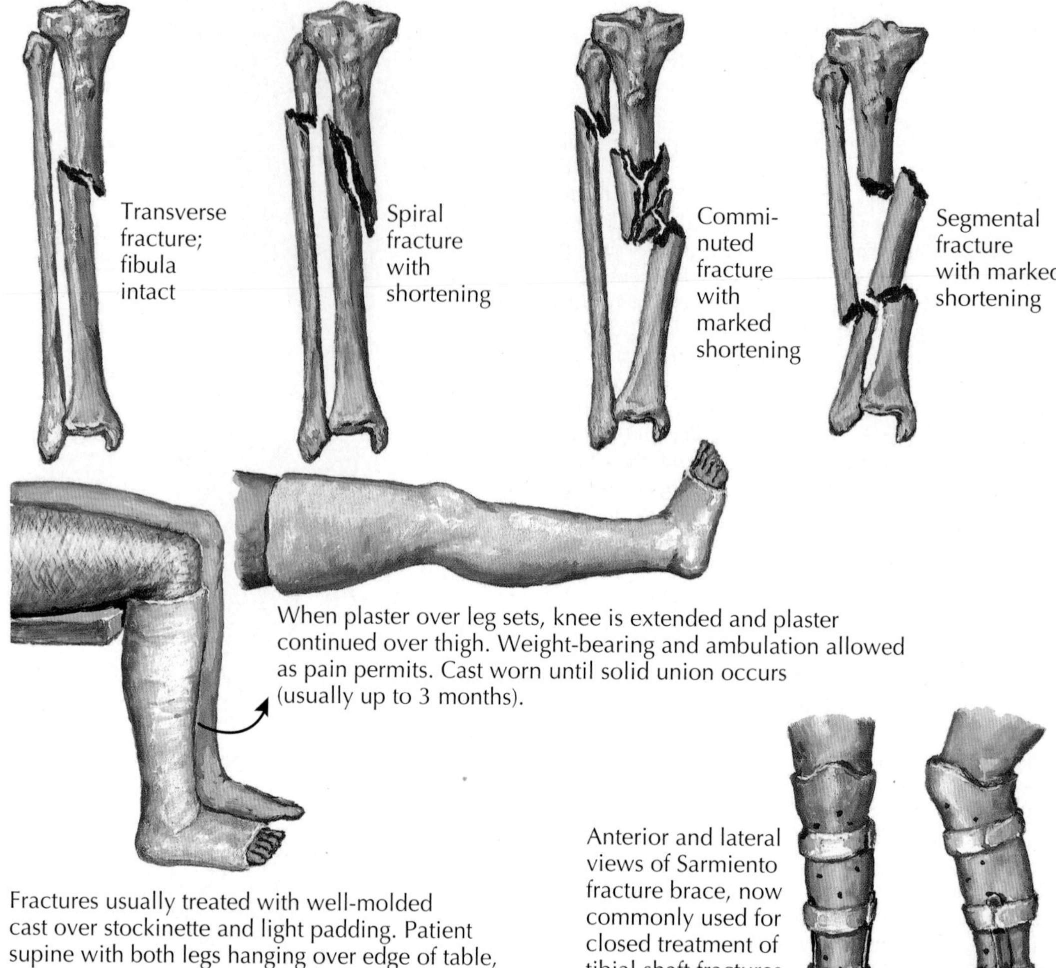

Transverse
fracture;
fibula
intact
Spiral
fracture
with
shortening
Commi-
nuted
fracture
with
marked
shortening
Segmental
fracture
with marked
shortening
When plaster over leg sets, knee is extended and plaster continued over thigh. Weight-bearing and ambulation allowed as pain permits. Cast worn until solid union occurs (usually up to 3 months).
Anterior and lateral views of Sarmiento fracture brace, now commonly used for closed treatment of tibial shaft fractures
Fractures usually treated with well-molded cast over stockinette and light padding. Patient supine with both legs hanging over edge of table, feet at right angle. After satisfactory visual and radiographic reduction and correction of angular and rotational deformities (compared with uninjured leg), cast applied from toes to knee.

Other treatment methods

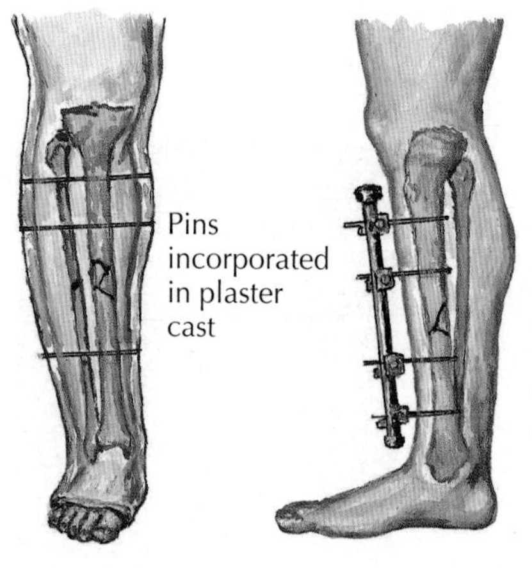

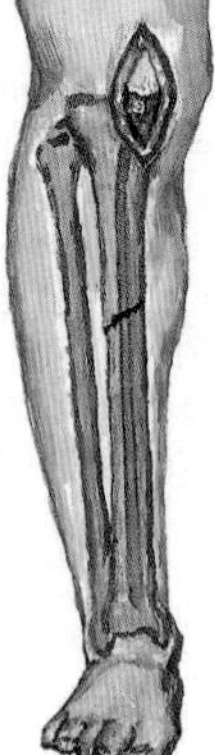

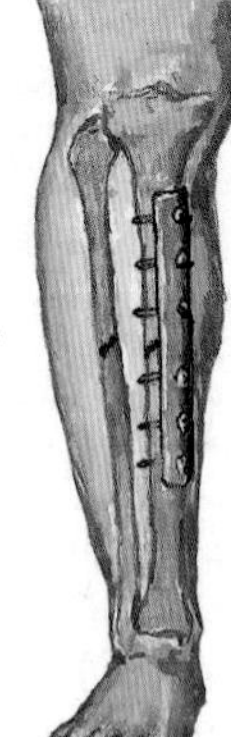

FRACTURE OF SHAFT OF TIBIA

Fractures of the tibial shaft are the most common fractures of a long bone. Because the tibia lies so close to the skin along the medial side of the leg, tibial shaft fractures are the most common open injuries. Many fracture patterns are seen in the tibia. As the amount of energy causing the fracture increases, so does the complexity of the fracture. Unlike the femur, this bone is not enveloped by thick muscles, and abnormalities of healing such as delayed union, malunion, and nonunion occur more frequently.

Stable fractures of the tibial shaft (i.e., fractures with little displacement and minimal comminution) can be managed with the use of a long-leg cast. When a long-leg cast is used for definitive fracture treatment, it remains in place for 10 to 12 weeks. For successful treatment, the patient must be able to place weight on the injured limb to stimulate fracture healing.

Sarmiento applied the concept of early weight-bearing to his development of a removable fracture brace or functional fracture brace. Treatment of a tibial shaft fracture with the functional brace is preceded by placing the patient in a cast until the acute soft tissue reaction subsides. Then the fracture brace is fitted and worn until the fracture has healed sufficiently and supplementary support is no longer required.

Several other methods are used to treat tibial fractures. Treatment with external fixators is generally reserved for more unstable and open tibial fractures or in the case of "damage control orthopedics" in which the patient's overall medical condition precludes more invasive surgical treatments. The external fixator allows visualization of the open fracture site while providing sufficient bone stability to allow care of the soft tissues without displacing the fracture.

Significant improvements have been made throughout orthopedics in terms of implants, and the treatment of tibial shaft fractures has benefited from this as well. Intramedullary nailing and plate fixation are becoming more effective and more widely used in the treatment of tibial fractures. These devices provide more stable internal fixation of the fracture fragments than does a cast or a functional brace. However, the risk of infection after internal fixation is increased.

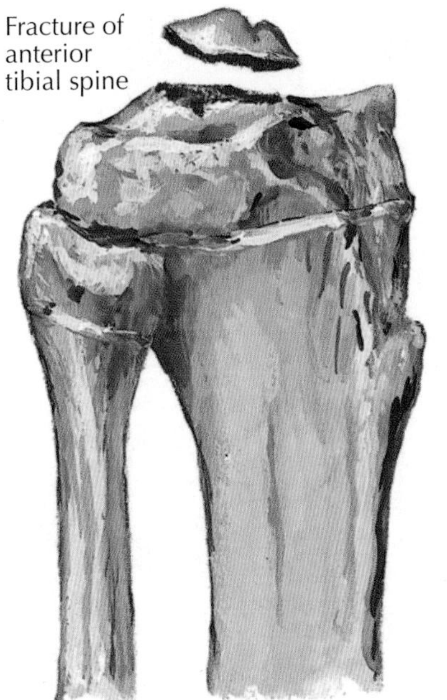

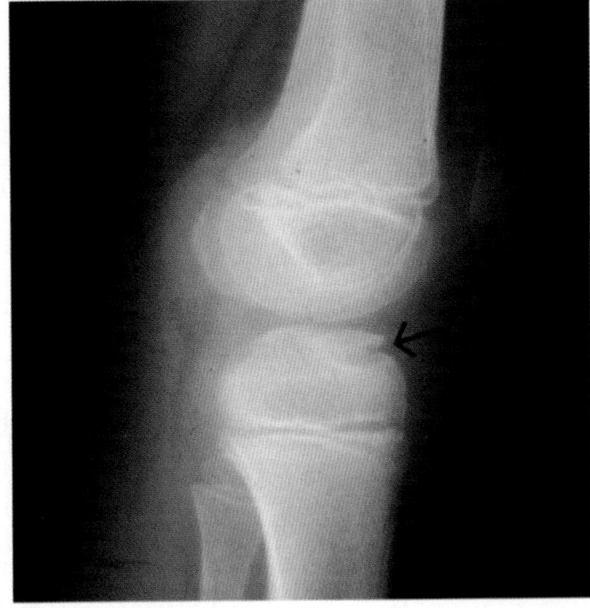

Valgus deformity after healing, possibly due to overgrowth of tibia relative to growth of fibula

Nondisplaced transverse fracture of metaphysis of proximal tibia

Anteroposterior radiograph. Healed transverse fracture with valgus deformity.

Fracture of Tibia in Children

The pediatric patient may suffer injuries similar to the adult patients mentioned previously. However, in the skeletally immature patient the ligamentous structures may be stronger than the physeal cartilage or even cancellous bone; consequently, injuries that commonly produce ligament damage in adults are more likely to cause fractures, particularly growth plate injuries, in growing children.

AVULSION OF ANTERIOR TIBIAL SPINE (INTERCONDYLAR EMINENCE)

Avulsion of the anterior tibial spine (intercondylar eminence) is typically due to a rotatory or extension type of injury that places excessive tension on the anterior cruciate ligament, which inserts into the anterior tibial spine. It may be necessary to obtain a radiograph in line with the anatomic posterior slope of the proximal tibia to see these fractures. The fragment of tibial spine may be nondisplaced (type I), elevated with an intact posterior hinge (type II), displaced (type III), or comminuted (type IV). Type I and II fractures can be treated by immobilizing the knee in full extension in a long-leg cast. Full extension of the knee joint tends to reduce the fragment and hold it in position during healing. Types III and IV require surgical treatment for anatomic reduction and fixation through either open or arthroscopic approaches.

FRACTURE OF THE PROXIMAL TIBIAL PHYSIS

These injuries may be due to direct or indirect trauma and typically present as pain, inability to bear weight, hemarthrosis, deformity, and tenderness distal to the joint line. The popliteal artery is tethered posteriorly behind the proximal tibia, and the peroneal nerve is tethered lateral to the fibula, so both are at risk of concomitant injury. Thus a careful neurovascular examination is important as well as examination of all four compartments of the lower leg for compartment syndrome due to damage to the recurrent anterior tibial artery and significant soft tissue injury associated with displaced fractures. Serial examinations of both compartments and vascular status should be performed, and additional testing such as angiography may be needed. Intimal arterial injuries may be present even with intact distal pulses initially but may cause delayed thrombosis. Nondisplaced fractures may be treated in a cast. Displaced or unstable fractures require operative treatment with temporary or permanent fixation depending on the pattern and relationship to the physis; in those fractures involving the articular surface, articular congruity must be restored.

FRACTURE OF SHAFT AND METAPHYSIS

Fractures of the tibial shaft, which occur fairly often in children, are often amenable to closed reduction and casting. Once satisfactory reduction is achieved, healing

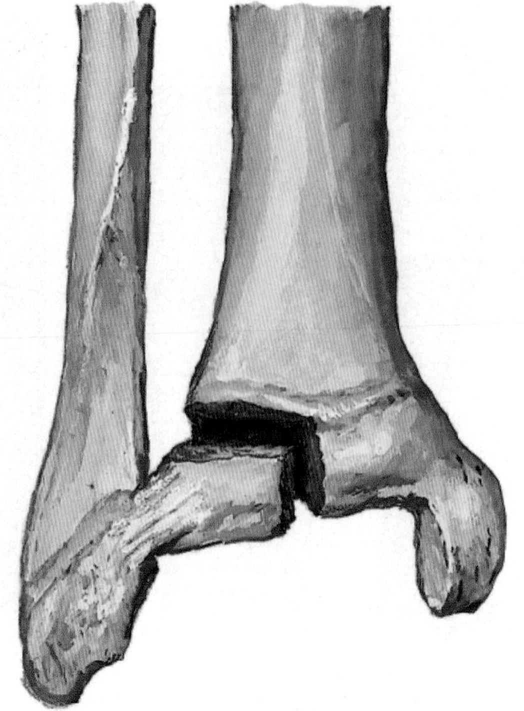

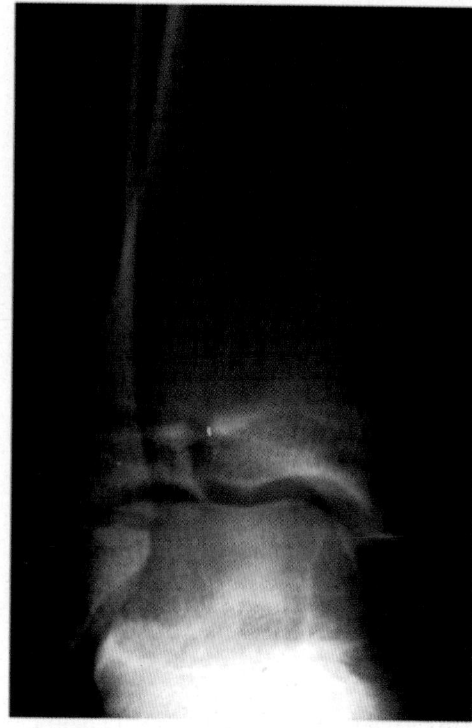

Tillaux (Salter-Harris type III) fracture of distal tibia.
Fracture line extends partially across growth plate and vertically through epiphysis. Medial portion of growth plate and epiphysis remain intact.

FRACTURE OF TIBIA IN CHILDREN (Continued)

typically proceeds well with few or no long-term complications. If an acceptable reduction cannot be obtained or the fracture pattern is unstable, operative intervention is warranted with either flexible titanium nails, a rigid intramedullary nail, or a plate and screws. One complication unique to young children occurs after fracture of the proximal tibial metaphysis. This fracture usually appears to be benign, with little or no angulation, but after healing has occurred, the limb tends to develop a progressive valgus angulation called a Cozen deformity. The cause of this deformity is not certain, but it may be from overgrowth of the tibia without concomitant overgrowth of the fibula because of increased vascularization from the healing response. Fortunately, as the child continues to grow, the valgus deformity partially corrects and usually does not require intervention. The recommended treatment consists of closed reduction and cast immobilization followed by close observation.

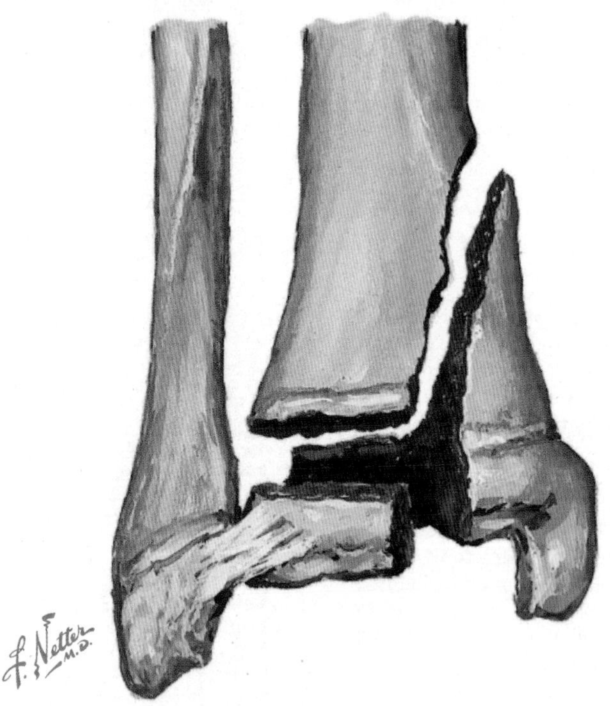

Triplane fracture. Three fragments: (1) anterior portion of epiphysis of distal tibia, (2) posteromedial portion of epiphysis with attached spike of metaphysis, and (3) shaft of tibia.

INJURY TO GROWTH PLATE

The growth plate (physis) of the distal tibia is very susceptible to injury. Twisting injuries, similar to those seen in adults, produce a variety of fracture patterns unique to the child's ankle because of the presence of the open growth plate. Injury pattern is dictated by what portions of the growth plate are still open; these injuries are called transitional ankle fractures. The distal tibial physis closes centrally first, then medially (anterior before posterior), and finally laterally. The Tillaux fracture, a Salter-Harris type III injury of the distal tibia, is common in children 12 to 15 years of age. An external rotation injury to the ankle joint causes the anteroinferior tibiofibular ligament to avulse the anterolateral portion of the epiphysis (last to close). Significantly displaced fragments require anatomic reduction and fixation to restore satisfactory function of the ankle joint.

The triplane fracture typically occurs in patients in a slightly younger age group than Tillaux fractures and has the appearance of Salter-Harris type II and type III fractures on anteroposterior and lateral radiographs. The three fracture fragments commonly are (1) the anterolateral portion of the epiphysis of the distal tibia (similar to the Tillaux fragment), (2) the tibial shaft, and (3) the large posterior fragment comprising the posterior and medial portions of the epiphysis plus a large metaphyseal fragment of variable size, although it may be seen as a two-part fracture in which the medial epiphysis remains attached to the tibia and the lateral portion has a metaphyseal fragment with it. Triplane fractures require anatomic reduction of the articular surface to ensure satisfactory function of the ankle joint after the fracture heals.

Bowleg and Knock-Knee

Bowleg (genu varum) and knock-knee (genu valgum) are angular deformities commonly seen in growing children. Although these conditions represent normal development (physiologic bowleg or knock-knee) in the majority of patients and resolve in time without treatment, it is important to differentiate between physiologic angular deformities and the variety of pathologic conditions that require special evaluation and treatment.

Clinical evaluation of the patient with angular deformities includes obtaining a family history and a description of the deformity, its onset, and its progression. The child should be observed ambulating, with particular attention paid to the stance phase of the gait to determine whether a lateral thrust (bowleg) or medial thrust (knock-knee) occurs immediately on weight-bearing. A thrust indicates that restraint of the knee by the medial or lateral ligaments is not adequate to resist the deformity. In children with physiologic bowleg or knock-knee, a thrust is not present. A thrust, however, is seen in patients with most of the pathologic conditions that cause varus or valgus deformities, indicating an incompetence of the knee ligaments and, most likely, a progressive deformity.

PHYSIOLOGIC BOWLEG AND KNOCK-KNEE

The natural history of physiologic bowleg and knock-knee was defined by Salenius and Vankka, who studied the development of the tibiofemoral angle, measured clinically and radiographically, in 1480 normal children (Plate 4.18). In the newborn, the tibiofemoral angle is 15 degrees varus. When the child is 18 months of age, the limbs appear to straighten, and when the child is between 2 and 4 years of age, the tibiofemoral angle changes to marked valgus (12 degrees). By 8 years of age, the limb straightens to the slightly valgus alignment that will remain throughout adulthood.

Clinical Manifestations. The normal infant usually stands with the legs apart, and early physiologic varus bowing of the lower limbs may be masked by fat. Internal tibial torsion often accompanies physiologic bowleg, accentuating the bowing when the child stands or walks. Physiologic knock-knee usually becomes evident at 2.5 to 3 years of age, with maximum physiologic valgus seen around 4 years of age. Flatfoot (pes planus) and external tibial torsion may also be present and accentuate knock-knee appearance.

Treatment. Reassurance and observation are sufficient for the patients with physiologic bowing of the lower limbs. Use of sleeping splints, corrective shoes, and active and passive exercises effects no apparent changes in the lower limbs that would not occur with normal growth and development. In children younger than 8 years of age, knock-knee may be safely ignored, unless it is excessive (tibiofemoral angle >15 degrees) or asymmetric. Correction of excessive physiologic valgus after 8 years of age, generally using a hemiepiphysiodesis technique, is indicated in cases of gait disturbance, patellofemoral maltracking, ligamentous instability, or cosmetic concerns.

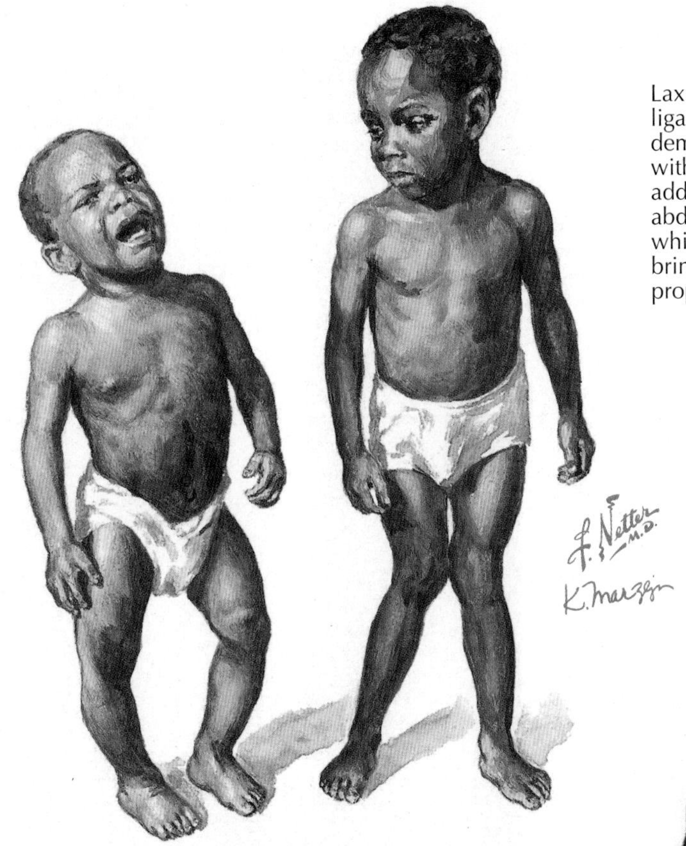

PATHOLOGIC BOWLEG AND KNOCK-KNEE

Blount Disease

The most common cause of pathologic bowleg, or tibia vara, is Blount disease (Plate 4.19). The etiology remains unclear. Some studies have suggested that the pathologic bowing is caused by a primary disturbance in growth with faulty ossification of the medial part of the epiphysis and metaphysis of the proximal tibia. Results of more recent studies indicate that the condition is secondary to mechanical stress of weight-bearing on the medial tibiofemoral compartment, delaying the growth of the medial tibial growth plate. In later stages of infantile Blount disease, bony bridge formation may be present, causing a "tether" on medial-sided growth.

Blount disease is divided into three types: (1) infantile, (2) juvenile, and (3) adolescent forms. The *infantile form* (up to age 4 years), which is usually bilateral and progressive, is associated with significant internal tibial torsion. Those affected frequently exceed the 95th percentile in weight, with an obvious lateral "thrust" present on examination. The *juvenile form* (4–10 years) has similar prognosis compared with the infantile form. The *adolescent form* is less common, usually unilateral in a patient with obesity, and carries with it a lower recurrence rate.

Two brothers, younger (left) with bowleg, older (right) with knock-knee. In both children, limbs eventually became normally aligned without corrective treatment.

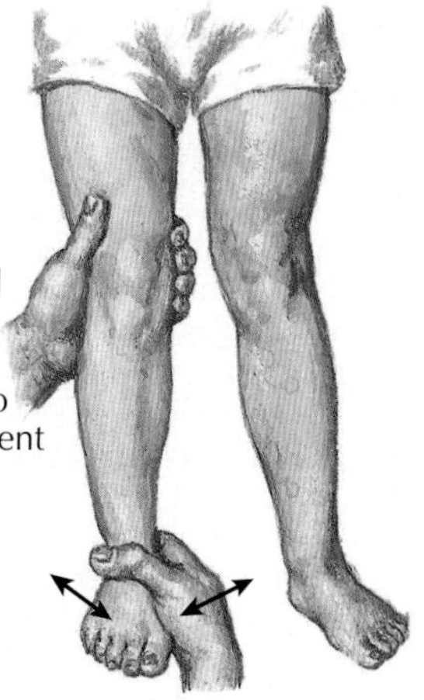

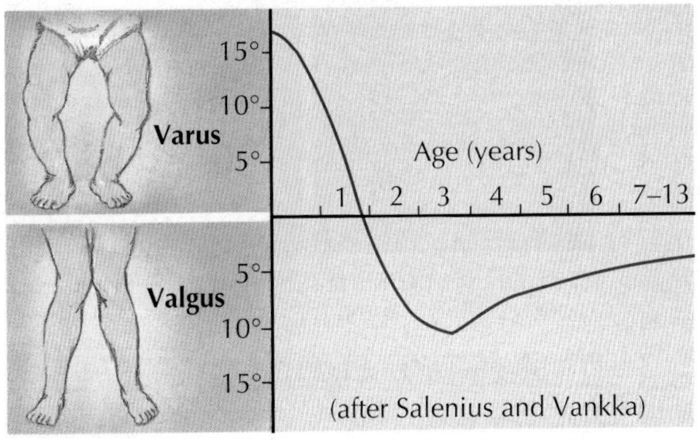

Graph depicts normal developmental changes in tibiofemoral angle. Substantial deviation suggests pathologic cause such as rickets, Blount disease, or other disorders requiring specific treatment.

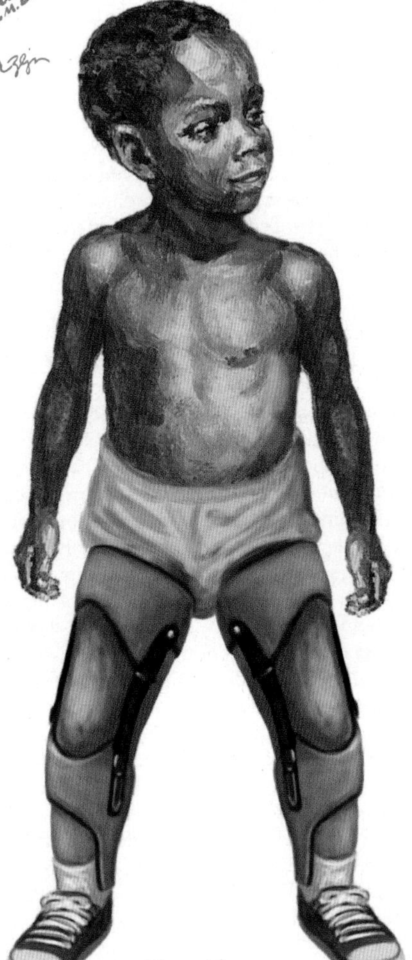

Bowleg and Knock-Knee (Continued)

Bony bridging is rarely present in the adolescent form, with the resulting deformity being less severe.

Plate 4.19 shows six stages of infantile Blount disease (Langenskiöld classification) based on radiographic evidence of the degree of epiphyseal depression and metaphyseal fragmentation of the medial proximal tibia. Prominent medial metaphyseal "beaking" is noted. Prognosis has been shown to correlate with the stage, with stages I and II allowing for restoration of anatomic alignment, in contrast to stages V and VI being associated with a high rate of recurrence after surgical realignment.

Rarely can infantile Blount disease be diagnosed radiographically before 18 months of age. The proximal metaphyseal-diaphyseal angle on radiographic analysis may be used to predict which cases of physiologic bowleg will progress to Blount disease. On the anteroposterior radiograph, a horizontal line is drawn parallel through the widest portion of the tibial metaphysis and an intersecting vertical line is drawn parallel to the lateral border of the tibia. A third line is drawn perpendicular to the line on the metaphysis, and the angle between the perpendicular line and the vertical line on the lateral border of the tibia is measured. In general, when the angle is less than 11 degrees, the bowleg deformity tends to resolve; an angle greater than 11 degrees is predictive of progression to Blount disease. Limb malrotation abnormalities may skew proximal metaphyseal-diaphyseal angle measurements and must be considered. In addition, if a child with bowleg exhibits a lateral thrust on weight-bearing, the prognosis is poor.

Treatment. The degree of deformity and the patient's age determine the treatment plan for Blount disease. In the infantile form, progression is usually rapid in the first 4 years and then slows for the remainder of the growth period. Observation is usually sufficient until the patient is 18 months of age, because a definitive diagnosis of infantile Blount disease is difficult before this age. If the varus deformity does not follow typical physiologic progression and improve by the time the child is 18 to 24 months of age and is in its early stages (I or II), it is treated with an orthosis, such as the elastic Blount brace (knee-ankle-foot orthosis), until the child is 3 years of age (see Plate 4.18).

Children older than 3 years with persistent bowleg and a tibiofemoral angle greater than 15 degrees of varus and stage III to VI Blount disease cannot be successfully treated with bracing, and an overcorrective proximal tibial osteotomy with or without bony bridge resection is required (see Plate 4.19). Recurrence is common in children with stage IV disease, obesity, and ligamentous laxity. Investigation for a physeal bar should be started in patients who have recurrent deformity after brace or surgical treatment. Premature physeal arrest of the medial tibial physis can occur and should be monitored to manage the child's varus deformity and potential leg-length discrepancy.

A child who undergoes a tibial osteotomy is at risk for serious sequelae and should be closely monitored for signs of compartment syndrome after surgery.

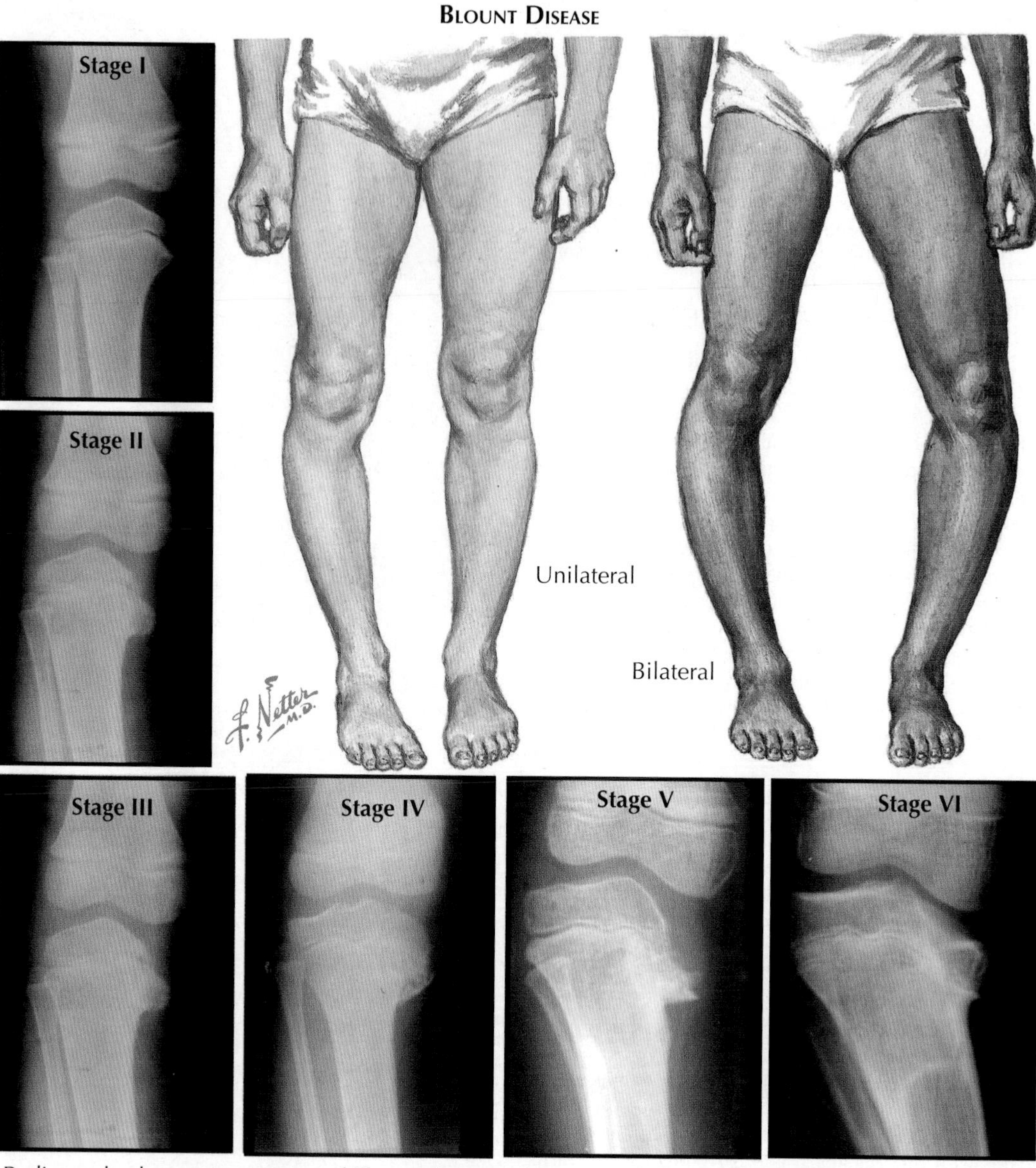

Radiographs demonstrate stages of Blount disease: progressive deformity of medial side of proximal tibial epiphysis and development of metaphyseal beak.

Schema of U-shaped osteotomy

Neurovascular compromise, anterior compartment syndrome, undercorrection or overcorrection, and failure to correct internal tibial torsion are potential problems.

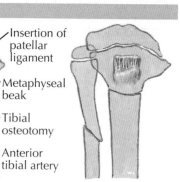

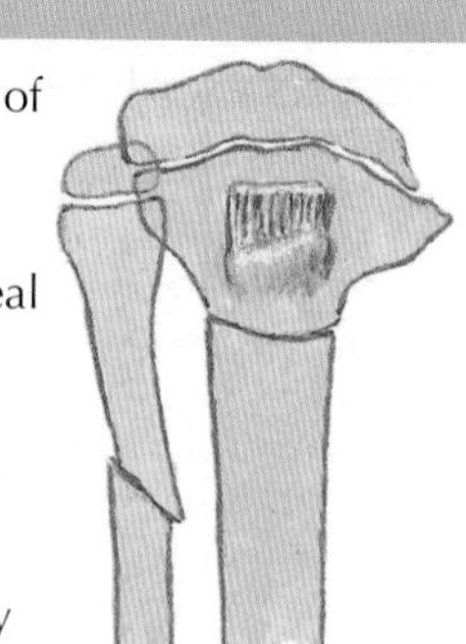

Other Causes of Pathologic Bowleg and Knock-Knee

Rickets can cause bowleg or knock-knee deformities. Vitamin D–dependent and Vitamin D–resistant rickets, generally occurring in early childhood. Conversely, rickets due to chronic renal insufficiency (renal osteodystrophy), which has a later onset, is now a common cause of knock-knee. Treatment with renal dialysis and kidney transplantation has improved the life expectancy of patients with this disorder, and surgical correction of severe valgus deformities is often required. It is important that children with rickets who undergo osteotomy receive proper medical management to ensure reliable healing.

Unilateral bowleg or knock-knee may be associated with trauma, surgery, tumors, congenital knee deformity, metaphyseal chondrodysplasia, osteocartilaginous exostosis, hemihypertrophy, paraxial fibular hemimelia, multiple epiphyseal dysplasia, Morquio syndrome, rickets, osteogenesis imperfecta, and fibrous dysplasia.

TOEING IN: METATARSUS ADDUCTUS AND INTERNAL TIBIAL TORSION

Metatarsus adductus

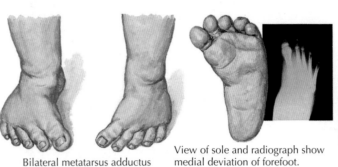

Bilateral metatarsus adductus

View of sole and radiograph show medial deviation of forefoot.

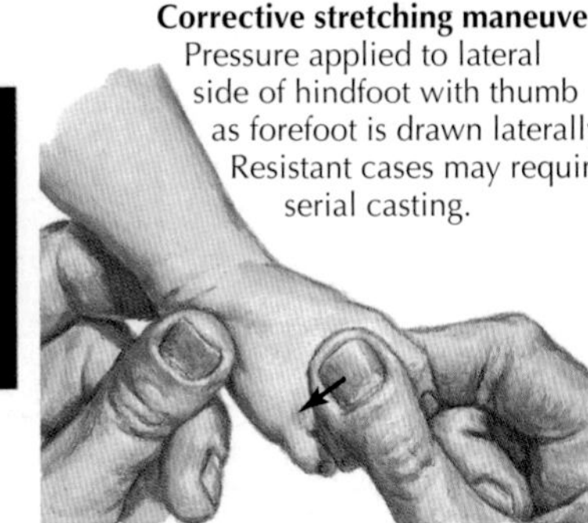

Corrective stretching maneuver. Pressure applied to lateral side of hindfoot with thumb as forefoot is drawn laterally. Resistant cases may require serial casting.

Internal tibial torsion

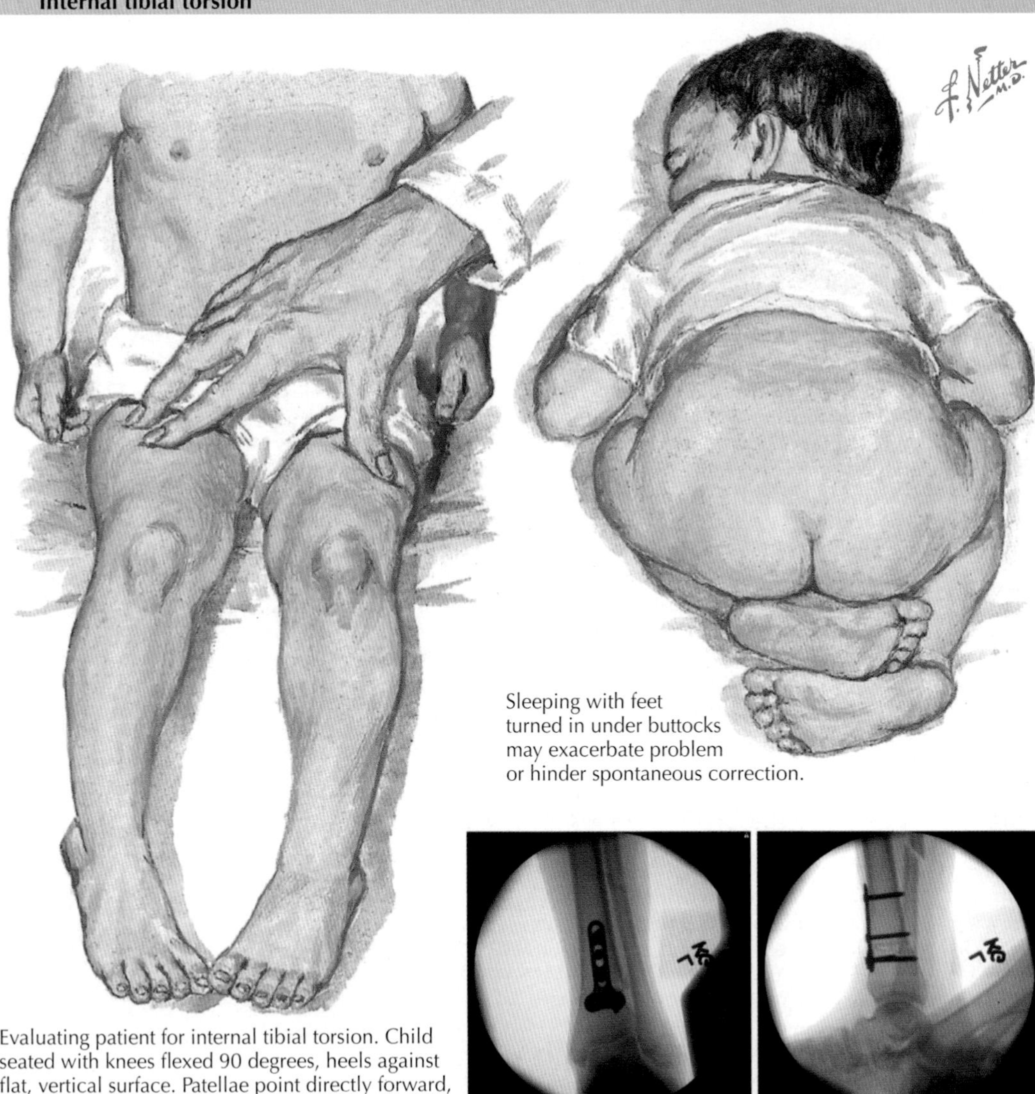

Evaluating patient for internal tibial torsion. Child seated with knees flexed 90 degrees, heels against flat, vertical surface. Patellae point directly forward, indicating that femurs are in neutral position, but feet point inward, indicating internal tibial torsion.

Sleeping with feet turned in under buttocks may exacerbate problem or hinder spontaneous correction.

Surgical correction of tibial rotational abnormality

ROTATIONAL DEFORMITIES OF LOWER LIMB

Rotational abnormalities in the lower limbs are common, particularly in the child's first several years. The abnormality may be at one level in the lower limb—the femur, tibia, or foot—or at several levels. Because the position of the feet is the most obvious clinical manifestation, these rotational problems are commonly referred to as toeing-in and toeing-out.

All rotational abnormalities in children should be evaluated to rule out a pathologic condition such as cerebral palsy, myelodysplasia (see Plate 1.45), diastematomyelia, or subtle onset of a neurologic problem such as peroneal muscular atrophy. Asymmetric findings and a history of progression, which are not characteristic of the usual rotational problem, strongly suggest a pathologic cause.

To obtain a proper and thorough evaluation, the child must be cooperative. First, the lower limb is examined in a sequential fashion, with the foot, tibia, and femur isolated in turn. Ambulatory children are observed standing and walking, both with and without shoes, to evaluate the coordination of walking, gait, and stance.

ABNORMALITIES OF THE FOOT

Metatarsus Adductus

In the newborn, the forefoot may turn in because of intrauterine positioning. Diagnosis is best made by inspecting the sole of the foot (Plate 4.20); a footprint can be made for documentation. Normally, the lateral border of the foot is straight. In the patient with metatarsus adductus, the lateral border of the forefoot is convex, with the curve beginning at the base of the fifth metatarsal.

When metatarsus adductus is suggested, the foot is tested for stiffness or suppleness by holding the heel firmly and attempting to push the foot laterally into an overcorrected position. In many children, the inward-turning foot can be corrected with the simple passive stretching exercise shown. Feet with mild deformity and good mobility typically do not require treatment. Spontaneous resolution of flexible deformity can occur up to 4 years of age, and minor residual deformity does not cause disability. Treatment of moderately deformed feet with some loss of mobility (passively correctable but not actively correctable) is controversial. Passive stretching and straight-last shoes can be helpful. Parents should perform the abduction exercise (see Plate 4.20) 10 times with every diaper change. An outward-flaring shoe (straight-last or reverse-last shoe) is sometimes used at this stage to keep the foot in an overcorrected position between exercises.

For a nonflexible, resistant, and symptomatic deformity, serial casting may be warranted. If serial casting fails to achieve proper alignment, then operative intervention is warranted. For younger children, surgical release of the abductor hallucis and first tarsometatarsal joint may be indicated. For older children, many operative interventions are described, including metatarsal osteotomies, opening wedge medial navicular osteotomy, and closing wedge cuboid osteotomy.

Calcaneovalgus

In the child with this common neonatal condition, the foot and ankle seem unusually lax and dorsiflex nearly to the shin (see Plate 5.38). Plantar flexion is restricted, and the heel is in valgus position.

Simple calcaneovalgus usually responds quickly to passive stretching exercises. Taping or casting of the foot in inversion and plantar flexion is effective for resistant deformities. Operative intervention is rarely ever required. Persistent deformity should be investigated to rule out congenital vertical talus.

ROTATIONAL DEFORMITIES OF LOWER LIMB (Continued)

ABNORMALITIES OF THE TIBIA

Internal Tibial Torsion

In this condition, the tibia is internally rotated on its long axis, causing the foot to point inward (see Plate 4.20). Internal tibial torsion is usually first noticed when the child is between 6 and 18 months of age and begins to walk.

Tibial torsion is best assessed with the child seated. The femurs are placed in neutral position with patellae pointing forward, the thighs directly in front of the hip joint, and the heels against the flat surface of the examining table. The feet are held in neutral position. Many examiners use the position of the medial malleolus relative to the lateral malleolus to determine the transmalleolar axis and its relationship to the long axis of the tibia or to a specific protuberance of the tibia, such as the tibial tuberosity. The malleoli are usually grasped by the examiner's fingers at the joint line either in the midportion or on the anterior aspect. The transmalleolar axis is then determined by observation or with a simple measuring device.

An alternative method is to use the thigh-foot angle, which reflects the difference in the angle between the axis of the thigh and that of the foot. With the patient prone and the knees flexed to 90 degrees, the foot and thigh are viewed from directly above.

The transmalleolar axis is normally in slight external rotation, about 5 degrees in the normal infant, increasing with growth to an average of 22 degrees in the adult. The greatest increase occurs in the first 18 months. Lateral bowing of the tibia, a common finding in children younger than 18 months of age, can accentuate internal tibial torsion.

Some controversy exists regarding the need for treatment. Internal tibial torsion often improves spontaneously, and in most children and adults, toeing-in due to internal tibial torsion is seldom a significant handicap.

Brace treatment has been a common form of treatment in the past. This treatment has proven to be ineffective and does not tend to change the natural history of gradual improvement. Additionally, treatment with the Denis-Browne bar can lead to genu valgum or excessive external tibial torsion.

Operative intervention is rarely required for internal tibial torsion. This would be reserved for patients older than the age of 8 years with significant internal tibial torsion that is limiting function. Frequent tripping because the feet catch behind the contralateral leg is a common difficulty for those patients with significant rotational deformity. For those with persistent difficulties, a supramalleolar tibial derotational osteotomy with internal fixation can be performed (see Plate 4.20). Proximal tibial osteotomies have a higher risk of compartment syndrome and late valgus deformity (Cozen phenomenon in younger children).

TOEING IN: INTERNAL FEMORAL TORSION

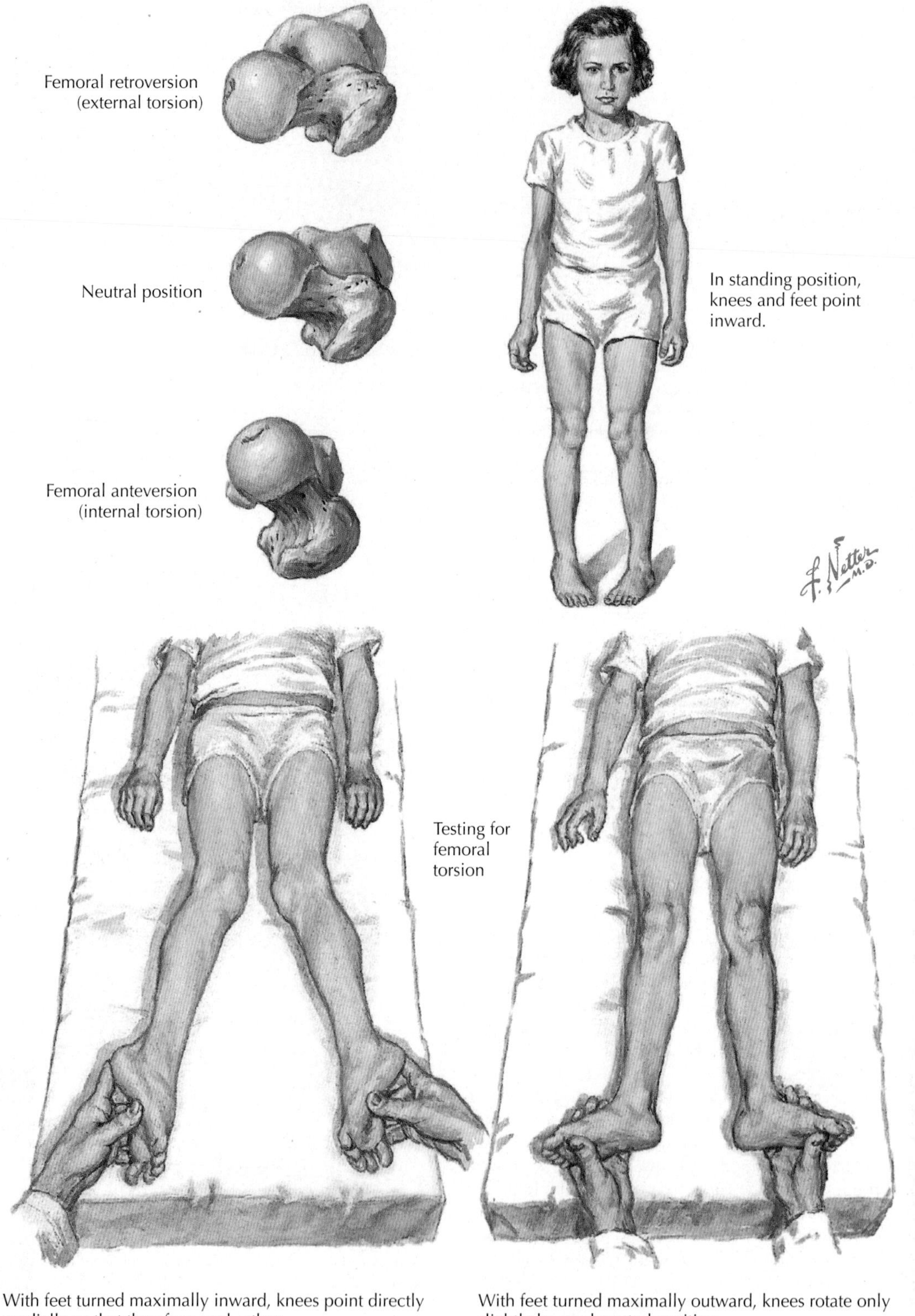

Femoral retroversion (external torsion)

Neutral position

Femoral anteversion (internal torsion)

In standing position, knees and feet point inward.

Testing for femoral torsion

With feet turned maximally inward, knees point directly medially so that they face each other.

With feet turned maximally outward, knees rotate only slightly beyond neutral position.

External Tibial Torsion

Less common than internal rotation, external tibial torsion is seldom a clinical problem in the child's first few years (Plate 4.22). Most children whose lower limbs appear to be externally rotated are found to have external rotation of the femur and therefore of the entire limb. Excessive external tibial torsion may limit push-off power during the stance phase. If treatment is indicated, a supramalleolar tibial derotational osteotomy with internal fixation can be performed.

ABNORMALITIES OF THE FEMUR

Internal Femoral Torsion (Anteversion)

This condition is the most common cause of toeing-in in children 3 to 12 years of age (Plate 4.21) and occurs because of the relationship of the femoral diaphysis and condyles to the femoral head and neck (femoral anteversion). The thighs can be rotated internally to a marked degree, but external rotation is quite limited. In patients who are severely affected, internal rotation may be as great as 90 degrees, whereas external rotation is

Toeing Out and Postural Torsional Effects on Lower Limbs

Toeing Out

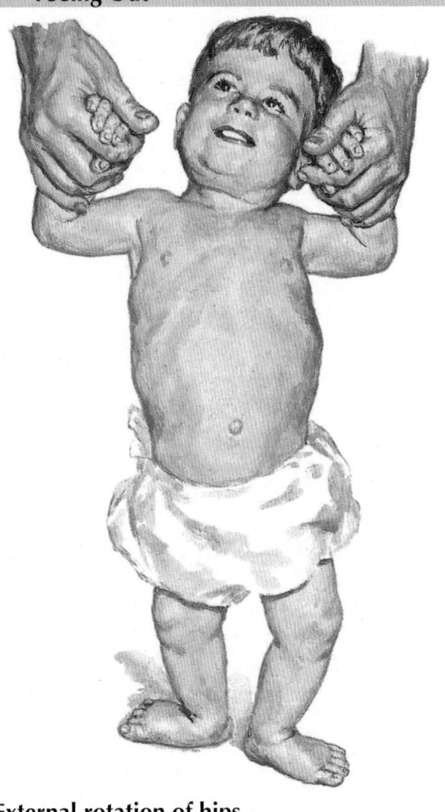

External rotation of hips. Knees and feet point laterally, indicating femoral origin of toeing-out deformity. Common in newborns but usually corrects spontaneously when child begins to walk.

In external rotation of hips, when feet are turned maximally inward, knees are in neutral position or, at most, in slight internal rotation.

External tibial torsion. Although feet are turned outward, knees point directly forward, showing that toeing out is due to tibial, not femoral, external torsion. This case resulted from overuse of Denis-Browne splint to correct internal femoral torsion.

Postural torsional effects on lower limbs

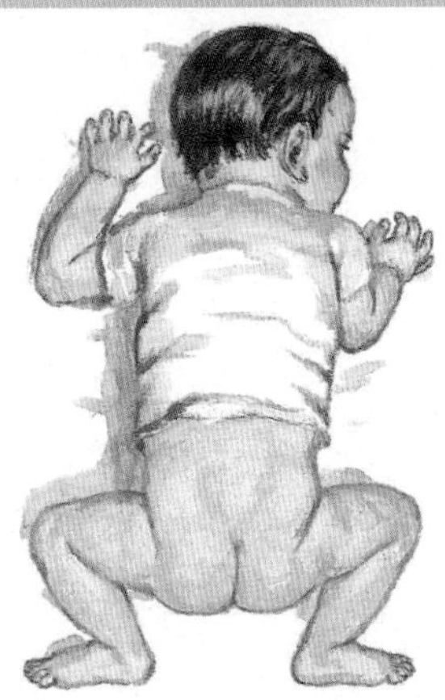

Spread-eagle or frog sleeping position may contribute to external rotation of hips.

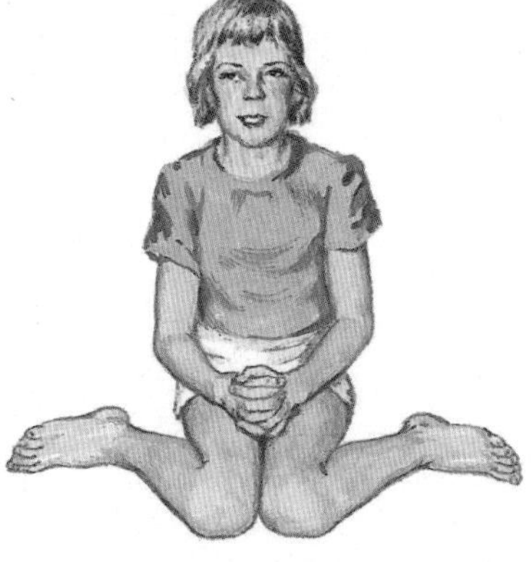

Reversed tailor position places internal torsional stress on femurs and external torsion on tibias. May delay correction of torsional deformities.

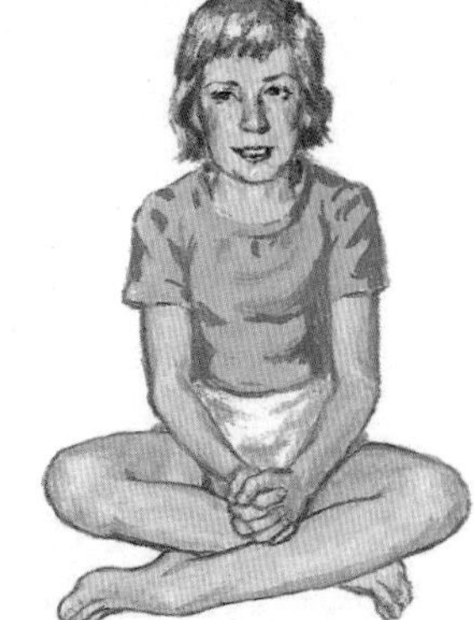

Sitting cross-legged (tailor position) applies external torsion on femurs and internal torsion to tibias. May help correct external tibial torsion.

Rotational Deformities of Lower Limb (Continued)

absent or very slight. With ambulation and stance, the patellae are noted to be pointed internally.

Although this condition is often referred to as a problem in hip rotation, the cause lies in the orientation of the femur itself. It is important to reassure parents that there is nothing wrong with the child's hip joint.

Femoral rotation is best assessed with the child recumbent, either supine or prone, and the hips in extension. With the patient supine, the physician rotates the entire limb. The position of the legs is observed in both internal rotation and external rotation. Marked internal rotation and limited external rotation of the femur strongly suggest internal femoral torsion.

Alternatively, with the patient prone, the pelvis is maintained level and the knees are flexed. Medial rotation refers to the angle between vertical and the axis of the tibia when the hips are maximally rotated inward. The internal hip rotation is accomplished by allowing the legs to fall outward by gravity alone. External rotation is also measured, with the patient in the same position, by allowing the legs to cross. The pelvis needs to remain flat on the table.

Although it may be tempting to do this type of examination with the patient sitting, the patient *must* be examined with the hips in extension, because this position tightens the anterior joint capsule. When the hips are flexed, these ligaments are relaxed, thus permitting a greater range of external rotation and resulting in an inaccurate evaluation.

Internal femoral torsion may also be measured using biplane radiography, axial tomography, fluoroscopy, magnetic resonance imaging, or computed tomography. Radiography is only appropriate if surgical correction is contemplated. Newer computed tomographic studies can help provide measurement for femoral rotation.

In the newborn, internal femoral torsion is at most 40 degrees. This usually decreases rapidly in the child's first 2 years and then continues to decrease more slowly, reaching a plateau at age 8 to 9 years and decreasing to about 16 degrees in adulthood.

Until the child is 2 years of age, the total range of rotation in the hip is about 120 degrees; thereafter, it is 90 to 110 degrees. Ideally, the ranges of internal rotation and external rotation are about equal (45–50 degrees).

No conservative treatment has been found to correct internal femoral torsion. Twister cables, braces, and orthopedic shoes have no effect and may produce abnormal external tibial torsion (see Plate 4.22) and a knock-kneed gait.

Fortunately, internal femoral torsion tends to improve with normal growth. However, many affected children prefer to sit in the reversed tailor or W-sitting position (Plate 4.22). This sitting position was once thought to cause harm to the hip socket and previously was actively discouraged. It is now known to have no detrimental effects.

In their teens, many children no longer toe in, although the degree of internal femoral torsion has not changed. This suggests an adaptive process in the lower limbs, most likely in the joint capsule and soft tissues about the joint. Occasionally, a child is seen with severe internal femoral torsion associated with little or no external rotation. The patient has trouble walking and running or is clumsy. In these patients, derotational femoral osteotomy should be considered.

External Rotatory Contracture of Hips

This condition is a common finding in children in the first few months of life and seldom represents true external femoral rotation (retroversion). Rather, it is related to the changes in the joint capsule and soft tissue structures about the hip that are in part due to the position of the fetus. In these patients, treatment with simple internal rotation stretching exercises is sufficient. The condition usually resolves by the time the child begins to walk. If not, use of a Denis-Browne splint with the feet set in neutral position or in slight internal rotation is the treatment of choice.

ANKLE AND FOOT

Surface Anatomy and Muscle Origins and Insertions

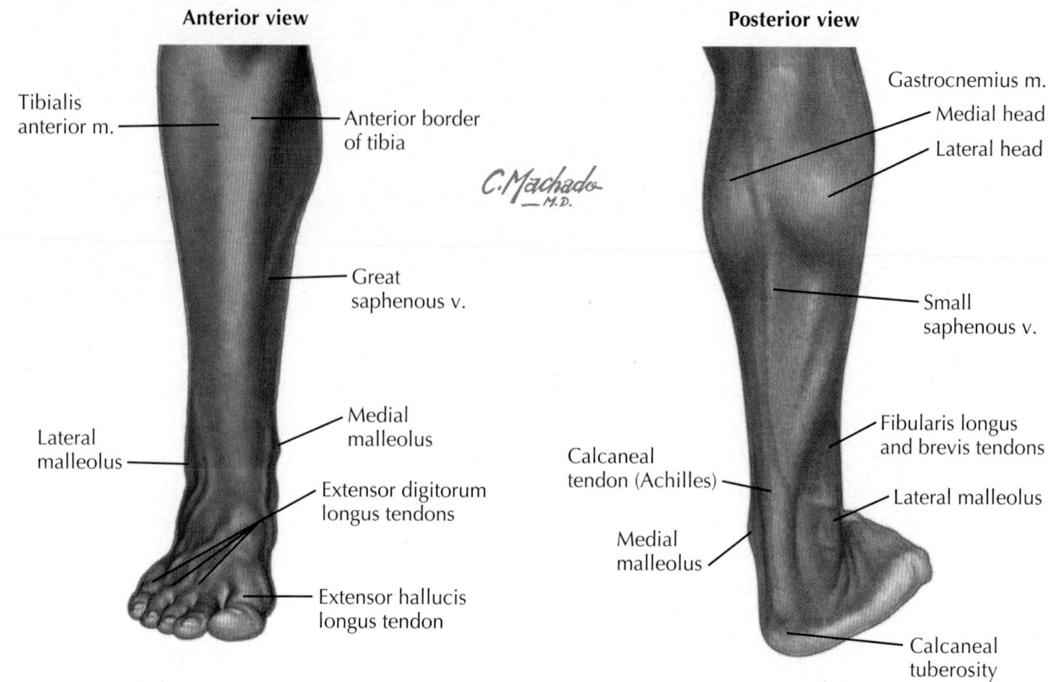

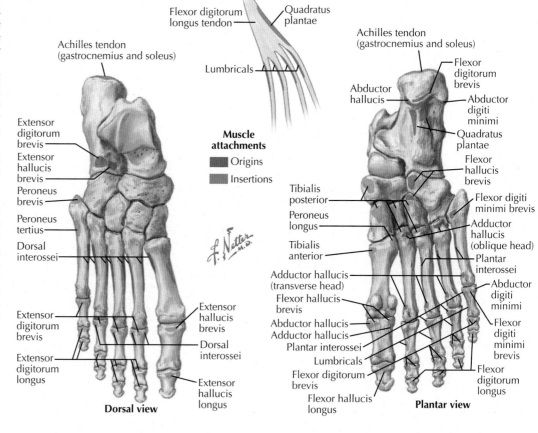

Flexor digitorum longus tendon
Quadratus plantae
Lumbricals
Achilles tendon (gastrocnemius and soleus)
Extensor digitorum brevis
Extensor hallucis brevis
Peroneus brevis
Peroneus tertius
Dorsal interossei
Extensor digitorum brevis
Extensor digitorum longus
Extensor hallucis brevis
Dorsal interossei
Extensor hallucis longus
Dorsal view
Muscle attachments
Origins
Insertions
Achilles tendon (gastrocnemius and soleus)
Abductor hallucis
Flexor digitorum brevis
Abductor digiti minimi
Quadratus plantae
Flexor hallucis brevis
Tibialis posterior
Flexor digiti minimi brevis
Peroneus longus
Adductor hallucis (oblique head)
Tibialis anterior
Plantar interossei
Adductor hallucis (transverse head)
Abductor digiti minimi
Flexor hallucis brevis
Abductor hallucis
Adductor hallucis
Flexor digiti minimi brevis
Plantar interossei
Lumbricals
Flexor digitorum brevis
Flexor digitorum longus
Flexor hallucis longus
Plantar view

Anatomy of the Ankle and Foot

TENDON SHEATHS AT ANKLE

The extrinsic tendons of the foot originate as muscles in the leg, and, as the tendons cross the ankle, they must change their orientation. The retinaculum and the corresponding bony anatomy account for the pulley system that allows this to occur and to generate a mechanical advantage for transmission of force. The retinaculum also prevents bowstringing by holding the tendons, vessels, and nerves against the bone as they transverse the ankle joint.

The *superior extensor retinaculum* is a reinforcement of the crural fascia just above the ankle. It is attached laterally to the lower end of the fibula and medially to the tibia, and it covers the structure of the anterior compartment of the leg. A strong septum runs from its deep surface to the tibia, separating a medial compartment for the tendon of the tibialis anterior muscle from a lateral compartment for the tendons of the long extensor muscles.

The *inferior extensor retinaculum* is a well-defined, Y-shaped band overlying the dorsum of the foot and the front of the ankle. The stem of the Y arises from the upper surface of the calcaneus and is in the form of two laminae, one superficial and one deep to the tendons of the peroneus tertius and extensor digitorum longus muscles. At the medial border of the latter tendon, the two laminae merge and the limbs of the Y begin to diverge. One limb is directed upward and medialward to attach to the medial malleolus. It passes over the tendon of the extensor hallucis longus muscle, the dorsalis pedis vessels, and the deep peroneal nerve but splits to form a separate canal for the tendon of the tibialis anterior muscle. The lower limb of the Y passes medialward across the medial border of the foot and is lost in the deep fascia of the sole.

The *flexor retinaculum* stretches from the medial malleolus to the medial tubercle of the calcaneus. From its deep surface, septa pass to the back of the lower end of the tibia and the capsule of the ankle joint. The four canals defined by these septa transmit, beginning medially, the tendon of the tibialis posterior muscle, that of the flexor digitorum longus muscle, the posterior tibial vessels and the tibial nerve, and the tendon of the flexor hallucis longus muscle. The upper border of the flexor retinaculum is continuous with the transverse intermuscular septum. Its lower border is continuous with the deep fascia of the sole and gives origin to the fibers of the abductor hallucis muscle.

The peroneal retinacula are thickenings of the fascia on the lateral side of the ankle. The *superior peroneal retinaculum* extends from the lateral malleolus into the fascia of the back of the leg and to the lateral surface of the calcaneus. The *inferior peroneal retinaculum* is a thickening of fascia, both ends of which attach to the lateral surface of the calcaneus. It is continuous superiorly with the stem of the Y of the inferior extensor retinaculum. Deep to the peroneal retinacula pass the tendons of the peroneus longus and peroneus brevis muscles; the peroneus brevis tendon is anterior, behind the medial malleolus and superior to the tendon of the peroneus longus muscle beneath the inferior peroneal retinaculum.

ANKLE JOINT

This tibiotalar articulation is a synovial joint of the hinge (ginglymus) type. The ankle joint appears as a mortise and tenon structure from architectural design

Tendon Sheaths of Ankle

Lateral view

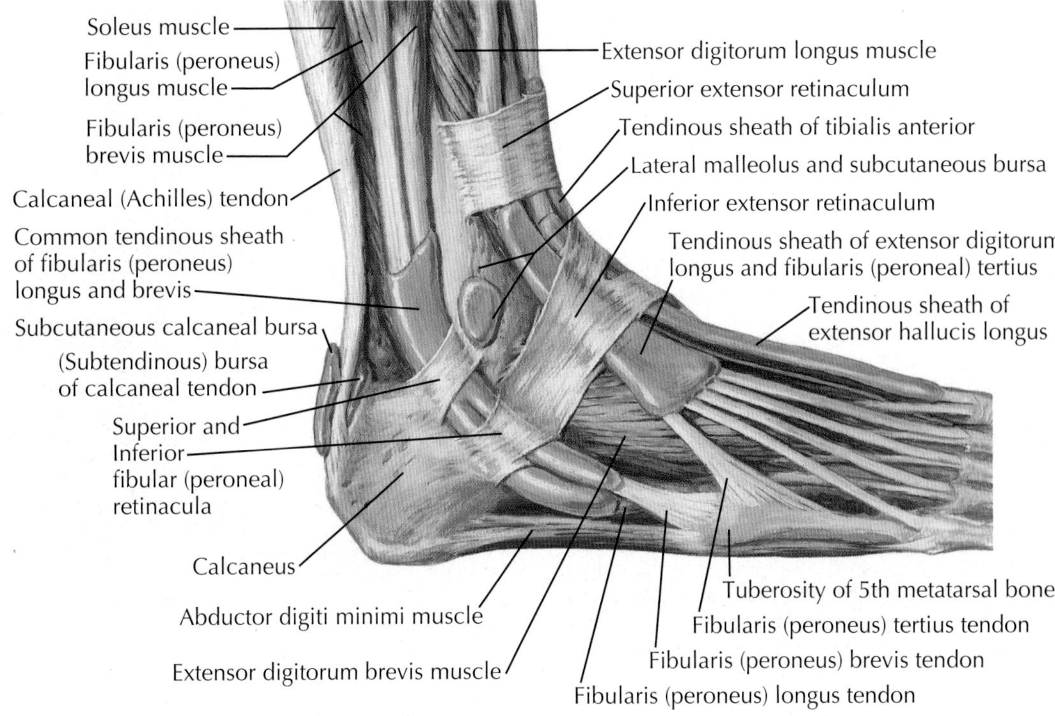

Medial view

Tibialis anterior tendon and sheath
Tibia
Sheath of tibialis posterior tendon
Superior extensor retinaculum
Medial malleolus and subcutaneous bursa
Inferior extensor retinaculum
Tibialis posterior tendon and sheath
Tibialis anterior tendon and sheath
Tendinous sheath of extensor hallucis longus
1st metatarsal bone
Tendinous sheath of flexor hallucis longus
Medial plantar nerve
Tendinous sheath of flexor digitorum longus
Calcaneal (Achilles) tendon
Tendinous sheath of flexor digitorum longus
Posterior tibial artery and tibial nerve
Tendinous sheath of flexor hallucis longus
Subcutaneous calcaneal bursa
(Subtendinous) bursa of calcaneal tendon
Flexor retinaculum
Calcaneus
Lateral plantar nerve
Abductor hallucis muscle (*cut*)
Plantar aponeurosis (*cut*)
Flexor digitorum brevis muscle (*cut*)

ANATOMY OF THE ANKLE AND FOOT (Continued)

and construction. The distal tibial plafond and medial malleolus along with the lateral malleolus from the distal fibula form the mortise for the body of the talus, which is the tenon.

The trochlea of the talus is convex from anterior to posterior and slightly concave from medial to lateral. The talar body is slightly larger anteriorly than posteriorly owing to the oblique nature of the lateral side. The medial side of the talar body articulates with the tibia via the medial malleolus, whereas the lateral side articulates with the distal fibula through the lateral malleolus.

The *articular capsule,* conforming to the requirements of free movement in flexion and extension at the ankle, is weak anteriorly and posteriorly. However, the joint has exceedingly strong collateral ligaments. The thin anterior and posterior parts of the capsule are attached above to the margins of the tibia and fibula and below to the talus both in front and behind the superior surface of its trochlea. The capsule blends with the deltoid ligament on the medial side of the ankle and with the anterior and posterior talofibular ligaments on the lateral side. The *deltoid ligament* is a strong triangular ligament, attached at its anterior and posterior borders and the tip of the medial malleolus. The ligament broadens inferiorly to form a continuous attachment to the bones of the foot; its four parts are designated by their separate distal attachments. The most anterior fibers compose the *anterior tibiotalar ligament.* These are adjacent to the superficial *tibionavicular ligament* to the upper and medial part of the navicular. Below, this ligament blends with the medial margin of the plantar calcaneonavicular ligament. Next, the fibers of the *tibiocalcaneal ligament* descend almost vertically to the whole length of the sustentaculum tali of the calcaneus. The posterior and thickest part of the deltoid is the *posterior tibiotalar ligament;* its fibers run lateral and posterior to the medial side of the talus and to the medial tubercle of its posterior process.

The lateral collateral ligament consists of three separate bands that are weaker than the stout deltoid ligament. The *anterior talofibular ligament* passes from the anterior border and tip of the lateral malleolus to the neck of the talus. The *calcaneofibular ligament* is a narrow, rounded cord that descends from the tip of the lateral malleolus to a tubercle at the middle of the lateral surface of the calcaneus. The almost-horizontal *posterior talofibular ligament* is strong and thick. It arises in the malleolar fossa of the lateral malleolus and passes medial and posterior to the upper surface of the posterior process of the talus.

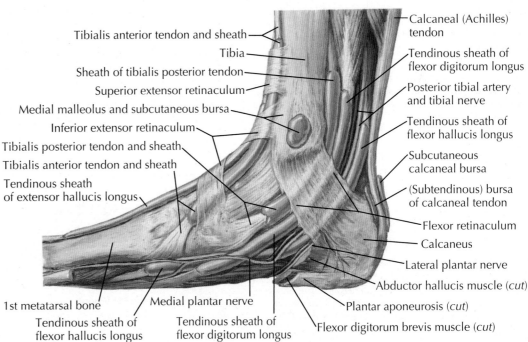

The *synovial membrane* of the ankle extends proximally, between the apposed surfaces of the ends of the tibia and fibula, as far as the interosseous ligament of the tibiofibular syndesmosis. The ankle joint receives its blood supply from the four malleolar branches of the anterior tibial, posterior tibial, and peroneal arteries. Its *nerve supply* is provided by branches from the tibial nerve and the lateral branch of the deep peroneal nerve.

MOVEMENTS

The primary motions attributed to the tibiotalar joint are dorsiflexion and plantar flexion through a normal range of approximately 90 degrees. In dorsiflexion, the broader anterior portion of the trochlea occupies and completely fills the mortise of the joint, and stability of the foot is greatest in this position. During this time, the fibula externally rotates slightly and the intermalleolar distance increases to accommodate the larger

ANATOMY OF THE ANKLE AND FOOT (Continued)

anterior surface. Conversely, in full plantar flexion, the narrowest part of the trochlea engages in the mortise and stability is markedly decreased; small amounts of side-to-side gliding movements, rotation, and abduction-adduction are permitted. The muscles entering the foot behind the malleoli, those of the lateral and both posterior compartments of the leg, produce plantar flexion at the ankle, and dorsiflexion follows contraction of the muscles of the anterior compartment of the leg.

DORSAL FOOT

Skin, Subcutaneous Tissue, and Fascia

The majority of the structures passing over the dorsum of the foot are continuations of the anterior compartment of the leg. The skin here is thin, and there is relatively little subcutaneous fat. The deep fascia is continuous with the extensor retinacula and curves over the margins of the foot to become the fascia of the sole. The fascia of the dorsal foot encloses the extensor tendon, with the extensor retinaculum being the primary checkrein to bowstringing and acting as a pulley to alter the orientation of motion of the extrinsic tendons.

Muscles

The *extensor digitorum brevis muscle* is broad and thin. It arises from the distal part of the superior and lateral surfaces of the calcaneus and the stem of the inferior extensor retinaculum. The muscle divides into four tendons for the medial four toes. The largest and most medial tendon, together with its belly, is often separately designated as the *extensor hallucis brevis muscle.* It inserts into the base of the first phalanx of the great toe. The other three tendons join the lateral sides of the tendons of the extensor digitorum longus muscle to the second, third, and fourth toes and assist in forming the extensor expansions on these digits. The muscle assists the long extensor muscle in extending the proximal phalanges of the medial four toes.

Arteries

The *dorsalis pedis artery* is the continuation of the anterior tibial artery at the ankle joint. It is directed forward across the dorsum of the foot to the proximal end of the first metatarsal space. Here, it divides into the deep plantar and first dorsal metatarsal arteries. The dorsalis pedis artery lies against the bones and ligaments of the dorsum, with the medial branch of the deep peroneal nerve lateral to it. It is accompanied by two venae comitantes. Its branches are the lateral tarsal, medial tarsal, arcuate, first dorsal metatarsal, and deep plantar arteries.

The *lateral tarsal artery* arises over the navicular bone and passes lateral and distal. It supplies the extensor digitorum brevis muscle and the tarsal articulations and anastomoses with branches of the arcuate, anterior lateral malleolar, and the perforating branch of the peroneal arteries. The dorsalis pedis artery is absent or greatly reduced in about 5% of cases, and this lateral anastomosis is greatly enlarged, taking over the main supply that usually comes down medially on the dorsum of the foot. In such variations, the peroneal artery is the principal source of blood supply. The *medial tarsal arteries* are two or three small branches that spread over the medial border of the foot, anastomosing with the medial malleolar arteries. The *arcuate artery* arises at the level of the bases of the metatarsals

LIGAMENTS AND TENDONS OF ANKLE

Right foot: lateral view

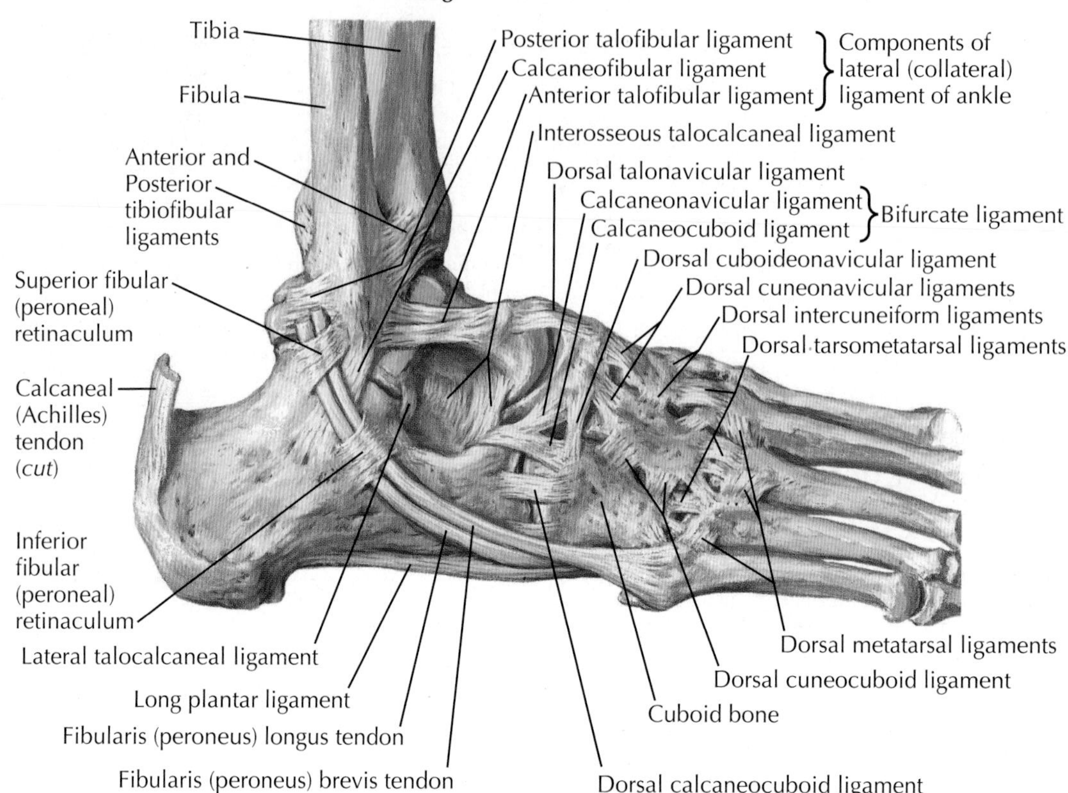

Right foot: medial view

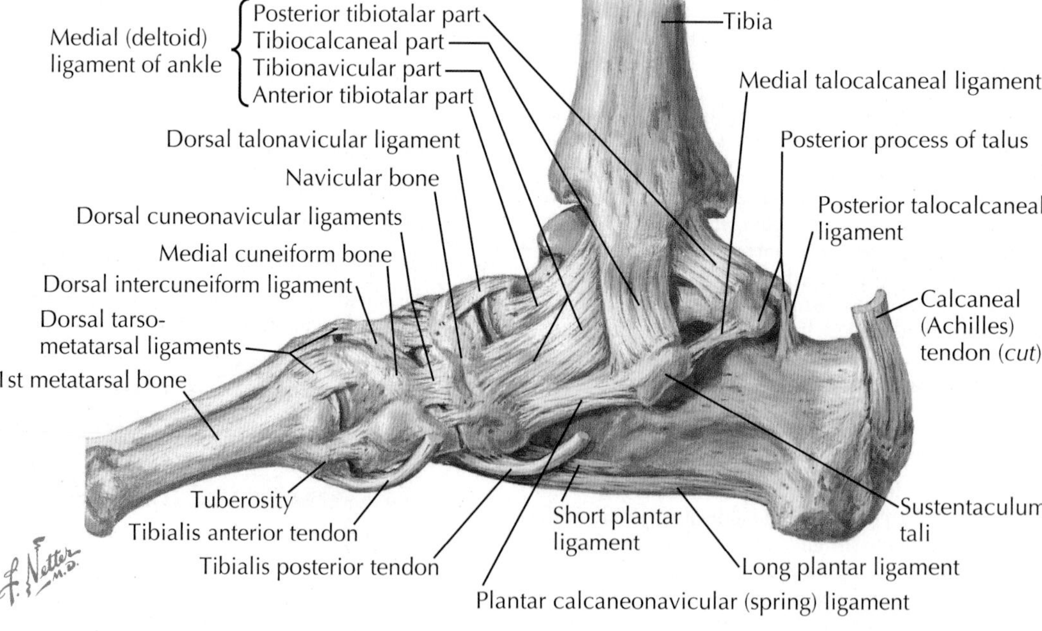

Dorsal Foot: Superficial Dissection

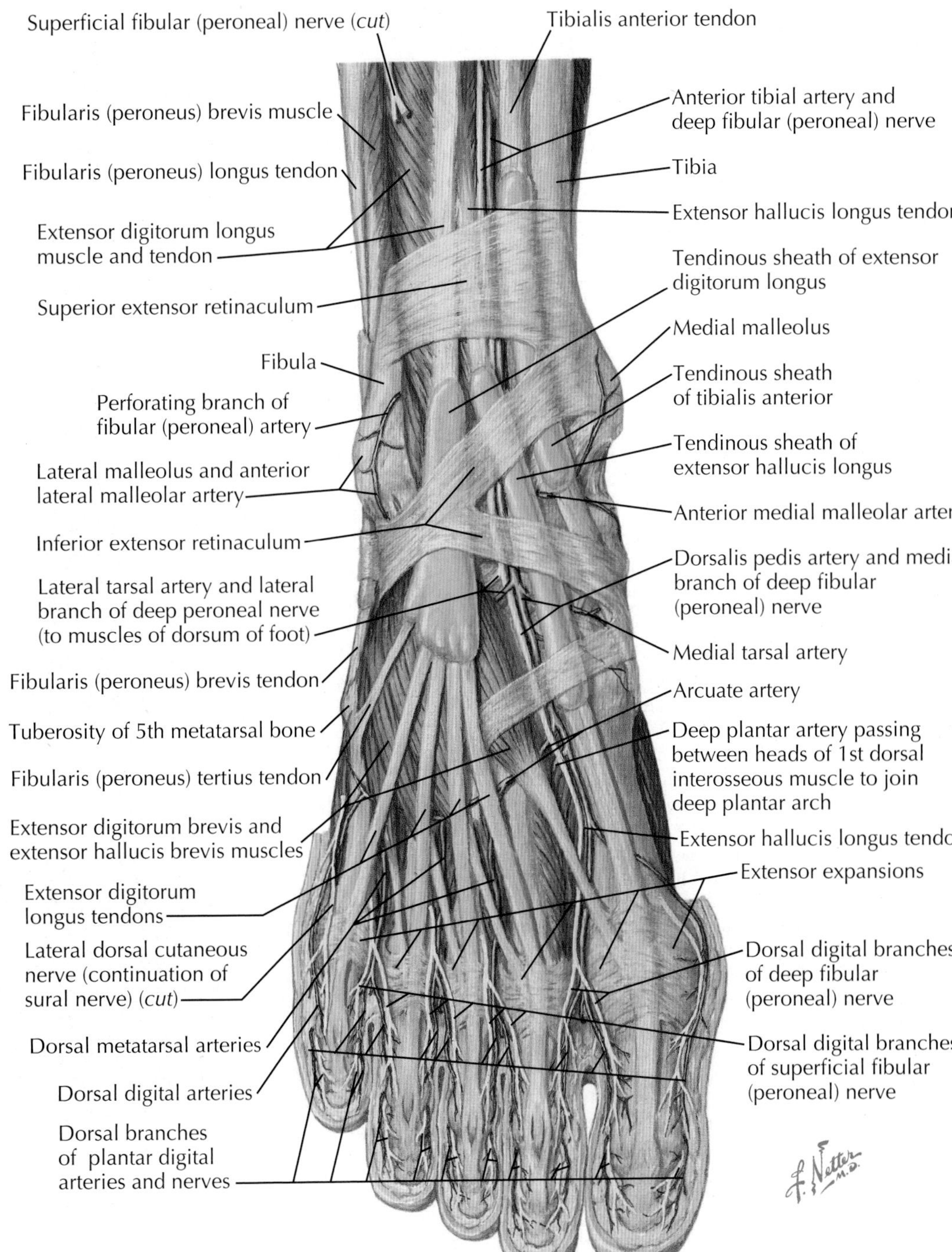

Anatomy of the Ankle and Foot (Continued)

and runs lateral across the proximal ends of these bones beneath the extensor tendons. Laterally, it ends by anastomosing with the lateral tarsal and lateral plantar arteries. Three *dorsal metatarsal arteries* arise from the arcuate artery and pass distally over the dorsal interosseous muscle to the clefts of the toes. Here, each divides into two *dorsal digital arteries* for the adjacent sides of the toes on either side of the cleft. Like the dorsal digital arteries of the fingers, they do not reach the distal phalanx. The fourth dorsal metatarsal artery has an additional dorsal digital branch for the lateral side of the small toe.

The metatarsal arteries have posterior and anterior perforating arteries proximally and distally in the interosseous space, which perforate to anastomose with corresponding plantar metatarsal arteries. The *first dorsal metatarsal artery* is like the other dorsal metatarsal arteries in its course and division into two dorsal digital arteries to the adjacent sides of the first and second toes. It also gives off an extra dorsal digital artery for the medial side of the great toe. The *deep plantar artery* is the much-enlarged posterior perforating branch of the first dorsal metatarsal artery. Passing proximally between the two heads of origin of the first dorsal interosseous muscle of the sole of the foot, it unites with the lateral plantar artery to form the plantar arterial arch (see Plate 5.10). It behaves like the radial artery in the hand, as that artery completes the deep palmar arterial arch.

Nerves

The *deep peroneal nerve* (S1, S2) divides into its medial and lateral terminal branches at the lower border of the inferior extensor retinaculum. As noted, the lateral branch supplies the extensor digitorum brevis muscle and the tarsal joints. The medial branch passes distally lateral to the dorsalis pedis artery. It divides into two dorsal digital nerves to the adjacent sides of the great and second toes. Other small branches supply the metatarsophalangeal and interphalangeal articulations of the great toe, and one supplies the first dorsal interosseous muscle.

Plantar Foot

Skin, Subcutaneous Tissue, and Fascia

The structures of the plantar region are shown in Plates 5.7 to 5.9. The *skin* of the foot is thin on the toes and instep. It is thickened over the heel and the heads of the metatarsals in response to friction and weight-bearing. There is much fat in the subcutaneous tissue of the sole and plantar aspects of the toes. Intermingled with fibrous connective tissue, the firmly supported fat over the sole and heel forms a cushioning pad for the weight-bearing parts of the foot. The *plantar fascia* is continuous with the deep fascia of the dorsum of the foot after attachments to the periosteum of the sides of the first and fifth metatarsals. Thinner membranous sheets medially and laterally enclose the compartments of the great and little toes, and a thickened plantar aponeurosis covers the central compartment. This *plantar aponeurosis* (comparable to the palmar aponeurosis in the hand) consists of longitudinally arranged bands of fibrous connective tissue, which diverge toward the toes from the medial process of the tuberosity of the calcaneus. Five digital slips pass to the plantar surface of the toes. Deeper-lying transverse fibers form a reinforcing band, the *superficial transverse metatarsal ligament,*

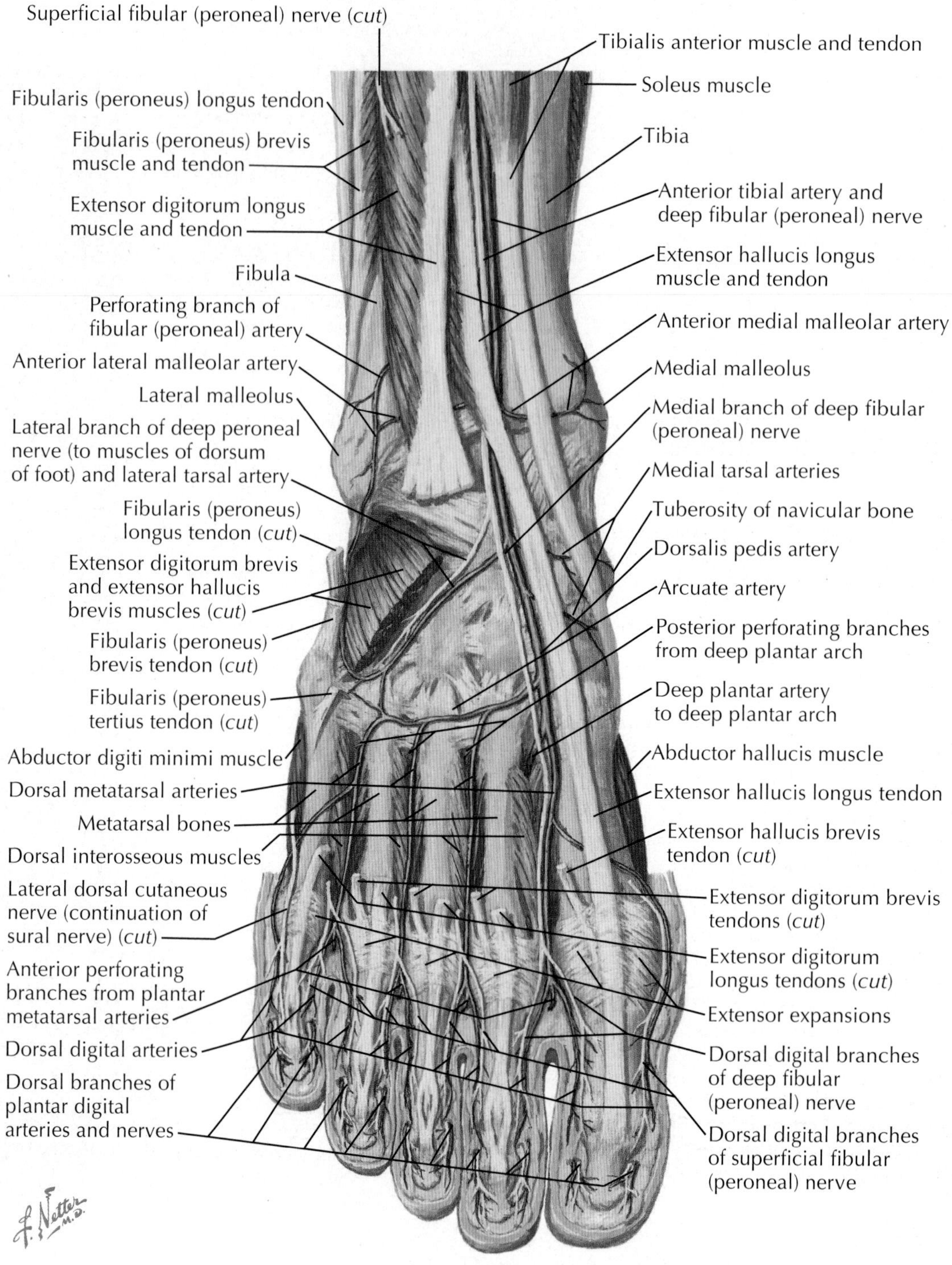

Anatomy of the Ankle and Foot (Continued)

over the heads of the metatarsals. *Transverse fasciculi* reinforce the webs of the toes.

Marginal fibers of the digital slips pass deeply to blend with the proximal ends of the fibrous sheaths of the flexor tendons and attach to the deep transverse metatarsal and plantar ligaments. The superficial central fibers of the digital slips end largely in the skin of the flexion creases between the toes and the sole. At the lateral and medial margins of the plantar aponeurosis, fibers radiate onto the thinner membranous fascia of the side compartments and deep intermuscular septa penetrate the soft parts of the sole of the foot and separate the central compartment from the others. These septa reach the plantar interosseous fascia and the bones and ligaments deep in the foot. The *lateral plantar fascia* is thick and well developed near the heel and thinner toward the small toe. A *calcaneometatarsal ligament* extends within it from the lateral process of the tuberosity of the calcaneus to the tuberosity of the fifth metatarsal. The thinner *medial plantar fascia* covers the intrinsic muscles of the great toe.

Compartments

The number of compartments that make up the plantar foot has been debated. Most believe that there are four clinically relevant compartments, namely, medial, lateral, central, and interosseous. Some research has identified nine compartments, including a separate calcaneal compartment that is continuous with the deep posterior compartment of the leg. The *medial compartment* contains the abductor hallucis and flexor hallucis brevis muscles, the tendon of the flexor hallucis longus, and the medial plantar nerve and vessels. The *lateral compartment* consists of the abductor digiti minimi and flexor digiti minimi brevis. The *central compartment* includes the flexor digitorum brevis, the tendon of the flexor hallucis longus and lumbricals, the adductor hallucis, the quadratus plantae, and the lateral plantar nerve and vessels. Finally, the *interosseous compartment* contains the interosseous muscles, the plantar arterial arch, the deep branch of the lateral plantar nerve, and the dorsal metatarsal branches of the dorsalis pedis artery.

Muscles

The *flexor hallucis brevis* is a two-bellied muscle; between its bellies, the tendon of the flexor hallucis longus muscle passes to its insertion on the base of the distal phalanx of the great toe. The muscle arises from the plantar aspect of the cuboid and the adjacent part of the lateral cuneiform, the tibialis posterior tendon, and the medial side of the first metatarsal. The two muscle bellies have an intermediate tendinous raphe, and the medial belly blends with the abductor hallucis muscle to insert into the medial side of the base of the proximal phalanx of the great toe. The lateral belly, combining with the tendon of the adductor hallucis muscle, inserts into the lateral side of the base of the same phalanx. A sesamoid in each tendon of the short flexor muscle acts as a bearing and plays against the underside of the head of the first metatarsal. The flexor hallucis brevis acts in flexion of the hallux through the metatarsophalangeal joint.

The *abductor hallucis muscle* arises superficially from the medial process of the tuberosity of the calcaneus, the flexor retinaculum, and the intermuscular septum separating it from the flexor hallucis brevis muscle. It inserts into the medial side of the base of the proximal phalanx of the great toe, partly blending with the

Dorsal Foot: Deep Dissection

Superficial fibular (peroneal) nerve (*cut*)
Fibularis (peroneus) longus tendon
Fibularis (peroneus) brevis muscle and tendon
Extensor digitorum longus muscle and tendon
Fibula
Perforating branch of fibular (peroneal) artery
Anterior lateral malleolar artery
Lateral malleolus
Lateral branch of deep peroneal nerve (to muscles of dorsum of foot) and lateral tarsal artery
Fibularis (peroneus) longus tendon (*cut*)
Extensor digitorum brevis and extensor hallucis brevis muscles (*cut*)
Fibularis (peroneus) brevis tendon (*cut*)
Fibularis (peroneus) tertius tendon (*cut*)
Abductor digiti minimi muscle
Dorsal metatarsal arteries
Metatarsal bones
Dorsal interosseous muscles
Lateral dorsal cutaneous nerve (continuation of sural nerve) (*cut*)
Anterior perforating branches from plantar metatarsal arteries
Dorsal digital arteries
Dorsal branches of plantar digital arteries and nerves
Tibialis anterior muscle and tendon
Soleus muscle
Tibia
Anterior tibial artery and deep fibular (peroneal) nerve
Extensor hallucis longus muscle and tendon
Anterior medial malleolar artery
Medial malleolus
Medial branch of deep fibular (peroneal) nerve
Medial tarsal arteries
Tuberosity of navicular bone
Dorsalis pedis artery
Arcuate artery
Posterior perforating branches from deep plantar arch
Deep plantar artery to deep plantar arch
Abductor hallucis muscle
Extensor hallucis longus tendon
Extensor hallucis brevis tendon (*cut*)
Extensor digitorum brevis tendons (*cut*)
Extensor digitorum longus tendons (*cut*)
Extensor expansions
Dorsal digital branches of deep fibular (peroneal) nerve
Dorsal digital branches of superficial fibular (peroneal) nerve
F. Netter M.D.

PLANTAR FOOT: SUPERFICIAL DISSECTION

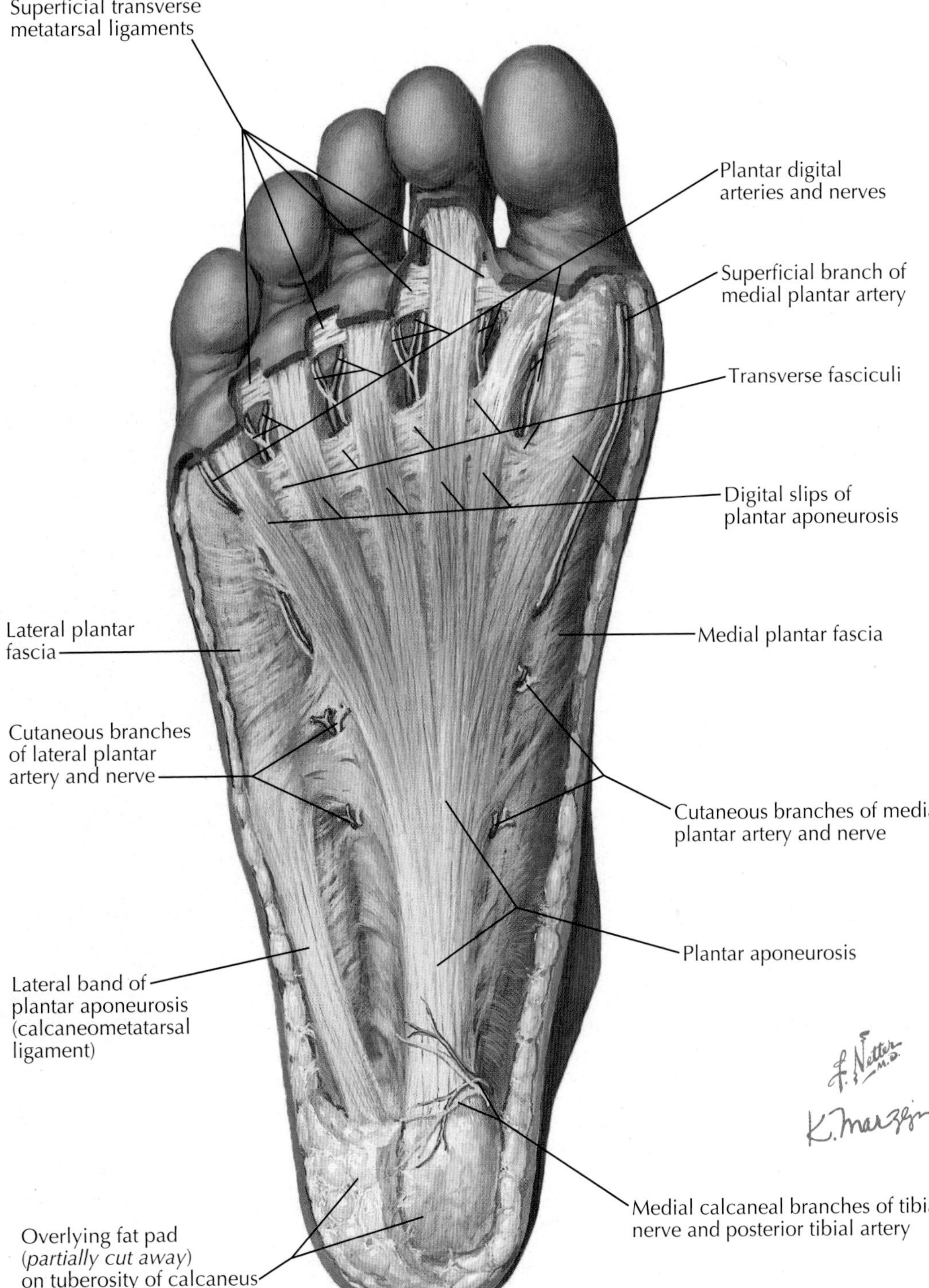

ANATOMY OF THE ANKLE AND FOOT (Continued)

medial head of the flexor hallucis brevis muscle. The abductor hallucis abducts the great toe from the axis of the second ray.

The *abductor digiti minimi muscle* arises from both the medial and lateral processes of the tuberosity of the calcaneus, from the lateral plantar fascia, and from the intermuscular septum between it and the flexor digitorum brevis muscle. Its tendon inserts on the lateral side of the base of the proximal phalanx of the fifth toe. The abductor digiti minimi abducts the fifth toe from the axis of the second ray.

The *flexor digiti minimi brevis muscle* underlies and is medial to the abductor digiti minimi tendon. Its origin is the base of the fifth metatarsal and the sheath of the peroneus longus tendon. Its tendon inserts on the lateral side of the base of the proximal phalanx of the fifth digit. The flexor digiti minimi brevis flexes the fifth toe through the metatarsophalangeal joint.

The *flexor digitorum brevis muscle* immediately underlies the plantar aponeurosis. It arises from the medial process of the tuberosity of the calcaneus, the posterior third of the plantar aponeurosis, and the intermuscular septa on either side of it. The muscle divides into four tendons. Opposite each proximal phalanx, each tendon divides into two slips, between which passes the tendon of the flexor digitorum longus muscle. Turning under the tendon of the flexor digitorum longus, the two slips of each tendon of the flexor digitorum brevis unite and insert into the base of the middle phalanx. The flexor digitorum brevis muscle flexes the middle phalanges of the lateral four toes and assists in metatarsophalangeal flexion of the same digits.

The *tendon of the flexor hallucis longus muscle* passes through the lateralmost compartment under the flexor retinaculum and enters the foot under the sustentaculum tali of the calcaneus. Directed toward the great toe, it passes superior to the tendon of the flexor digitorum longus muscle (to which it contributes a tendinous slip) and then lies in the groove between the two bellies of the flexor hallucis brevis muscle. It inserts on the base of the distal phalanx. The flexor hallucis longus muscle flexes the great toe at the distal interphalangeal joint.

The *quadratus plantae muscle,* accessory to the long digital flexor, arises by two heads separated from one another by the long plantar ligament. Its tendinous lateral head arises from the lateral border of the plantar surface of the calcaneus and from the long plantar ligament. Its fleshy medial head takes origin from the medial surface of the calcaneus and the medial border of the long plantar surface of the calcaneus and the medial border of the long plantar ligament. The two parts join to form a flattened, muscular band inserting into the lateral margin and both surfaces of the tendon of the flexor digitorum longus muscle. The quadratus plantae muscle assists the tendons of the flexor digitorum longus muscle in flexing the toes and helps to bring the line of traction of those tendons more nearly parallel with the long axis of the foot.

The *lumbrical muscles,* as in the hand, are four small, cylindrical muscles arising from the four tendons of the flexor digitorum longus muscle. The tendons cross on the plantar side of the deep transverse metatarsal ligaments and end in the medial surface of the extensor expansion over the lateral four toes. The lumbrical muscles flex the proximal phalanges at the metatarsophalangeal joints and extend the middle and distal phalanges.

The *adductor hallucis muscle* arises by oblique and transverse heads. The oblique head arises from the

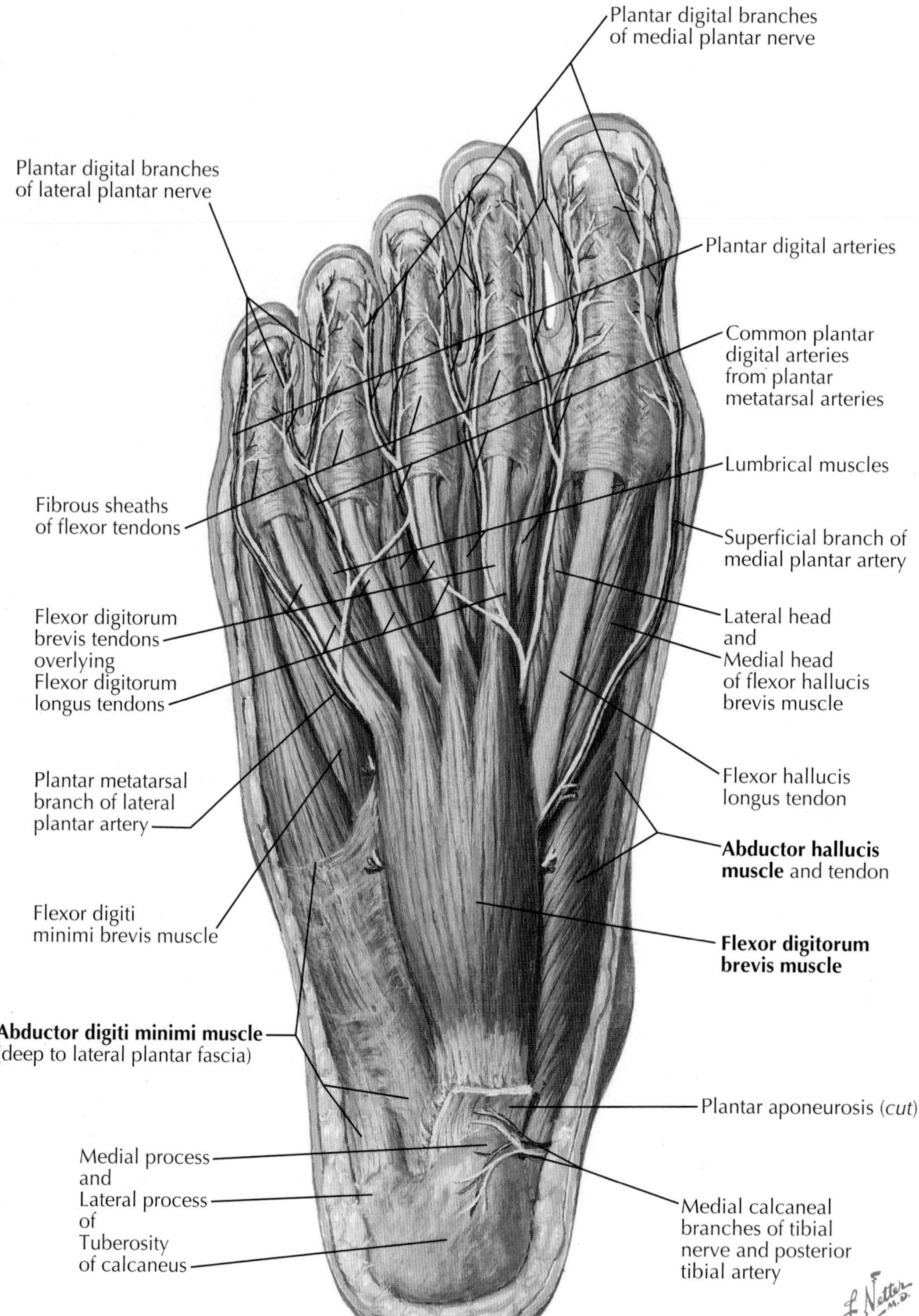

Anatomy of the Ankle and Foot (Continued)

bases of the second, third, and fourth metatarsals and from the sheath of the peroneus longus muscle, whereas the transverse head takes origin from the plantar metatarsophalangeal ligaments of the third, fourth, and fifth digits and from the deep transverse metatarsal ligament. The tendons of both the oblique and transverse heads and that of the lateral head of the flexor hallucis brevis muscle insert into the lateral side of the base of the proximal phalanx of the great toe. The adductor hallucis muscle adducts the great toe and aids in maintaining the transverse arch of the foot.

The *interosseous muscles of the foot* are very similar in structure and placement to the comparable muscles of the hand, except that, here, the plane of reference for abduction and adduction of the toes is through the second digit rather than the third. The four *dorsal interosseous muscles* are bipennate and arise from the adjacent sides of both metatarsals of the space in which they lie. They have a longer origin from the metatarsal of the digit into which they insert. The first and second dorsal interosseous muscles lie on the medial and lateral sides of the second metatarsal and insert into the same sides of the bases of the proximal phalanx. The third and fourth dorsal interosseous muscles lie on the lateral surfaces of the third and fourth metatarsals, respectively, and insert into the lateral sides of the bases of their proximal phalanges. Minor insertions occur into the dorsal extensor expansions. These muscles are abductors of the digits with reference to the midplane of the second digit. The three *plantar interosseous muscles* (adductors of the third, fourth, and fifth digits) are unipennate. They arise from the bases and medial sides of the third to fifth metatarsals and insert into the medial sides of the proximal phalanges. The interosseous muscles, as in the hand, are abductors and adductors of the digits and also serve in flexion of the metatarsophalangeal joints.

Digital fibrous sheaths begin over the heads of the metatarsals and extend to the bases of the distal phalanges. They arch over the tendons, attaching to the capsules of the joints and the margins of the proximal and middle phalanges. Over the shafts of these bones, the fibers of the sheath are transverse and strong, but over the joints, the sheaths are much thinner and most of their fiber bundles run obliquely from side to side. Slender transverse bands cross the joint intervals. The marginal fibers of the digital slips of the plantar aponeurosis terminate in the fibrous sheaths.

Synovial sheaths occupy the digital sheaths of the toes. They enclose the tendon of the flexor hallucis longus muscle and the tendons of the flexor digitorum longus and flexor digitorum brevis muscles of the lateral four toes. The synovial sheaths invest the tendons from just proximal to the openings of the digital fibrous sheaths to the bases of the distal phalanges. The *tendon of the flexor digitorum longus muscle* passes the ankle in the second compartment under the flexor retinaculum and enters the foot deep to the abductor hallucis muscle. Passing diagonally toward the center of the sole, it expands and receives from behind the broad insertion of the quadratus plantae muscle. The tendon now divides into four slips, which enter the digital fibrous sheaths surrounded by separate synovial sheaths, pass through the separation of the tendons of the flexor digitorum brevis muscle, and terminate in the bases of the distal phalanges.

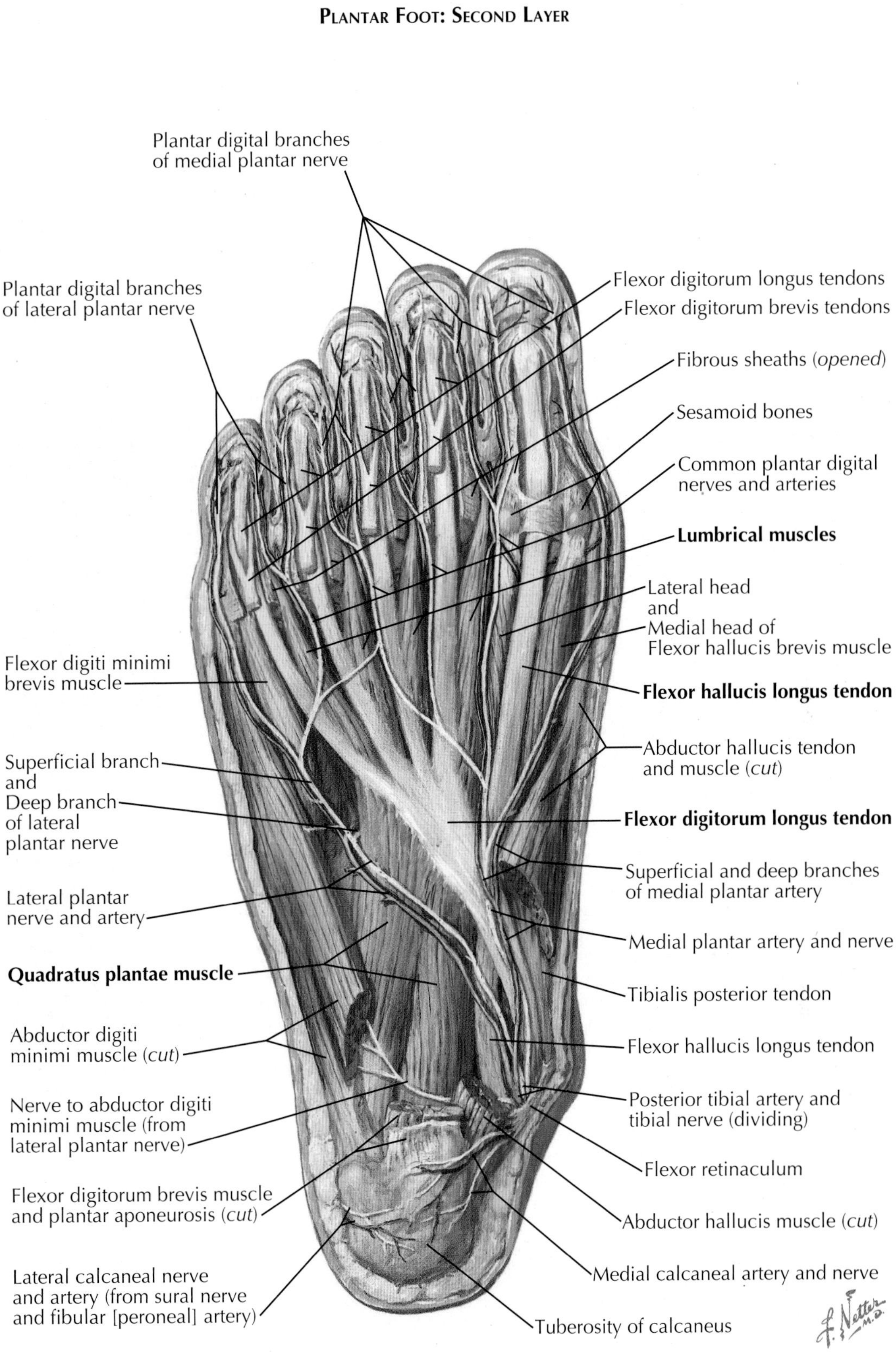

Plantar Foot: Second Layer

Anatomy of the Ankle and Foot (Continued)

Arteries

The *medial plantar artery* does not usually form an arch like the superficial palmar arch of the palm. The artery accompanies the medial plantar nerve and, like it, provides three digital branches. The branches anastomose with the three plantar metatarsal arteries of the plantar arch at the base of the interdigital clefts. These vessels are small and may be partially or completely absent.

The *lateral plantar artery* accompanies the lateral plantar nerve diagonally across the sole of the foot. Accompanied by venae comitantes, it turns around the margin of the quadratus plantae muscle and sinks into the deeper plane of the foot. Perforating the plantar interosseous fascia, it passes medially across the fourth to second metatarsals and interosseous muscles as the *plantar arterial arch.* In the proximal part of its course, the artery gives off calcaneal branches to the heel, muscular branches to the small toe, and cutaneous branches to the lateral side of the foot. The lateral plantar veins mirror the artery.

The *plantar arterial arch* crosses the sole medially under the plantar interosseous fascia. Its formation as an arch is due to the free anastomosis of the lateral plantar artery and the deep plantar branch of the dorsalis pedis artery. The plantar arch gives off four plantar metatarsal arteries, three perforating branches, and branches to the tarsal joints and muscles of the compartment.

The *plantar metatarsal arteries* run forward from the arch on the plantar surface of the interosseous muscles. Each artery divides into a pair of *proper plantar digital arteries,* which supply the adjacent sides of the toes. Each plantar metatarsal artery gives off, near its point of division, an anterior perforating branch that passes through the interosseous space to anastomose with a corresponding branch of a dorsal metatarsal artery. The proper plantar digital arteries, as in the fingers, provide terminal branches, which pass dorsally to supply the nail beds and skin of the distal phalanges. The perforating branches of the plantar arch anastomose with posterior perforating branches of the dorsal metatarsal arteries. The *deep branch of the lateral plantar nerve* passes into the interosseous-adductor compartment directly behind the plantar arterial arch. It supplies muscular branches to the lateral three lumbrical muscles, the interosseous muscles of each space (except the fourth space in some cases), and both heads of the adductor hallucis muscle. Articular branches reach the intertarsal and tarsometatarsal joints.

Nerves

The *medial plantar nerve* is the larger of the two plantar nerves. It arises from the division of the tibial nerve beneath the posterior part of the abductor hallucis muscle and passes forward, accompanied by the small medial plantar artery, in the medial intermuscular septum between the abductor hallucis and flexor digitorum brevis muscles. The muscular branches to the abductor hallucis and flexor digitorum brevis muscles arise here and enter the deep surfaces of the muscles, and articular branches supply the joints of the tarsals and metatarsals. The proper digital nerve for the great toe supplies the flexor hallucis brevis muscle, and a branch of the first common digital nerve supplies the first lumbrical muscle.

The *lateral plantar nerve,* smaller than the medial plantar, passes diagonally in the sole of the foot, between the flexor digitorum brevis and quadratus plantae muscles,

PLANTAR FOOT: THIRD LAYER

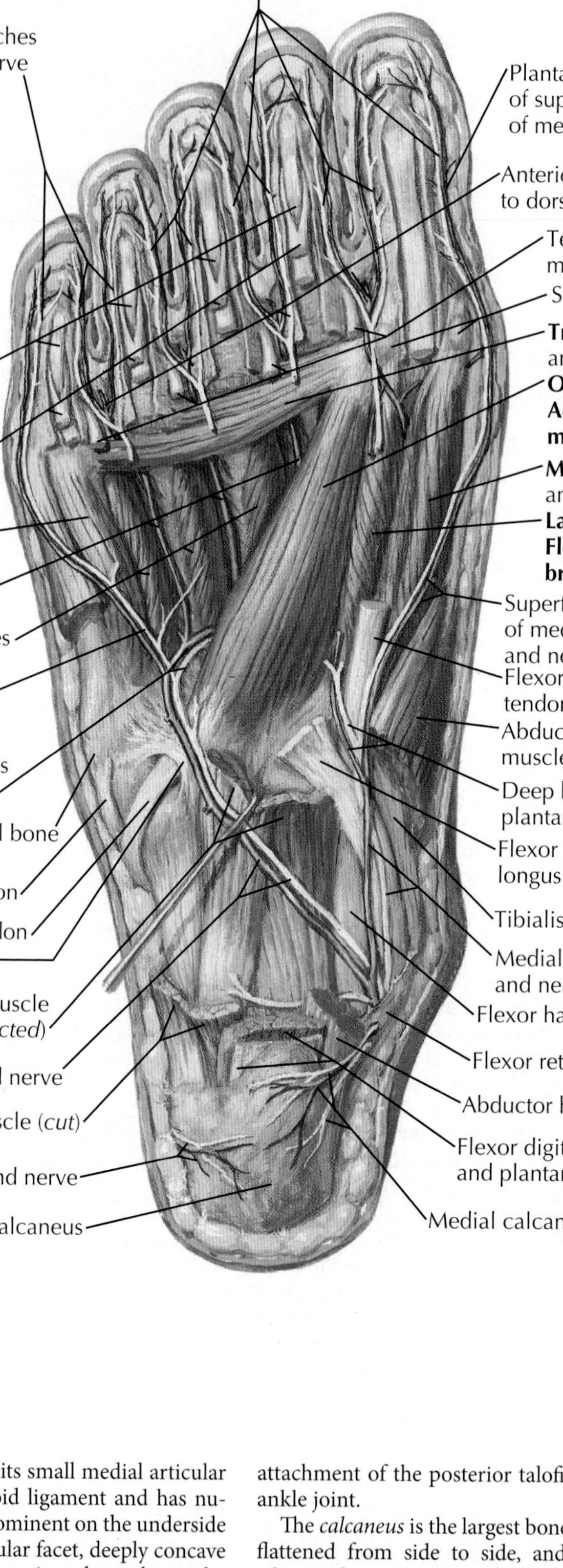

ANATOMY OF THE ANKLE AND FOOT (Continued)

and provides muscular branches to the abductor digiti minimi through Baxter's nerve and quadratus plantae muscles and articular branches to the calcaneocuboid joint. At the lateral margin of the quadratus plantae, the nerve divides and a deep branch sinks into the interosseous-adductor compartment of the sole. The remaining superficial branch splits into one common digital branch for adjacent sides of the fourth and fifth toes and into a nerve that supplies a proper digital branch for the lateral side of the fifth toe and muscular branches to the flexor digiti minimi brevis muscle and, occasionally, the two interosseous muscles of the fourth interosseous space.

BONES

There are seven tarsals, five metatarsals, and 14 phalanges within the foot. The tarsals are the talus, calcaneus, navicular, three cuneiforms (medial, intermediate, and lateral), and cuboid. The arrangement of the bones indicates a limited independence between the bones forming the medial three digits and those forming the lateral two digits. The talus receives the weight of the body at the ankle and constitutes the summit of the bony longitudinal arch of the foot.

The *talus articulates* with many bones: the tibia and the fibula above and on its sides, the calcaneus below, and the navicular in front; as such, the majority of the talus is covered with articular surface. No muscles insert into it, but it receives a number of ligaments. It has a head, a body, and a neck. The *head* of the talus is its rounded anterior extension; it is directed forward and medial and has three articular surfaces. The large *navicular surface* is rounded, convex, and oval; followed to its underside, it passes into a flat, triangular *anterior calcaneal articular surface.* Through this latter surface, the head of the talus bears on the anterior facet of the calcaneus and on the plantar calcaneonavicular ligament. The third and most posterior facet, the oval *middle calcaneal articular surface,* bears on the upper surface of the sustentaculum tali of the calcaneus. The *neck* of the talus is its somewhat-restricted part between the head and the body. On the upper side, it is rough for ligaments and shows a number of vascular foramina. Inferiorly, there is a deep groove, the *talar sulcus,* which forms the roof of the tarsal sinus, occupied by the interosseous talocalcaneal ligament. The *body* of the talus is roughly quadrilateral, with its upper portion, the trochlea, entering into the formation of the ankle joint. The region of the talus inferior to its small medial articular surface is rough for the deltoid ligament and has numerous vascular foramina. Prominent on the underside of the body is an oblong articular facet, deeply concave from side to side. This is the *posterior calcaneal articular surface.* The posterior process of the talus is grooved by the tendon of the flexor hallucis longus muscle. Medial to this groove is the medial tubercle for the medial talocalcaneal and posterior tibiotalar ligaments; on the lateral aspect of the groove is a lateral tubercle for the attachment of the posterior talofibular ligament of the ankle joint.

The *calcaneus* is the largest bone of the foot. It is long, flattened from side to side, and bulbous posteriorly where it forms the heel. The superior surface of the calcaneus exhibits, anteriorly, three articular facets for the talus. The largest is the *posterior talar articular surface,* which is triangular and convex from anterior to posterior. Anterior to it is a deep depression, which leads onto the sustentaculum tali as the *calcaneal sulcus,* the floor

Interosseous Muscles and Deep Arteries of Foot

Dorsal view

Fibularis (peroneus) longus tendon (*cut*)
Fibularis (peroneus) brevis tendon (*cut*)
Cuboid bone
Lateral tarsal artery
Tuberosity of 5th metatarsal bone
Fibularis (peroneus) tertius tendon (*cut*)
Posterior perforating branches (from deep plantar arterial arch)
Dorsal metatarsal arteries
Extensor digitorum longus tendons (*cut*)
Extensor expansions
Anterior perforating branches (from plantar metatarsal arteries)
Dorsal digital arteries
Navicular bone
Dorsalis pedis artery
Medial tarsal artery
Lateral
Intermediate
Medial
Cuneiform bones
Dorsal tarsometatarsal ligaments
Dorsal metatarsal ligaments
Arcuate artery
Deep plantar artery passes to contribute to deep plantar arch
Dorsal interossei muscles
Metatarsal bones
Extensor hallucis longus tendon (*cut*)
Extensor digitorum brevis and extensor hallucis brevis tendons (*cut*)

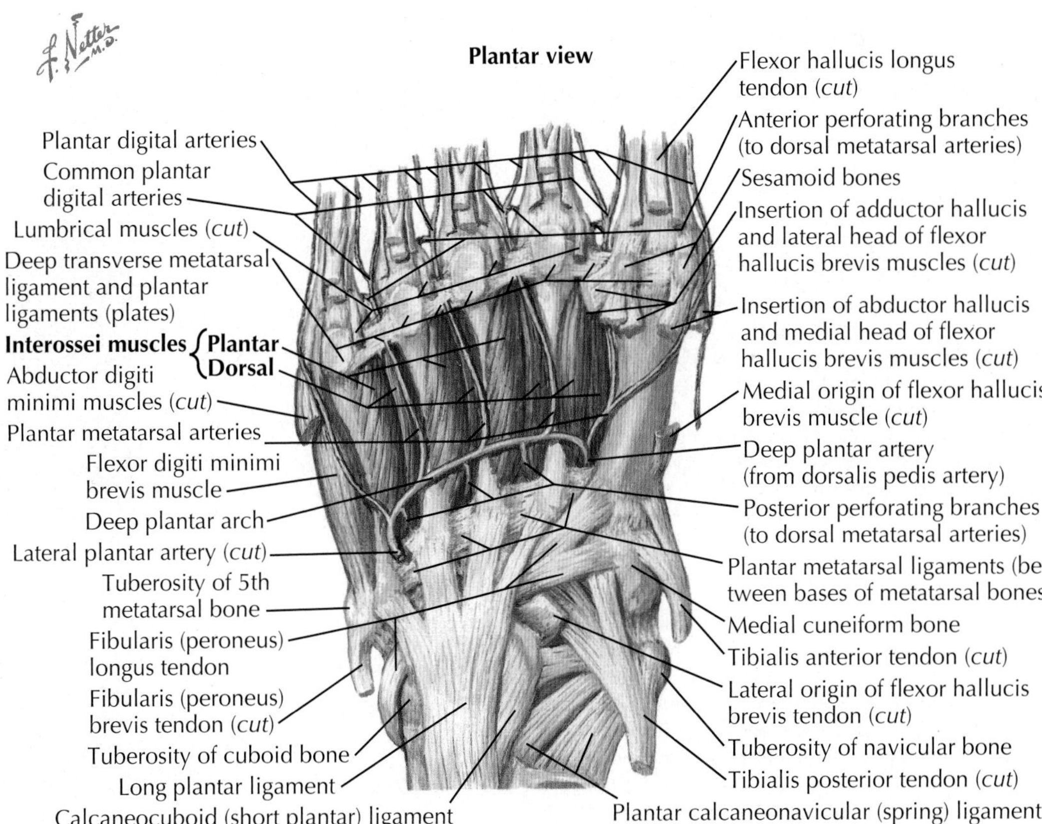

Anatomy of the Ankle and Foot (Continued)

of the tarsal sinus. The upper surface of the sustentaculum tali carries the *middle talar articular surface* for the posterior facet of the head of the talus. A small oval *anterior talar articular surface* characterizes the anterior end of the superior surface of the bone.

The inferior surface of the calcaneus is narrow and uneven. The long plantar ligament attaches here. The *tuberosity* is the posteroinferior part of the bone. It is rough and striated for the attachment of the Achilles tendon; toward its superior surface, it is smooth for the subtendinous bursa of the Achilles tendon. Two processes characterize the tuberosity inferiorly: the larger medial process gives origin to the abductor hallucis, flexor digitorum brevis, and abductor digiti minimi muscles, whereas the narrow lateral process gives origin to the abductor digiti minimi muscle. The *medial surface of the calcaneus* is smoothly concave and overhung by the prominent *sustentaculum tali;* the latter has a sulcus on its underside for the flexor hallucis longus muscle. The *lateral surface of the calcaneus* is rough and at about its middle has a small swelling for attachment of the calcaneofibular ligament; inferior to this is a *peroneal tubercle* that separates the tendons of the peroneus longus and peroneus brevis muscles, the peroneus longus tendon inferior to it. The anterior extremity of the calcaneus is the *cuboidal articular surface.* It is roughly triangular and carries a saddle-shaped articulation for the cuboid.

The *navicular* is a flattened oval bone located between the head of the talus and the three cuneiforms. It is characterized by a large, oval, concave articular facet on its posterior surface for the head of the talus and by a rounded eminence at its medial plantar extremity, the *tuberosity,* for the primary attachment of the tibialis posterior muscle. Three triangular facets separated by two vertical ridges occupy its anterior surface; they articulate with the three cuneiforms. The superior and inferior surfaces of the bone are rough for ligaments, and the lateral surface frequently exhibits a small articular facet for the cuboid.

The *cuneiforms* are all wedge shaped, but the broader side of the wedge faces plantarly on the medial cuneiform and dorsally on the other two. The posterior portion of each bone is concave and articulates with one of the facets of the navicular. The anterior aspect of each bone enters into the tarsometatarsal joint of the first, second, or third digit; there are articular surfaces between the adjacent cuneiforms and one between the lateral cuneiform and the cuboid. The dorsal and plantar surfaces of these bones are rough for the attachment of the ligaments and tendons. The medial cuneiform is the largest, and the middle bone is the shortest. This size difference forms a recess into which the second metatarsal is received. The articulation of the lateral cuneiform with the cuboid is by a large triangular or oval facet situated toward the posterosuperior aspect of its lateral surface.

The *cuboid* is interposed on the lateral side of the foot between the calcaneus and the fourth and fifth metatarsals. Its dorsal surface is rough and nonarticular; its plantar surface has a prominent ridge, which receives the long plantar ligament and ends laterally in the *tuberosity* of the bone. The tuberosity has a convex cartilage-covered facet over which the tendon of the peroneus longus muscle passes as it enters the foot. Laterally, the cuboid is short and concave for the peroneus longus

Cross-Sectional Anatomy of Ankle and Foot

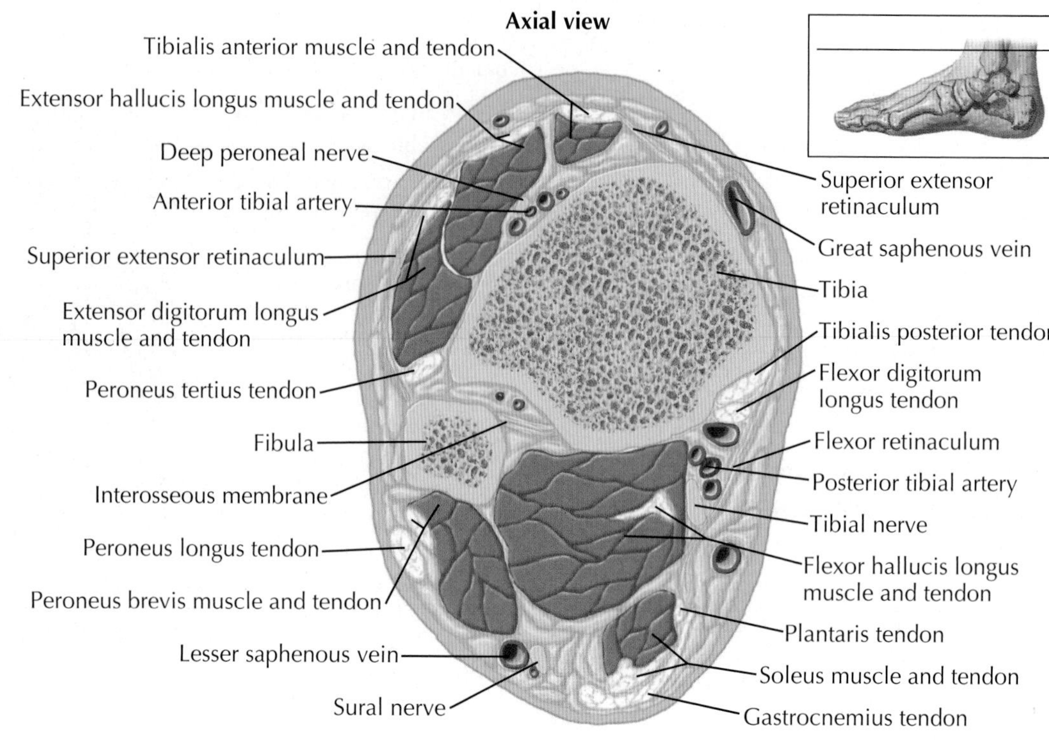

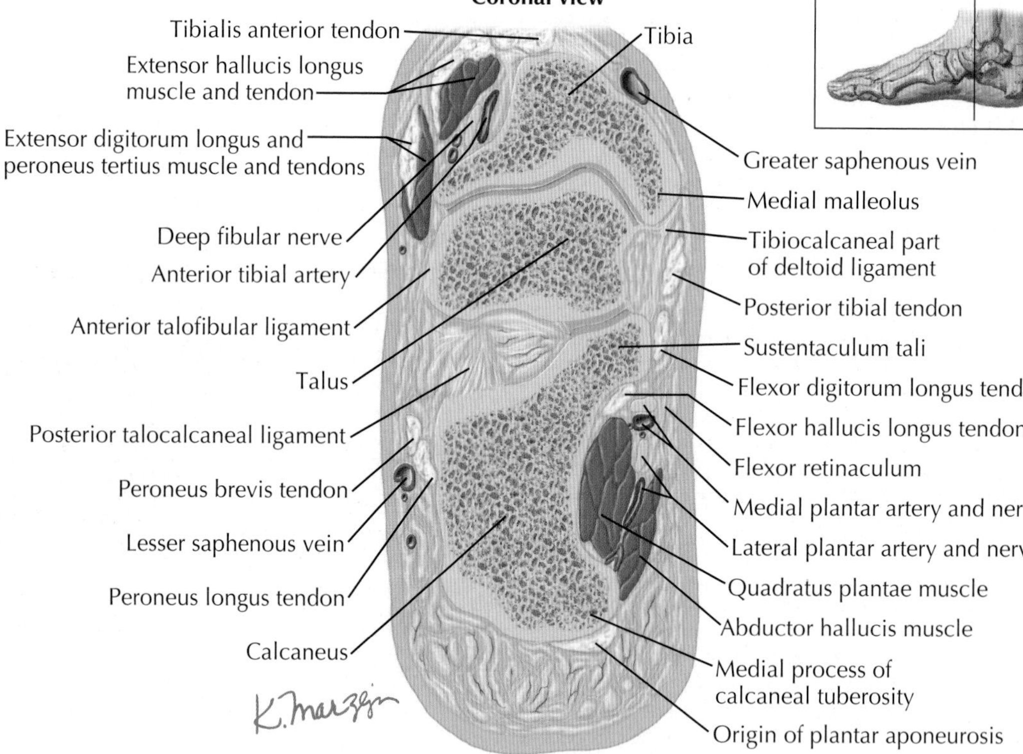

Anatomy of the Ankle and Foot (Continued)

tendon; its longer medial side bears either a large triangular or an oval facet for articulation with the lateral cuneiform. The posterior surface of the cuboid is entirely articular and is saddle shaped for participation in the calcaneocuboid joint. The distal surface of the cuboid has a small medial and a larger lateral facet. These slightly concave facets articulate with the bases of the fourth and fifth metatarsals, respectively.

The *metatarsals* are long bones each consisting of a base, a body, and a head. They are 6 to 8 cm long and are relatively flat dorsally but concave longitudinally on their plantar sides. The bases carry smooth articular surfaces for articulation with the cuneiforms and cuboid (and in most cases with each other) and show pits for ligaments on their sides. The bodies are narrow and tend to be triangular in cross section. The heads present convex articular surfaces, somewhat flattened from side to side, for articulation with the proximal phalanges; dorsally on their sides they exhibit tubercles for the attachment of the collateral ligaments of the metatarsophalangeal joints.

The *first metatarsal* is the broadest and most massive of the series. At its base, a tuberosity projects downward and laterally to receive the tendon of the peroneus longus muscle. The head of the bone is broad, and its plantar surface has two deep grooves separated by a ridge; in these grooves lie the sesamoids within the tendons of the flexor hallucis brevis muscle. The *second metatarsal* is the longest, and its base fits into the recess formed by the three cuneiforms. Thus the base of this bone has articular facets for all the cuneiforms and for the base of the third metatarsal. The *third metatarsal* articulates with the end of the lateral cuneiform and, by facets on the sides of its base, with the adjacent sides of the second and fourth metatarsals. The *fourth metatarsal* articulates with the medial of the two facets of the cuboid and with the adjacent third and fifth metatarsals. There may also be a facet for contact with the lateral cuneiform. The base of the *fifth metatarsal* is expanded laterally into a rough tuberosity for the insertion of the peroneus brevis tendon. It articulates with the lateral facet of the cuboid and, on its medial side, with the fourth metatarsal.

The *phalanges* of the toes consist of 14 bones: 3 for each digit except the great toe, which has 2. Except for that of the great toe, which is broad and thick, the *proximal phalanges* are broadened at their extremities and narrow throughout their bodies. The bases have single, round or oval, cup-like faces for reception of the heads of the corresponding metatarsals. The heads of the proximal phalanges present rounded pulley-like surfaces, grooved in the middle and raised at the edges, for articulation with the bases of the middle phalanges. The *middle phalanges* are short, but their bodies are proportionately broader than those of the proximal phalanges. Both ends of the middle phalanges have trochlear surfaces. The *distal phalanges* are also short. They exhibit broadened bases with trochlear surfaces and rough, broadened distal tuberosities for support of the nails and pulp of the toes.

OSSIFICATION

The *tarsals* are ossified from a single center for each bone, except the calcaneus, which has a separate epiphysis for its tuberosity. The principal ossification center for the calcaneus appears at the sixth fetal month; the talus, during the seventh fetal month; the cuboid, at the

Cross-Sectional Anatomy of Ankle and Foot (Continued)

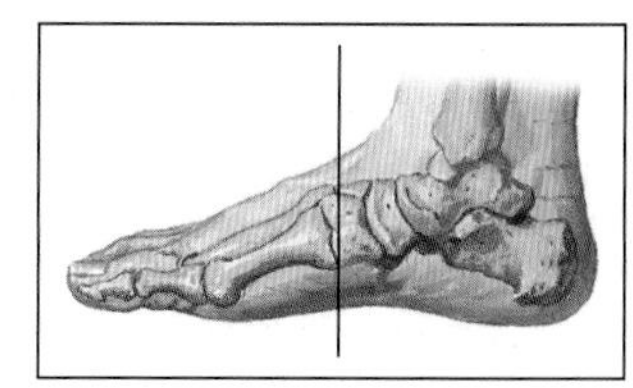

Anatomy of the Ankle and Foot (Continued)

time of birth; the lateral cuneiform, during the first year; and the medial cuneiform, during the third year. Ossification centers for the intermediate cuneiform and navicular appear in the fourth year. The epiphysis for the tuberosity of the calcaneus appears between ages 8 to 10 and is united with the rest of the bone at puberty. Ossification of all the tarsals is complete shortly after puberty.

In each of the *metatarsals,* a primary center of ossification for the body and the base (except the body and head for the first metatarsal) appears about the ninth week of fetal life, and these bones are well ossified at birth. A secondary center for each of the heads (base of first metatarsal) appears in the third year and fuses to the shaft between ages 14 to 17 years. The *phalanges* are each ossified from two centers: one for the body and head and one for the base. Those for the bodies and heads appear from between the 10th fetal week to the time of birth. The distal phalanges appear first and the middle phalanges appear last. The secondary ossification centers for the bases appear during the third year of life and unite with the shafts from ages 14 to 17 years.

JOINTS

The intertarsal joints are the subtalar, talocalcaneonavicular, calcaneocuboid, transverse tarsal, cuneonavicular, and intercuneiform. To maintain the foot against the weight of the body, the plantar ligaments are stronger and more extensive than the dorsal ligaments. Blood vessels are supplied from adjacent branches of the dorsalis pedis, medial plantar, and lateral plantar arteries, whereas the nerve supply comes from the deep peroneal and medial and lateral plantar nerves.

The *subtalar joint* is formed between the large concave facet on the underside of the body of the talus and the convex posterior articular surface of the superior aspect of the calcaneus. A loose, thin-walled articular capsule unites the bones, attaching to the margins of the articular surfaces. Somewhat stronger portions are designated as the posterior, medial, and lateral talocalcaneal ligaments. The *medial talocalcaneal ligament* connects the medial tubercle of the posterior process of the talus with the posterior margin of the sustentaculum tali; the *lateral talocalcaneal ligament* is parallel to, and deeper than, the calcaneofibular ligament. The *posterior talocalcaneal ligament* is a short band, its fibers radiating from a narrow attachment on the lateral tubercle of the talus to the upper and medial parts of the calcaneus. The *interosseous talocalcaneal ligament* is located in the tarsal sinus. It is a strong band, composed of several layers of fibers interspersed with fatty tissue, which connects the adjacent surfaces of the talus and calcaneus along their oblique grooves. Support for the subtalar joint is also derived from those ligaments of the ankle joint that, passing from the tibia and fibula to the calcaneus, span the talus.

The *talocalcaneonavicular* joint is formed between the articular surfaces of the head of the talus and the navicular, the plantar calcaneonavicular ligament, the sustentaculum tali, and the adjacent part of the anterior articular surface of the calcaneus. The thin articular capsule encloses this common articular cavity. The capsule is reinforced between the neck of the talus and the dorsal surface of the navicular by the broad *dorsal talonavicular ligament.* Supporting the joint below is

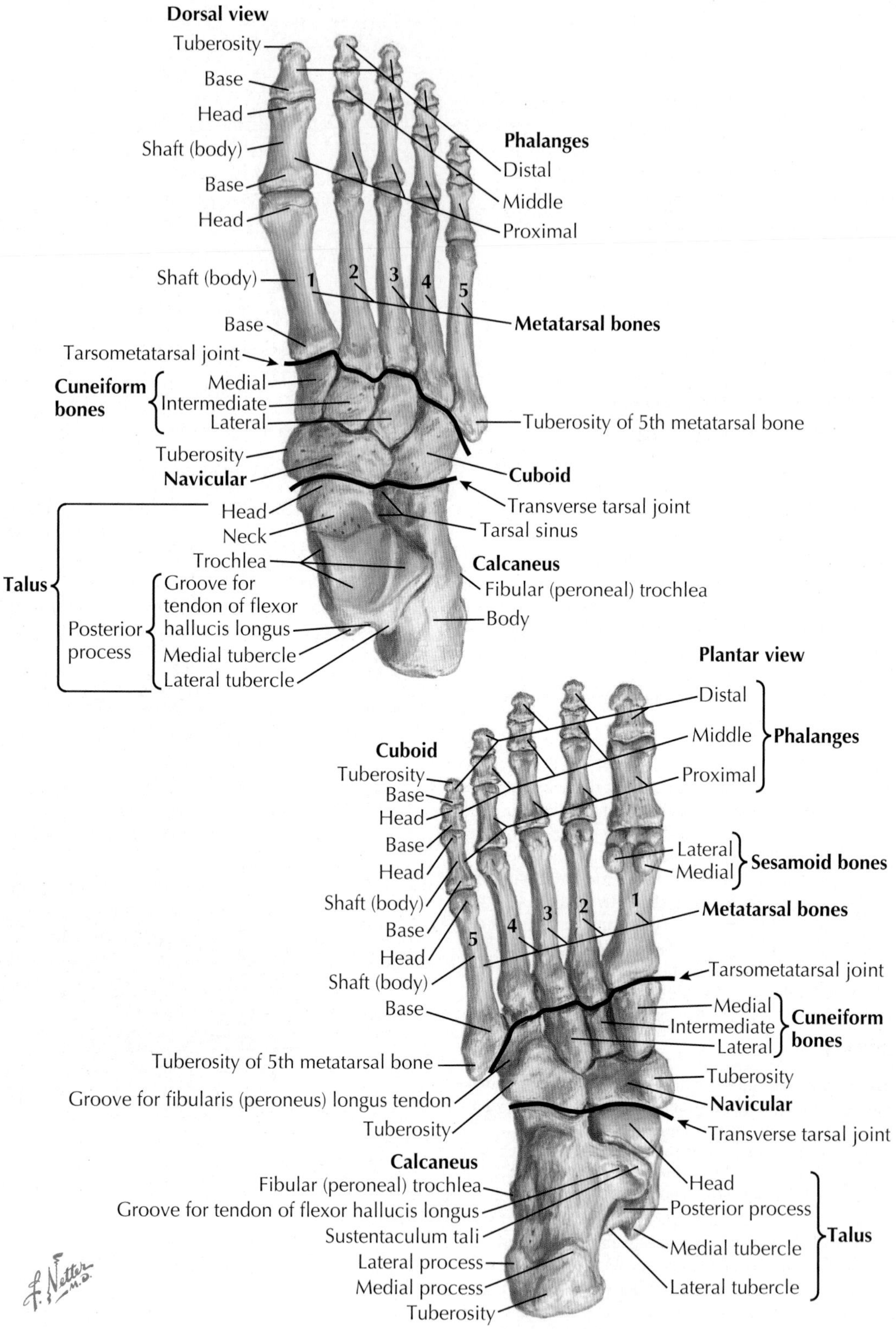

Anatomy of the Ankle and Foot (Continued)

the thick, dense, fibroelastic *plantar calcaneonavicular ligament.* This ligament extends from the sustentaculum tali and the distal surface of the calcaneus to the entire width of the inferior surface of the navicular and to its medial surface behind its tuberosity. Medially, it blends with the deltoid ligament and, laterally, with the lower border of the calcaneonavicular portion of the bifurcate ligament. Its upper surface is smooth and contains a fibrocartilaginous plate on which the head of the talus bears. The *calcaneonavicular portion of the bifurcate ligament* completes the socket on the lateral side. Its short fibers pass from the upper surface of the anterior end of the calcaneus to the adjacent lateral surface of the navicular.

The *calcaneocuboid joint* unites the saddle-shaped articular surfaces of the calcaneus and the cuboid. Its joint cavity is separate from adjacent cavities, and an articular capsule encloses it. The thin, broad *dorsal calcaneocuboid ligament* reinforces the capsule dorsally. The *bifurcate ligament,* also involved in the talocalcaneonavicular joint through its calcaneonavicular portion, has a calcaneocuboid band that ends on the dorsomedial angle of the cuboid and is one of the main connections between the first and second rows of tarsals. The calcaneocuboid joint takes much of the thrust of the body weight onto the lateral side of the foot and the lateral part of its longitudinal arch. It is therefore supported by strong plantar ligaments: the plantar calcaneocuboid and the long plantar ligaments.

The *plantar calcaneocuboid ligament* is attached to the rounded eminence at the anterior end of the inferior surface of the calcaneus and to the plantar surface of the cuboid behind its tuberosity and oblique ridge. The fibers of this wide ligament are short and strong, and the ligament is partially covered by the long plantar ligament. The *long plantar ligament* stretches from the plantar surface of the calcaneus in front of the tuberosity of the cuboid, its more superficial fibers spreading forward to the bases of the third, fourth, and fifth metatarsals.

The *transverse tarsal joint* is a name given to the irregular articular plane crossing the foot from side to side. It is composed of the talonavicular articulation medially and the calcaneocuboid joint laterally. These separate joints combine functionally to contribute primarily to the inversion/eversion action of the foot.

Bones of Foot

The subtalar and talocalcaneonavicular joints combine to allow for the ability to adapt to uneven or irregular surfaces. These provide movement around an axis passing through the tarsal sinus. Additional ligaments unite the navicular and the cuboid. The *dorsal cuboideonavicular* and *plantar cuboideonavicular ligaments* unite adjacent surfaces of the two bones, and a strong *interosseous cuboideonavicular ligament* connects the rough nonarticular portions of their adjacent surfaces. There may be a small joint cavity between the posterior medial angle of the cuboid and the lateral margin of the navicular; it will be continuous with the cuneonavicular joint in front of it.

Distal intertarsal joints are the *cuneonavicular, intercuneiform,* and *cuneocuboid articulations.* These are united by a common articular capsule enclosing a common articular cavity, which also extends downward to

Anatomy of the Ankle and Foot (Continued)

include the tarsometatarsal joint between the intermediate cuneiform and the second and third metatarsals, and the intermetatarsal joints between the second and third and the third and fourth metatarsals. Adjacent bones are united by weak *dorsal cuneonavicular ligaments* for each of the cuneiforms, *dorsal intercuneiform ligaments,* and a *dorsal cuneocuboid ligament. Plantar ligaments* correspond in names to the dorsal ligaments, and there are also *intercuneiform and cuneocuboid interosseous ligaments.* Slight gliding motions at these distal joints contribute to the adaptability and flexibility of the foot.

The *tarsometatarsal joints* are plane joints between the distal row of tarsals and the metatarsals (the medial three metatarsal bases with the cuneiforms and the lateral two with the cuboid). There are three tarsometatarsal joint cavities. Medially, there is a separate joint cavity between the first metatarsal and the medial cuneiform. The intermediate articulation includes articulations of the second and third metatarsals and is an extension of the distal intertarsal joint space. The lateral articulation includes the contact of the fourth and fifth metatarsals with the cuboid. Weak *dorsal* and somewhat stronger *plantar tarsometatarsal ligaments* connect adjacent borders of the cuneiforms and the second and third metatarsals.

Intermetatarsal joints are interposed between the bases of the lateral four metatarsals, mostly as forward extensions of the tarsometatarsal joints. *Dorsal, plantar, and interosseous metatarsal ligaments* close these joint spaces; these interosseous ligaments are strong and help maintain the transverse arch of the foot. These joints provide slight gliding movements contributing to the flexibility of the foot, although the first joint also permits slight rotary movements of the great toe.

The *metatarsophalangeal joints* are condyloid joints between the rounded heads of the metatarsals and the cupped proximal extremities of the proximal phalanges. They are very similar to the metacarpophalangeal joints of the fingers; each joint is enclosed by an articular capsule, reinforced by plantar and collateral ligaments. The articular capsule is loose and reinforced dorsally by fibers from the extensor tendon expansions. The *plantar ligament,* like its palmar counterpart, is a dense, fibrocartilaginous plate that is firmly attached to the proximal plantar border of the phalanx and serves as part of the bearing surface for the head of the metatarsal. At the sides, it is attached to the collateral ligaments and the deep transverse metatarsal ligaments. For the great toe, the sesamoids and their interconnecting ligaments replace the plantar ligament. The strong *collateral ligaments* pass from the tubercles on each side of the head of the metatarsal to the sides of the proximal end of the phalanx and the plantar ligament. The plantar ligaments are interconnected by the *deep transverse metatarsal ligament,* which connects the heads and the joint capsules of all the metatarsal heads. The movements allowed at the metatarsophalangeal joints are dorsiflexion, plantar flexion, abduction, adduction, and circumduction.

The *interphalangeal joints* are similar to the metatarsophalangeal joints, but their trochlear surfaces permit only dorsiflexion and plantar flexion. Each joint has an articular capsule and plantar and collateral ligaments. Blood vessels and nerves to these and to the metatarsophalangeal joints are branches of digital vessels and nerves.

Bones of Foot (Continued)

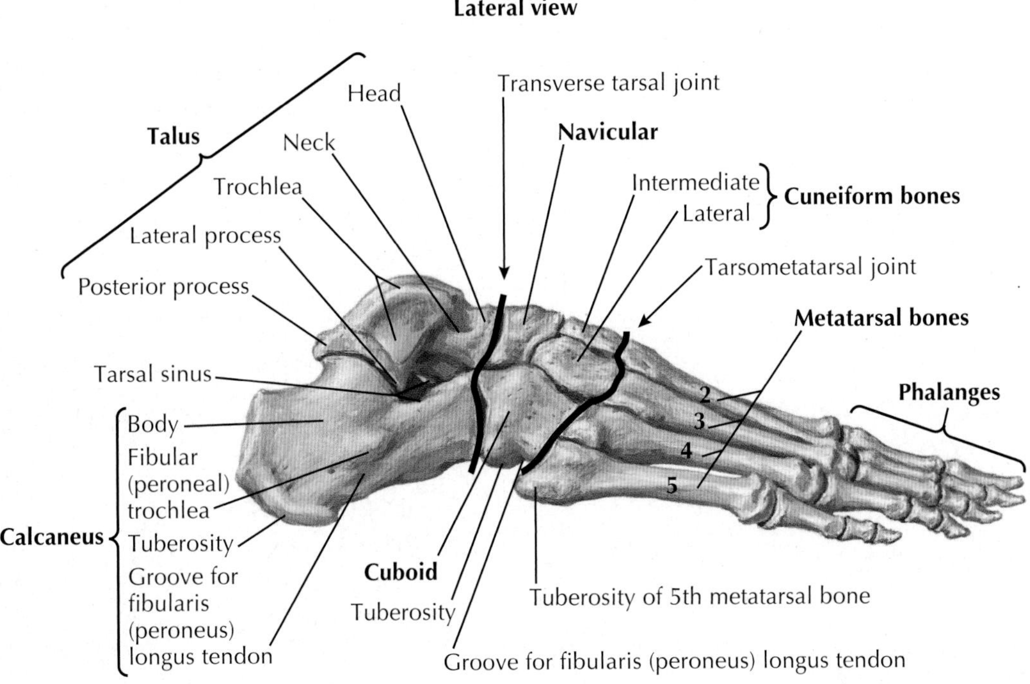

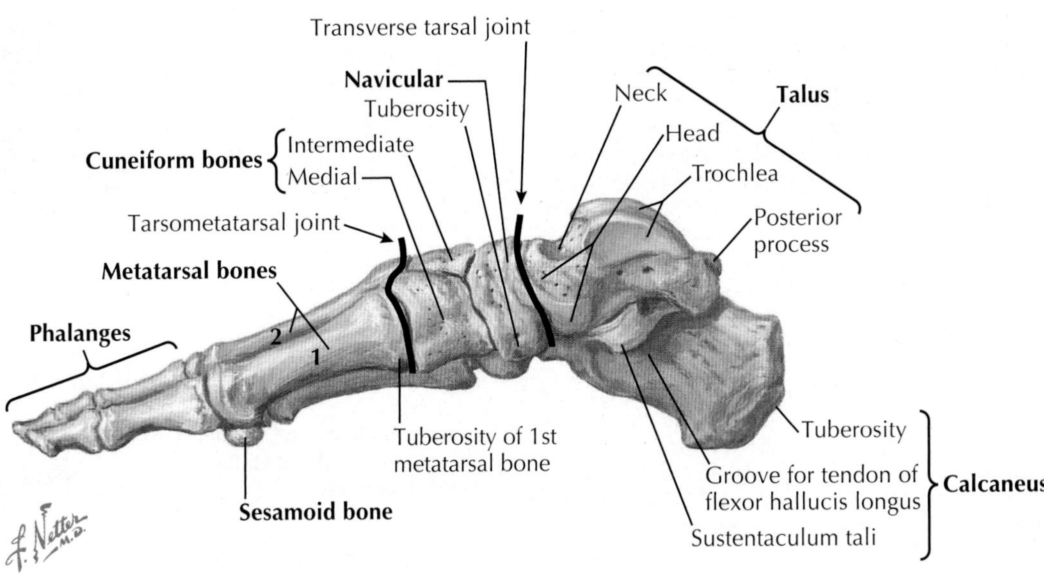

Ligaments and Tendons of Foot: Plantar View

Distal phalanx of great toe
Flexor digitorum longus tendon to 2nd toe (*cut*)
Flexor digitorum brevis tendon to 2nd toe (*cut*)
Flexor hallucis longus tendon (*cut*)
4th distal phalanx
Interphalangeal (IP) joint
4th middle phalanx
Proximal phalanx of great toe
Deep transverse metatarsal ligaments
Flexor hallucis brevis tendon (medial and lateral heads)
5th proximal phalanx
4th lumbrical tendon (*cut*)
Metatarsophalangeal (MP) joint
Abductor digiti minimi and flexor digiti minimi brevis tendons (*cut*)
Sesamoid bones
Abductor hallucis
Plantar ligaments (plates)
Adductor hallucis
Interosseous muscles (*cut*)
1st metatarsal bone
5th metatarsal bone
Plantar tarsometatarsal ligaments
Plantar metatarsal ligaments
Medial cuneiform bone
Tuberosity of 5th metatarsal bone
Tibialis anterior tendon (*cut*)
Fibularis (peroneus) brevis tendon
Plantar cuneonavicular ligament
Cuboid bone
Plantar cuboideonavicular ligament
Fibularis (peroneus) longus tendon
Tuberosity of navicular bone
Tuberosity of cuboid bone
Plantar calcaneonavicular (spring) ligament
Long plantar ligament
Tibialis posterior tendon
Plantar calcaneocuboid (short plantar) ligament
Flexor digitorum longus tendon (*cut*)
Calcaneus
Sustentaculum tali
Medial process and Lateral process of Tuberosity of calcaneus
Flexor hallucis longus tendon (*cut*)
Posterior process of talus (medial and lateral tubercles)

Anatomy of the Ankle and Foot (Continued)

FOOT DYNAMICS

The foot is a unique structure. Through the combined actions of multiple joints, it can act as a rigid platform for push-off during the gait cycle, yet also be flexible enough to absorb the force of heel strike. It is strong enough to withstand body weight and the increasing force seen during walking and running, yet also is flexible enough to accommodate uneven ground. Skeletally, it has an arched structure composed of a number of bones linked together by joints and ligaments. The bones of the foot are arranged in longitudinal and transverse arches. The longitudinal arch is supported posteriorly on the tuberosity of the calcaneus; anteriorly, it rests on the heads of the five metatarsals. The transverse arch results from the shape of the distal tarsals and the bases of the metatarsals. These are generally broader dorsally so that, as they fit against one another, a domed configuration results. The talus is at the summit of the foot and is primarily related to the navicular, the three cuneiforms, and the medial three metatarsals. These bones constitute the medial column of the longitudinal arch. Laterally, the calcaneus relates anterior to the cuboid and to the lateral two metatarsals, forming the lateral column of the longitudinal arch. The medial segment shows a much higher arch and considerable elasticity, whereas the lateral segment is flatter, is more rigid, and makes the initial contact with the ground in weight-bearing.

This is a body part of considerable stability and resistance to deformation coupled with the capacity for elastic recoil and the development of strong dynamic responses. In standing, the weight of the body is distributed equally between the heel and the ball of the foot and is shared between the feet, depending on posture. The ligaments are primary in relaxed standing, and the action of muscles is not normally induced except in flatfoot, imbalance, or the initiation of movement.

The plantar ligaments of the foot are the strongest ligaments, and their support function is enhanced by robust interosseous ligaments that keep the bones from spreading apart. Notable on the sole of the foot are the long plantar and plantar calcaneonavicular and calcaneocuboid (short plantar) ligaments. The elasticity of the plantar calcaneonavicular ligament and its reception of the head of the talus have led to its being called the *spring ligament.* The plantar aponeurosis may be thought of as a *tie rod* for the longitudinal arch, resisting spread of its two ends. The toes add to the *grasp* of the foot on the ground, and the great toe is of special importance. The foot is raised against the contact of the great toe with the ground, and its bones and muscles contribute much to the *push-off.* The stresses of standing are borne at the ball of the foot between the head of the first metatarsal and those of the second to fifth metatarsals in a ratio of 1:2.

The gait cycle and the biomechanics of the foot are much more complex than what can be covered in this section. However, it is essential to understand the anatomy of the foot and the resulting interactions between the numerous small joints that allow for such complex actions. Regardless of what research defines as the human gait cycle and the role of the foot, the one constant remains anatomy.

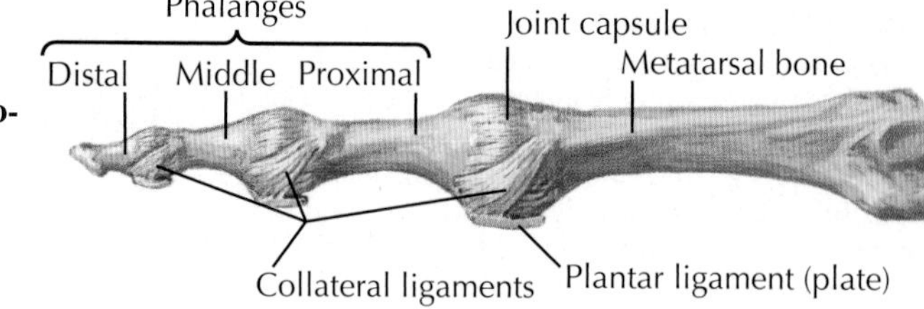

Capsules and ligaments of metatarsophalangeal and interphalangeal joints: lateral view

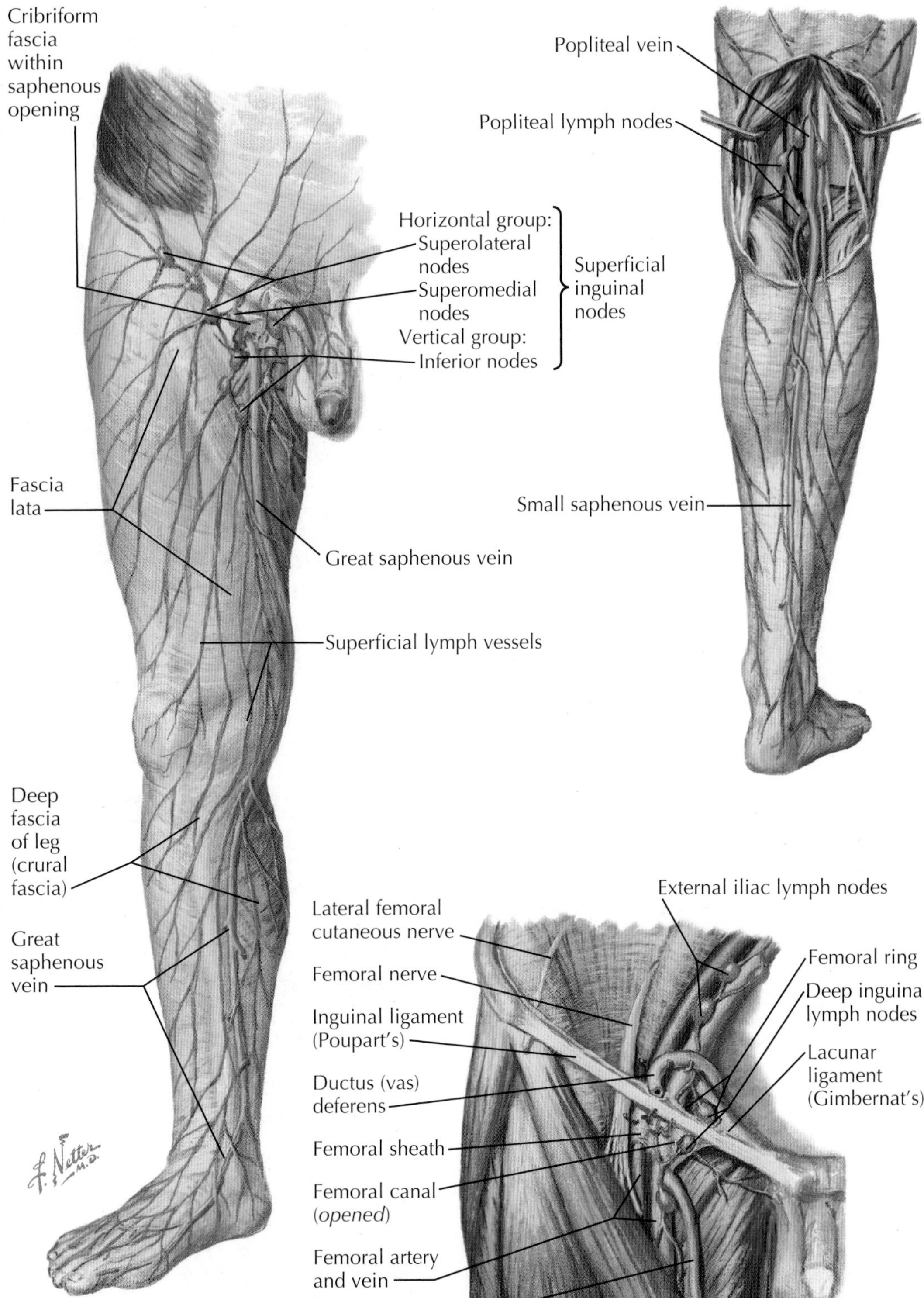

LYMPHATIC DRAINAGE

SUPERFICIAL LYMPHATIC VESSELS

These vessels, which have a similar arrangement to the superficial lymphatic vessels of the hand, arise in plexuses on the plantar side of the toes and foot. Collecting vessels pass through interdigital clefts to the dorsum of the foot, to join there with collecting vessels from the dorsum of the toes. Collecting vessels from the medial and dorsal parts of the foot accompany the greater saphenous vein like those from the lateral part of the foot accompany the lesser saphenous vein.

The larger stream of ascending vessels is with the greater saphenous vein, toward which also converge vessels from the lateral and medial borders and the front and back of the leg and thigh. These ascending vessels end above in the superficial inguinal lymph nodes, to which also pass collecting vessels from the lower abdomen and perineum, scrotum/penis or the vulvar region, and the gluteal region. The area of drainage of the lesser saphenous vein provides lymph vessels that accompany that vein, pierce the popliteal fascia with it, and end in the popliteal lymph nodes.

The *superficial inguinal lymph nodes,* 12 to 20 in number, are arranged in the form of a T in the subcutaneous tissue of the groin. Most of the nodes lie in the horizontal part of the T in a chain parallel to, and about 1 cm below, the inguinal ligament. They receive lymph from the lower abdominal wall, the buttocks, the penis/scrotum or vulvar region, and the perineum. The fewer, larger nodes of the vertical limb of the T lie along the termination of the greater saphenous vein. These nodes principally receive afferent vessels superficially from the limb below them but also from the penis/scrotum or vulva, perineum, and buttocks. The superficial inguinal lymph nodes send their efferent channels through the femoral sheath to the external iliac nodes. Only a few of these channels end in the deep inguinal nodes.

DEEP LYMPHATIC VESSELS

These vessels accompany the deep blood vessels of the limb. In the leg, they follow the anterior and posterior tibial and peroneal vessels to the popliteal nodes. Certain lymph vessels of the gluteal region follow the superior and inferior gluteal vessels to the internal iliac nodes. The *popliteal nodes* are usually small, six to seven in number, and lie in the fat of the popliteal fossa. One lies at the termination of the lesser saphenous vein and receives the lymph channels accompanying that vein. Another node usually lies between the popliteal artery and the capsule of the knee joint and is especially concerned with the lymphatic drainage of the knee. Other nodes of the popliteal group receive the channels that follow the deep blood vessels of the leg. The efferent vessels of the popliteal nodes follow the femoral vessels to the deep inguinal nodes.

The *deep inguinal nodes* are from one to three in number, lying on the medial side of the femoral vein. If three are present, one is usually located in the femoral canal, one at its upper end (femoral ring), and one below the junction of the greater saphenous and femoral veins. These nodes receive the deep lymphatic drainage of the lower limb, some channels from the penis or clitoris, and a few of the efferent channels from the superficial inguinal nodes. They discharge to the external iliac nodes. Drainage from the external iliac nodes is through the common iliac and lateral lumbar lymph node groups to the thoracic duct.

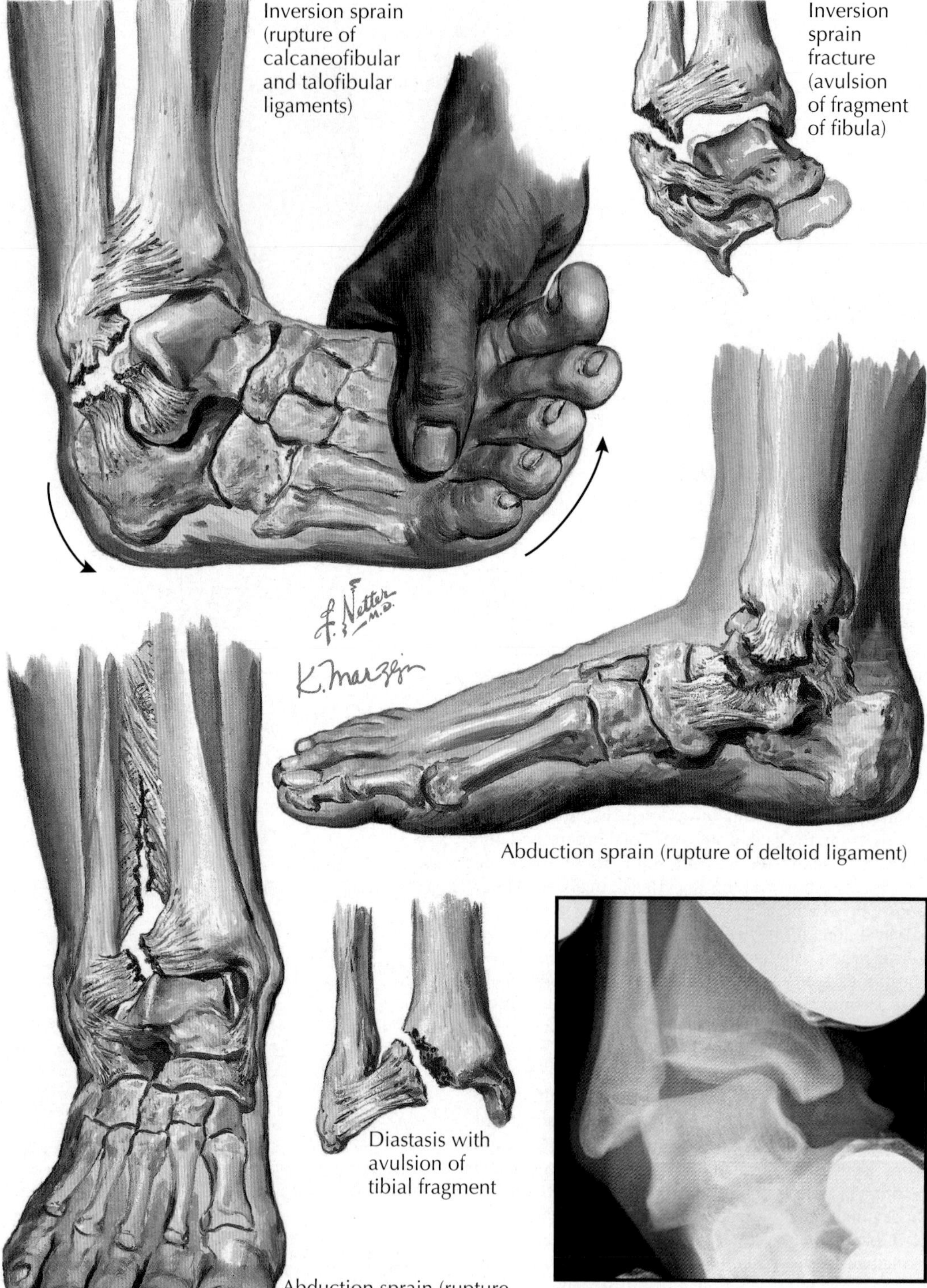

Stress radiograph demonstrating laxity of the calcaneofibular ligament and chronic ankle instability

ANKLE SPRAINS

Ankle sprains are the most common lower extremity injury in athletic and active individuals. Sprains of the ankle occur when a forceful inversion of the foot occurs, producing tearing of the ligaments on the lateral side of the ankle. These ligaments primarily include the anterior talofibular ligament and the calcaneofibular ligament. A "high" ankle sprain occurs when the foot is externally rotated on the leg, injuring the syndesmosis.

The vast majority of ankle sprains will heal uneventfully with appropriate nonsurgical treatment. A minority of patients will go on to have chronic symptoms characterized by recurrent ankle sprains and pain.

Physical Examination. The acutely sprained ankle is invariably swollen, tender, and ecchymotic over the lateral ankle and hindfoot, and, because of this, an examination can be difficult in the first few days after injury. Most patients are able to bear weight, but it is often uncomfortable. It is important to both examine the foot and ankle to rule out other areas of pain.

In the setting of chronic ankle instability, the examination is focused more on pain and ligamentous laxity. In these cases, tenderness is more localized over the anterolateral ankle where the anterior talofibular ligament is located. Tenderness may also be present in the retrofibular area if the peroneal tendons are injured or inflamed. Likewise, the anterolateral corner of the talus may be tender if an osteochondral lesion is present.

Stability testing is critical to making the diagnosis of chronic ankle instability. The anterior drawer maneuver tests the laxity of the anterior talofibular ligament and is performed with the ankle in the plantar flexed position. One hand stabilizes the leg, and the other grasps the heel and pulls the foot forward on the leg in an attempt to translate the talus anteriorly. A normal anterior talofibular ligament will resist this, and little motion will be observed. A chronically attenuated anterior talofibular ligament will allow up to a centimeter or more of anterior translation.

MECHANISMS OF ANKLE SPRAINS

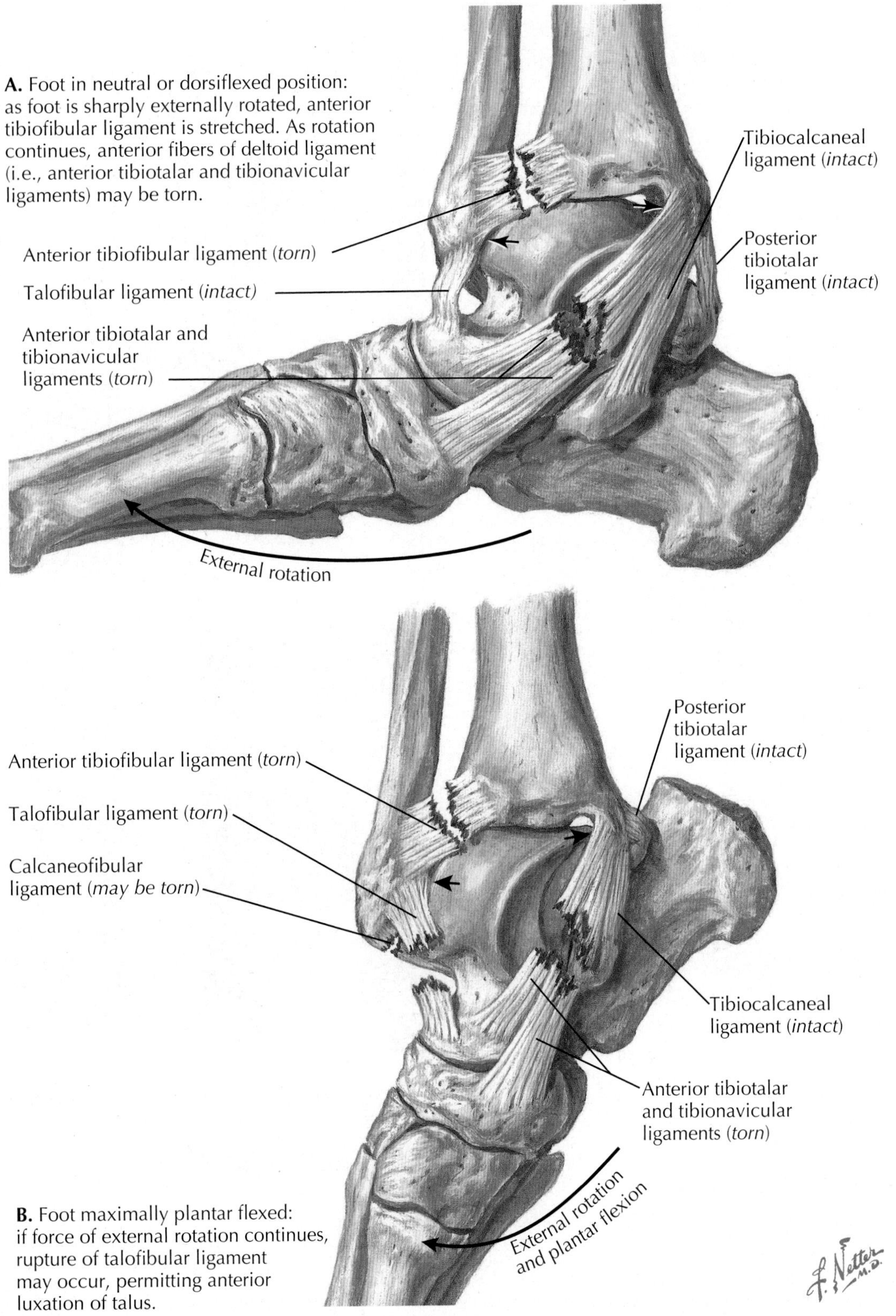

ANKLE SPRAINS (Continued)

The calcaneofibular ligament is tested using a maneuver called the talar tilt. The calcaneofibular ligament is tested with the ankle in neutral dorsiflexion. Again, the leg is stabilized and the heel grasped, followed by an inversion stress applied to the ankle. A normal calcaneofibular ligament will resist inversion stress, whereas an injured one will allow lateral opening during this maneuver. This must be distinguished from normal subtalar motion, which occurs when the foot is slightly more plantar flexed.

Radiographic Findings. Weight-bearing plain films of the foot and ankle are important to obtain in the setting of an acute sprain, to rule out fractures or other injuries. In the chronic setting, radiographs may also reveal lucency within the corners of the talus if an osteochondral lesion of the talus is present. Stress radiographs while performing anterior drawer and talar tilt maneuvers may be useful in demonstrating and quantifying chronic ankle instability.

Magnetic resonance imaging (MRI) is not mandatory but is frequently helpful to evaluate associated soft tissues such as the talar articular cartilage and peroneal tendons. A normal anterior talofibular ligament will appear as a tight black band on axial T1-weighted MR images. An injured anterior talofibular ligament will appear thickened and irregular or may be difficult to visualize on MRI.

Treatment. Acute sprains are best treated with functional rehabilitation. This involves early weight-bearing, bracing, and supervised physical therapy aimed at improving strength, balance, proprioception, and range of motion as well as decreasing pain. Restoring the eversion strength of the peroneal tendons is critical to restoring the proprioceptive ability of the ankle. Full recovery from a severe sprain may take 3 to 6 months.

The treatment of chronic instability involves surgical tightening of the lateral ankle ligaments. The ligaments are cut and then reattached at the appropriate tension, thus restoring stability to the ankle. Severely attenuated ligaments may require tissue augmentation with local or free tendon grafts. Postoperative rehabilitation is critical to achieving a good outcome.

ROTATIONAL FRACTURES

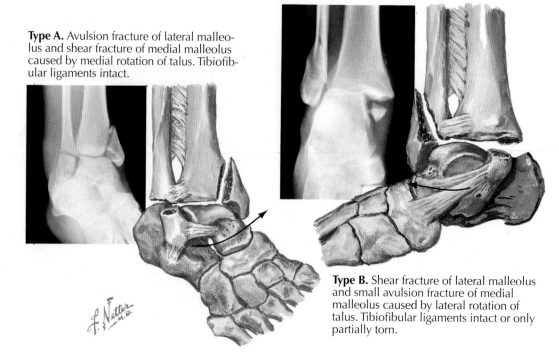

Type A. Avulsion fracture of lateral malleolus and shear fracture of medial malleolus caused by medial rotation of talus. Tibiofibular ligaments intact.

Type B. Shear fracture of lateral malleolus and small avulsion fracture of medial malleolus caused by lateral rotation of talus. Tibiofibular ligaments intact or only partially torn.

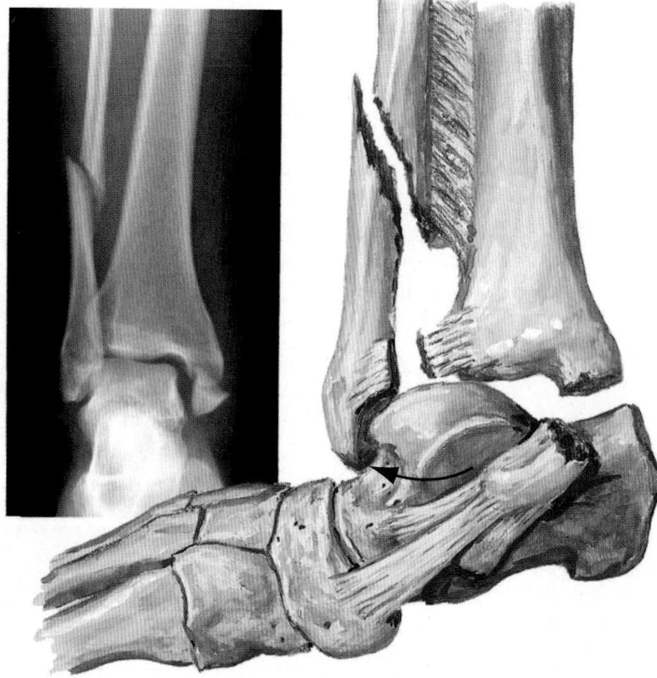

Type C. Disruption of tibiofibular ligaments with diastasis of syndesmosis caused by external rotation of talus. Force transmitted to fibula results in oblique fracture at higher level. In this case, avulsion of medial malleolus has also occurred.

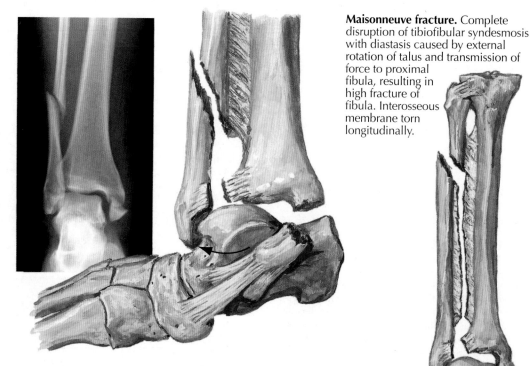

Maisonneuve fracture. Complete disruption of tibiofibular syndesmosis with diastasis caused by external rotation of talus and transmission of force to proximal fibula, resulting in high fracture of fibula. Interosseous membrane torn longitudinally.

Torn deltoid ligament

ANKLE FRACTURES

Ankle fractures are increasing in number as the population ages. Although not exclusive to the elderly population, they account for up to 5% of fractures in the elderly. Numerous studies have attempted to classify and categorize ankle fractures to better understand the mechanism of injury. This section focuses on ankle fractures caused by rotational injury, which is the most common mechanism.

CLASSIFICATION

Two of the main classifications used are the Danis-Weber classification, which has commonly been simplified to discuss the level of fibula fracture, and the Lauge-Hansen classification, which attempts to organize the injury based on mechanism.

Danis-Weber Classification

- Infrasyndesmotic fibula fracture ± medial malleolus, posteromedial fracture
- Fibula fracture at the level of the ankle joint ± medial malleolus, posterolateral fracture
- Fibula fracture above the level of the ankle joint ± medial malleolus fracture

Lauge-Hansen Classification

- *Supination-adduction:* infrasyndesmotic fibula fracture ± vertical fracture of the medial malleolus
- *Supination-external rotation:* posterior-oblique fibula fracture ± transverse medial malleolus, posterior malleolus fracture
- *Pronation-abduction:* comminuted fibula fracture at the level of the ankle joint ± transverse medial malleolus fracture
- *Pronation-external rotation:* fibula fracture above the level of the joint ± distal medial malleolus avulsion fracture

Physical Examination. Patients report tenderness to palpation on the lateral side of the ankle with a maximal point of tenderness at the level of the fracture. With more severe injuries, patients also report tenderness to palpation over the medial aspect of the ankle. This is due to progression of injury to the medial side, either causing a fracture of the medial malleolus or injury to the deltoid ligament. This is an important clinical examination finding because it can influence the treatment plan.

Ecchymosis and swelling are common examination findings, and in the case of surgical intervention, these can guide the timing of surgery. Instability may be

Repair of Fracture of Malleolus

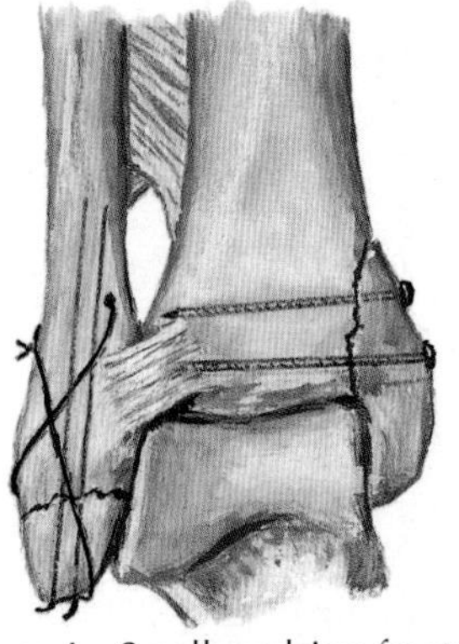

Type A. Small avulsion fracture of fibula fixated with Kirschner wires plus tension band wire; larger fracture of medial malleolus with two screws.

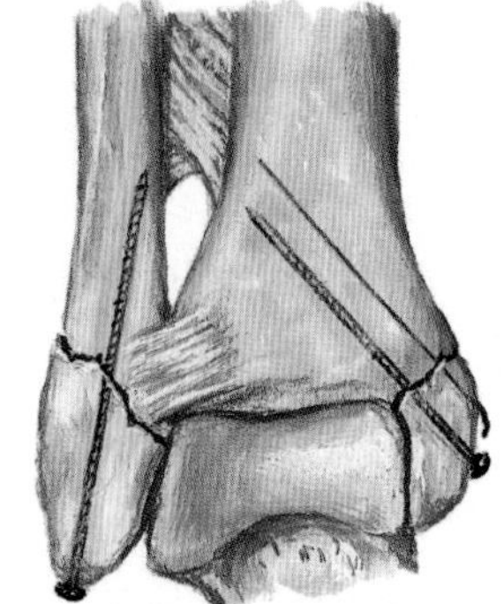

Larger fracture of lateral malleolus fixated with long, obliquely placed screw; small fracture of medial malleolus with Kirschner wire plus screw

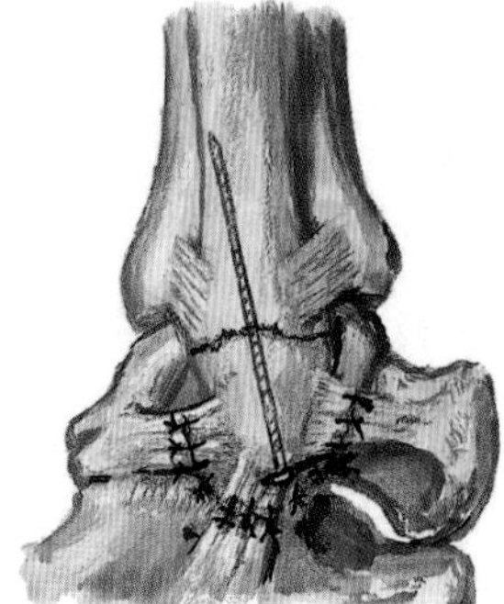

Torn lateral collateral ligament and joint capsule sutured

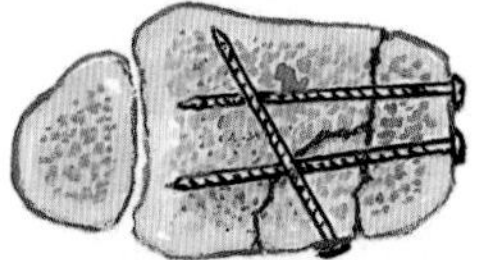

Sectional view shows fracture of medial malleolus and posteromedial tibia fixated with screws.

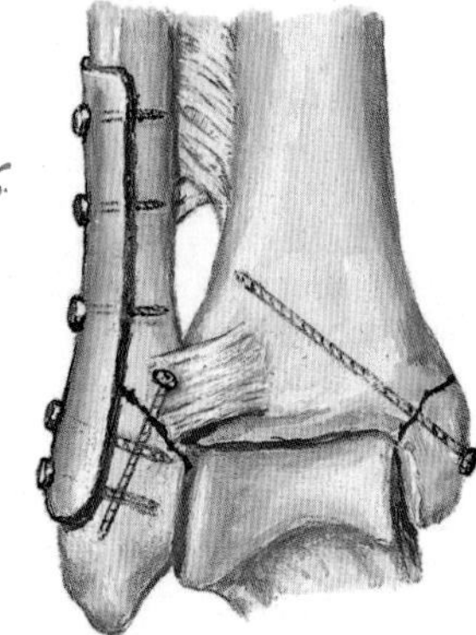

Type B. Fracture of fibula fixated with obliquely placed screw and plate; fracture of medial malleolus with screw.

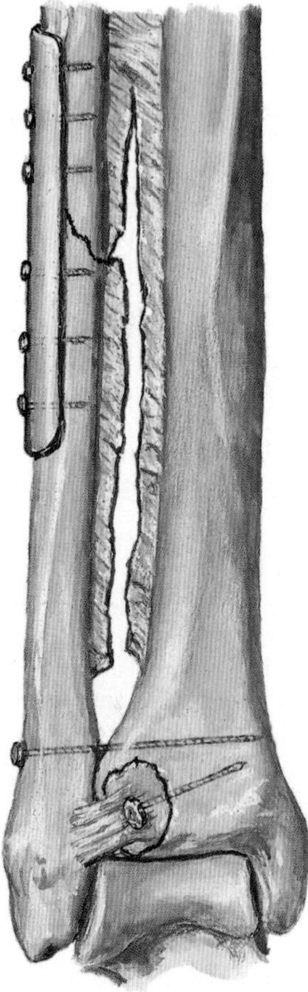

High fracture of fibula fixated with plate; avulsion of tibiofibular ligament with lag screw. Correction of diastasis with transfixion screw necessitated by extensive tear of interosseous membrane.

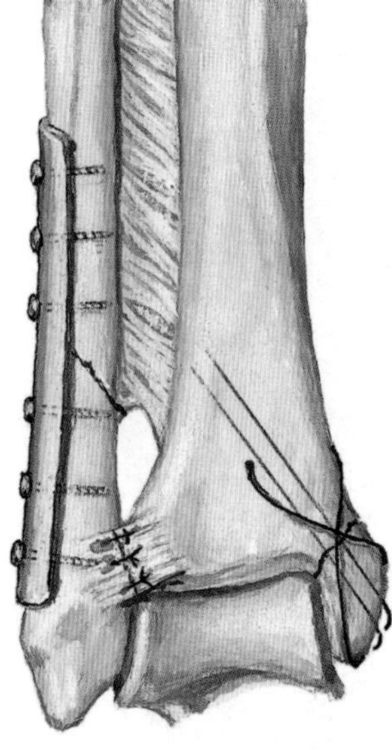

Type C. Fibula fixated with plate; small fracture of medial malleolus with Kirschner wires plus tension band wire. Tibiofibular ligaments sutured.

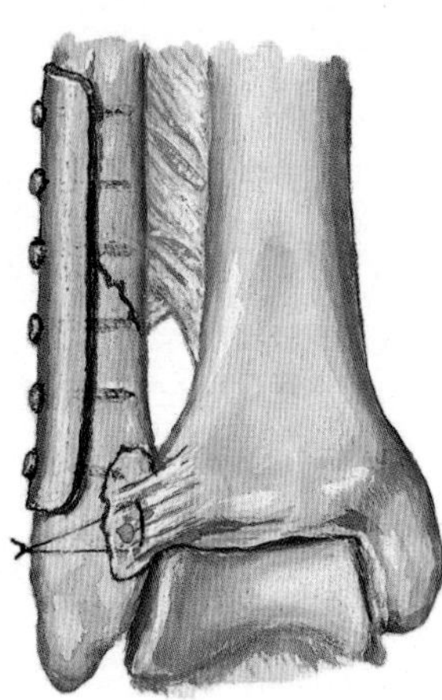

Avulsion fracture of tibiofibular ligament fixated with wire through bone

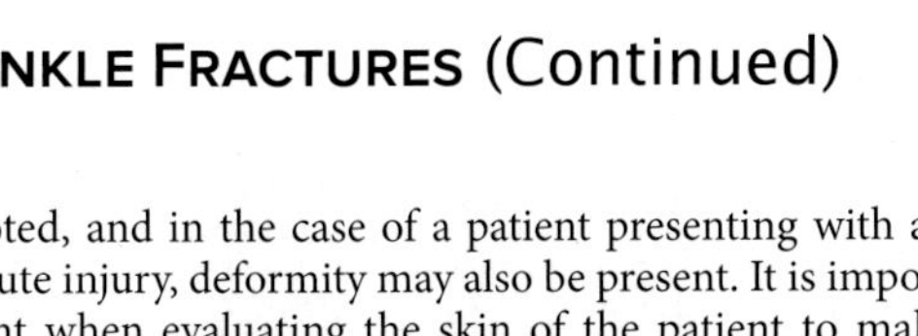

Ankle Fractures (Continued)

noted, and in the case of a patient presenting with an acute injury, deformity may also be present. It is important when evaluating the skin of the patient to make sure that there are no areas under tension from an underlying deformity. Strength testing and range-of-motion testing are often deferred owing to significant pain as well as the standing examination. The neurovascular examination, however, is critical for evaluation.

Imaging. Standard anteroposterior, lateral, and mortise radiographs are the main diagnostic modalities required for the average patient and are often all that is necessary to determine a treatment plan. Patients who have a questionable injury to the medial side of the ankle may be evaluated with an external rotation stress radiograph to evaluate the stability of both the syndesmosis and ankle. All ankle fractures treated operatively should undergo a stress view radiograph intraoperatively to evaluate the syndesmosis after fixation.

If there is concern for intraarticular extension of fracture lines, radiographs may not be sufficient to evaluate the injury. Computed tomography (CT) is used for detailed evaluation of the bony injury, including fractures of the posterior malleolus, anterolateral fractures of the tibia, and pilon fractures. There is limited role for MRI in ankle fractures except for the case of suspected stress fractures.

Treatment. Nondisplaced fractures of the lateral malleolus can be treated with cast immobilization in situations in which there is no ankle instability noted or injury to the medial side. Patients are kept non-weight-bearing for 6 to 8 weeks during the course of immobilization to maintain the fracture in appropriate alignment. Weight-bearing is progressed over time with the use of a fracture boot.

Displaced fractures of the lateral malleolus or fractures with associated medial injury are often unstable and require surgical fixation. Treatment includes open reduction and internal fixation with plates and screws. Other techniques are available, including percutaneous fixation; however, those are patient-specific procedures. Patients who have an injury to the syndesmosis require fixation. There is debate as to the number of screws and the screw size for syndesmotic fixation, but the value of treatment is *not* debatable.

All treatment is highlighted by some period of immobilization and non–weight-bearing. Advances in implants and fixation techniques have allowed physicians to attempt early weight-bearing, but 6 to 8 weeks of non–weight-bearing remains standard.

PILON FRACTURE

Pilon fractures represent a subset of fractures about the ankle due to a high-energy axial load. They are more correctly categorized as tibial plafond fractures with a pilon-type mechanism. *Pilon,* meaning hammer, defines fractures sustained from an axial load impacting the talar body into the distal tibial plafond. These fractures include combinations of injuries to the tibial articular surface, the fibula, the tibial metaphysis, and often the diaphysis. Patients often are victims of motor vehicle accidents or falls from height. They may report significant pain and swelling with an inability to ambulate. Because of the mechanism, there should be a high index of suspicion for other injuries and potential risks, including compartment syndrome and compression fractures of the lumbar spine.

Physical Examination. In the acute setting, patients will present with a painful, swollen leg with or without an obvious deformity. It is essential, as with any trauma, to assess the neurovascular status of the patient. The amount of swelling and skin changes are also important to note. Some patients, as many as 20% to 30%, may present with an open wound and therefore should be treated emergently. While assessing the patient it is important to note whether a deformity is present and whether it is causing any compromise to the neurovascular structures of the soft tissue. If so, this should be addressed urgently.

The remainder of the examination is often deferred, owing to the amount of pain these patients will be experiencing. In the office setting it is again essential to document the neurovascular status and to compare this to the initial examination. Importantly with pilon injuries, the splint or cast should be removed to assess the soft tissue. This will be critical to surgical planning as well as to continued immobilization management.

Imaging. Standard anteroposterior, lateral, and mortise view radiographs are obtained as well as full-length tibia films. If there are any other complaints at the time of injury, or in the office, associated with other areas of the body, it is necessary to evaluate those due to the mechanism. Traction radiographs may be helpful but also difficult to obtain owing to pain and skin compromise.

Pilon fractures, by definition, affect the distal tibial plafond and therefore the articular surface. To completely evaluate the extent of the intraarticular fracture lines it may be necessary to obtain a CT scan. There are some occasions when a CT scan may be deferred if it will not influence treatment; however, the majority of tibial plafond fractures should be evaluated with advanced imaging. Although the CT scan may not change the plan to operate, it will give more information for preoperative planning.

Treatment. There is little room for nonoperative management in the treatment algorithm for pilon fractures. However, nondisplaced fractures with little joint involvement and patients who are not surgical candidates will require nonoperative treatment with immobilization and a period of non–weight-bearing.

The majority of pilon fractures are treated with operative fixation. Although there are many techniques to fix the fractures, the strategy for appropriate reduction remains constant. Rüedi and Allgöwer defined a stepwise approach to treating pilon fractures: (1) fixation of fibula, (2) tibial joint reduction, (3) bone grafting of metaphyseal defects, and (4) buttress plating.

Because of the risk of wound healing complications and the potential for significant swelling, there is a role for staged treatment. One technique involves early internal fixation of the fibula with temporary external fixation of the tibia until swelling resolves enough to allow for the approaches necessary to treat the tibia. This may involve a period of 10 to 14 days until definitive fixation is performed.

The role of percutaneous fixation and limited internal fixation as well as thin wire external fixation is evolving; however, anatomic articular reduction remains the mainstay of treatment.

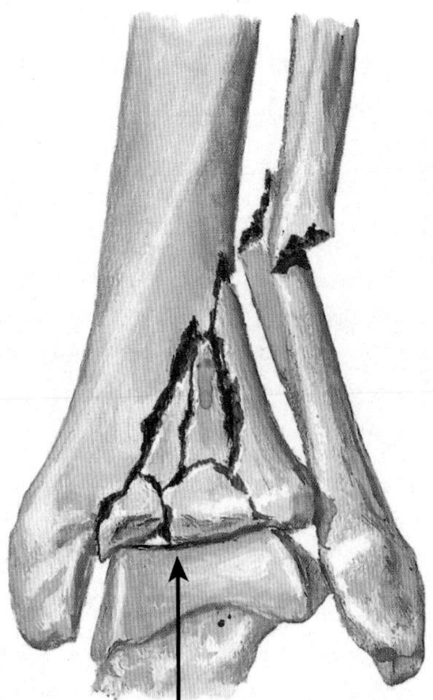

Usual cause is vertical loading of ankle joint (e.g., falling from a height and landing on heel, usually with ankle dorsiflexed). Fracture and compression of articular surface of tibia plus separation of malleoli and fracture of fibula.

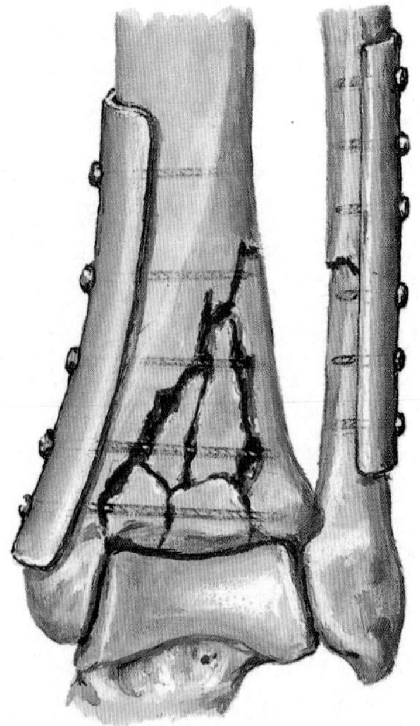

Fibula restored to correct length (determined from opposite limb) and fixed with 1/3 tubular plate. Articular surface of tibia reconstructed and stabilized with medial plate.

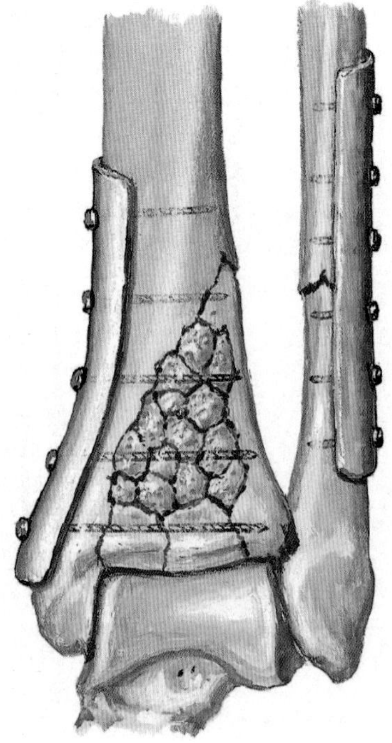

Residual bone defect filled with cancellous bone autograft from ilium

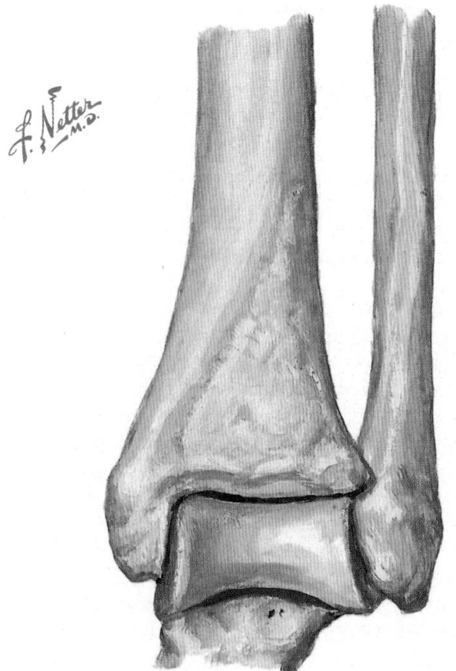

Bone graft well incorporated and fractures healed; plates removed about 1 year later with good functional result.

Osteochondral fracture of talar dome

If fragment is small, it may be removed; if large, it should be pinned in good apposition to restore congruity of articular surface.

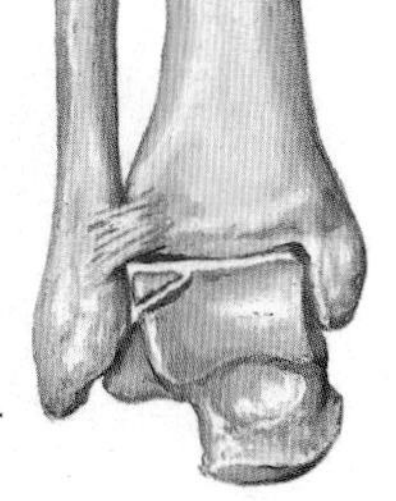

Type II. Fracture of talar neck with subluxation or dislocation of subtalar joint.

Fracture of talar neck

Usual cause is impact on anterior margin of tibia due to forceful dorsiflexion.

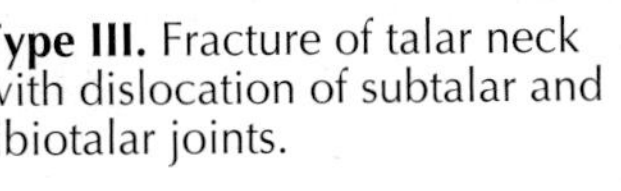

Type III. Fracture of talar neck with dislocation of subtalar and tibiotalar joints.

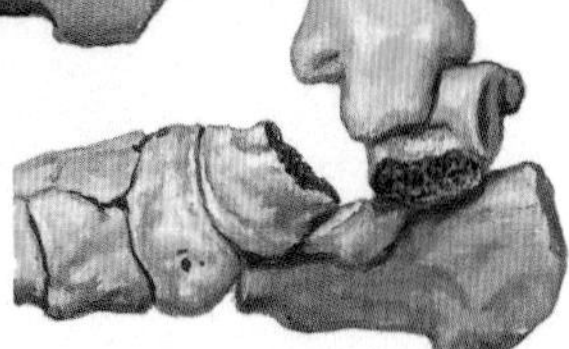

Type I. No displacement.

Fracture of talar processes

Large fracture of lateral process fixed with Kirschner wire and lag screw.

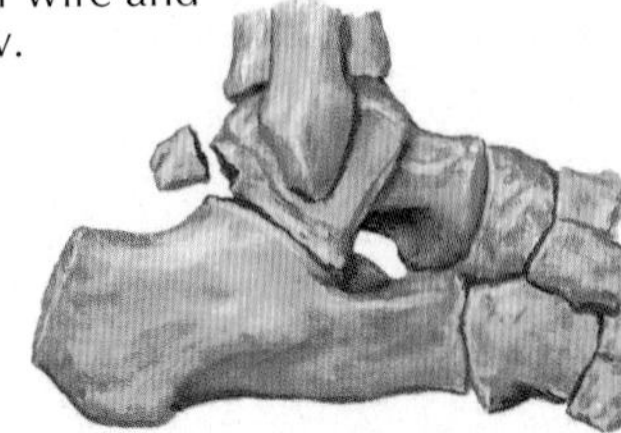

Fracture of posterior process. Irregularity of fracture line and comparison with other foot help differentiate it from congenital os trigonum.

Position of foot and x-ray beam for anteroposterior visualization of talar neck fracture

75°

Open repair of talar neck fracture. Anteromedial incision made with ankle in extension. Bone fragments apposed and aligned, and joints reduced. Compression screw inserted across fracture line. Alternatively, fracture fixed with two threaded pins.

Anterior tibial a.
Perforating branch of peroneal a.
Anterior lateral malleolar a.
Posterior tibial a.
Dorsalis pedis a.
Anterior lateral tarsal a.
Artery of tarsal sinus
Deltoid a.
Artery of tarsal canal

Blood supply of talus. Because of profuse intraosseous anastomoses, avascular necrosis commonly occurs only when surrounding soft tissue is damaged, as in types II and III fractures of talar neck.

Avascular necrosis of talar body is evidenced by increased density (sclerosis) compared with other tarsal bones.

TALUS FRACTURE

Talus fractures represent severe injuries to the ankle. Different portions of the talus may be injured based on the mechanism of injury. High-energy falls from a height or motor vehicle accidents may produce a forced dorsiflexion injury that results in fracture of the talar neck or body. These are the most severe talus injuries and carry the most significant morbidity owing to the disruption of the blood supply to the talus that occurs. Within this group of injuries, the severity increases depending on the amount of displacement present. Type I fractures are essentially nondisplaced and have the best prognosis. Type II fractures are displaced and are much more likely to involve disruption of the intraosseous blood supply of the talus. Type III fractures are displaced and also dislocated, which in most cases results in avascular necrosis of the talar body. This classification scheme is known as the Hawkins classification.

Inversion injuries can result in an osteochondral fracture of the talus, usually involving the anterolateral talar dome. Snowboarders are susceptible to fracture of the lateral process of the talus.

Forced plantar flexion can result in a fracture of the posterior process of the talus.

Physical Examination. A patient with a talus fracture will present with significant pain and swelling about the ankle. Bruising medially and laterally may be noted, and the normal skin wrinkles present about the hindfoot may be obliterated by the swelling. If dislocation is present, obvious deformity will be visible.

In high-energy injuries, fracture blisters may be noted. These may be partial-thickness (clear) or full-thickness (bloody) blisters.

Imaging. Three views of both the foot and ankle should be obtained to evaluate for a possible talus fracture. Each of the potentially injured portions of the talus should be scrutinized for fracture. The specialized Canale view is particularly helpful in visualizing the talar neck. To perform this view, the foot and leg are internally rotated and the beam is angled about 75 degrees relative to the floor. All suspected talus fractures should be evaluated with a fine-cut CT scan to determine displacement and comminution.

Treatment. Most talar neck and body fractures should be treated with open reduction and internal fixation. The goal is anatomic reduction and stable fixation. This is best achieved using both anteromedial and anterolateral approaches. If only the anteromedial approach is used, malreduction may occur. Fixation is usually achieved with anterior to posterior screws placed across the fracture site.

Nondisplaced lateral process fractures can be treated with immobilization. But fractures that are displaced require open reduction and internal fixation, usually with minifragment screws.

Nondisplaced osteochondral fractures may also be treated nonsurgically. But any displacement or instability of the fracture requires either fixation or excision, depending on the size of the fragment. These injuries are frequently amenable to arthroscopic treatment.

EXTRAARTICULAR FRACTURE OF CALCANEUS

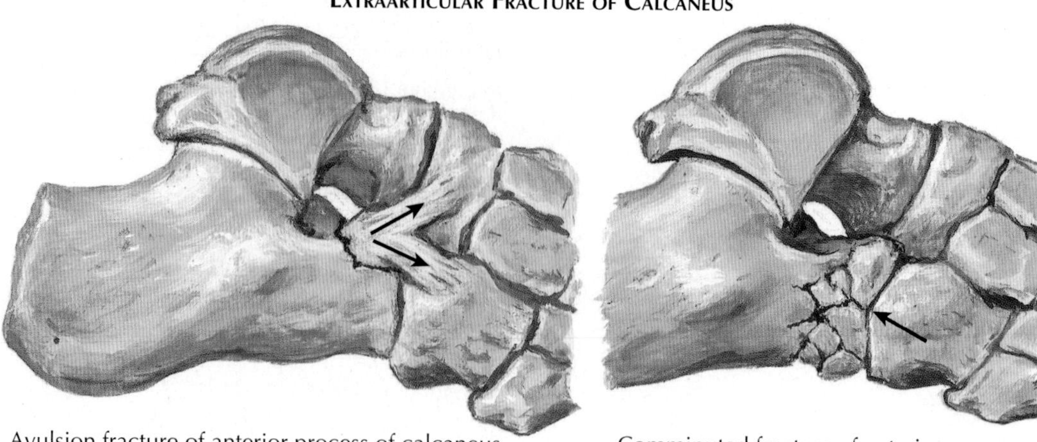

Avulsion fracture of anterior process of calcaneus caused by tension on bifurcate ligament

Comminuted fracture of anterior process of calcaneus due to compression by cuboid in forceful abduction of forefoot

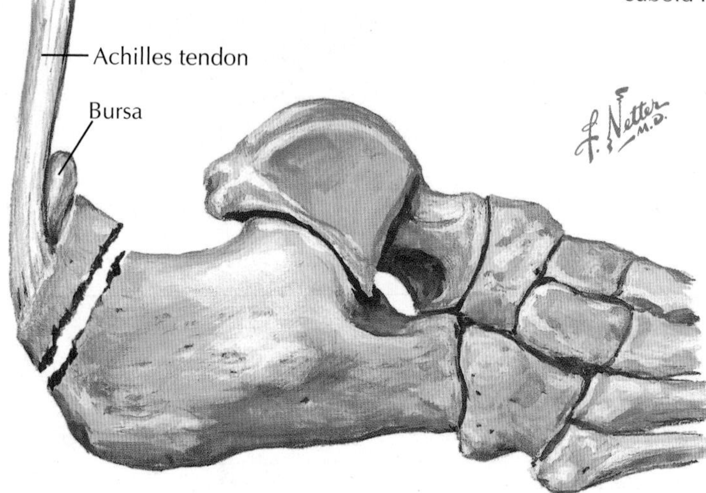

Avulsion fracture of tuberosity of calcaneus due to sudden, violent contraction of Achilles tendon

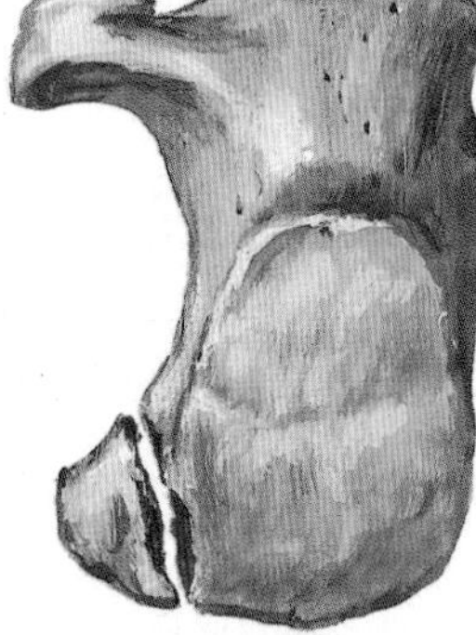

Fracture of medial process of tuberosity of calcaneus

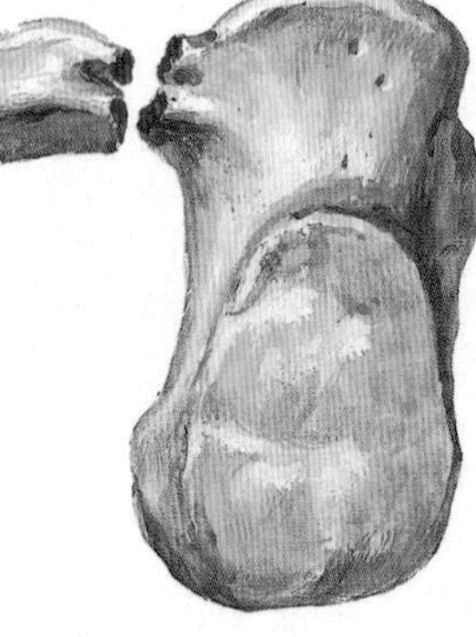

Fracture of sustentaculum tali

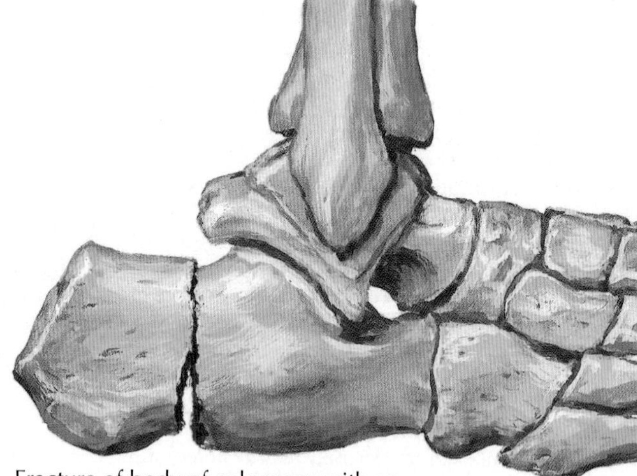

Fracture of body of calcaneus with no involvement of subtalar articulation

CALCANEUS FRACTURE

Fractures of the calcaneus represent a heterogeneous group of injuries. The severity and mechanism of injury that produces a fracture of the calcaneus vary based on where specifically the fracture is located. Calcaneal body fractures occur when a significant force is transmitted up through the bottom of the heel, such as after a fall from a height or motor vehicle accident. Rarely, these fractures may spare the posterior facet of the subtalar joint. Unfortunately, most calcaneal body fractures are intraarticular. These are very severe injuries, and the subtalar joint can be profoundly damaged and displaced.

Inversion injury similar to what occurs in an ankle sprain can produce a fracture of the anterior process of the calcaneus. This fracture variant occurs due to the pull of the bifurcate ligament that attaches to the anterior process.

Conversely, forced abduction injuries of the foot may produce a compression fracture of the anterior calcaneus. These injuries may also involve the cuboid bone and have been called "nutcracker" fractures, owing to the compression mechanism of injury.

The pull of the Achilles tendon may produce a fracture of the tuberosity of the calcaneus. This also represents a severe injury because the function of the gastrocsoleus complex is rendered incompetent. Moreover, the thin skin over the posterior heel is vulnerable to ischemic necrosis and breakdown with this fracture pattern.

Lower-energy falls may produce small fractures of the medial process of the calcaneal tuberosity.

However, with higher-energy trauma, the sustentaculum tali may be fractured. This injury pattern may be difficult to detect on standard radiographs.

Physical Examination. A patient with a calcaneus fracture will present with significant pain and swelling about the hindfoot. In virtually all cases, ecchymosis medially and laterally will be noted and the normal skin wrinkles present about the hindfoot will be obliterated by the swelling.

In high-energy injuries, fracture blisters may be noted. These may be partial-thickness (clear) or full-thickness

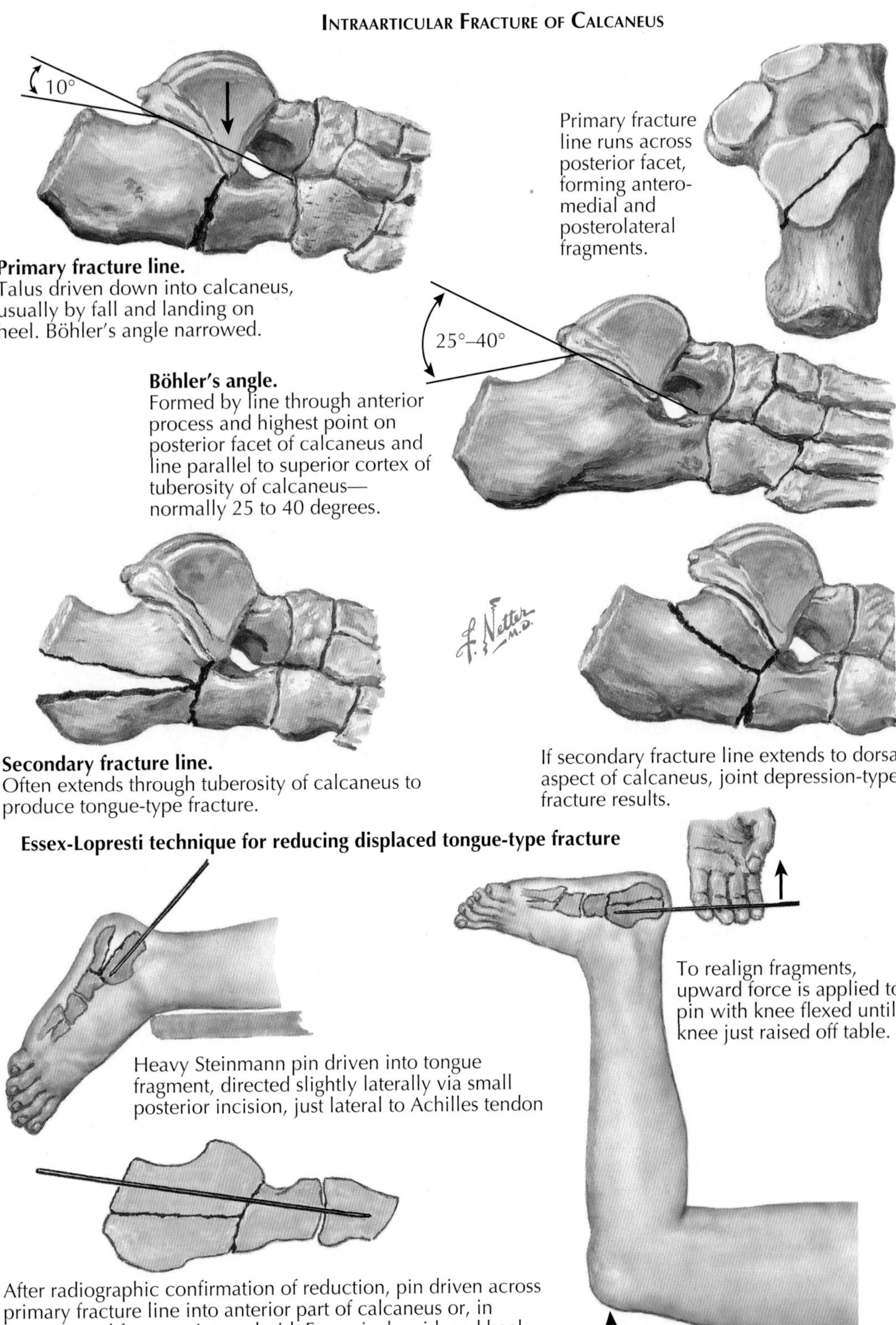
Intraarticular Fracture of Calcaneus
10°
Primary fracture line runs across posterior facet, forming anteromedial and posterolateral fragments.
Primary fracture line.
Talus driven down into calcaneus, usually by fall and landing on heel. Böhler's angle narrowed.
25°–40°
Böhler's angle.
Formed by line through anterior process and highest point on posterior facet of calcaneus and line parallel to superior cortex of tuberosity of calcaneus—normally 25 to 40 degrees.
Secondary fracture line.
Often extends through tuberosity of calcaneus to produce tongue-type fracture.
If secondary fracture line extends to dorsal aspect of calcaneus, joint depression-type fracture results.
Essex-Lopresti technique for reducing displaced tongue-type fracture
To realign fragments, upward force is applied to pin with knee flexed until knee just raised off table.
Heavy Steinmann pin driven into tongue fragment, directed slightly laterally via small posterior incision, just lateral to Achilles tendon
After radiographic confirmation of reduction, pin driven across primary fracture line into anterior part of calcaneus or, in comminuted fracture, into cuboid. Excessively widened heel may be corrected with manual compression. Pin incorporated into short leg, non–weight-bearing cast.

CALCANEUS FRACTURE (Continued)

(bloody) blisters. Attention should be paid to determine whether the Achilles tendon is intact. The foot should be evaluated for neurologic compromise as well. Compartment syndrome of the foot can complicate fracture of the calcaneus.

Imaging. Three views of both the foot and ankle should be obtained as well as an axial view of the heel to evaluate the calcaneus. Each of the potentially injured portions of the calcaneus should be scrutinized for fracture. With displaced intraarticular fractures of the calcaneus, the angle between a line drawn from the anterior process to the posterior facet and a line from the tuberosity to the posterior facet will be flattened. This angle is referred to as Bohler's angle. All suspected calcaneus fractures should be evaluated with a fine-cut CT scan. CT will accurately assess the severity of the injury by allowing determination of displacement and joint involvement.

Treatment. Nondisplaced extraarticular fractures are most commonly treated nonsurgically with immobilization and protected weight-bearing. Displaced fractures of the tuberosity require surgical treatment. Large anterior process fractures that are displaced significantly are treated with open reduction and internal fixation. However, if the fragment is small or minimally displaced, anterior process fractures can be treated nonsurgically. Chronically symptomatic anterior process fractures can be excised.

Displaced intraarticular calcaneus fractures are best treated surgically with open reduction and internal fixation using a plate and screws. Surgery allows restoration of joint congruity and calcaneal morphology, which decreases the risk for future problems such as subtalar arthritis and peroneal impingement. However, patients with significant medical comorbidities may be more safely treated with immobilization and non–weight-bearing. Certain fracture patterns may be amenable to percutaneous fixation. The tongue-type fracture occurs when the major fracture line extends posteriorly to include the calcaneal tuberosity. With these fractures, the Essex-Lopresti maneuver can allow reduction using a minimally invasive approach.

Fifth Metatarsal Fractures

Patients presenting with lateral foot pain after a twisting injury of the foot and ankle need to be considered for a fifth metatarsal fracture. There is a wide spectrum of fracture possibilities with the fifth metatarsal, but most discussion revolves around fractures of the base of the metatarsal. The fifth metatarsal fracture, or Jones fracture, is actually a spectrum of injury of the fifth metatarsal, with a true Jones fracture representing a small population of these fractures. Patients will often complain of difficulty with ambulation and altered gait due to pain. The location of pain and the mechanism of injury will often lead the physician to the diagnosis. There is a select population of patients who present with injury during athletic activity, and, although the mechanism is often similar, it is necessary to mention this group because this injury can be treated differently in the elite athlete.

As with most fractures, patients with fifth metatarsal fracture present after a trauma. The exact mechanism of injury is usually an inversion sprain that is accompanied by a powerful contraction of the peroneus brevis, resulting in a fracture. Although this is the most common injury, it is possible that a patient can sustain this injury by a direct blow to the lateral foot, in addition to any complex foot trauma. Another version of this injury is a stress injury that is a result of a cavus foot that increases the pressure seen over the fifth metatarsal. It is possible that people with subtle cavus feet, as described by Manoli, have a stronger propensity to these types of fractures.

Physical Examination. While examining the patient with a suspected fifth metatarsal fracture, it is important to examine the entire lateral foot and ankle along with the medial side for associated injuries. There are many bony prominences that must be palpated. The entire lateral foot may demonstrate swelling and ecchymosis, or it may be entirely absent. The patient will complain of tenderness along the fifth metatarsal, and the location of the tenderness will help determine the type of fracture. Patients will often have pain with resisted eversion as the peroneus brevis pulls on the injured area. Weight-bearing and gait analysis are often difficult due to pain and can be deferred in these patients. If the patient can bear weight, it is important to look at the alignment of the foot to see whether the patient has a cavus foot. These patients will have a peek-a-boo heel when looking from anterior to posterior.

Imaging. With acute injuries, standard radiographs are often sufficient to make the diagnosis. Patients will often have difficulty with weight-bearing, and in these patients non–weight-bearing radiographs are adequate. The anteroposterior radiograph is the most useful radiograph to view the fracture. The next step is to proceed to CT or MRI if radiographic findings are inconclusive. CT is used to evaluate potential nonunions and delayed healing, whereas MRI is useful with a suspected stress injury. Bone scanning can be used, but the other modalities are more useful.

Treatment. Fracture of the fifth metatarsal, and, more importantly, the Jones fracture, is a hotly debated topic. It is currently believed that most patients are best treated nonoperatively, whereas the elite athlete is best treated with surgery, owing to the long healing and high nonunion rate. The difficulty is the definition of an elite athlete and who should be treated surgically.

The nonoperative treatment includes protected weight-bearing in a postoperative shoe or walking boot depending on the patient's symptoms. It is also appropriate to place the foot in a cast. The patient is treated with protected weight-bearing for 6 to 8 weeks as symptoms dictate. As healing occurs, weight-bearing is progressed in normal shoes. If the patient continues to demonstrate symptoms and the radiographs show delayed healing, it may be necessary to prolong the length of protected weight-bearing.

Surgical management for Jones fractures is open reduction and internal fixation with an intramedullary screw. There is considerable debate about the specific details of the screw fixation, but the underlying method remains the same.

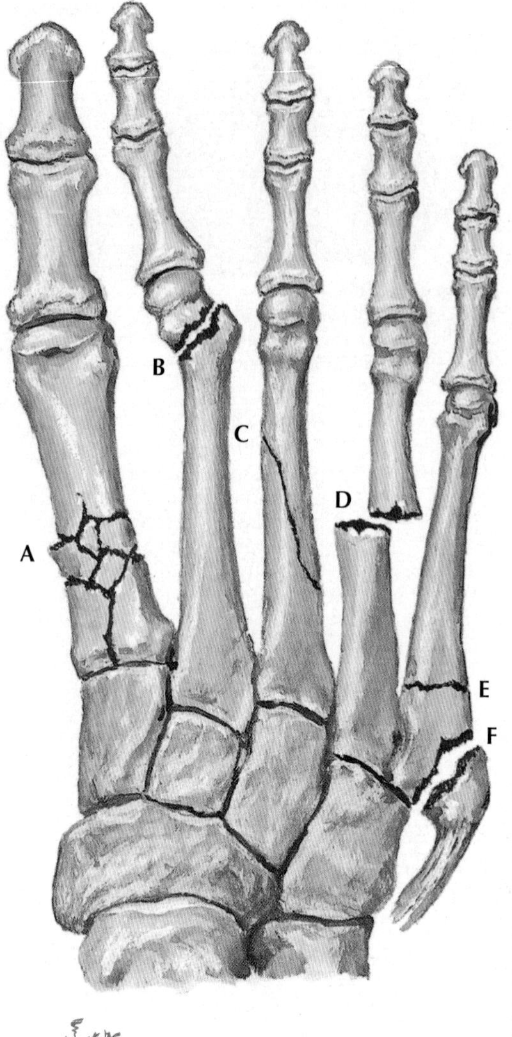

Types of fractures of metatarsal:
A. Comminuted fracture
B. Displaced neck fracture
C. Oblique fracture
D. Displaced transverse fracture
E. Fracture of base of 5th metatarsal
F. Avulsion of tuberosity of 5th metatarsal

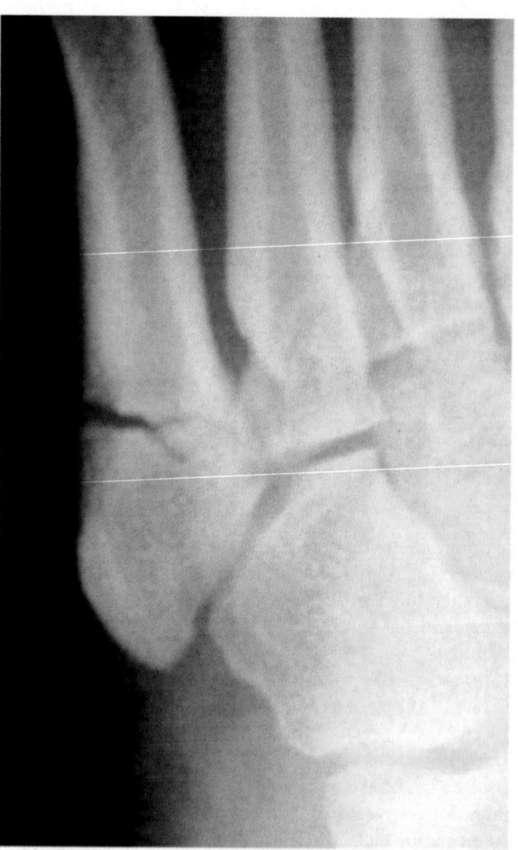

Jones fracture

Lisfranc Injury

Any patient with an acute injury with foot pain should be evaluated or at least considered for a Lisfranc injury. Midfoot sprains, fractures, and dislocations represent commonly missed injuries in the emergency department and office settings. The Lisfranc injury represents any combination of injury, whether fracture or ligamentous injury, to the tarsometatarsal joints. Patients will report midfoot pain, with or without midfoot swelling and plantar ecchymosis. In most patients, there is an acute event that represented the onset of symptoms. In the patient with diabetes or, more specifically, the patient with neuropathy, no specific event may be noted.

The tarsometatarsal joints are by nature a strong stable complex. There is a combination of bony architecture and strong plantar ligaments that create a stable midfoot. The medial cuneiform and second metatarsal have a strong plantar ligament known as the Lisfranc ligament that is thought to be the main stabilizer of the tarsometatarsal joints. In addition, the recessed second tarsometatarsal joint creates a keystone that enhances stability. These anatomic factors as well as the biomechanics of the foot contribute to the large amount of force necessary to injure the Lisfranc complex.

Motor vehicle accidents and sporting injuries represent the major causes of Lisfranc injuries. The position of the foot while on the gas pedal along with an axial load to the foot is the most likely cause of injury to this area in a motor vehicle accident. With sporting injuries, it is often the result of a player who is at the toe-off portion of the gait cycle when a player steps on, or lands on, the foot, imparting an axial load to the foot. Patients with neuropathy may have no inciting cause of their injury and often no significant examination findings, with the exception of a change in the foot position.

Physical Examination. Because of the nature of these injuries, the patient often presents with significant swelling and ecchymosis of the midfoot. There may be a bony prominence to the midfoot if there is significant dorsal dislocation of the Lisfranc complex. Patients will have difficulty standing, and thus gait analysis and a standing examination may be deferred. Tenderness to palpation over the midfoot is present, although this may be absent in the neuropathic patient. Gross instability of the tarsometatarsal joints may be observed in significant injuries. It is important to perform a thorough neurovascular examination because of the significant trauma and a complete examination of surrounding structures in the foot due to the force imparted during injury.

Imaging. Lisfranc injuries have pathognomonic radiographic findings that are often described. On an anteroposterior radiograph, the alignment of the second ray will demonstrate disruption of a straight line along the medial border of the second metatarsal and intermediate cuneiform. With an internal rotation oblique radiograph of the foot, the fourth metatarsal should form a straight line with the cuboid, and this may also be disrupted. Any number of fracture combinations may be seen with the metatarsals and cuneiforms along with ligamentous disruptions that may or may not be evident on plain radiographs. The lateral radiograph of the foot may also show dorsal subluxation or gross dislocation of the tarsometatarsal joints.

In patients with suspected Lisfranc injury but without obvious radiographic findings, it is necessary to proceed with advanced imaging. CT will evaluate the bony injury and help show any widening within the Lisfranc complex, and MRI should be used in those patients with suspected ligamentous injury without obvious bony injury.

Treatment. The debate among surgeons is not whether to fix a displaced Lisfranc injury but whether to perform an open reduction and internal fixation or whether to fuse the tarsometatarsal joints involved. Studies have demonstrated that nonoperative management of displaced Lisfranc injuries has poor results with long-term sequelae. Fractures involving the Lisfranc complex require fixation, whereas ligamentous disruption also requires repair by realignment of the normal anatomy. Further research has shown that people who sustain purely ligamentous Lisfranc injuries may do better with fusion, whereas those who have a bony component may be best treated with open reduction and internal fixation. Either treatment option is acceptable based on the current literature, with the underlying management premise being realignment of the disrupted Lisfranc complex. Postoperative management requires a period of immobilization and non–weight-bearing.

Patients with nondisplaced injuries or those who are not surgical candidates may be treated with a course of non–weight-bearing with cast immobilization.

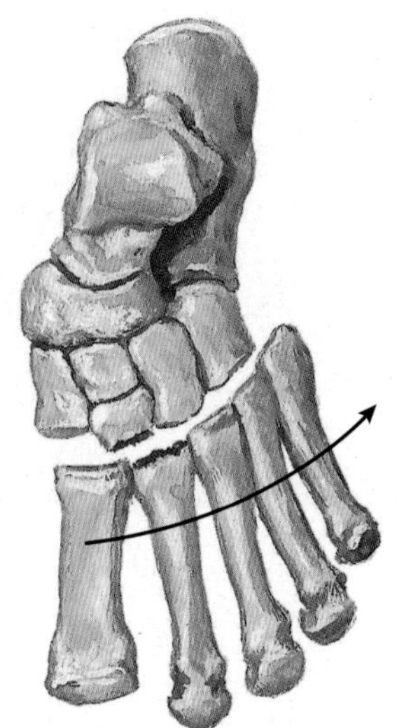

Homolateral dislocation. All five metatarsals displaced in same direction; fracture of base of 2nd metatarsal.

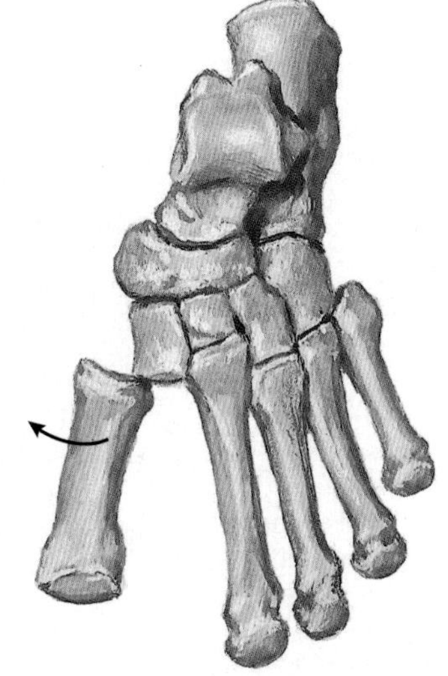

Isolated dislocation. One or two metatarsals displaced; others in normal position.

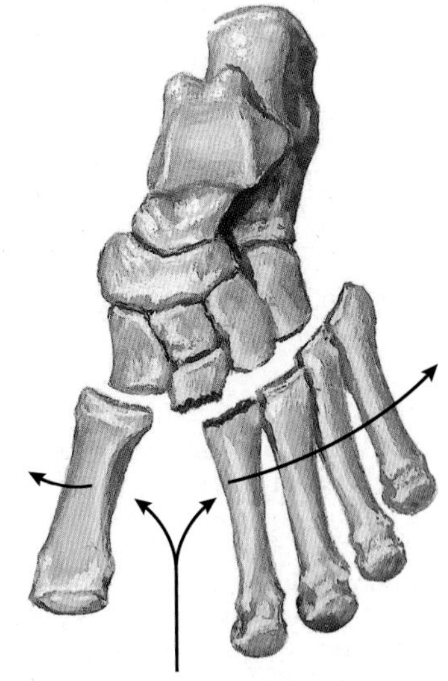

Divergent dislocation. 1st metatarsal displaced medially, others superolaterally.

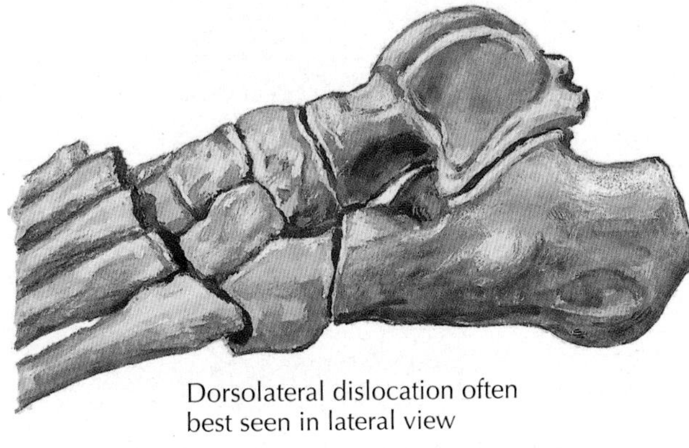

Dorsolateral dislocation often best seen in lateral view

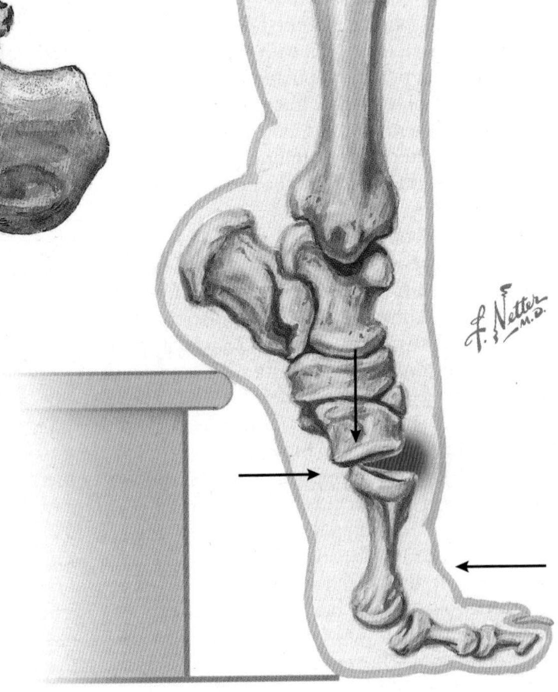

Injury may occur from seemingly trivial event (e.g., misstep into a hole with axial compression and abduction force on plantar flexed foot).

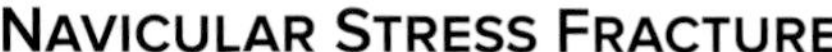

Navicular Stress Fracture

Although uncommon in the general population, the active individual, especially runners, can present with vague midfoot pain related to a navicular stress fracture. Often the individual describes soreness and pain that occur over a prolonged period of time without improvement of symptoms. Initially the pain occurs with activity, and, as the condition progresses, the patient will describe pain earlier in activity and then pain with activities of daily living. The hallmark symptom is pain occurring with activity. Pain that originates at rest and is relieved with activity or pain that occurs at the beginning of the day and improves as the day progresses suggests other conditions.

Stress fractures occur with repetitive trauma, and navicular stress fractures are no different. Athletes and active individuals involved in sports requiring running and explosive push-off seem to be at risk. It is likely that the increased load seen at the talonavicular joint as well as the increased force seen with explosive athletic movement are what put this population at an increased risk for this type of injury. Stress fractures occur as the normal balance of microfractures, and repair is tipped toward injury. These microscopic injuries, or microfractures, accumulate over time to form the progressive symptoms of stress fractures.

Physical Examination. A general foot and ankle examination is paramount in any patient presenting with vague pain. Often palpation of the foot is the most important examination in this population. The location of tenderness will lead the physician to a specific constellation of problems. Patients with a navicular stress fracture will describe tenderness dorsally over the navicular or talonavicular joint. The location of the tenderness can be confusing because it is often close to the ankle joint. It is important to determine whether the location of tenderness is the anterior ankle joint or just distal at the talonavicular joint or the navicular itself. Provocative tests have been described, including hopping on the affected foot; however, the general examination is often best. Tenderness can also occur along the medial arch and sometimes on the plantar part of the foot. The remaining findings of the examination are often normal, including those of the neurovascular examination, strength testing, and range of motion.

Imaging. Obtaining standard radiographs is common with a new problem or new patient, but a navicular stress fracture is not often seen on initial radiographs. There is a delay in diagnosis with stress fractures, and it is often attributed to the lack of radiographic findings. The next step in diagnosis is advanced imaging. Two common modalities are bone scanning and CT. Three-phase bone scanning is an inexpensive option without exposure to radiation. The gold standard remains CT of the foot, which can reach a sensitivity of close to 100%, but the high exposure to radiation remains a major drawback. Early detection can also be made with MRI, but the lower cost of and ease in obtaining a CT make it the first-line examination, in addition to the high sensitivity.

Injury to Midtarsal (Chopart) Joint Complex

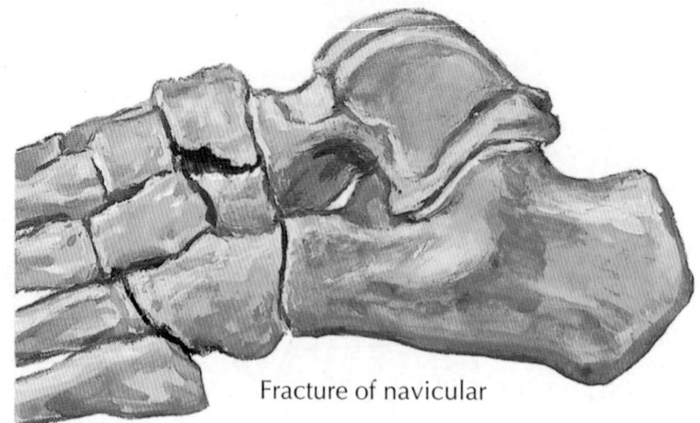

Fracture of navicular

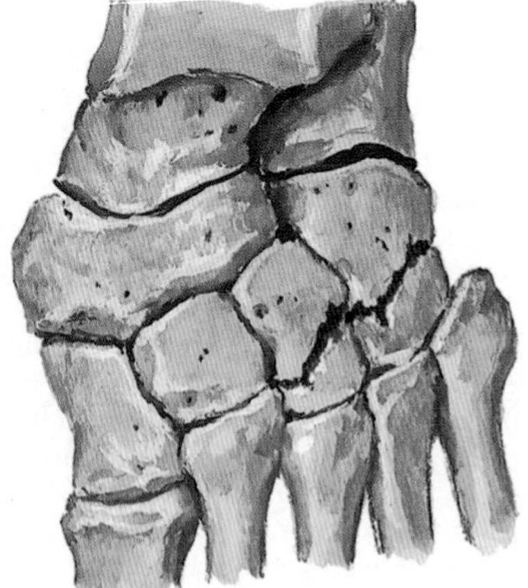

Fracture of cuboid and lateral cuneiform

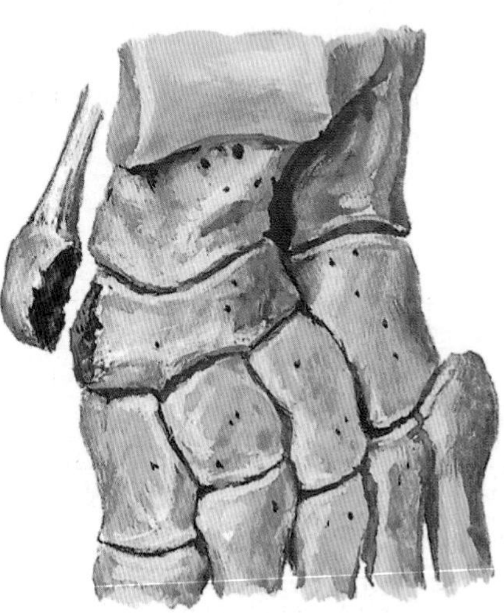

Avulsion of tuberosity of navicular by tibialis posterior tendon

Dorsal dislocation of navicular reduced and fixed with pin through 1st metatarsal, medial cuneiform, and talus

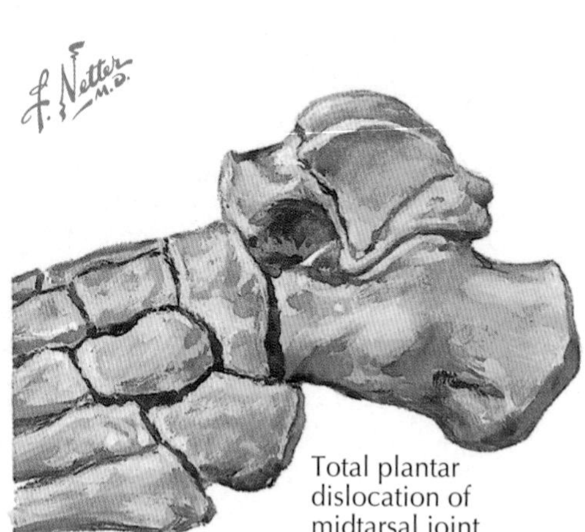

Total plantar dislocation of midtarsal joint

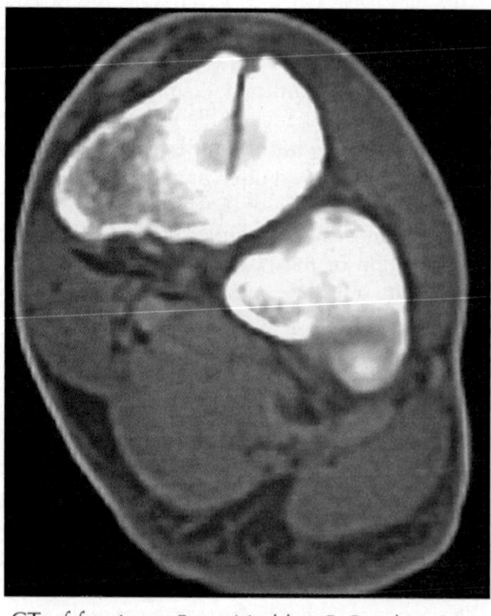

CT of fracture. *From Madden C, Putukian M, Young C, McCarly E. Netter's Sports Medicine. Elsevier; 2009.*

Treatment. Treatment is divided based on the presentation of symptoms and the radiographic findings. Nondisplaced fractures or suspected navicular stress fractures are treated with protected weight-bearing and rest. Initial treatment involves a non–weight-bearing cast for 6 to 8 weeks followed by advancing weight-bearing in a protective boot along with assistance. If symptoms persist despite non–weight-bearing, then prolonged non–weight-bearing can be attempted.

Displaced navicular fractures as well as fractures that fail nonoperative treatment require open reduction and internal fixation. Bone grafting can be used based on patient factors and radiographic findings. A standard anterior approach over the navicular is used to access the fracture. The talonavicular joint may need to be opened to obtain accurate reduction and joint congruity.

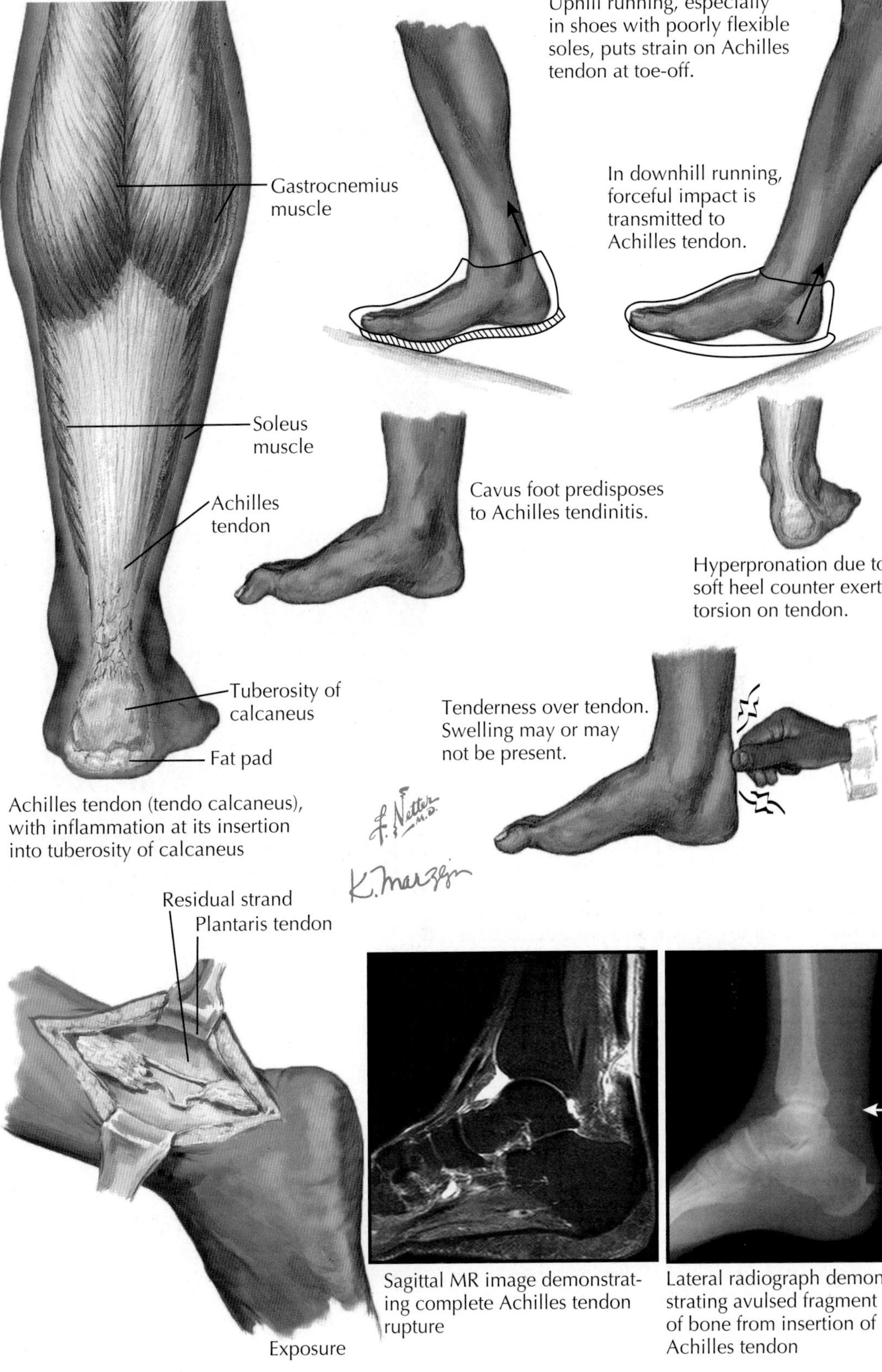
Uphill running, especially in shoes with poorly flexible soles, puts strain on Achilles tendon at toe-off.
Gastrocnemius muscle
In downhill running, forceful impact is transmitted to Achilles tendon.
Soleus muscle
Achilles tendon
Cavus foot predisposes to Achilles tendinitis.
Hyperpronation due to soft heel counter exerts torsion on tendon.
Tuberosity of calcaneus
Fat pad
Tenderness over tendon. Swelling may or may not be present.
Achilles tendon (tendo calcaneus), with inflammation at its insertion into tuberosity of calcaneus
Residual strand
Plantaris tendon
Exposure
Sagittal MR image demonstrating complete Achilles tendon rupture
Lateral radiograph demonstrating avulsed fragment of bone from insertion of Achilles tendon

Achilles Tendon Rupture

Achilles tendon ruptures occur frequently in the middle-aged athlete. The rupture commonly occurs 4 to 5 cm proximal to the insertion on the calcaneus. This location corresponds to a relatively avascular area within the Achilles that likely predisposes it to injury. Achilles tendon ruptures most frequently occur when the gastrocsoleus muscle complex is subjected to an excessive force that requires strong eccentric contraction. This commonly occurs during activities that require abrupt change of direction, jumping, or sprinting. Classically, individuals will describe a sensation of being struck in the back of the leg with a bat. They may also report hearing or feeling a distinct pop. Many are unable to ambulate after injury, but some are still able to walk with a limp.

Physical Examination. Physical examination of a ruptured Achilles tendon reveals swelling and ecchymosis over the posterior aspect of the distal leg with tenderness localized to this area. The patient is best examined prone with the other leg exposed for comparison. Palpation along the Achilles tendon reveals a palpable gap at the site of the rupture. When the patient bends both knees while prone, the resting position of the injured ankle is usually noted to be in increased dorsiflexion compared with the contralateral side. Passive manual dorsiflexion also reveals increased motion on the injured side compared with the normal side. The Thompson test involves manual compression at the gastrocsoleus junction, looking for passive ankle plantar flexion. This is also best performed with the patient prone or kneeling. On the injured side, squeezing of the calf will not result in passive ankle plantar flexion. This is an abnormal finding of the Thompson test.

Imaging. A lateral radiograph of the ankle should be obtained to rule out the presence of an avulsion fracture at the insertion of the Achilles tendon on the calcaneus. If the diagnosis of an Achilles rupture is in doubt, then MRI is the test of choice. A sagittal MR image will reveal discontinuity of the normally low-intensity signal of the Achilles tendon. A gap consisting of high-intensity fluid signal is usually visible.

Treatment. Achilles ruptures can be treated both nonsurgically as well as surgically, and each mode of treatment has specific advantages and disadvantages. Nonsurgical treatment avoids all surgical risks but historically has involved longer periods of immobilization and a higher incidence of weakness and rerupture. Newer nonsurgical treatment protocols have shown promising results addressing these shortcomings. It remains an excellent option for the patient with low demands or medical comorbidities that make the risks of surgical treatment prohibitive.

Surgical treatment involves using strong sutures to directly repair the torn ends of the Achilles. This restores the anatomic length and tension of the gastrocsoleus complex, which facilitates return of strength. Surgical treatment also seems to decrease the risk of rerupture. These advantages are counterbalanced against an increased incidence of wound breakdown and infection.

The outcomes after both surgical and nonsurgical treatment are good, but both are dependent on effective and thorough rehabilitation.

Peroneal Tendon Injury

Injury to the peroneal tendons may occur in association with lateral ankle sprains. The same inversion mechanism that results in tearing of the lateral ankle ligaments can produce varying degrees of tears in the peroneal tendons. The peroneus brevis is the most frequently injured, owing to its location directly behind and against the fibular groove. When the foot and ankle are forcefully inverted, the brevis tendon is stretched and compressed against the fibular groove, which may result in a longitudinal tear. These tears may be less than full thickness or extend fully through the width of the tendon and extend for several centimeters.

Acute inversion can also injure the superior peroneal retinaculum, which holds the tendons behind the fibula. If this occurs, the tendons may subluxate or frankly dislocate from behind the fibula.

The peroneus longus is less frequently injured from an acute sprain or inversion. Rather, it is more commonly subject to chronic, repetitive stress. This is particularly true in the patient with a high arch or cavovarus foot. This biomechanical situation produces significant additional strain on the peroneus longus and can produce chronic tearing and tendinopathy.

Physical Examination. Peroneal tendon injuries produce pain and swelling in the retrofibular area. Often the strength of active eversion may be compromised and should be compared with the contralateral side. Evidence of peroneal subluxation can be elicited by having the patient actively evert the foot while the ankle is moved from plantar flexion to dorsiflexion. When injury to the superior peroneal retinaculum has occurred, the tendons can be visualized to come out of the groove, subluxate over the anterolateral aspect of the fibula, and then spontaneously reduce back into the groove.

The integrity of the ankle ligaments should be evaluated because peroneal tendon injuries often accompany ankle sprains and instability.

It is critical to observe the patient stand and ambulate to detect abnormalities of alignment, specifically cavovarus. The patient with cavovarus will demonstrate a high arch and walk on the lateral border of the foot. The heel may appear to be inverted when viewed from behind.

Imaging. Weight-bearing radiographs should be obtained to assess alignment and to look for associated fractures about the distal fibula. In some cases of superior peroneal retinaculum injury, a thin rim of bone may be avulsed off the posterolateral fibula.

MRI is the study of choice to evaluate the peroneal tendons. The axial T1- and T2-weighted views demonstrate the position of the tendons within the groove and will readily demonstrate any subluxation that is present. Injured peroneal tendons will also have increased fluid surrounding them, as demonstrated on the T2-weighted sequences. Longitudinal tears are best visualized on the axial views and appear as if the affected tendon has been divided in two. Chronic tearing or tendinopathy results in heterogeneous signal within a grossly enlarged tendon.

Treatment. Small peroneal tears may respond to activity modification, rest, and rehabilitation, but most require surgical treatment. Small tears are best excised leaving the normal tendon intact. Intrasubstance tearing can be debrided and repaired using a tubularizing stitch. Severe tendinosis may require excision of the affected area and tenodesis to the intact other tendon. If the superior peroneal retinaculum is avulsed, it is repaired back to bone using drill holes or suture anchors. If subluxation is long-standing, the fibular groove may require deepening through a fibular osteotomy. All associated problems such as ankle instability and cavovarus alignment must be corrected at the same time to prevent recurrence.

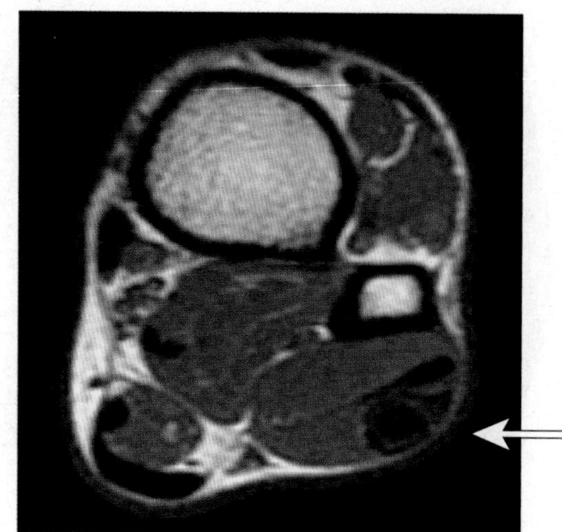

Axial MR image demonstrating chronic tendinopathy of the peroneus longus (*arrow*)

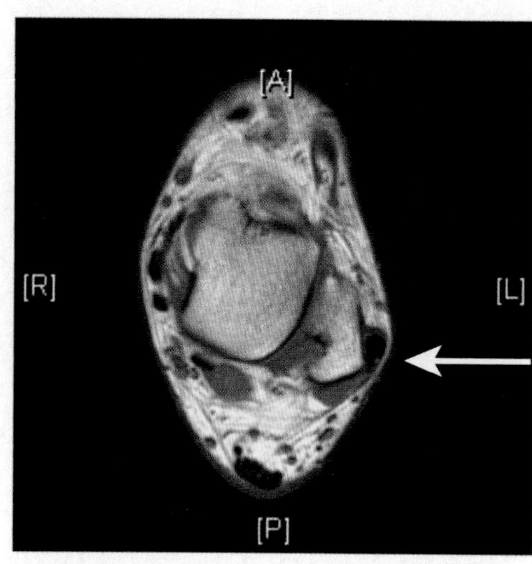

Axial MR image demonstrating dislocation of peroneal tendons from retrofibular groove (*arrow*)

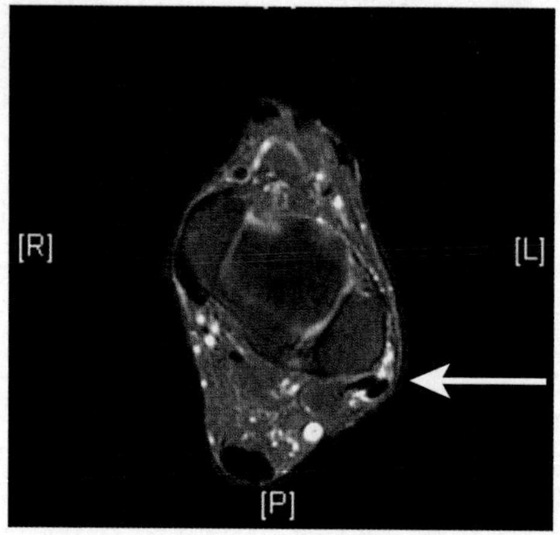

Axial MR image demonstrating injury to superior peroneal retinaculum and subluxation of peroneal tendons (*arrow*)

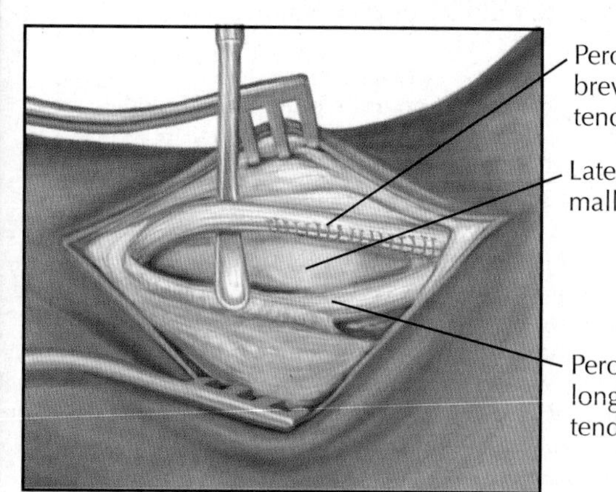

Surgical repair of torn peroneus brevis tendon with tubularizing whip stitch

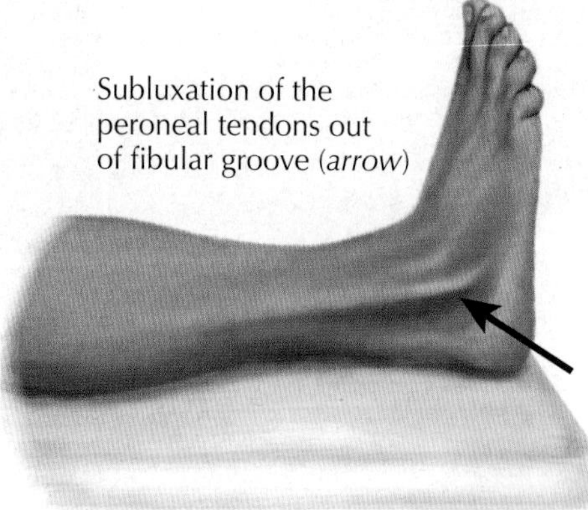

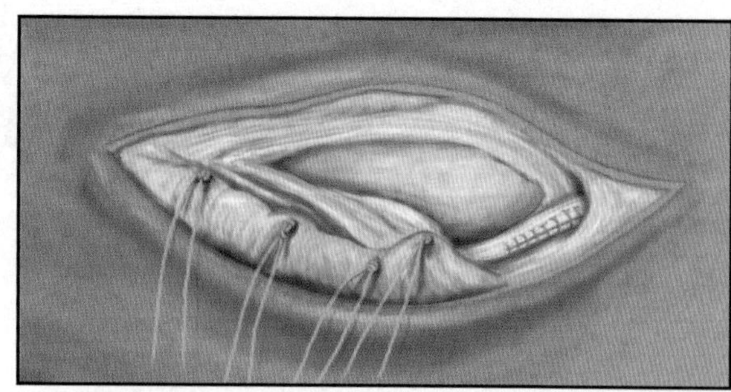

Surgical repair of superior peroneal retinaculum with suture anchors to correct subluxating peroneal tendons

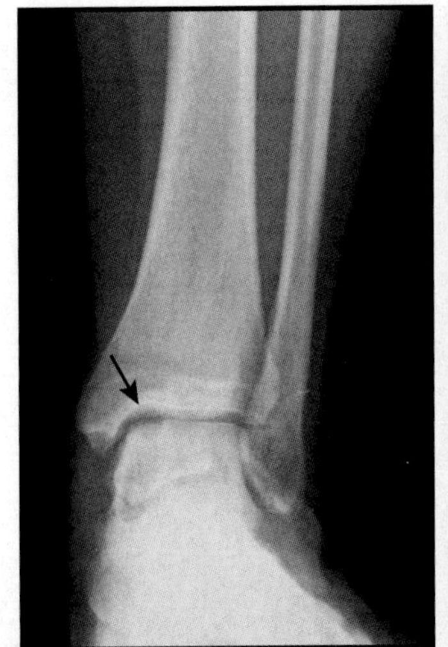

AP radiograph demonstrating lucency of medial talar dome in patient with osteochondral lesion of talus (*arrow*)

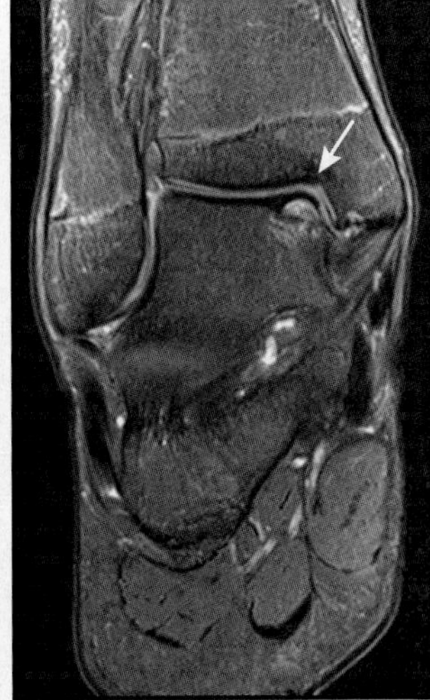

MRI of medial talar osteochondral lesion of talus (*arrow*)

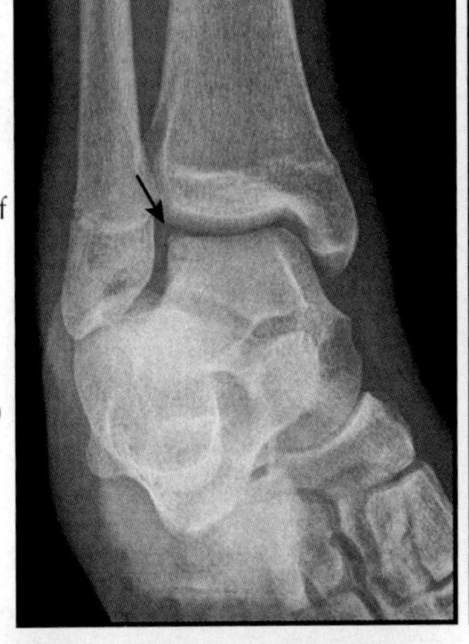

Radiograph of acute displaced lateral talar osteochondral lesion (*arrow*)

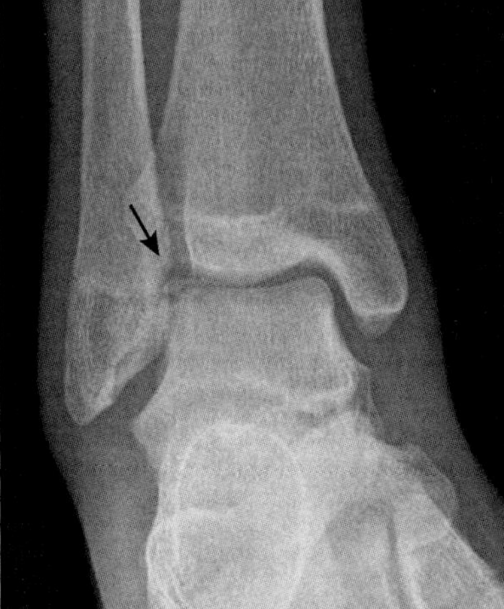

Radiograph of acute displaced lateral talar osteochondral lesion (*arrow*)

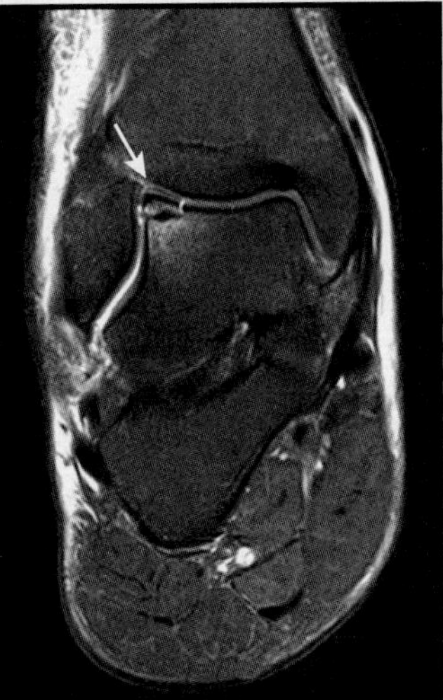

MRI of acute displaced lateral talar osteochondral lesion (*arrow*)

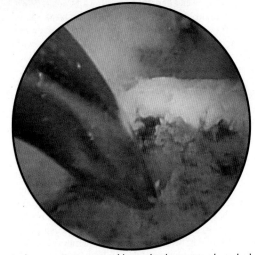

Arthroscopic image of lateral talar osteochondral lesion being treated with microfracture

OSTEOCHONDRAL LESIONS OF THE TALUS

Osteochondral lesions of the talus occur when a focal area of the talar dome is injured. The injured portion of the talus involves the articular cartilage that forms the ankle joint surface, along with a variable amount of underlying subchondral bone. Osteochondral lesions occur over a spectrum of severity from nondisplaced lesions to completely displaced loose bodies. Most lesions occur in either the posteromedial talar dome or the anterolateral talar dome. Historically, most anterolateral lesions were observed to result from a traumatic event such as an ankle sprain. Conversely, posteromedial lesions more frequently occurred without a traumatic event. In adolescents, these posteromedial lesions may occur without any discernible cause, in which case they are referred to as *osteochondritis dissecans* lesions.

Symptoms of an osteochondral lesion of the talus include pain localized to the ankle, swelling, and, occasionally, mechanical symptoms.

Physical Examination. Physical examination may reveal swelling about the ankle or crepitus with range of motion. With anterolateral lesions, the lateral shoulder of the talus may be tender to palpation.

Imaging. Weight-bearing radiographs of the ankle should be obtained. An osteochondral lesion may not be well visualized if the bone portion of the lesion is small. However, if there is significant bone involvement, an area of lucency will be visible at either the medial or lateral shoulder of the talus. An osteochondral lesion of the talus should be further evaluated by CT and/or MRI. These studies provide much greater information regarding the lesion's size, location, and stability.

Treatment. Initial treatment in most cases is nonsurgical, including activity modification, antiinflammatory medication, and sometimes immobilization. If symptoms persist or if the lesion is displaced or unstable, surgical treatment is indicated. Arthroscopy of the ankle remains the most common surgical treatment for osteochondral lesions of the talus. Arthroscopy allows the surgeon to directly inspect the articular cartilage and to remove loose or damaged osteochondral fragments. Most osteochondral lesions of the talus that are not acute will require debridement of all unstable bone and cartilage. It is important once all damaged material has been removed to stimulate bleeding within the underlying bone. This bleeding is achieved using a technique known as "microfracture" and is necessary for the formation of fibrocartilage over the injured area.

Acute osteochondral lesions may be amenable to fixation. This can be attempted arthroscopically but usually requires arthrotomy to anatomically reduce the fragment and stabilize it with pins or screws.

Particularly large osteochondral lesions or lesions that remain symptomatic despite arthroscopic treatment can be treated with osteochondral transplant. This procedure involves removing the damaged portion of the talus and replacing it with a plug of bone and overlying cartilage either from the knee or from a cadaver talus. Osteochondral transplantation is more invasive than arthroscopy and may require osteotomy of the medial or lateral malleolus to achieve the necessary exposure.

TURF TOE

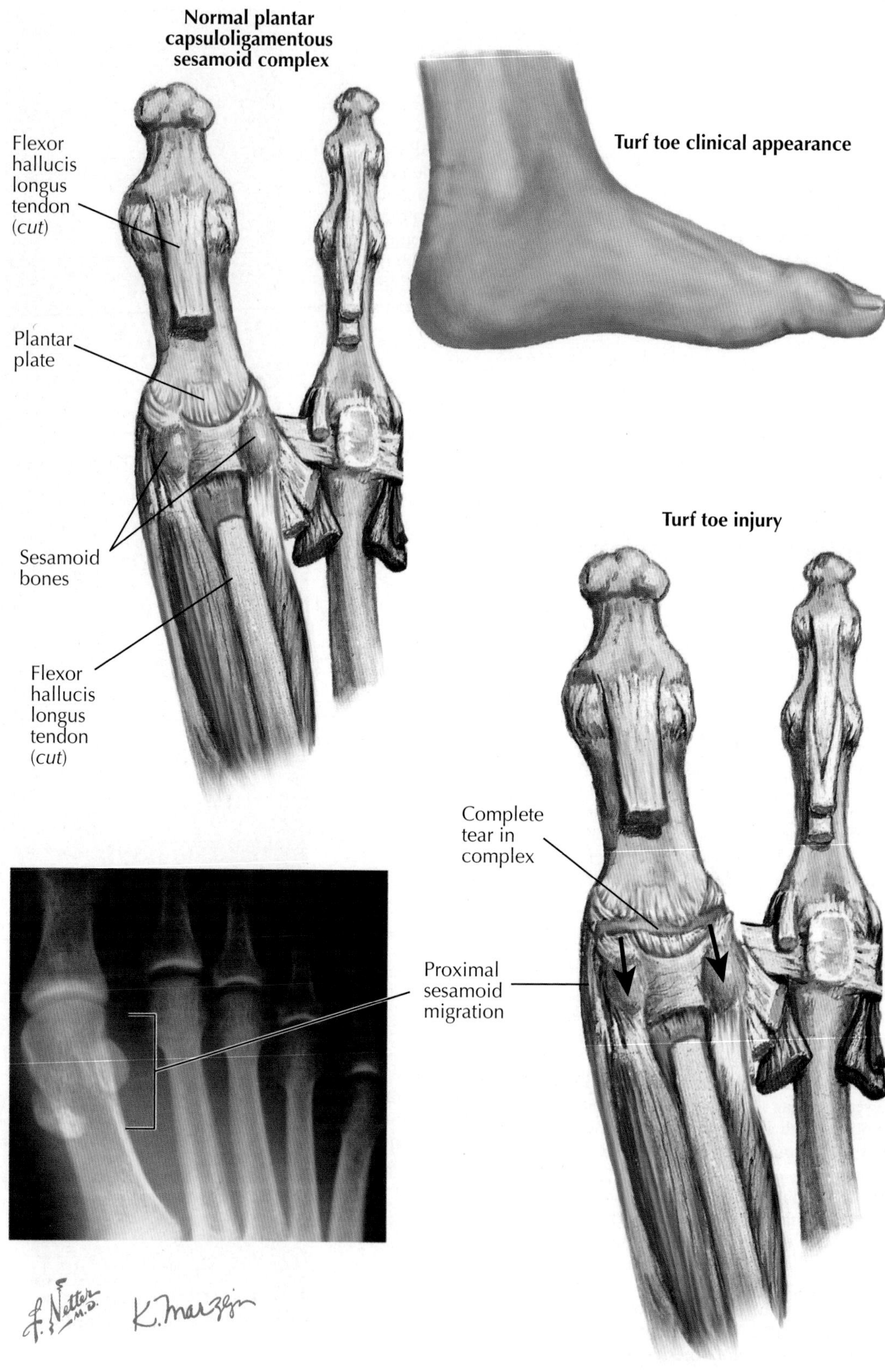

Turf toe is an injury almost exclusively seen in athletes. Although theoretically possible to occur in everyday activity, the typical patient presents after a repetitive or violent hyperdorsiflexion injury to the great toe. The patient reports plantar pain located at the first metatarsophalangeal joint and also pain with ambulation, especially with push-off.

As described, the mechanism of injury involves some variety of dorsiflexion through the first metatarsophalangeal joint. The athlete often presents after a dorsiflexion moment as the patient is pushing off, whereas another athlete steps on the foot or lands on the foot, driving the first metatarsophalangeal joint into sudden hyperdorsiflexion. Patients who present with chronic pain along the plantar aspect of this joint often describe repetitive running and cutting. As the name implies, it was originally thought that the firm nature of the artificial turf accentuated this condition. Studies have failed to demonstrate a higher incidence of injury in athletes playing on artificial turf. It is also possible that the improved construction of the newer artificial surfaces allows for more forgiveness as with real grass surfaces. Whatever the mechanism, the injury involves the plantar sesamoid complex, capsule, and plantar plate.

Physical Examination. Patients with turf toe will have a very specific constellation of findings centered on the plantar first metatarsophalangeal joint. There may be swelling and ecchymosis as with any acute injury. The tenderness may be more medial or lateral if the injury only involves part of the complex. The patient will also complain of pain with range of motion, especially dorsiflexion and hyperdorsiflexion. In the acute setting, there may also be pain with plantar flexion, but that is most likely related to the swelling rather than injury to the dorsal capsule.

Imaging. The history and physical examination are often all that is needed to make the diagnosis. Most injuries will not demonstrate any findings on plain radiographs, especially in the chronic injuries or the minor acute injuries. Those patients who present with significant acute injuries will have findings on plain radiographs. It is important to get comparison films of the contralateral foot to evaluate the sesamoid complex. When evaluating the anteroposterior radiograph of the foot, the sesamoids may be proximally migrated compared with the uninjured side. This is often subtle, but when it is seen it is extremely helpful in confirming the diagnosis. The next step in imaging is to check a stress view image under fluoroscopic imaging to see whether the sesamoids continue to move with normal range of motion of the first metatarsophalangeal joint. When the capsule and plantar plate are disrupted, the sesamoids will not move. If further imaging is necessary to confirm the diagnosis, MRI is the study of choice. There will be edema along the plantar plate and sesamoids. It may be possible to observe a tear in the plantar capsule as well.

Treatment. The majority of patients will be treated nonoperatively. Most injuries involve some degree of stretching or tearing of the plantar complex, and simple immobilization will be sufficient. A select group of patients who have a complete tear and elite athletes will be candidates for surgical repair.

Those patients with minor injuries without radiographic findings may be treated with protected weight-bearing and observation. Those with more severe injuries are treated with cast immobilization of the foot with a good toe box. It may be helpful to add slight plantar flexion to the toe box to allow for better approximation of the capsule to bone. The length of treatment depends on the severity of injury, but 6 weeks may be necessary. After a 3- to 4-week period in a cast, the patient's foot may be placed in a boot. Throughout the immobilization the patient may bear weight in the cast or boot. After the immobilization period, the patient should begin gradual return to play on an individualized basis.

Patients with a severe injury may undergo primary repair of the plantar complex by an open approach. The decision to use a one-incision technique or two-incision technique depends on surgeon preference. In patients with chronic injuries that are unresponsive to nonoperative management and who are undergoing surgical repair, an augmentation of the plantar capsule may be needed.

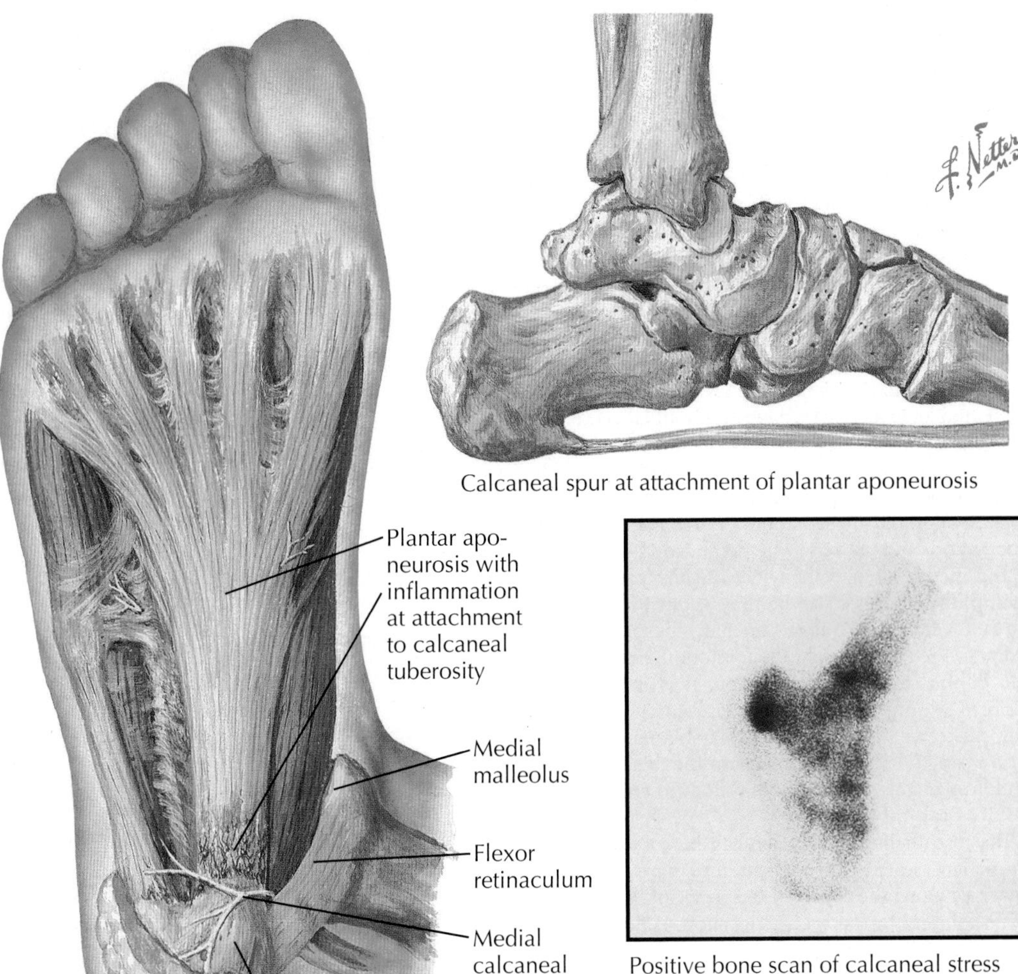

Calcaneal spur at attachment of plantar aponeurosis

Positive bone scan of calcaneal stress fracture

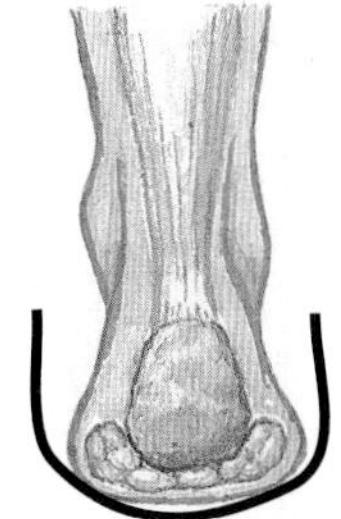

Loose-fitting heel counter in running shoe allows calcaneal fat pad to spread at heel strike, increasing transmission of impact to heel.

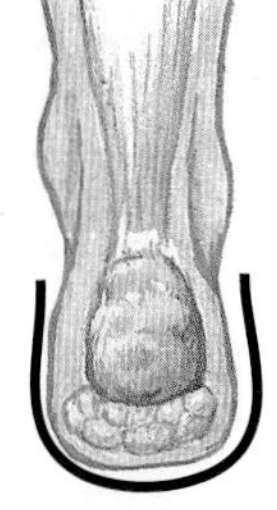

Firm, well-fitting heel counter maintains compactness of fat pad, which buffers force of impact.

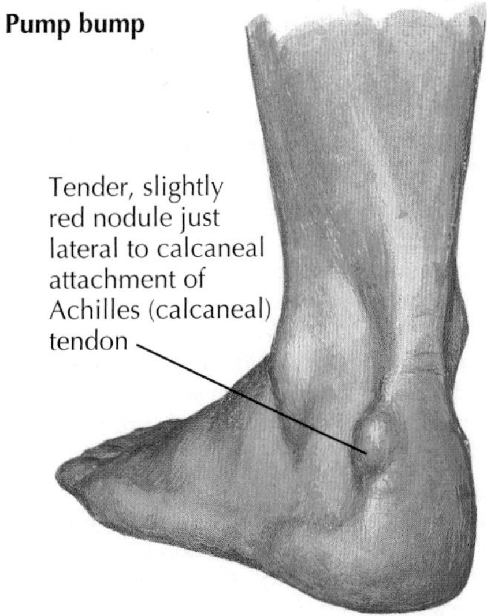

Plantar Fasciitis

Plantar fasciitis is a common condition seen in the office of the orthopedic surgeon as well as by primary care physicians. Most often, patients report intense plantar heel pain, often located along the medial border, although atypical pain can be located anywhere along the plantar fascia. Patients describe pain that is worse in the morning, especially affecting the first steps of the day as they get out of bed. As activity is increased or the foot is stretched, the pain improves. As the condition progresses, patients may experience pain throughout the day. Some patients will report changing activities recently, increasing activity, or participating in a prolonged activity that initiated symptoms.

Physical Examination. Heel pain is a common presenting symptom; therefore it is important to identify the specific location of the heel pain. Patients with plantar fasciitis will most commonly have pain localized to the plantar medial heel, although pain may be present anywhere along the course of the plantar fascia. Also, many patients will often have tightness of the Achilles tendon and pain with dorsiflexion of the toes. The results of the rest of the examination may be normal, including range-of-motion testing throughout the foot and a neurovascular examination. There may be swelling along the plantar heel, but skin changes are not common.

Imaging. Radiographs are often negative. Occasionally, a patient will have a plantar "heel spur." This exostosis is most likely an effect of the inflammation or an incidental finding and not a cause of the pain. If the radiographs are negative, this does not exclude the diagnosis of plantar fasciitis. If pain continues after initial treatment, MRI can be done to look for localized edema along the plantar fascia or edema in the calcaneus. MRI can also be used to exclude calcaneal stress fractures while examining the plantar fascia.

Treatment. Appropriate nonoperative treatment is always the initial course of action. Aggressive stretching centered around the Achilles tendon is the key component to treatment. Stretching of the plantar fascia is also included. Often, gel heel cups can be prescribed to soften the impact along the plantar heel, but adequate stretching is paramount. If it is suspected that the patient will not be able to perform the home therapy, organized physical therapy can be given.

If an exhaustive nonoperative program has been followed without relief, a few other options exist. Some physicians offer corticosteroid injections in the plantar heel, but a large number of physicians believe that this injection may weaken the plantar fascia and lead to rupture. The last course of action if nonoperative management fails is surgical intervention. Plantar fascia release has been described in both open and endoscopic techniques. Current research suggests that surgical lengthening of the gastrocnemius-soleus complex can relieve symptoms, but long-term studies have yet to be published.

Posterior Tibial Tendonitis/ Flatfoot

Patients who present with the early symptoms of posterior tibial tendonitis report pain along the posterior tibial tendon, or medial arch pain. As the condition progresses, failure of the posterior tibial tendon leads to collapse of the medial arch. At this point, the patient may also begin to report lateral foot pain as the lateral structures begin to impinge under the distal fibula. Many patients may have asymptomatic flatfoot that may not necessitate treatment.

Physical Examination. Findings of the physical examination of patients with posterior tibial tendonitis vary based on the severity of deformity. A standing examination and analysis of gait are paramount in the examination of the patient with suspected posterior tibial tendonitis. Observation of the patient during ambulation and at rest will demonstrate a collapse of the medial arch. When viewing the patient from behind, the hindfoot will be in a valgus position, and the foot will demonstrate a "too many toes" sign, which is due to the abduction of the forefoot. Before completion of the standing examination, it is important to perform a single-leg heel-rise examination. Patients with posterior tibial tendonitis may be unable to perform a single-leg heel rise because the posterior tibial tendon is unable to lock the hindfoot to create a rigid foot for push-off.

The rest of the examination can be concluded with the patient seated. The patient may have tenderness anywhere along the course of the posterior tibial tendon corresponding to the specific location of degeneration or inflammation. The flexibility of the flatfoot deformity is examined by looking for re-creation of the medial arch when non–weight-bearing. Strength testing reveals weakness with inversion and plantar flexion. Finally it is important to examine the tightness of the Achilles tendon because it may contribute to the flatfoot deformity.

Imaging. The diagnosis of posterior tibial tendonitis and adult acquired flatfoot is based largely on physical examination and plain radiographs. Advanced imaging is rarely needed for diagnosis, but CT and MRI can be used for surgical planning. Weight-bearing radiographs are essential for proper evaluation because the deformity may be flexible and only re-created with weight-bearing. Anteroposterior images of the foot will demonstrate talar head uncovering as the navicular shifts laterally relative to the talus. Additionally on these views, deformity through the midfoot and forefoot with abduction may be seen. Lateral radiographs will show a loss of the normal alignment of the foot with plantar flexion of the talar head, sag of the midfoot, and possible gapping of the joints on the plantar side. It is also important to obtain a radiograph of the ankle because presence of tibiotalar tilt may change surgical management.

Treatment. Treatment of posterior tibial tendonitis depends mostly on the stage of the disease. In the early stages when pain and weakness are the main symptoms, the treatment of choice is nonoperative. Management is aimed at protecting the posterior tibial tendon. Bracing and orthotics are the first-line treatment. In addition to these assistive devices, stretching of the Achilles tendon and the gastrocsoleus complex may be helpful. Nonoperative management is also appropriate for patients in advanced-stage disease in the early presentation.

If nonoperative treatment fails to provide relief, surgical management is appropriate. In the early stages of the condition, simple debridement of the inflamed posterior tibial tendon and repair or reconstruction is an option.

Posterior Tibial Tendon Dysfunction

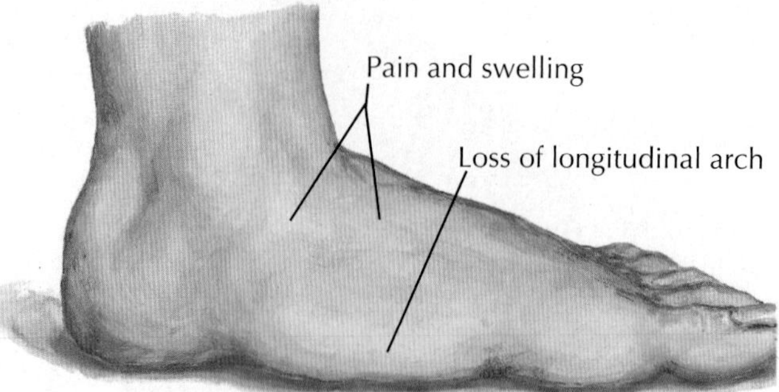

Medial view of pronated foot reveals flattened longitudinal arch.

Dysfunction of posterior tibial tendon (PTT) may result from tenosynovitis or tendinosis. Symptoms include pain and swelling over course of tendon, and loss of tendon function results in loss of longitudinal arch.

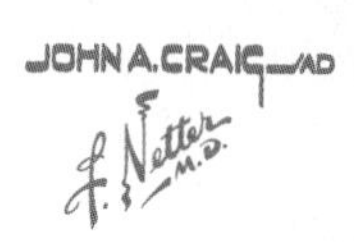

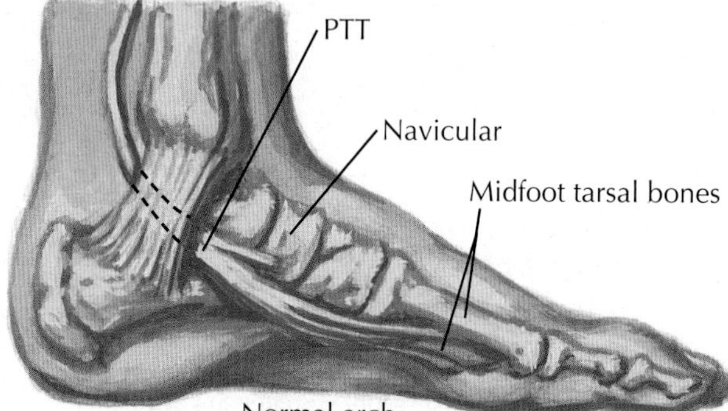

Insertion of PTT extends beyond navicular to all midtarsal bones of foot and is the major supporting structure of midfoot.

Posterior view reveals hyperpronation in left foot. In normal foot, midlines of calcaneus and leg are aligned or deviate less than 2 degrees.

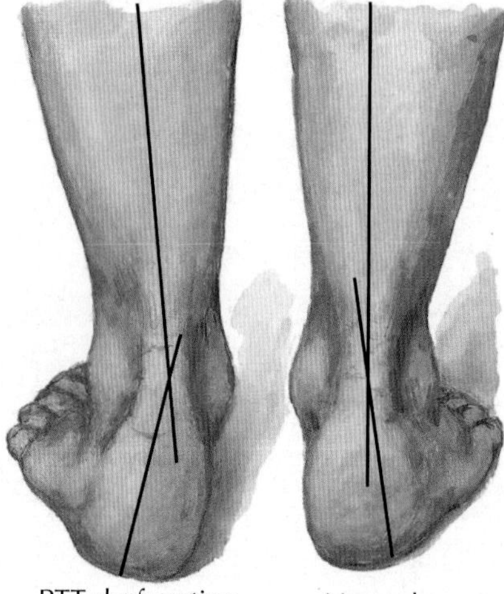

Standing. In the standing position, increased heel valgus and "too many lateral toes" may be observed on posterior view.

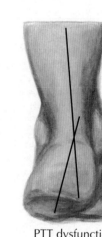

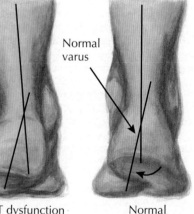

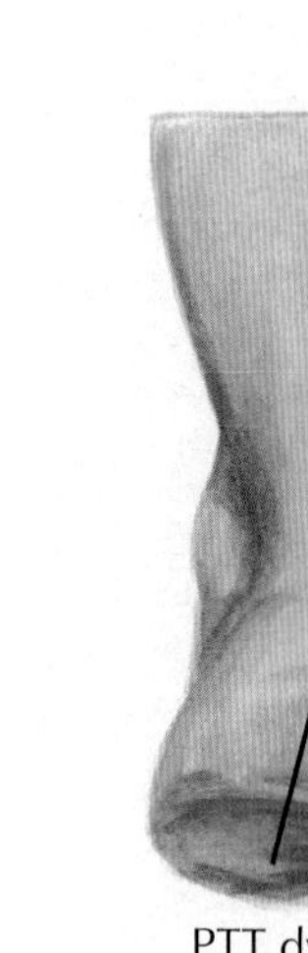

Heel rise. On toe standing, normal PTT function pulls heel into varus. PTT dysfunction allows heel to remain in valgus position.

In more advanced stages, this simple procedure fails to address the underlying deformity. If the flatfoot deformity is flexible, then a reconstructive option is the treatment of choice. The surgeon has multiple procedures available for correction of a flexible deformity, including medial displacement calcaneal osteotomy, posterior tibial tendon reconstruction, flexor digitorum longus transfer, small joint fusions or osteotomies, lateral column lengthening, and Achilles tendon lengthening. The choice of which combination of procedures to use is based on the location and degree of deformity as well as surgeon preference.

Patients with rigid flatfoot deformities are typically treated with fusions of the hindfoot, namely, fusions of the subtalar joint, talonavicular joint, and possibly the calcaneocuboid joint. Adult acquired flatfoot deformity can also involve changes to the tibiotalar joint, in the form of tibiotalar tilt, and this must be addressed during surgical treatment of the flatfoot.

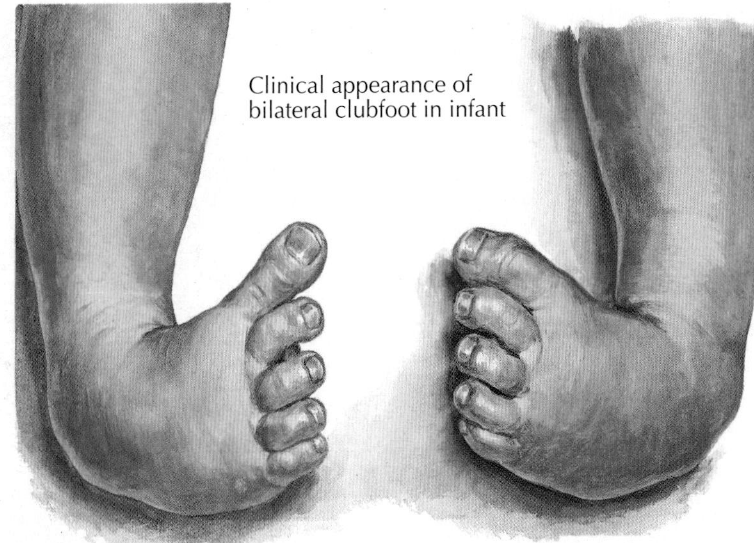

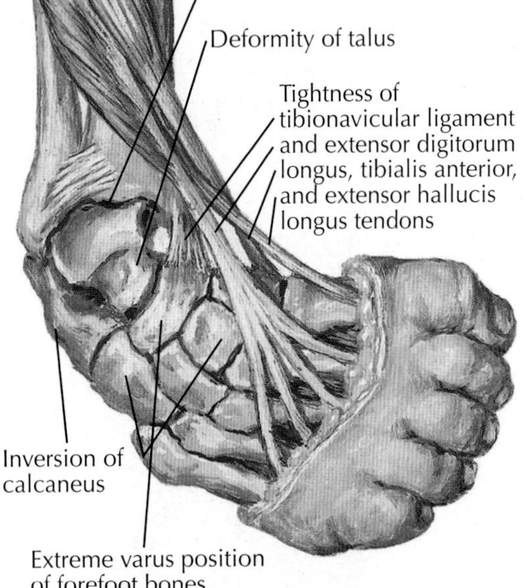

CONGENITAL CLUBFOOT

Congenital clubfoot (congenital equinovarus) is a structural foot deformity that is present at birth. The entire foot is plantar flexed (equinus), and both forefoot and hindfoot are inverted (varus). The deformity, which may be unilateral or bilateral, occurs in about 1 in 800 births and is more common in male than in female infants. There is a strong genetic tendency, as seen in the increased incidence in the children and grandchildren of affected persons.

Three categories of congenital clubfoot have been described. *Postural clubfoot* is not a true structural abnormality and usually responds rapidly to conservative management. In the so-called *true clubfoot,* the degree of severity varies widely. *Arthrogrypotic* or *teratologic clubfoot* is a severe deformity that often requires early, radical surgery to achieve correction.

Etiology and Pathology. The etiology of congenital clubfoot is not known, but a genetic mode of inheritance is well established. Although females are less often affected than males, their deformity is often more severe and more difficult to treat, especially if bilateral.

Congenital clubfoot is characterized by bones that are abnormal not only in their relationship to each other but also in shape and size. Thus even after correction, the true clubfoot is smaller than normal and some signs of the deformity persist. In addition, the ligaments connecting the bones and the musculotendinous structures acting on the bones and joints are contracted and foreshortened.

One of the most consistent and important pathologic manifestations is a pronounced medial angulation of the head and neck of the talus, a deformity that persists to some degree even after acceptable correction has been achieved. The ossification centers of the tarsal bones demonstrate varying degrees of abnormal endochondral growth and development.

Treatment. Because the pathologic features of congenital clubfoot vary in severity, the types and results of treatment also vary substantially. In some patients, correction can be achieved and maintained with simple surgical methods, whereas in other patients, complex and sophisticated surgery is required, followed by postoperative bracing.

Lateral radiograph demonstrates severe clubfoot complicated by extreme plantar flexion of forefoot in newborn.

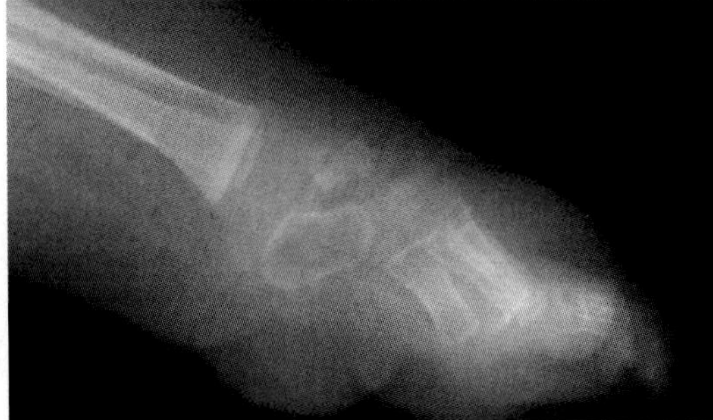

Anteroposterior (*above*) and lateral (*below*) radiographs show congenital clubfoot in newborn.

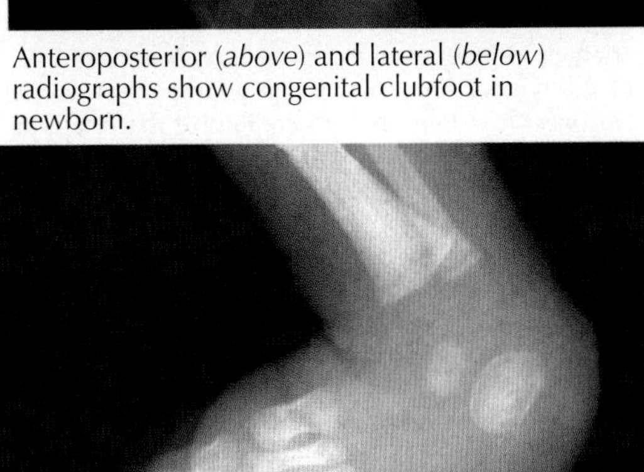

Corrective Manipulation. Treatment of congenital clubfoot should be started as soon as possible after birth. In recent years, the Ponseti method of manipulation and casting of clubfeet has revolutionized the treatment of this disorder, with a 95% success rate in avoiding major corrective surgery. The manipulation technique and the care with which casts are applied are extremely important. Ponseti described a four-step sequence consisting of (1) correction of the cavus deformity by dorsiflexing the first ray; (2) correction of the adductus deformity by abducting the forefoot; (3) correction of the varus deformity by continued supination of the midfoot and overcorrection of the forefoot into an abducted position, thus allowing the hindfoot to evert through the subtalar joint; and (4) correction of the equinus deformity through dorsiflexion of the foot or percutaneous Achilles tenotomy. When abducting the forefoot, it is critical to use the lateral aspect of the talar head and not the

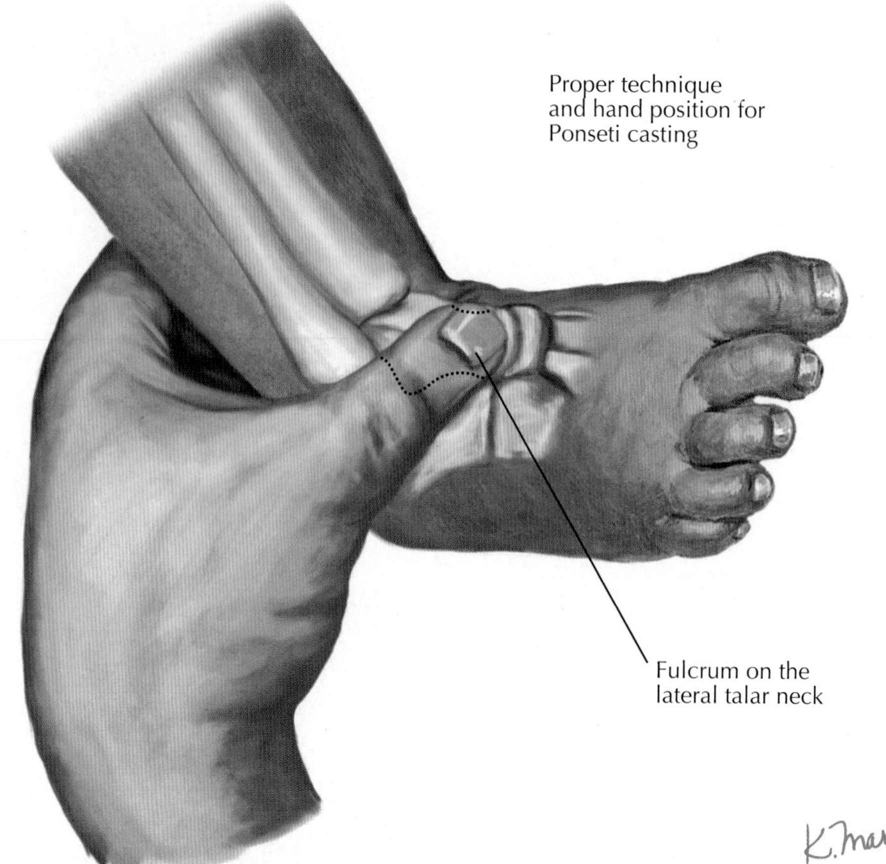

Abduction of the forefoot (**A**) creates valgus of the hindfoot by eversion of the calcaneus through motion of the subtalar joint (**B**).

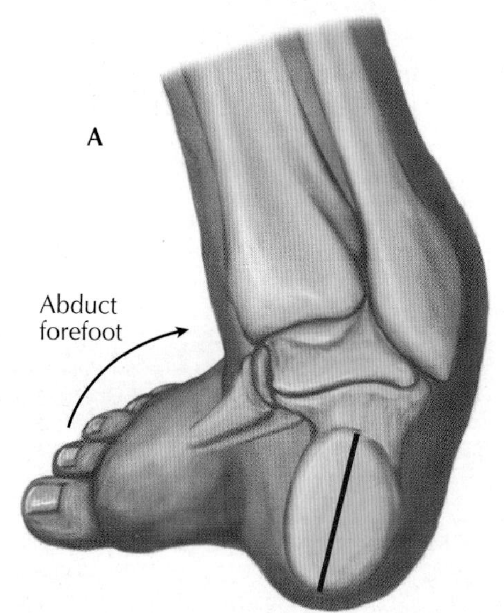

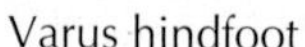

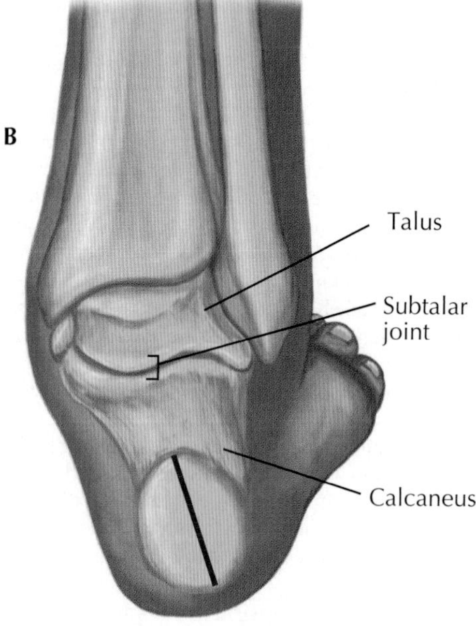

Congenital Clubfoot (Continued)

calcaneocuboid joint as the fulcrum, because the latter will block the eversion of the calcaneus required to achieve valgus alignment of the hindfoot. Casts are applied weekly for 3 to 8 weeks until full correction is achieved. An abduction brace consisting of straight-last shoes externally rotated 60 degrees on a Denis-Browne bar is then worn full time for 3 months and then at night only until age 4 years.

Surgical Procedures. If the feet fail to correct after 8 weeks of casting, surgical correction is required. The age at which surgery should be performed is controversial. The minimum age is 3 or 4 months, but some surgeons prefer to wait until the patient is at least 1 year old. Surgery revises the bone and joint relationships by elongating the contracted ligaments and tendons. A variety of techniques and surgical approaches are used, but the type of procedure is not as important as the principles. It is important to emphasize that the type and amount of surgical correction required vary with the degree of resistance to manipulation and the severity of the deformity.

In the foot, the structures that most commonly require elongation are the tibionavicular portion of the deltoid ligament, the tibialis posterior tendon, the talonavicular joint capsule, and the talocalcaneal joint capsule and interosseous ligament. The long toe flexors may also require elongation. The procedure to lengthen these structures is called a medial release. If the foot has a significant cavus deformity as well, the contracted plantar muscles may also require release; this combined operation is called a plantar medial release.

A posterior release is performed to correct the equinus deformity at the ankle: the calcaneal (Achilles) tendon is lengthened; the ankle joint capsule and all posterior tibiotalar, talofibular, and calcaneofibular ligaments are severed; and the tibiofibular syndesmosis is released posteriorly. It is often necessary to combine posterior and medial release procedures in what is called a posteromedial release.

After surgical correction, the foot and ankle are immobilized in a well-padded above-knee cast. The cast is changed 1 week and 2 weeks after surgery to allow inspection of the wound and verification of the correction. Then, a more snug, well-molded cast with very little padding is applied. After 6 to 12 weeks, casts are replaced with retentive splints and braces, which are required for several months (years for resistant cases, especially the arthrogrypotic clubfoot). All patients must be observed throughout their growth period to assess and ensure that the correction is maintained.

In some patients, the deformity tends to relapse or recur. Recurrent clubfoot must be corrected with whatever means are appropriate. After correction is achieved, a number of patients require transfer of the tibialis anterior tendon to the dorsum of the foot to correct persistent muscle imbalance, which manifests as dynamic swing-phase varus causing a lateral foot strike.

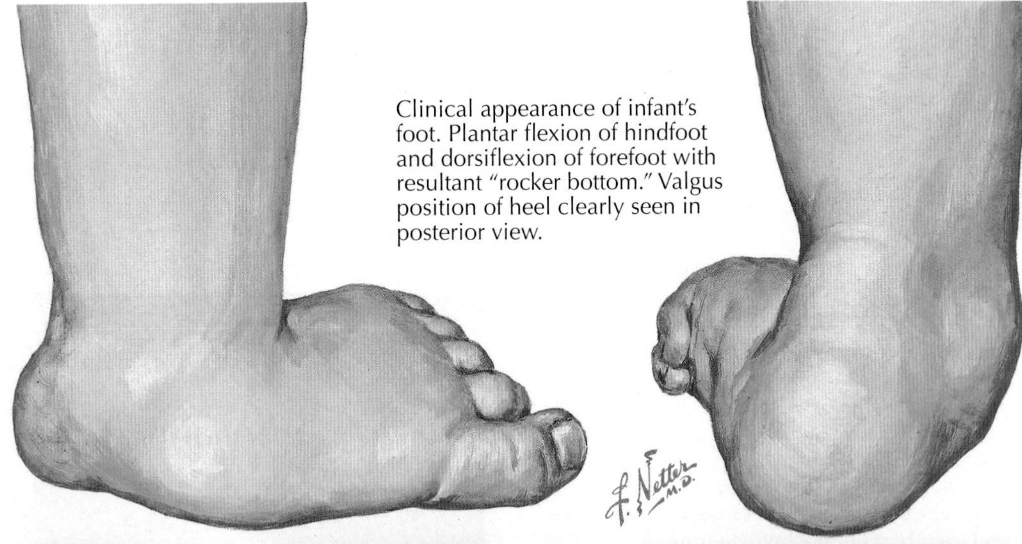

Clinical appearance of infant's foot. Plantar flexion of hindfoot and dorsiflexion of forefoot with resultant "rocker bottom." Valgus position of heel clearly seen in posterior view.

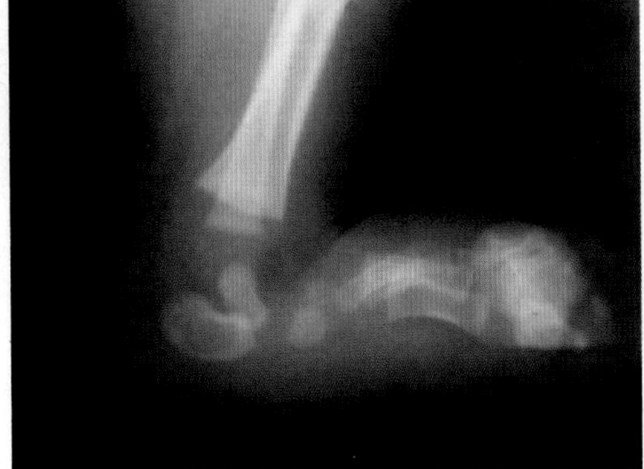
Lateral radiograph shows vertical position of talus, plantar flexion of hindfoot, and dorsiflexion of forefoot.

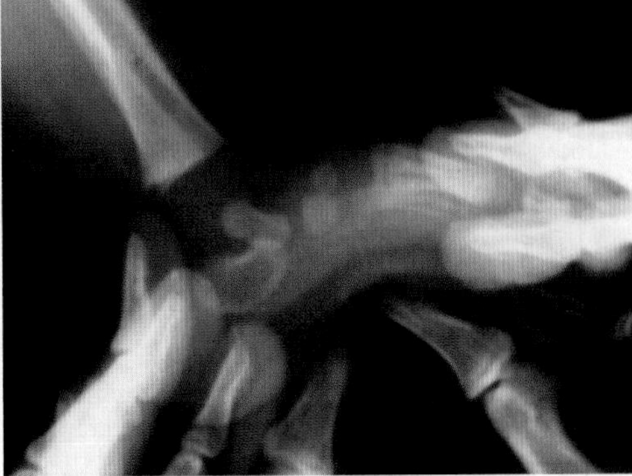
Radiograph demonstrates that forced plantar flexion of forefoot fails to correct abnormal position of hindfoot.

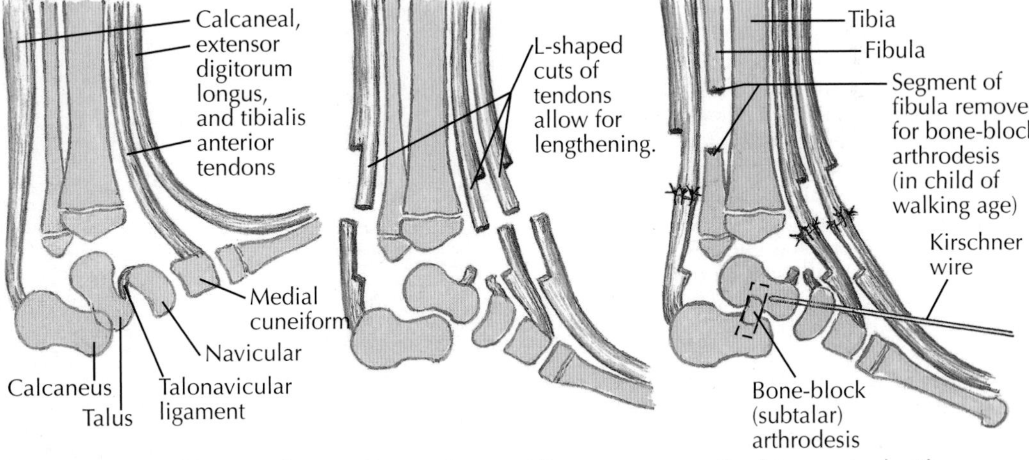

Typical abnormal bone and joint relationships. Vertical talus, hindfoot equinus, dorsiflexion of forefoot.

Taut tendons and ligaments sectioned to permit bones to assume proper relationships.

Tendons repaired with lengthening procedure. Talonavicular joint stabilized with Kirschner wire.

Congenital Vertical Talus

Although congenital vertical talus is a deformity present at birth, often the diagnosis is not made because of its superficial resemblance to infantile calcaneovalgus. The heel is in valgus position and the sole of the foot is convex, a clinical appearance that led to the synonyms "congenital convex pes valgus" and "rocker-bottom" foot. True congenital vertical talus is much less common than clubfoot, and there is almost always a coexisting congenital abnormality such as clubfoot, syndactyly, neuromuscular syndrome, or lumbosacral agenesis.

The etiology of the deformity is not yet understood, but because it is a structural congenital deformity, some genetic abnormality must exist.

Clinical Manifestations. As in congenital clubfoot, the bones not only have an abnormal relationship with one another but also are abnormal in size and configuration, with abnormal articulating surfaces. The ligamentous and musculotendinous structures about the foot and ankle are contracted and rigidly hold the bones in position.

This paradoxical deformity consists of plantar flexion (equinus) of the hindfoot and ankle and dorsiflexion of the midfoot and forefoot. The navicular is held in fixed dorsal subluxation or dislocation on the top of the head and neck of the talus. This abnormal position of the navicular can be identified readily in a lateral radiograph of the foot because there is an area of increased density in the superior aspect of the talar neck that corresponds to the location of the talonavicular articulation.

Treatment. The unique combination of forefoot dorsiflexion and hindfoot plantar flexion in congenital vertical talus almost always requires correction. Corrective measures should be started as soon as the diagnosis is made. Dobbs described a minimally invasive approach to the correction of vertical talus that consists of serial casting followed by percutaneous pinning of the talonavicular joint. Every week, the foot is manipulated gently into plantar flexion and inversion, using the medial talar head as the fulcrum, and a cast is applied until maximum plantar flexion and inversion has been achieved. The talonavicular joint is then pinned percutaneously in a retrograde fashion from the navicular into the talus. A percutaneous tenotomy of the Achilles tendon is performed to correct the hindfoot equinus. Surgery should be planned as soon as the manipulation program has been completed and the child is at least 3 months of age.

Traditional surgery to correct congenital vertical talus may be done in one or two stages. The sequence of procedures is less important than the concepts of correction. The forefoot must be aligned with the hindfoot, which means that the talonavicular and subtalar (talocalcaneal) joints must be reduced and stabilized. The posterior structures of the ankle are released to bring the entire foot out of the equinus position.

In children of walking age, it is often necessary to perform a subtalar extraarticular (bone block) arthrodesis to achieve and maintain stability of the talocalcaneal joint. Bone block arthrodesis is rarely needed in patients too young to walk.

After surgery, the foot is immobilized in a cast for 3 months, after which it is protectively splinted in a well-molded ankle-foot orthosis for several months.

CAVOVARUS FOOT

The cavovarus foot deformity is unique, largely because it has a variety of causes. Although it is not rare, the incidence is not well established. Seldom present at birth, the deformity gradually becomes apparent as the child's foot grows and matures.

Etiology and Pathology. Three distinct etiologic categories have been identified: (1) paralytic muscle imbalance, (2) residuals of congenital clubfoot, and (3) unknown, or idiopathic. Whenever possible, it is important to identify the exact cause so that proper treatment can be administered. In this regard, the diagnosis of cavovarus foot, especially in a previously normal foot, necessitates a thorough search for an underlying neurologic cause, particularly if it is unilateral. If a neurologic problem is suspected, radiographs of the lumbosacral spine are indicated, and MRI of the lumbosacral spine and electromyography may also be necessary.

Clinical Manifestations. The term *cavovarus* refers to the two distinguishing clinical features: a varus hindfoot and a heightened longitudinal arch (cavus). The forefoot—particularly the first metatarsal—is excessively plantar flexed. In fact, in children and young adolescents, the plantar flexed first metatarsal is the most significant feature, not only because it is responsible for the cavus appearance of the foot but also because on weight-bearing it forces the heel into varus position, and weight is thus transferred primarily onto the lateral border of the foot. Claw toe deformity is another characteristic feature.

Radiographic Findings. The weight-bearing radiograph reflects some of the same clinical manifestations seen on physical examination. The metatarsals are excessively plantar flexed, the midfoot is elevated, and the hindfoot is in varus position (seen in the reduced plantar flexion of the talus). Dorsiflexion of the metatarsophalangeal joints is also apparent.

Treatment. If the deformity results from an underlying neurologic problem that is amenable to surgery, this should be treated before the foot deformity is corrected. Cavovarus foot always requires surgery. Casts and orthoses are not effective for correcting or preventing the progression of the deformity.

Before surgical correction, the flexibility of the forefoot and hindfoot must be assessed, which can be done in several ways. The Coleman block test provides the best documentation of foot flexibility and involves having the patient stand on a block of wood 1 to 1.5 inches high. The heel and fifth metatarsal are placed on the block, and the first metatarsal is allowed to "fall" to the floor. This eliminates the effect of fixed forefoot pronation on the hindfoot (tripod effect). If the heel goes into valgus position, the hindfoot is supple; if the heel remains in varus, the hindfoot is considered rigid. In most children and young adolescents, the hindfoot is flexible, and thus forefoot pronation is the principal problem.

In younger children with the earliest stage of the disease, treatment of cavovarus deformity may require only a radical plantar release. Deformity due to residual clubfoot is treated with a plantar medial release. These procedures are followed by sequential manipulations and cast applications.

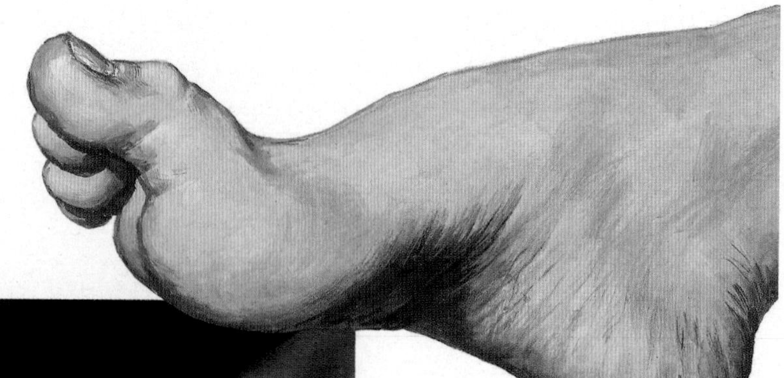

Cavovarus foot with characteristic high arch extending upward from ball of foot and cock-up deformity of toes

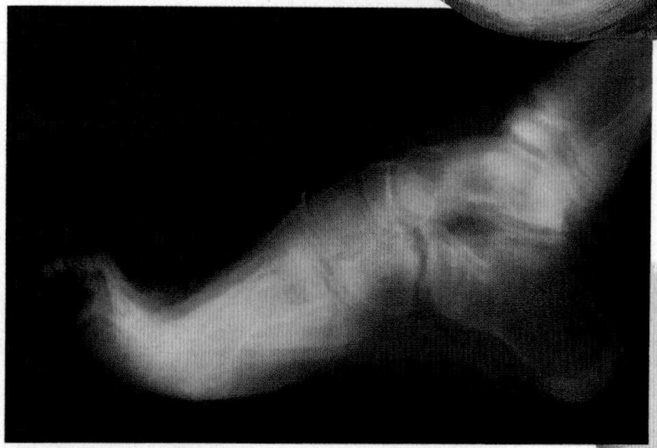

Radiograph of foot shown above reveals fixed bony configuration, dorsiflexion of hindfoot, and sharp plantar flexion of forefoot.

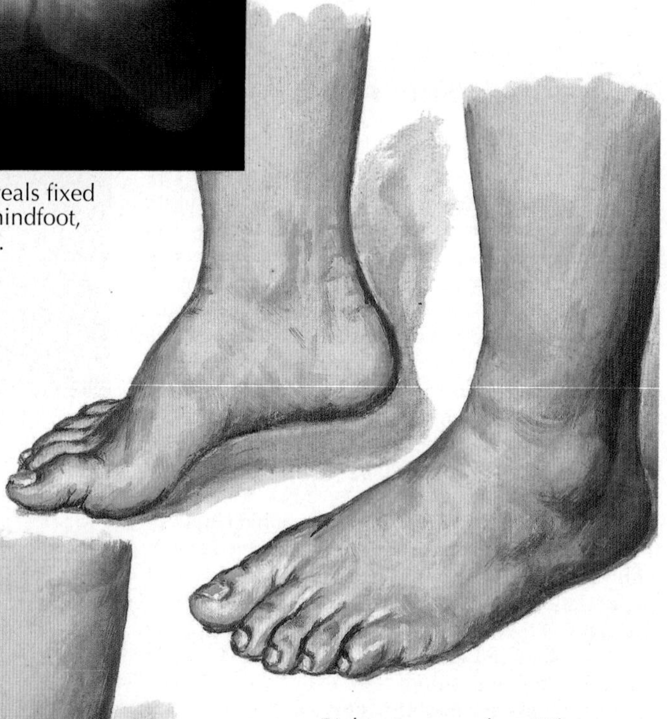

Right cavovarus foot. When patient stands, weight is on ball of foot and heel is elevated.

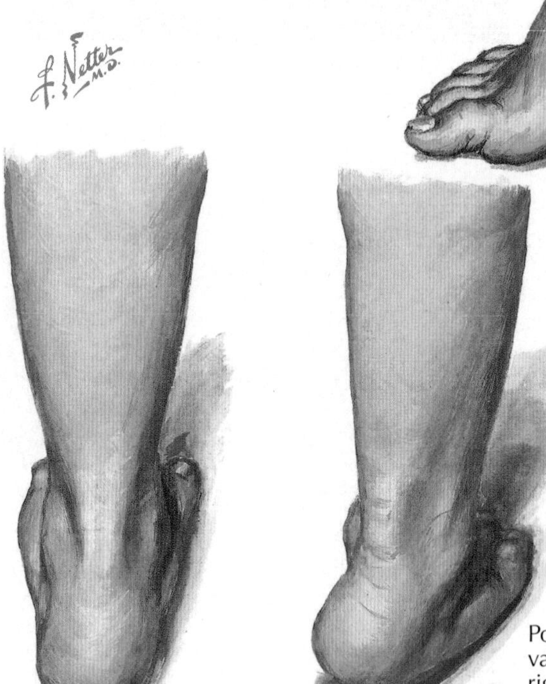

Posterior view clearly shows varus deformity of affected right foot.

Tendon transfers are indicated for deformity due to an identified neurologic disorder with demonstrable muscle imbalance. In many cases, the best balancing procedure includes transfer of the posterior tibial tendon to the dorsolateral aspect of the foot as well as transfer of the peroneus longus to the peroneus brevis. To correct associated claw toe deformities, the long toe extensors are moved to the metatarsals (Jones technique) or to the tarsals (Hibbs technique).

In older children and adolescents, simple soft tissue releases are usually inadequate because adaptive bony changes have occurred. In the child with a flexible hindfoot, soft tissue release must be accompanied by dorsiflexion osteotomy of either the first metatarsal or the medial cuneiform. In addition, older adolescents with a rigid hindfoot require a sliding osteotomy of the calcaneus to restore the valgus alignment of the heel and decrease its inclination.

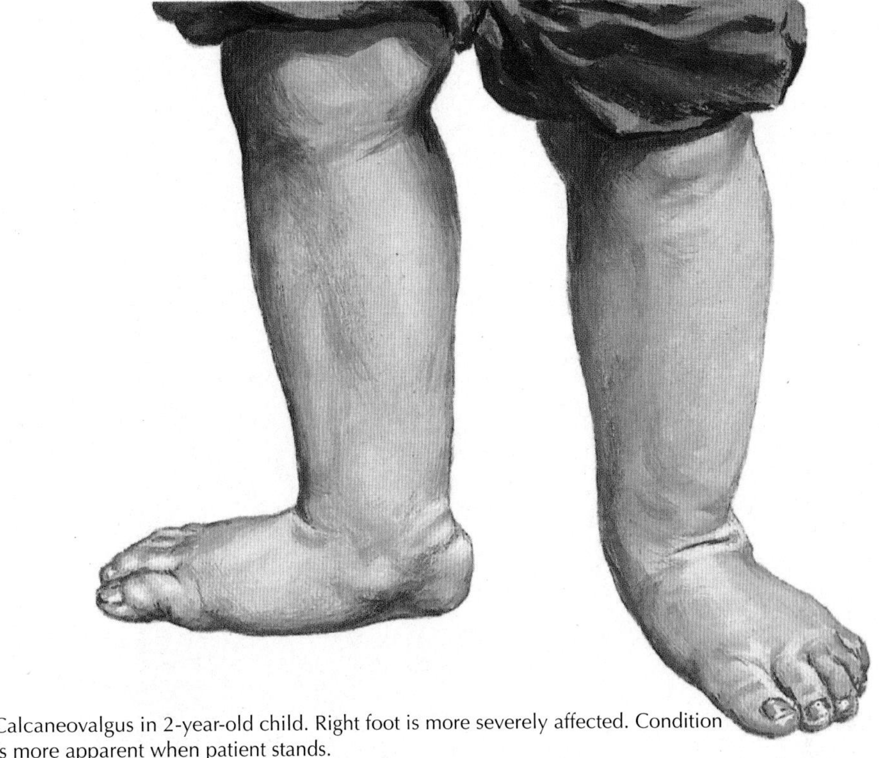

Calcaneovalgus in 2-year-old child. Right foot is more severely affected. Condition is more apparent when patient stands.

CALCANEOVALGUS AND PLANOVALGUS

The major distinguishing feature of these two foot deformities is the age at onset. Calcaneovalgus (congenital calcaneovalgus) refers to a flexible flatfoot in infants and young children, whereas planovalgus is a similar deformity that occurs in older children and adolescents. Both are nonstructural, flexible, and postural abnormalities of unknown etiology and prevalence. Although by definition the abnormality consists of flatfoot, the clinical criteria used in diagnosis are highly subjective.

Clinical Manifestations. The physical findings are distinctive in very young infants and children. When the foot and ankle are dorsiflexed, the dorsal aspect of the foot can be apposed to the anterior aspect of the tibia. The plantar surface of the foot is flat, the hindfoot is in valgus position, and the forefoot is abducted. Superficially, this deformity strongly resembles congenital vertical talus. The flexibility of the calcaneovalgus foot is one of several features that allow differentiation of the two disorders. However, some cases require radiographic evaluation for definitive diagnosis.

During weight-bearing, the planovalgus foot is characterized by a flattened longitudinal arch, valgus hindfoot, and plantar flexion and medial rotation of the talus on the calcaneus. The midfoot and forefoot are abducted and, in some patients, the calcaneal (Achilles) tendon is contracted. However, in a non–weight-bearing position, the foot assumes a normal configuration. Also, when the patient walks on the toes or on the ball of the foot, the longitudinal arch appears normal.

Radiographic Findings. In both calcaneovalgus and planovalgus deformities, the ossification centers of the foot bones are normal. The only radiographic abnormalities are in the relationships of the bones, which can be easily reduced by positioning or non–weight-bearing. Lateral radiographs reveal a substantial divergence in the long axes of the talus and calcaneus; a similar decrease in these axes is seen in anteroposterior radiographs of the weight-bearing foot.

Treatment. In most patients, flexible flatfeet are asymptomatic, and it is impossible to predict which calcaneovalgus or planovalgus feet will become painful in adulthood. A small number of truly flexible flatfeet become substantially rigid if the feet do not correct with growth, and permanent adaptive changes occur.

Treatment of calcaneovalgus and planovalgus is controversial for the following reasons: (1) it is impossible to *quantitate* what constitutes a flexible flatfoot; (2) no device has been developed that predictably alters the growth, development, or final adult configuration of a flexible flatfoot; (3) it is difficult to determine how much pain or excessive shoe wear should be tolerated; (4) the results of surgery in the treatment of flexible flatfoot are extremely difficult to assess; and (5) it has not been proven that the mere presence of a flexible flatfoot requires any form of treatment.

In a few patients, excessive shoe wear, symptoms, or severe deformity justifies the use of a supportive device. The best is a soft longitudinal arch cushion that can be used with any shoe. If this is unsuccessful in relieving symptoms, a durable plastic foot orthosis may be considered.

Surgery is never justified for asymptomatic, *flexible* calcaneovalgus or planovalgus deformity in a young child. In adolescents with persistent, symptomatic flatfeet who have a substantial problem with wearing shoes, a calcaneal lengthening osteotomy combined with a plantar-based closing wedge osteotomy of the medial cuneiform may be considered.

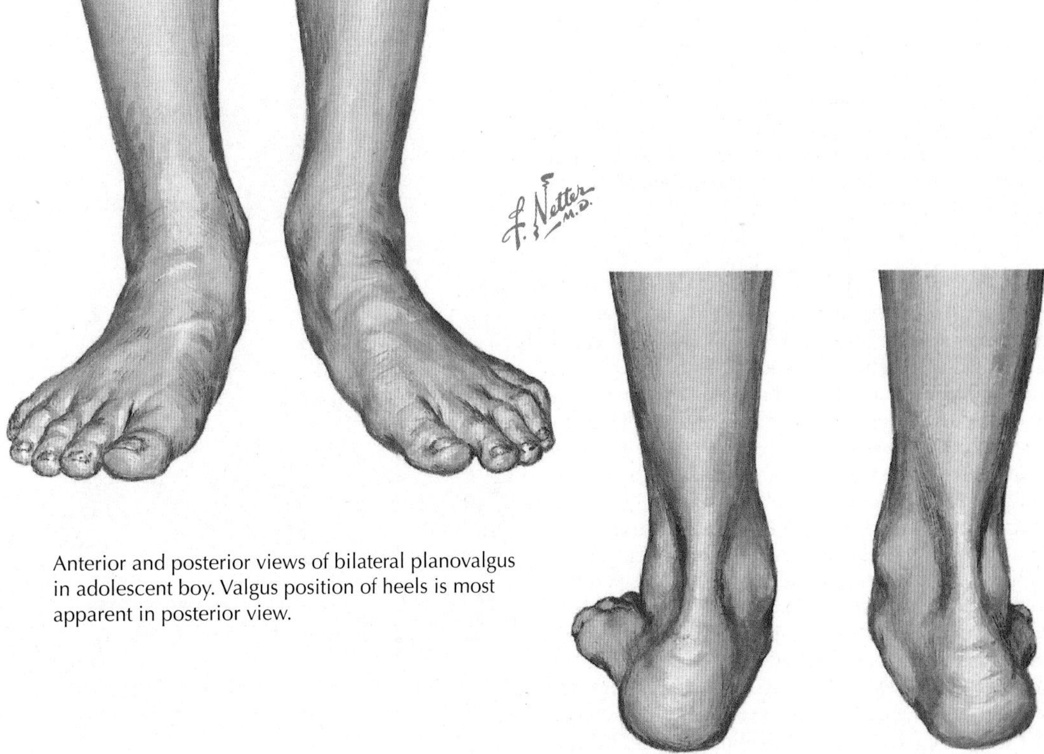

Anterior and posterior views of bilateral planovalgus in adolescent boy. Valgus position of heels is most apparent in posterior view.

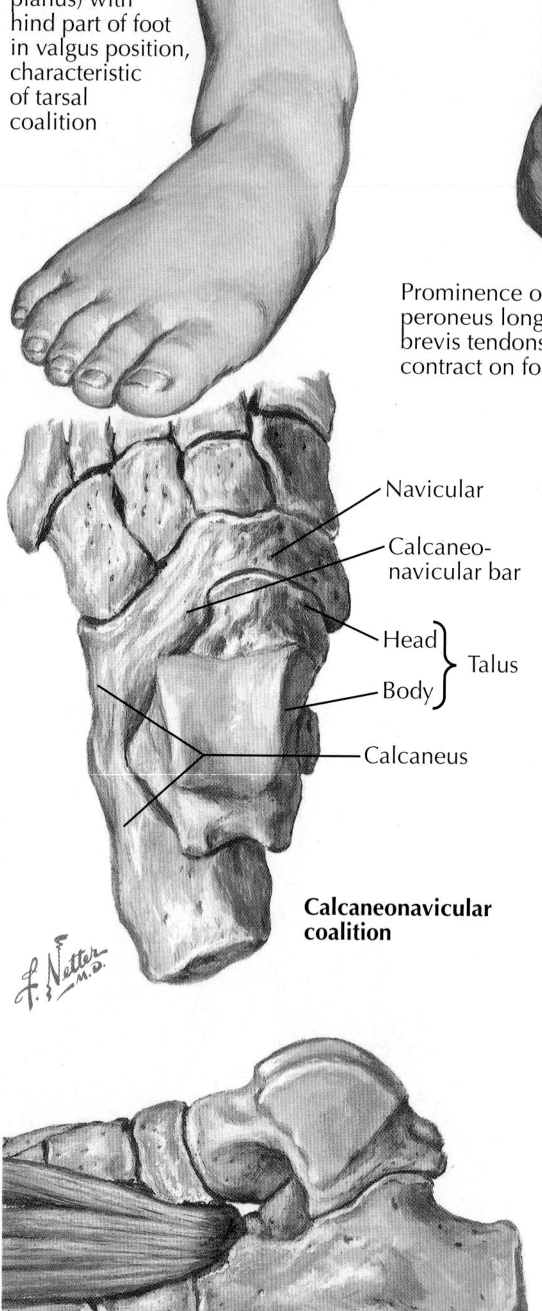

Rigid, painful flatfoot (pes planus) with hind part of foot in valgus position, characteristic of tarsal coalition

Calcaneonavicular coalition

Calcaneonavicular bar resected and extensor digitorum brevis muscle interposed to prevent re-formation of coalition

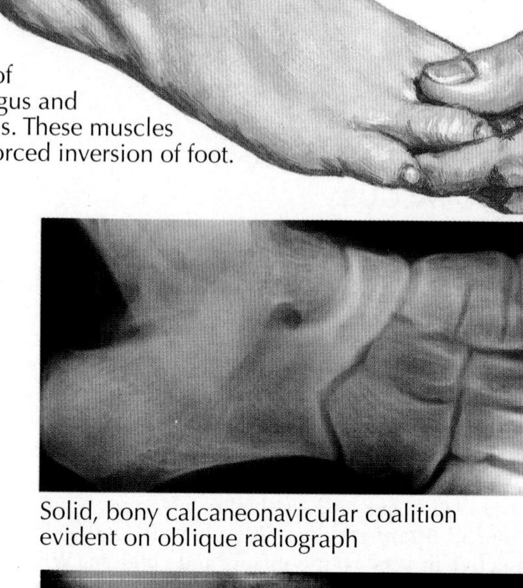

Prominence of peroneus longus and brevis tendons. These muscles contract on forced inversion of foot.

Solid, bony calcaneonavicular coalition evident on oblique radiograph

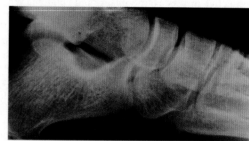

Cartilaginous calcaneonavicular coalition visible but poorly defined on lateral radiograph

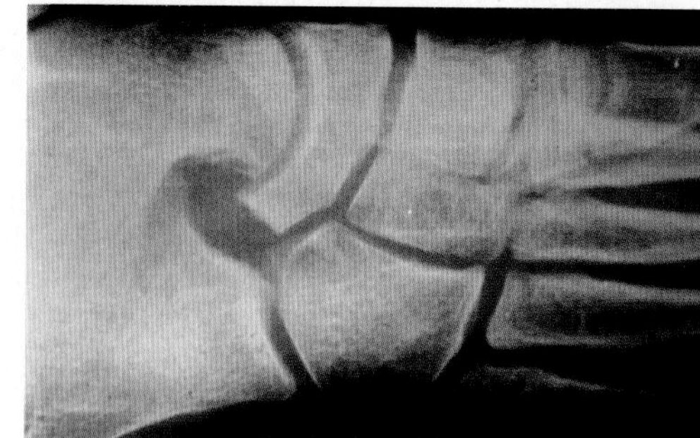

Postoperative radiograph

TARSAL COALITION

Coalition between the tarsal bones is a frequent cause of painful flatfoot (pes planus) in the older child or adolescent. Rigid flatfoot, a valgus heel with limited subtalar motion, and pain in the subtalar area are the major clinical findings. Coalition may develop between any of the tarsal bones, but the most common coalitions are between the calcaneus and the navicular and the talus and the calcaneus. Although a single coalition is most common, more than one are occasionally found in the same foot.

CALCANEONAVICULAR COALITION

Clinical Manifestations. Coalition between the calcaneus and the navicular usually becomes apparent in patients between 8 and 12 years of age when the cartilaginous coalition that results from an embryologic failure of tarsal segmentation undergoes ossification. Symptoms occur because the ossification limits subtalar motion, which is required for normal walking. When the foot is placed on the ground in normal gait, the subtalar joint rotates externally to compensate for internal rotation of the tibia on the femur with full extension at the knee. If subtalar motion is restricted, the navicular is displaced dorsally on the talus and the calcaneus is forced into valgus position with each step. The peroneus longus and peroneus brevis tendons adaptively shorten. The limited subtalar motion and tendon shortening create the clinical picture of the rigid flatfoot. When inversion of the foot is attempted, the shortened peroneal tendons contract, pulling the foot into eversion. This contraction of the tendons also protects the subtalar area when it is painful.

Radiographic Findings. Calcaneonavicular coalition is most clearly seen on the oblique radiograph. Although visible on both anteroposterior and lateral views, the coalition is much more difficult to recognize in these projections.

Treatment. An asymptomatic calcaneonavicular coalition does not require surgical treatment. For symptomatic coalitions before degenerative changes have occurred (usually seen in patients younger than 14 years), immobilization for 6 weeks in a below-knee walking cast may relieve symptoms.

Patients whose symptoms are not sufficiently relieved by casting are candidates for surgical resection of the coalition. This procedure is not appropriate if degenerative changes have occurred or if coalition between the talus and calcaneus is also present. The resection is performed through a lateral incision. The extensor digitorum brevis muscle is freed from its insertion and reflected distally, with care to preserve the nerve supply. The coalition is located and the talocalcaneal, talonavicular, calcaneocuboid, and cuneonavicular joints are identified. A rectangular section of the coalition is removed, and the extensor digitorum brevis muscle is then placed into the defect.

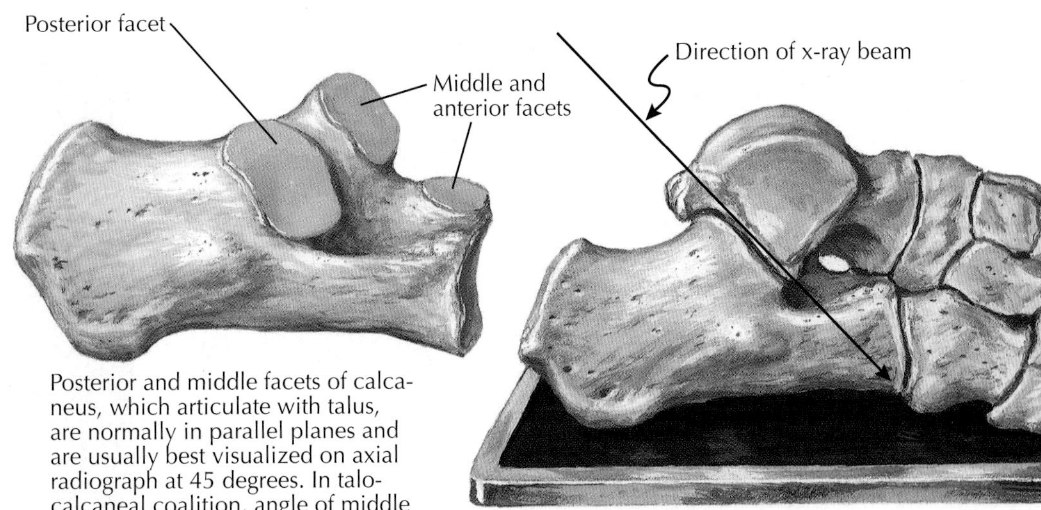

Posterior and middle facets of calcaneus, which articulate with talus, are normally in parallel planes and are usually best visualized on axial radiograph at 45 degrees. In talocalcaneal coalition, angle of middle facet may vary. Additional axial view taken at angle of sustentaculum tali (determined with lateral view). Anterior facet is in a different plane and cannot be seen on axial view because it is obscured by head of talus.

Axial (Harris) technique. Patient stands on cassette; x-rays projected at 45-degree angle.

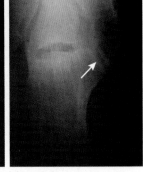

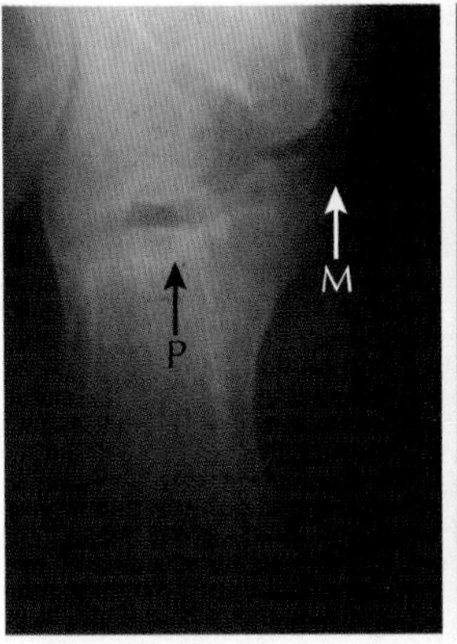

Axial radiographs. In normal foot (*left*), posterior (*P*) and middle (*M*) facets are open and in parallel planes. Cartilaginous coalition of middle facet (*right*), which is angled (*arrow*) in relation to posterior facet. When coalition ossifies, joint line is obliterated by bone.

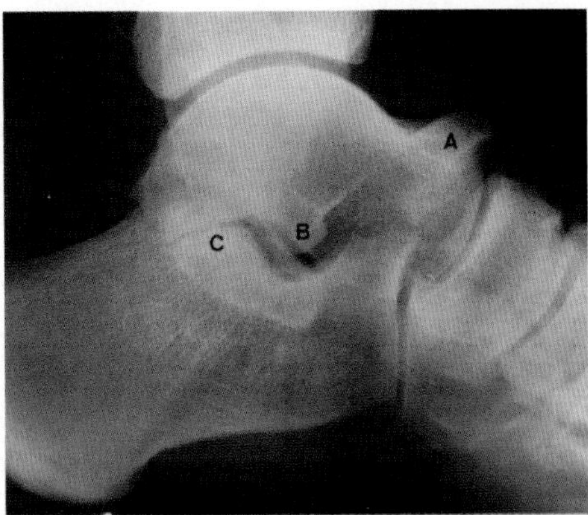

Secondary signs of talocalcaneal coalition. *A*, Beaking of talus; *B*, broadening of lateral process of talus; *C*, narrowing of subtalar joint.

Tarsal Coalition (Continued)

The patient wears a below-knee cast for 7 to 10 days, after which subtalar motion is begun. Weight-bearing is not allowed until the amount of subtalar motion reaches that obtained during the operation (at 3–4 weeks).

In patients older than 14 years who have degenerative changes, a below-knee weight-bearing cast, a Plastazote insert for the shoe, or an ankle-foot orthosis may relieve the pain. Failure to respond to these conservative measures and the presence of degenerative changes indicate the need for triple arthrodesis.

TALOCALCANEAL COALITION

Clinical Manifestations. Although coalition between the calcaneus and the talus may occur in any of the three facets, the middle facet is the one most commonly involved. The anatomic configuration of the middle and anterior facets varies from person to person. At least four different patterns are seen: (1) a single, small middle facet; (2) a single middle facet that extends posteriorly and is almost as large as the posterior facet; (3) a middle facet that extends anteriorly; and (4) two facets—the middle and anterior facets—in the medial compartment. Coalition may be seen in any of these facets.

Talocalcaneal coalition generally becomes symptomatic in the early teenage years when the preexisting cartilaginous coalition ossifies.

Radiographic Findings. Coalition between the talus and calcaneus may be difficult to detect on plain radiographs. Because the normal posterior and middle facets are in parallel planes at approximately 45 degrees to the sole of the foot, these two areas can be identified on an axial (Harris) view. Cartilaginous coalition between the talus and calcaneus in the area of the middle facet may also be detected by an irregularity of the joint surfaces of the talus and calcaneus. However, CT or MRI is usually required to visualize the extent of the coalition.

Treatment. Use of a below-knee, weight-bearing cast for 6 weeks frequently relieves symptoms; thereafter, a Plastazote insert or an ankle-foot orthosis is prescribed. Recurrent symptoms are managed similarly. Symptoms often abate when the facet ossifies completely, particularly if the heel remains in a neutral position. In a few patients with a large middle facet, tarsal tunnel syndrome develops from pressure on the median plantar nerve; a large middle facet may also prevent full plantar flexion of the ankle, because it abuts the posterior portion of the ankle joint.

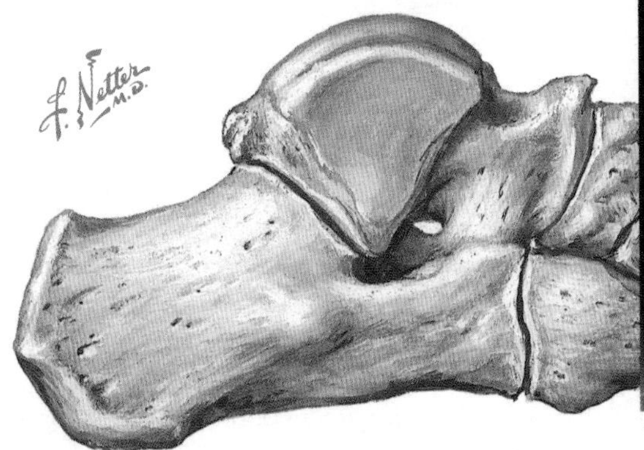

Bony coalition of anterior facet

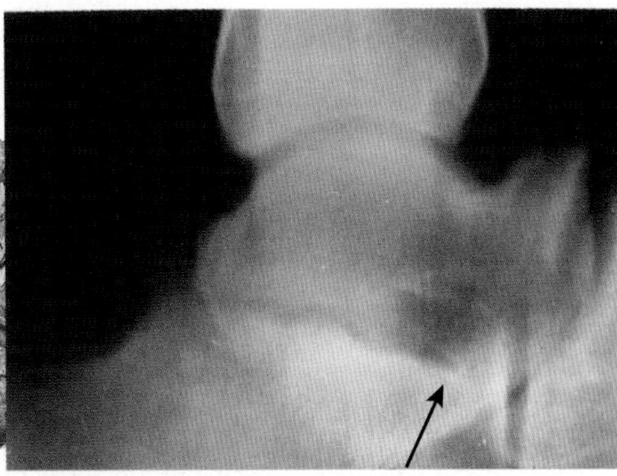

Tomogram reveals bony coalition of anterior facet (*arrow*). Beaking of talus is also evident.

Resection of the coalition is the treatment of choice in the patient younger than 16 years with no degenerative changes and with persistent pain after cast immobilization. Interposition of fat or the dorsal half of the flexor hallucis longus tendon decreases the risk of recurrence.

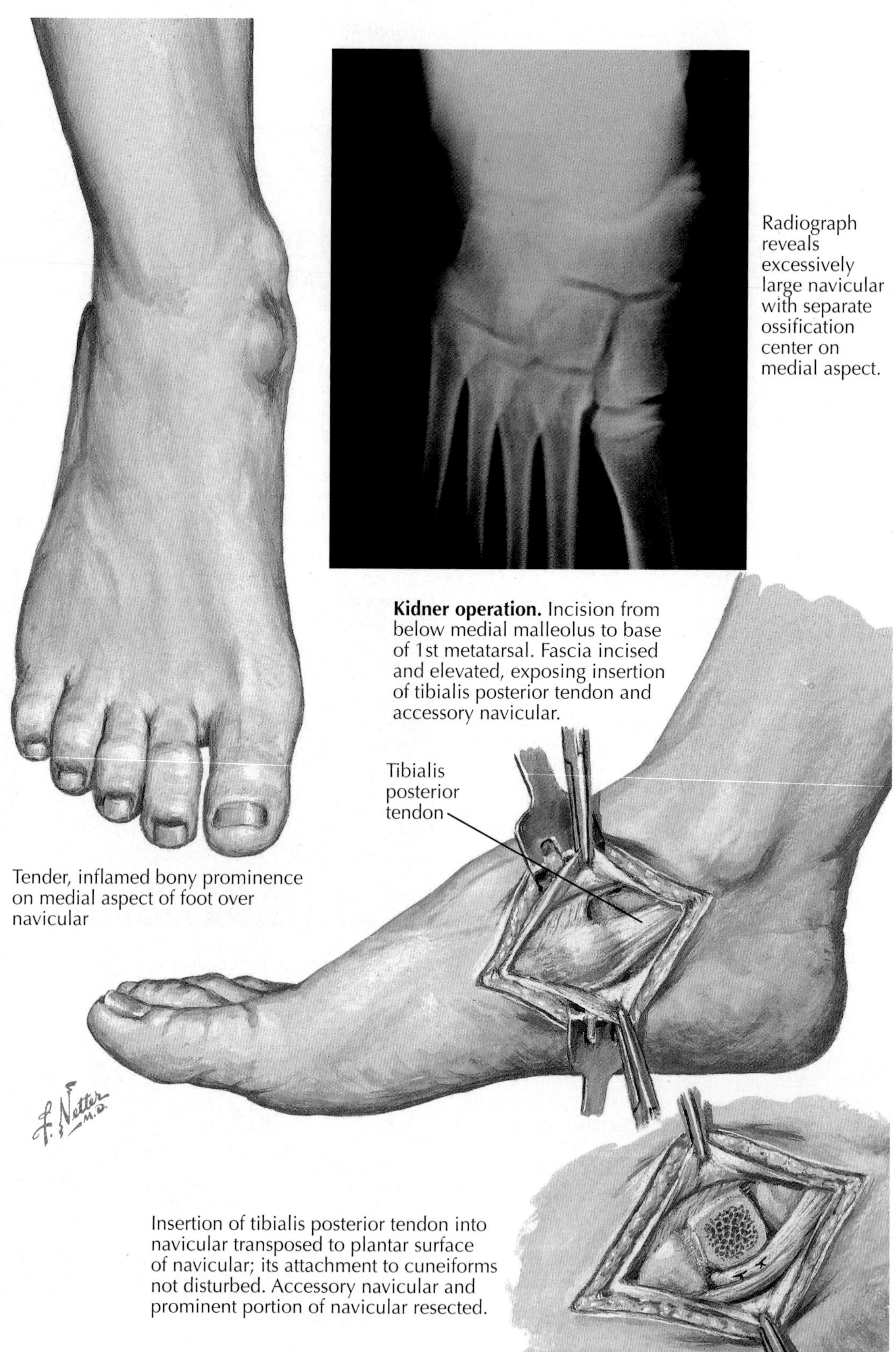

Radiograph reveals excessively large navicular with separate ossification center on medial aspect.
Kidner operation. Incision from below medial malleolus to base of 1st metatarsal. Fascia incised and elevated, exposing insertion of tibialis posterior tendon and accessory navicular.
Tibialis posterior tendon
Tender, inflamed bony prominence on medial aspect of foot over navicular
Insertion of tibialis posterior tendon into navicular transposed to plantar surface of navicular; its attachment to cuneiforms not disturbed. Accessory navicular and prominent portion of navicular resected.

Accessory Tarsal Navicular

The accessory tarsal navicular is located on the medial side of the foot, proximal to the navicular and in continuity with the tibialis posterior tendon. Although the accessory bone appears distinct from the navicular on radiographs, it is actually attached by fibrous tissue or cartilage.

Clinical Manifestations. The accessory navicular is frequently seen in conjunction with flatfoot. Pressure from the shoe on the prominence may cause pain, but the subtalar motion is adequate and the peroneus longus and peroneus brevis tendons do not become shortened.

Treatment. Pain and tenderness over the prominence can be relieved by altering the shoe or by placing a doughnut-shaped piece of moleskin on the skin around the prominence. If symptoms are not relieved with local measures, a short-leg cast may be used for 6 weeks. If symptoms recur after conservative measures are discontinued, excision of the accessory navicular may be indicated. Asymptomatic flatfoot with an accessory navicular is not an indication for surgery.

The incision is placed on the medial side of the foot dorsal to the prominence of the navicular because a painful scar may result if the incision is placed over the prominence. The tibialis posterior tendon is stripped away from the accessory navicular from dorsal to plantar, leaving the distal insertion of the tendon intact. The entire accessory navicular and the prominent portion of the navicular are removed by osteotomy so that no prominence remains on the medial side of the foot. The tibialis posterior tendon is reattached to the cut surface of the navicular using a suture anchor with the forefoot in slight inversion.

Congenital Toe Deformities

POLYDACTYLY (DUPLICATION OF PARTS)

As in the hand, additional or malformed digits are common, often familial, deformities. The primary goal of treatment is to produce a narrow foot and ensure satisfactory shoe fit. The decision as to which toe to remove is based primarily on which procedure will result in the best appearance; the most lateral or the most medial toe is usually the one removed.

Sophisticated surgical procedures used in the hand are not applicable in the foot, because they seldom result in good function. Simple removal of redundant skin and loosely attached toes restores a satisfactory foot contour. The traditional method of ligating the base of the toe in the newborn nursery is discouraged because it may leave an unsightly dimple and is upsetting to the parents.

Surgical procedures requiring use of a general anesthetic and a tourniquet should be delayed until the child is 12 to 18 months of age. For duplicated toes with deformed or duplicated metatarsals, complete removal of the ray is required. Duplication of the great toe coupled with a deformed and shortened first metatarsal is a special problem because it is often associated with hallux varus. A more extensive procedure that involves lengthening of the abductor hallucis tendon and plication of the adductor and medial soft tissues is required to realign the toe and prevent recurrence of the deformity.

MACRODACTYLY (OVERGROWTH)

Enlargement of the toes is not an uncommon deformity, and sometimes the foot or entire lower limb is enlarged as well. Although usually idiopathic, macrodactyly is frequently associated with neurofibromatosis.

Treatment is usually not necessary in the newborn, but, later, cosmetic problems related to poor shoe fit may require surgical procedures such as narrowing the foot by removing a ray, epiphysiodesis, or amputation of the large toe or the distal phalanx.

CURLY TOES

In this common deformity, one or more toes are bent or curled downward and overlap one another. The condition, which appears to have a high familial incidence, is believed to be due to congenital hypoplasia or absence of the intrinsic muscles of the affected toes. In some patients, the deformity improves with growth. If improvement does not occur, pressure from the shoe or weight-bearing may cause pain.

Conservative management such as strapping or taping is not effective. If surgical correction is necessary in a young child, simple flexor tenotomy usually suffices. In older children whose deformity has become more rigid, more extensive procedures such as surgical syndactyly and resection of the phalanx may be needed.

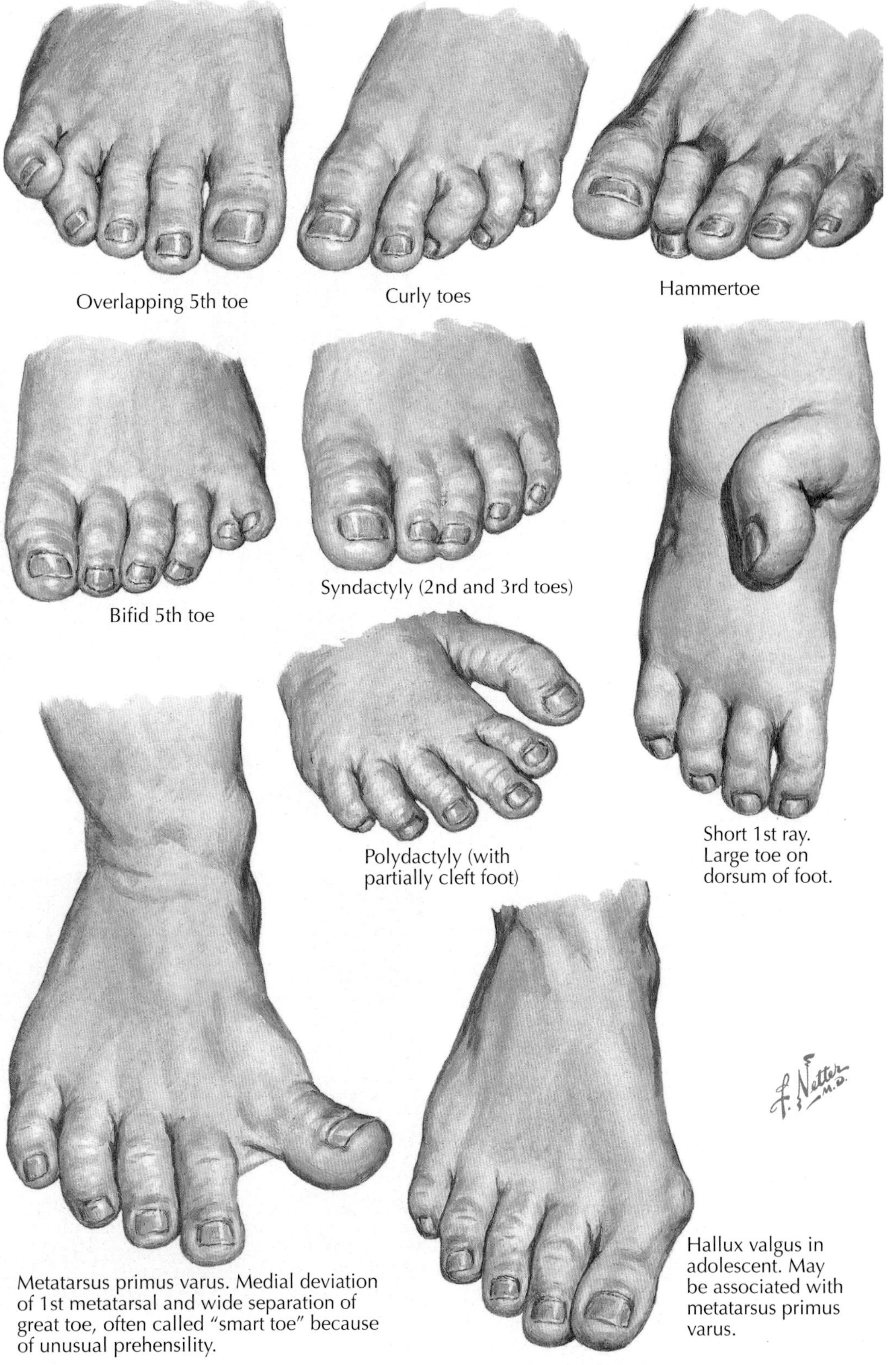

Overlapping 5th toe

Curly toes

Hammertoe

Bifid 5th toe

Syndactyly (2nd and 3rd toes)

Short 1st ray. Large toe on dorsum of foot.

Polydactyly (with partially cleft foot)

Metatarsus primus varus. Medial deviation of 1st metatarsal and wide separation of great toe, often called "smart toe" because of unusual prehensility.

Hallux valgus in adolescent. May be associated with metatarsus primus varus.

F. Netter M.D.

OVERLAPPING FIFTH TOE

A common familial deformity, the overlapping fifth toe is characterized by a contraction of both the skin over the dorsum of the toe and the dorsal capsule of the metatarsophalangeal joint. This makes the fifth toe excessively prominent and thus prone to irritation from the shoe. Although conservative measures such as passive stretching and strapping have traditionally been recommended for infants, these procedures are not very successful. If a significant malalignment persists in an older child, surgical correction may be necessary.

SYNDACTYLY

This webbing deformity, which also occurs in the hand, requires treatment only if it leads to angular deformity.

CLEFT FOOT

This deformity, which is transmitted as an autosomal dominant trait, is usually bilateral. It is often associated with a cleft hand and other anomalies, such as urinary tract abnormalities, deafness, and cleft lip and palate. Because foot function remains good, treatment consists of surgery to narrow the foot and produce a better appearance.

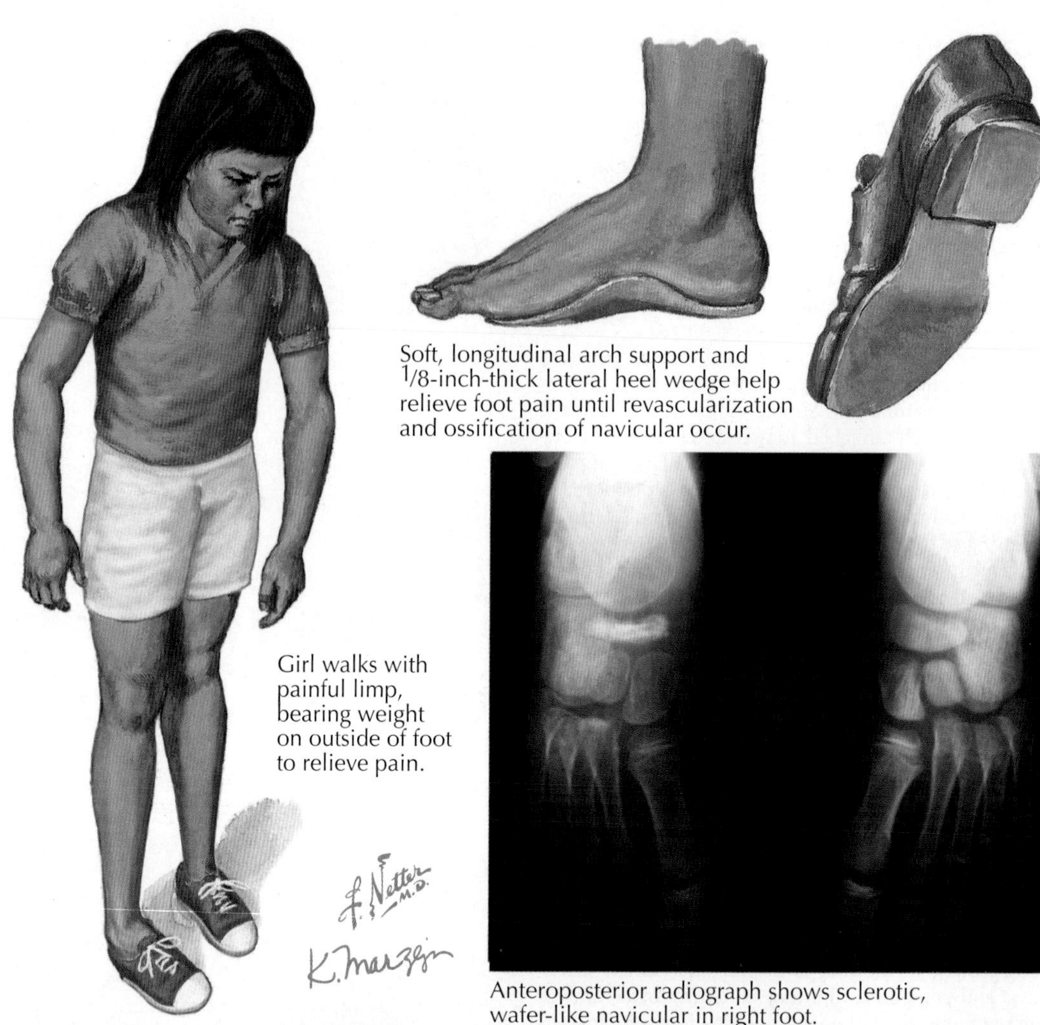

Soft, longitudinal arch support and 1/8-inch-thick lateral heel wedge help relieve foot pain until revascularization and ossification of navicular occur.
Girl walks with painful limp, bearing weight on outside of foot to relieve pain.
F. Netter M.D.
K. Marzen
Anteroposterior radiograph shows sclerotic, wafer-like navicular in right foot.

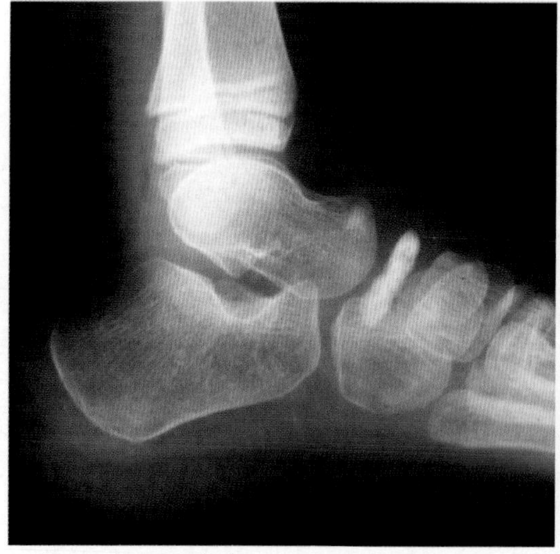

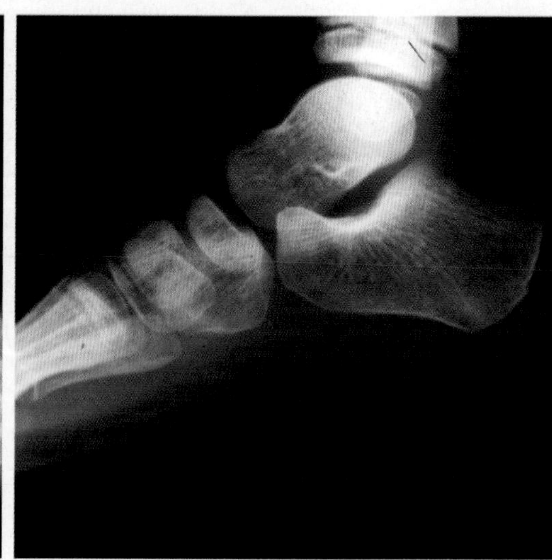

Radiographs reveal characteristic changes in navicular of involved right foot (*left*) compared with normal left foot (*right*).

KÖHLER DISEASE

Köhler disease is a self-limiting avascular necrosis of the tarsal navicular. It is usually unilateral and most often affects boys around age 4 and girls around age 5 years. The navicular is located at the apex of the longitudinal arch of the foot, where it is subjected to repetitive compressive forces during weight-bearing. Normally, the navicular is the last bone in the foot to ossify, and irregular ossification is not uncommon, especially in boys. The navicular ossifies later in boys than in girls, and delayed ossification appears to make the navicular more vulnerable to compressive damage.

It has been speculated that compression of the spongy ossification center of the navicular at a critical phase in its growth causes the irregular ossification. The compressive forces can occlude the vessels of the soft ossification center, rendering it avascular. Histologic studies show the typical changes of avascular necrosis: areas of necrosis, resorption of dead bone, and formation of new bone.

Clinical Manifestations. The child with Köhler disease walks with a painful limp, shifting weight to the lateral edge of the foot to relieve pressure on the longitudinal arch. Pain, tenderness, and swelling develop in the region of the tarsal navicular.

Radiographic Findings. In most patients, the navicular appears on radiographs as a thin wafer of bone with patchy areas of sclerosis and rarefaction and loss of its normal trabecular pattern. These radiographic findings produce the appearance of navicular collapse. In some patients, the navicular maintains its normal shape, although with a uniform increase in density and minimal fragmentation. This may represent a normal, sometimes familial, variant of ossification that is occasionally seen on the opposite, asymptomatic foot in children with Köhler disease as well as in asymptomatic individuals.

Treatment and Prognosis. Because the disease is self-limiting, the prognosis is excellent, and no long-term disability or deformity results. The vascularity of the navicular is adequately supplied by a circumferential leash of vessels, allowing rapid revascularization. The affected navicular regains its normal shape before the foot completes growth, and normal ossification is usually completed in 2 years. Symptomatic treatment is needed for the pain and swelling. Soft, longitudinal arch supports; a medial heel wedge; and limitation of strenuous activity usually relieve the symptoms. If the pain is severe or persists, a short-leg walking cast may be used for 4 to 6 weeks, followed by use of a stiff-soled shoe.

COMMON FOOT INFECTIONS

The foot exists in an environment that unfortunately can be conducive to infection. Primarily, the use of shoes constricts the foot and produces a warm, moist environment that encourages bacterial growth. Foot infections can occur in all individuals. However, patients with diabetes are particularly susceptible to foot infection due to the loss of protective sensation. Even trivial trauma either from a poorly fitting shoe or from barefoot walking can result in violation of the skin and lead to severe infection. Poor blood supply and diminished immune function further compromise the diabetic patient's ability to fight foot infection. Common locations for foot infections include the paronychial (nail) area and the deep spaces of the foot.

PARONYCHIAL INFECTION

Onychocryptosis is the formal name for the common condition referred to as ingrown toenail. The great toe is most frequently affected. Both medial and lateral sides of the nail may be involved. Three patterns of ingrown toenail can be observed. In the first, incorrect nail trimming technique results in a fishhook-shaped spur that digs into the lateral nail groove. In the second type, the nail develops an inward curvature of the lateral margin that also produces impingement with the tissue of the nail groove. In the last type, hypertrophy of the paronychial tissue at the margin of the nail produces the impingement. Wearing tight shoes that pinch the lateral skinfold between the shoe and the underlying toenail often precipitates or aggravates the problem. In each of these instances, the resulting impingement produces inflammation where the nail meets the nail fold. This inflammation can then lead to secondary infection.

Ingrown toenails are best prevented with proper toenail-trimming technique. The toenail should be allowed to grow beyond the lateral skinfold and should be cut straight across, not rounded at the corners. The risk of ingrown toenail is minimized by making sure that the square edge of the nail extends just slightly beyond the skinfold and by wearing well-fitting shoes.

An inflamed, ingrown nail is treated initially with removal of all compressive shoes and stockings and warm soaks in Epsom salts and water. Oral antibiotics can be started if significant erythema consistent with cellulitis develops along the affected border of the toe. If the inflammation or infection fails to resolve with these measures, particularly if purulence persists beneath the paronychial fold, then surgical treatment may be required. The most common surgical treatment involves a hemiresection of the nail plate. This is usually performed under digital block. An elevator is used to lift the lateral nail margin from underneath the hypertrophied paronychium. Scissors are used to make a longitudinal cut in the nail plate, and the lateral quarter of the nail plate is removed. After partial excision of the toenail and the surrounding granulation tissue, the patient may be given oral antibiotics and encouraged to soak the toe twice a day in warm water. The excised area heals by secondary intention.

COMMON INFECTIONS OF FOOT

Ingrown toenail

Area of excision

En bloc excision includes nail matrix

Broken lines show lines of incision for excision of lateral 1/4 of toenail, nail bed, and matrix.

En bloc excision of lateral part of toenail, nail bed, and matrix

After excision, wound allowed to granulate

Fungal infection of toenail

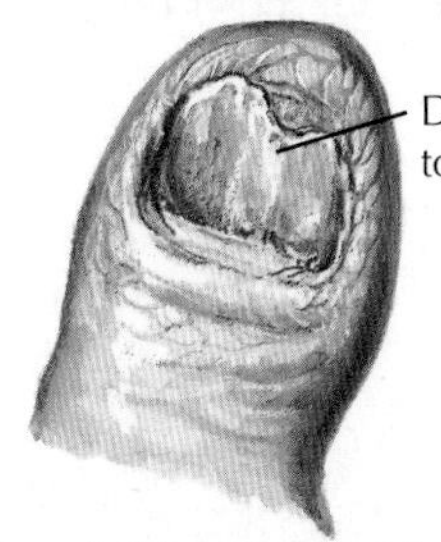

Toenail deformity caused by chronic fungal infection

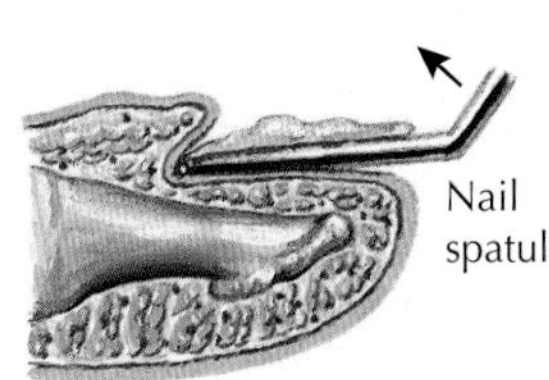

Toenail plate freed from nail bed and proximal nail fold

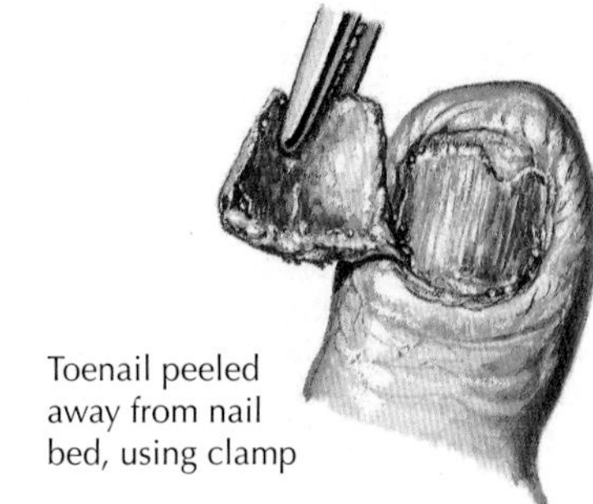
Toenail peeled away from nail bed, using clamp

Puncture wound

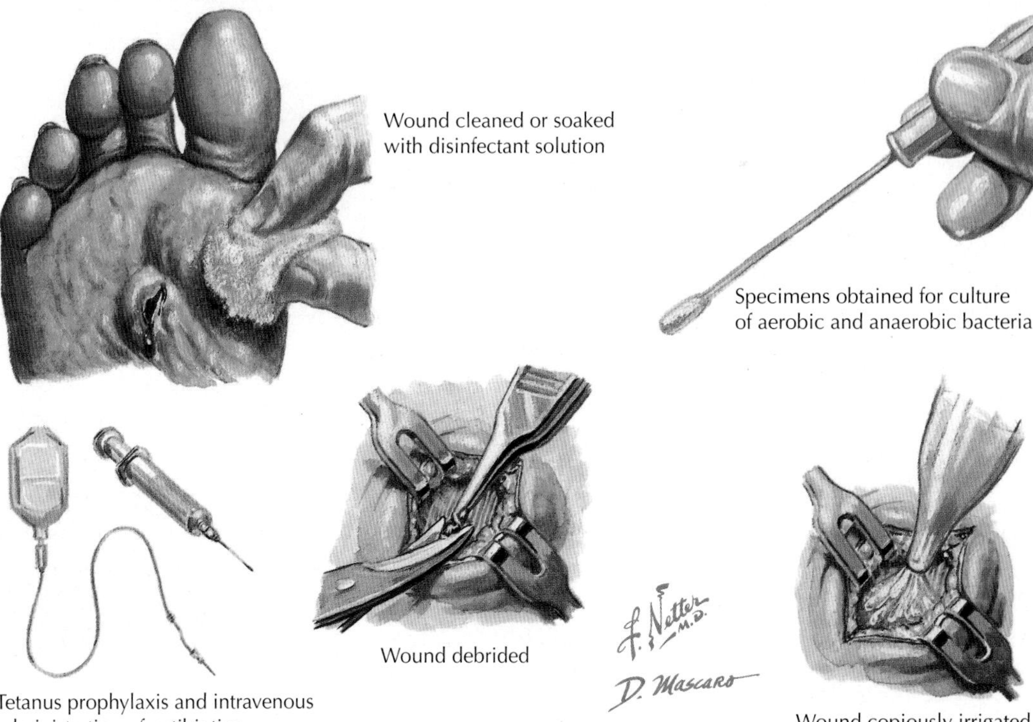

Wound cleaned or soaked with disinfectant solution

Specimens obtained for culture of aerobic and anaerobic bacteria

Tetanus prophylaxis and intravenous administration of antibiotics

Wound debrided

Wound copiously irrigated

FUNGAL INFECTION OF TOENAIL

Chronic fungal infection of the nail is called onychomycosis. The fungal infection causes the toenail to become hypertrophic, deformed, yellow, and friable. Once established, a fungal infection is extremely difficult to eradicate.

Conservative treatment includes simple trimming of the toenail to maintain an essentially normal shape and appearance. When the toenail becomes severely deformed and thickened, it may cause painful pressure on the adjacent skin. Occasionally, pressure from large, deformed nails creates secondary low-grade cellulitis around the periphery of the nail. Removal of the toenail may be necessary to decrease the pain and inflammation.

Under a digital block, the surgeon may elevate the toenail from its bed and remove it entirely. Necrotic debris that has accumulated beneath the nail is then debrided. Performed in isolation, nail removal provides only temporary relief of mechanical symptoms because when the nail regrows, the fungus is still present and the nail deformity recurs. Administering antifungal

COMMON FOOT INFECTIONS (Continued)

topical medications after nail removal can significantly improve the success rate. Currently, the most effective means of definitively treating this infection involves the use of powerful oral antifungal antibiotics.

PUNCTURE WOUND

Puncture wound of the foot remains one of the most common presenting injuries seen in hospital emergency departments and one of the most common causes of serious infection in the foot. The penetrating object frequently carries pathogens with it when it breaks the skin and deposits these organisms deep into the foot. Once the object is removed, the skin may close over the top, preventing drainage. This creates an ideal environment for abscess formation. Although shoes provide some protection to the foot, sharp objects such as nails can pierce the sole of the shoe and penetrate the foot. Although tetanus, which is caused by *Clostridium tetani,* is a theoretical complication of a puncture wound, such an infection is exceedingly rare because of widespread effective immunization. On the other hand, penetration of the sole of the foot may seed the foot with other aggressive bacteria that can produce serious local infection. Gram-positive cocci such as *Staphylococcus* and *Streptococcus* species remain common causes of foot infection after puncture wounds, but a large number of infections are due to gram-negative organisms, particularly *Pseudomonas aeruginosa. Pseudomonas* is believed to thrive within shoes and is delivered into the foot when the puncturing object penetrates both the shoe and the foot. Gram-negative infections can be quite aggressive, particularly if the puncture wound extends to bone, and can result in not only deep abscess formation but also bone infection known as osteomyelitis.

It is critical to take aggressive steps to prevent infection after puncture wound of the foot. Adequate anesthesia is required, often employing a tibial nerve or ankle block. The puncture wound is opened up widely to allow for removal of any foreign bodies or debris and to allow ample irrigation. The tract must be spread to the depth of the penetration. Once adequate debridement and irrigation have been performed, it is critical to leave the wound open to allow for drainage. This greatly decreases the risk of subsequent infection. The wound heals secondarily, usually in 1 to 2 weeks.

DEEP INFECTION

A neglected or improperly treated puncture wound may lead to a serious deep space abscess in the foot. An abscess is a focal collection of purulent material in a defined closed space. The foot possesses five distinct deep fascial compartments in which infection may occur. These compartments include the superficial posterior, plantar, central, posterior dorsal, and dorsal spaces. The central plantar space in particular is frequently involved when a deep foot abscess develops. Symptoms frequently include diffuse swelling, pain, and erythema of the foot, particularly along the instep. If untreated, deep space infection of the foot can extend along the flexor tendons to involve the deep fascial compartment of the leg.

Antibiotics alone are insufficient to treat a deep space infection. Once an abscess has developed in one of the closed spaces of the foot, it must be treated with surgical incision and drainage. The central space of the plantar aspect of the foot is best approached through a medial foot incision, which reflects the abductor hallucis muscle plantarly and allows both access to the central space and visualization of the critical neurovascular structures coursing to the toes. Alternatively, if the infection appears to be more dorsal, a dorsomedial and dorsolateral incision can be used to decompress the abscess. All necrotic and infected tissue must be debrided and the wound thoroughly irrigated and left open. Severe infection may require repeat surgical debridement. Wounds are usually allowed to heal by secondary intention, which may be facilitated by negative-pressure wound dressings.

Tissue specimens are obtained for culture, and broad-spectrum antibiotics are administered. Appropriate antibiotics are administered when cultures identify the specific organisms involved. The infection is often polymicrobial.

DEEP INFECTIONS OF FOOT

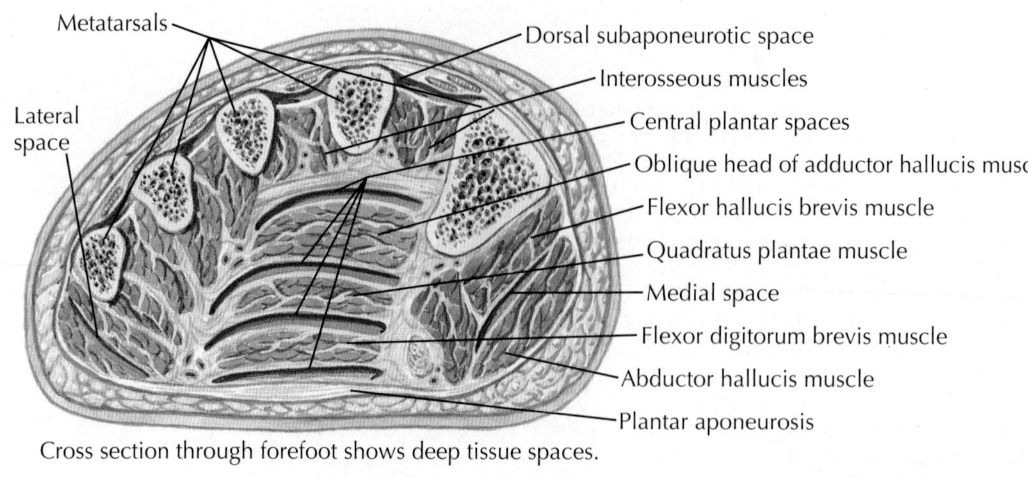

Cross section through forefoot shows deep tissue spaces.

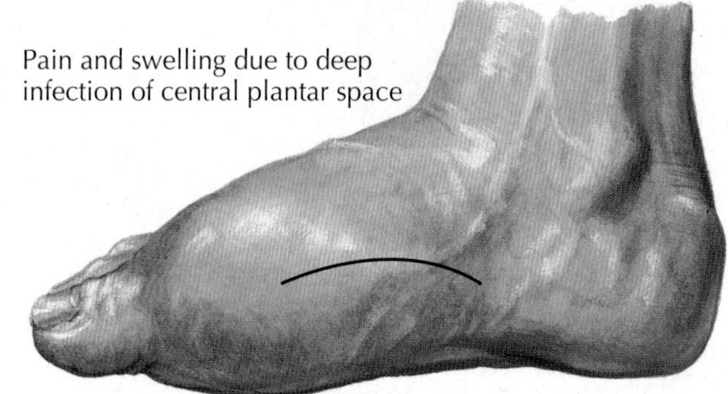

Pain and swelling due to deep infection of central plantar space

Incision site for drainage of central plantar spaces

Puncture wound or perforating ulcer may penetrate deep central plantar spaces, leading to abscess.

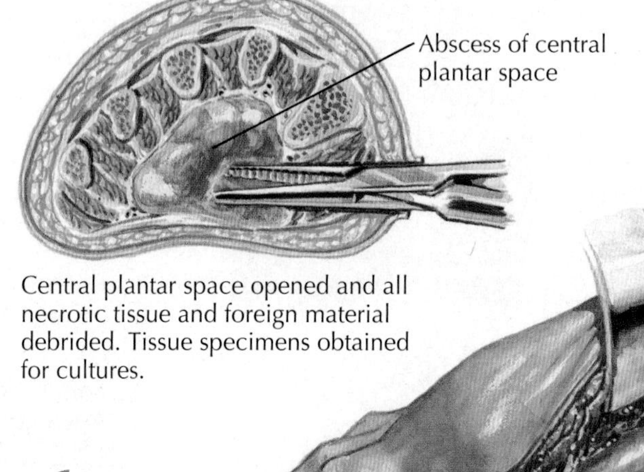

Central plantar space opened and all necrotic tissue and foreign material debrided. Tissue specimens obtained for cultures.

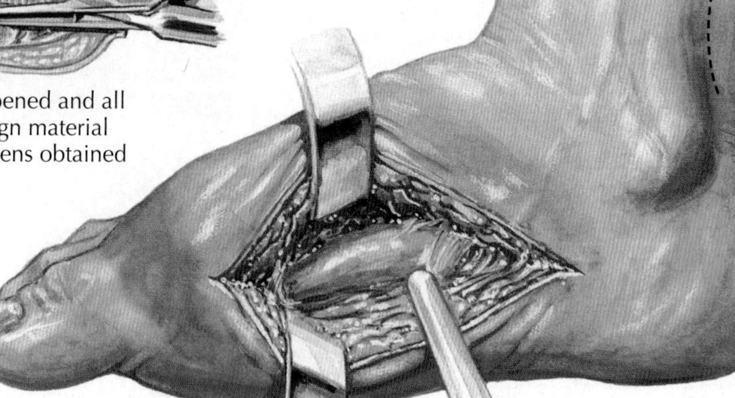

If proximal spread occurs, separate incision may be made for drainage.
F. Netter M.D.
D. Mascaro

Wound irrigated and drained

Lesions of the Diabetic Foot

Diabetic ulcer

Charcot joint

Ulcer

Atrophy of interosseous muscles

Clawfoot deformity

Corn

Injury and ulceration are result of diabetic neuropathy.

Callus

Typical locations of ulcers

Infection

Cross section through forefoot shows abscess in central plantar space. Infection due to impaired immune response, skin defects, and poor perfusion.

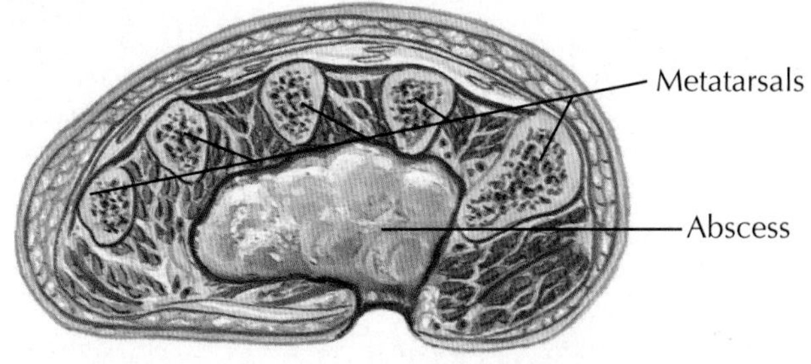

Gangrene

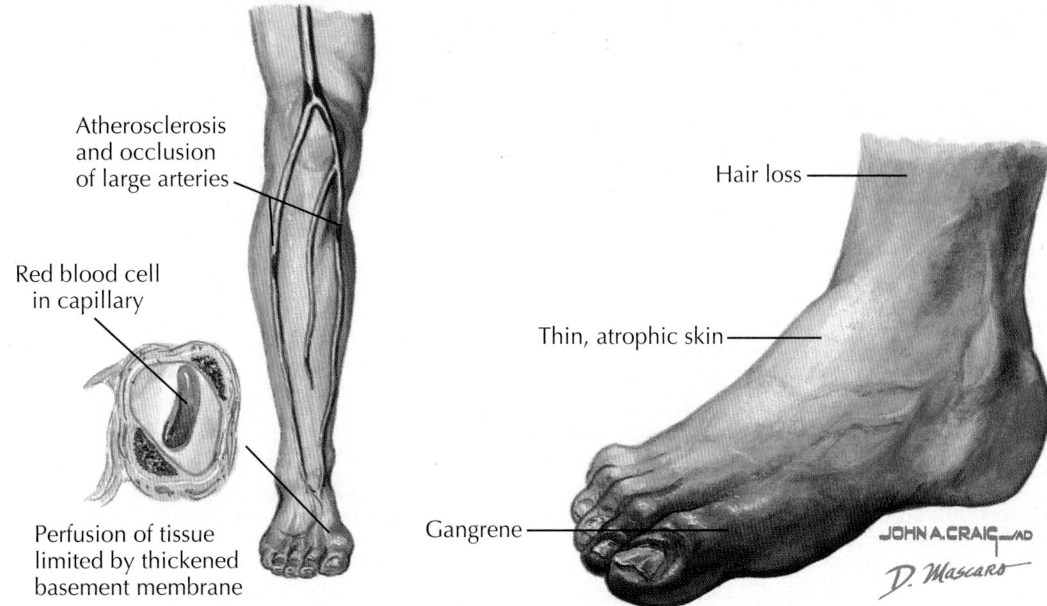

Diabetic Foot Ulceration

Patients with diabetes are susceptible to a host of foot-related problems. One of the most common and troublesome problems is ulceration and subsequent infection of the foot. Ulceration of the foot develops in the patient with diabetes primarily as a result of peripheral neuropathy and loss of the normal protective sensation. Whereas the individual with normal protective sensation would immediately sense minor trauma such as the rubbing of a shoe and take immediate steps to correct it, the individual with diabetes is not aware of the problem, allowing the pressure to continue unabated. Eventually, even minor repetitive trauma can result in formation of an ulcer. Ulcers occur most commonly on the weight-bearing plantar surface of the foot and over bony prominences. Once ulceration develops, it is also more likely to become infected in the patient with diabetes owing to diminished immune function and impaired circulation. Failure to sense the normal signs of infection due to neuropathy can result in progression to osteomyelitis and extensive, limb-threatening infection in the patient with diabetes.

Classification. Diabetic ulcerations are best characterized by evaluating the lesion's depth and the vascularity of the foot. Wagner popularized a classification of diabetic foot ulcers that included six categories. Grade 0 refers to a pressure area that has not yet ulcerated. Grade 1 describes superficial, noninfected ulcers. Grade 2 describes deep, noninfected ulcers, commonly with involved tendon. Grade 3 describes deep, infected ulcers usually with osteomyelitis. Grades 4 and 5 refer to the vascularity of the foot, with partial gangrene included as grade 4 and complete gangrene as grade 5.

Physical Examination. After assessing and classifying the depth and tissue involvement of the diabetic foot ulceration, the patient must be evaluated as a whole to determine the ulcer's healing potential. The ability to heal a diabetic foot ulcer is directly affected by the patient's vascular and nutritional status. Vascular assessment begins by recording the color and temperature of the feet and palpating for dorsalis pedis and posterior tibial pulses. If the pulses are absent or significantly diminished, formal evaluation by a vascular medicine specialist is indicated. This formal vascular evaluation often includes measurement of the ankle-brachial index (ABI) and transcutaneous oxygen saturation. The ABI assesses the blood pressure in the foot relative to the blood pressure in the arm. An ABI value less than 0.45 has been associated with decreased ability to heal a diabetic foot ulcer. Similarly, transcutaneous oxygen saturation reflects how well oxygenated the blood is that perfuses the foot. Transcutaneous oxygen pressures less than 30 mm Hg have also been associated with decreased healing potential.

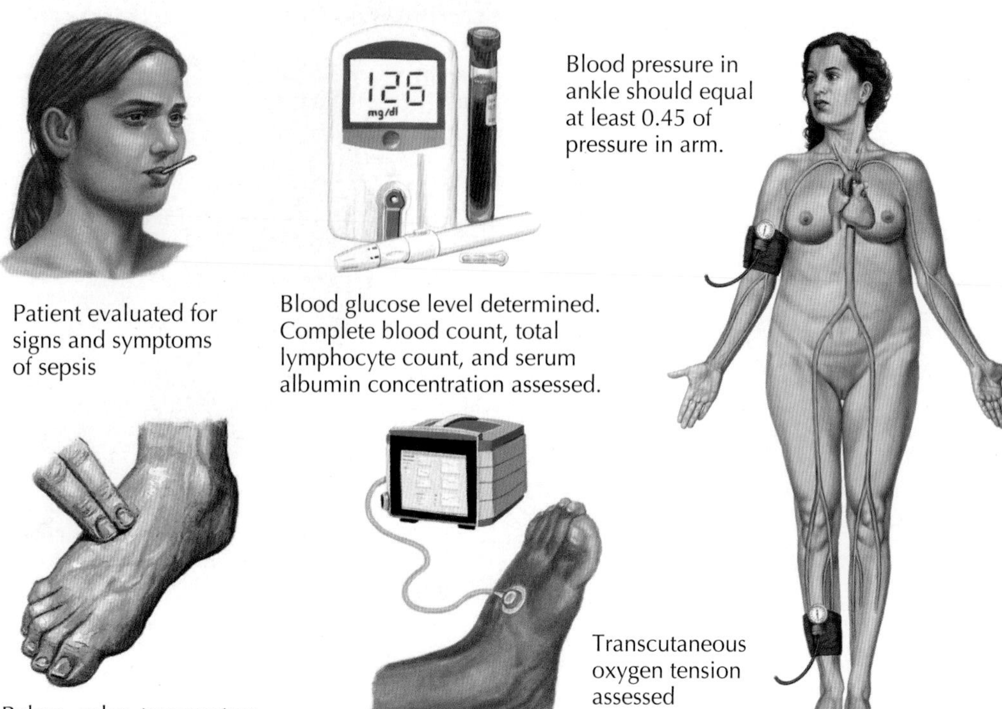
Clinical Evaluation of Patient With Diabetic Foot Lesion
126
mg/dl
Blood pressure in ankle should equal at least 0.45 of pressure in arm.
Patient evaluated for signs and symptoms of sepsis
Blood glucose level determined. Complete blood count, total lymphocyte count, and serum albumin concentration assessed.
Pulses, color, temperature, and skin status assessed
Transcutaneous oxygen tension assessed

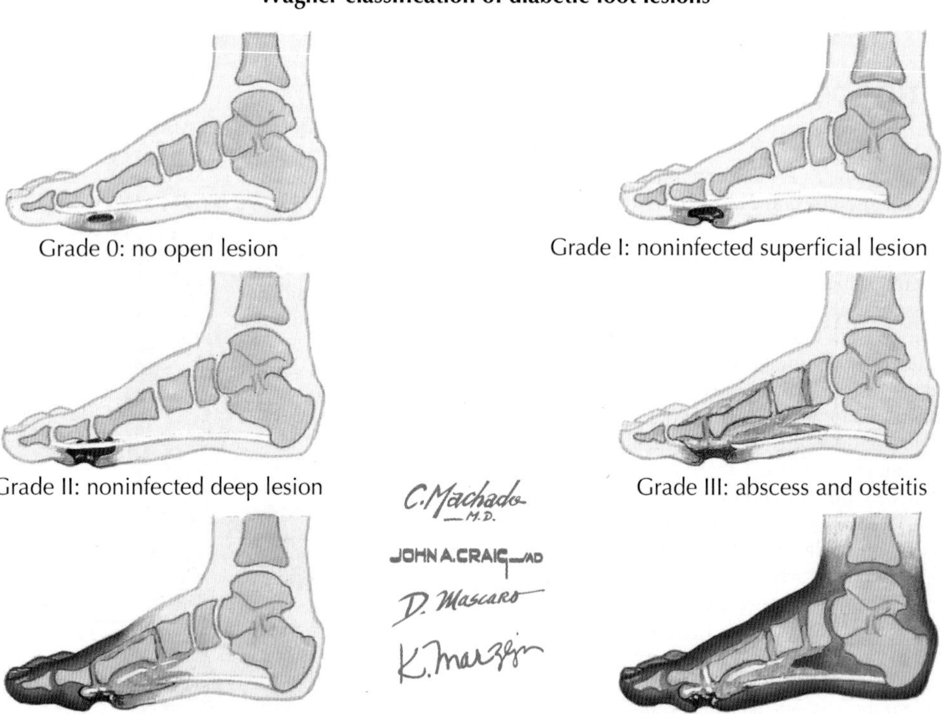
Wagner classification of diabetic foot lesions
Grade 0: no open lesion
Grade I: noninfected superficial lesion
Grade II: noninfected deep lesion
Grade III: abscess and osteitis
Grade IV: gangrene of forefoot
Grade V: gangrene of entire foot
C. Machado M.D.
JOHN A. CRAIG AD
D. Mascaro
K. Marzejon

Diabetic Foot Ulceration (Continued)

Patients with diabetes, although frequently overweight, may paradoxically be malnourished. Malnourishment can impair the patient's ability to heal foot ulceration. Nutritional status can be assessed through simple blood tests such as measuring the patient's albumin level and total lymphocyte count. A serum albumin level less than 3.0 g/dL or a total lymphocyte count less than 1500 cells/mm^3 suggest poor nutrition that may complicate healing of an ulcer.

Treatment. A successful treatment plan for diabetic foot ulceration must address all of the contributing factors in a comprehensive manner. If vascular supply is suboptimal, peripheral arterial stenting or bypass procedures may be indicated to improve blood supply to the foot. A vascular surgeon is needed to determine whether this is feasible and appropriate. Poor nutrition can be aggressively addressed by correcting dietary errors and augmenting with protein supplements. Blood glucose control should also be optimized because this improves healing and decreases the risk of infection. Ulcerations associated with infection must be aggressively debrided of all involved tissue, and appropriate antibiotic therapy is then instituted.

Most diabetic foot ulcerations develop as a result of abnormal pressure applied to the insensate foot. Thus the most critical part of treatment is removing the abnormal pressure. For plantar foot ulcerations, this often requires use of a total contact cast. A total contact cast is an intimately fitting cast applied to the leg and foot that distributes the load of weight-bearing across the entire bottom of the cast, effectively unloading the area of ulceration. A good total contact cast allows the patient with diabetes to remain mobile while the ulcer heals, usually in 6 to 8 weeks. Forefoot ulceration is often accompanied by tightness of the Achilles tendon, which is thought to increase pressure beneath the metatarsal heads, contributing to ulceration. Percutaneous lengthening of the Achilles tendon concomitantly with total contact casting has been demonstrated to decrease the likelihood of ulcer recurrence.

Once the ulcer has healed, casting can be discontinued and the patient transitioned into proper diabetic footwear. Good diabetic shoes should be wide and deep to accommodate the foot and decrease the risk of friction and subsequent ulceration. Patients with deformities or bone prominences may require custom shoes or custom orthotic inserts to further protect and unload these structures. In severe cases, surgery may be necessary to reduce deformity to prevent recurrence of ulceration.

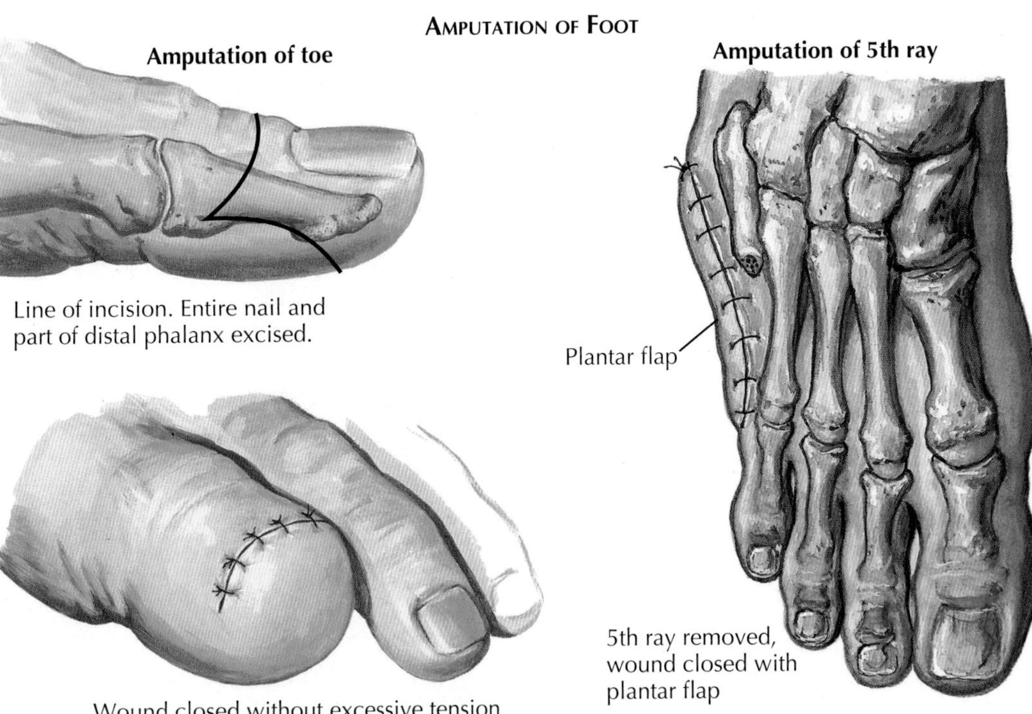

Amputations in the Foot

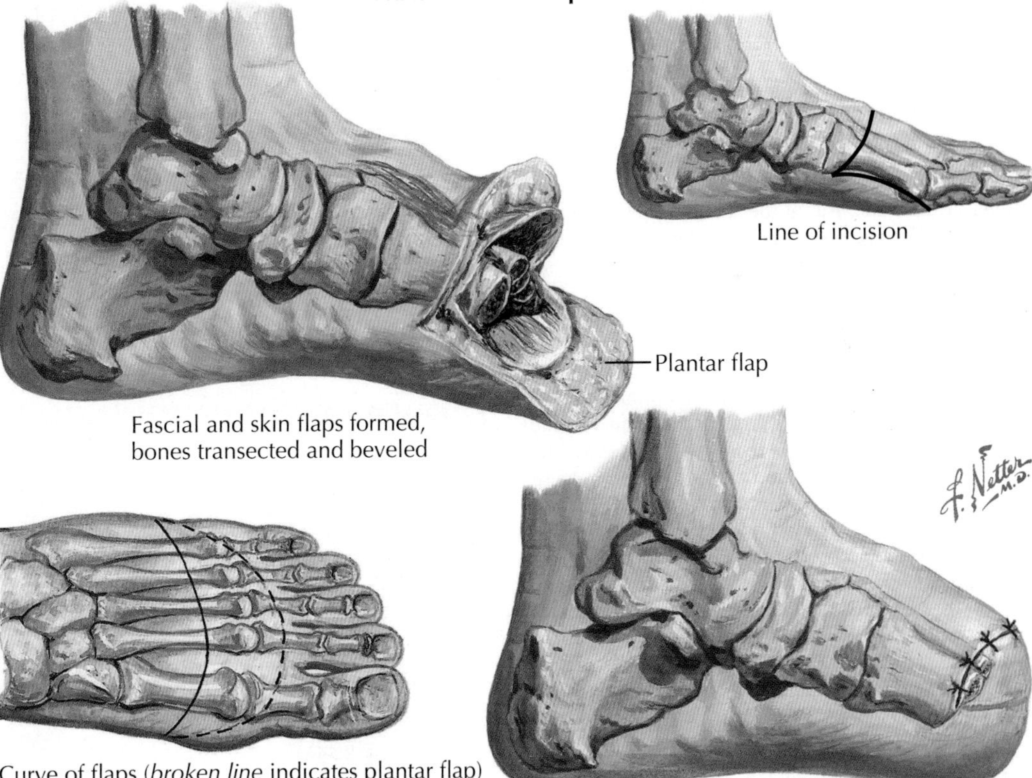

Amputation of all or a portion of the foot represents the most elemental form of foot surgery. Often it is disparaged by the surgeon, perhaps because it can be perceived as a failure of treatment. But when performed properly, amputation is truly a reconstructive procedure that can eradicate infection, correct deformity, decrease pain, and improve function.

Amputation in the foot can be indicated in the treatment of diabetes, peripheral vascular disease, trauma, infection, tumors, and congenital abnormalities. Foot amputation is especially common in the diabetic population. Peripheral neuropathy, poor blood supply, and impaired immune function all contribute to place the patient with diabetes at greater risk for limb-threatening infection.

TOE AMPUTATION

Both the great toe and the lesser toes may require amputation. Toe amputation is usually performed for the treatment of infection, ischemia, or posttraumatic deformity. The most distal level of great toe amputation is known as a terminal Syme amputation. This procedure is indicated for the treatment of posttraumatic nail deformity, onychomycosis, or recurrent infection of the great toenail. With the terminal Syme amputation, the nail plate, matrix, and eponychial folds are excised along with the distal portion of the distal phalanx. The skin edges are then approximated without tension.

When amputating the great toe more proximally, an effort should be made to maintain the base of the proximal phalanx if possible. This better preserves the weight-bearing and plantar flexion function of the first ray. It is also beneficial in the lesser toes to leave a portion of the proximal phalanx. This allows the toe to serve as a spacer and prevent migration of adjacent toes.

RAY AMPUTATION

When injury or infection involves an entire toe, resection of a single ray (the digit plus the head and shaft of the corresponding metatarsal) can effectively treat the problem while maximizing residual foot function. The most common ray amputations involve the first ray and the fifth ray. By virtue of being located on the medial and lateral borders of the foot, respectively, these are the technically easiest ray amputations to perform. First ray amputation does affect the push-off power of the foot, but this can be accommodated with a special orthotic shoe insert. Central ray amputations are less common and technically more difficult owing to the paucity of soft tissue flaps for closure.

When multiple rays are amputated, it is referred to as a partial forefoot amputation. Although partial forefoot amputations can be successful, the more rays that are resected, the greater the impact on the foot's balance and function.

Syme Amputation (Wagner Modification)

Stage I

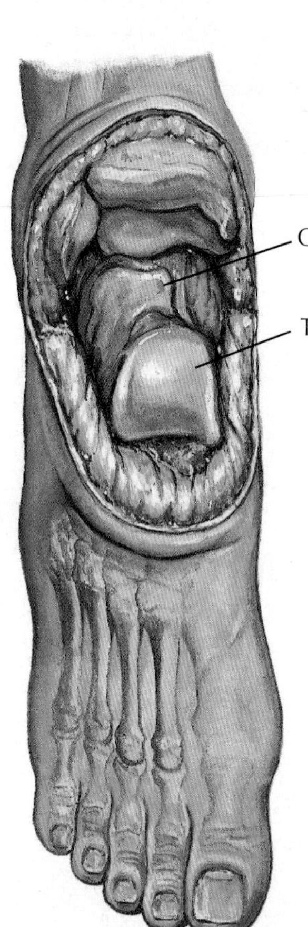

2. Talus dislocated and foot placed in plantar flexion to allow dissection of calcaneus.

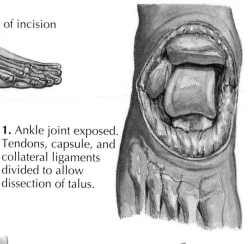

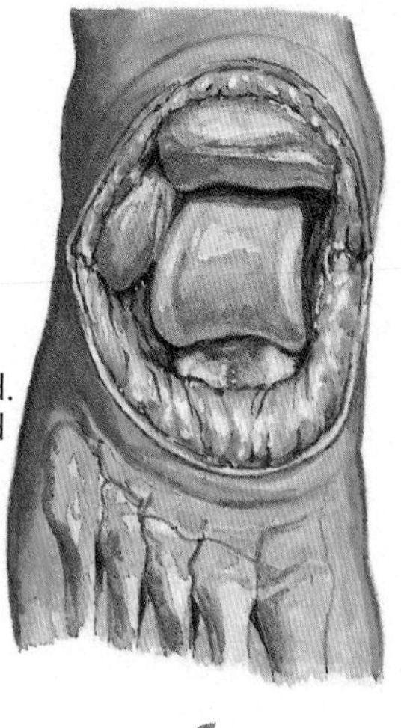

1. Ankle joint exposed. Tendons, capsule, and collateral ligaments divided to allow dissection of talus.

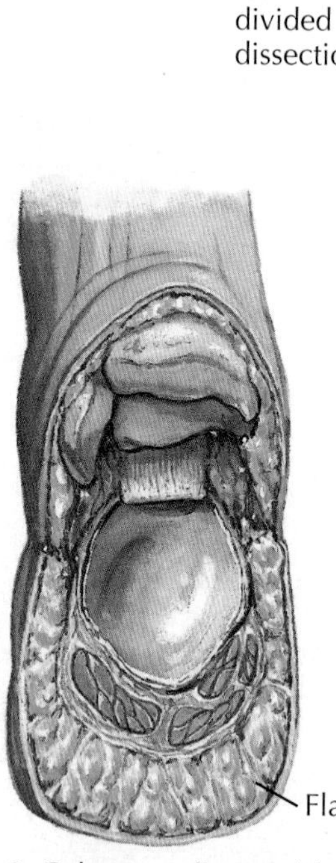

3. Calcaneus dissected free, leaving thick plantar pad flap.

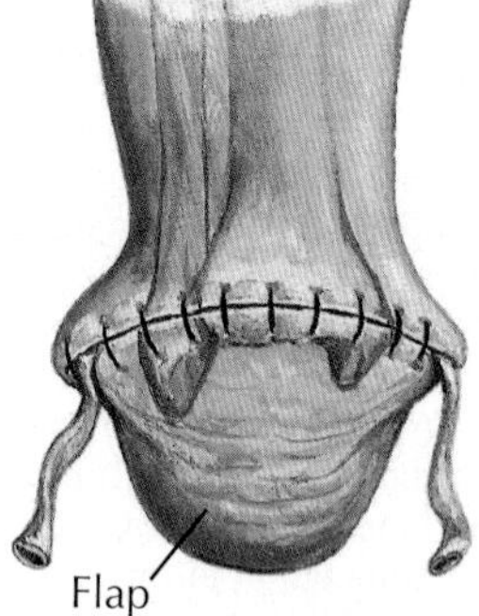

4. Heel pad flap rotated up over distal tibia and fibula and closed in layers over drain.

Stage II (delayed)

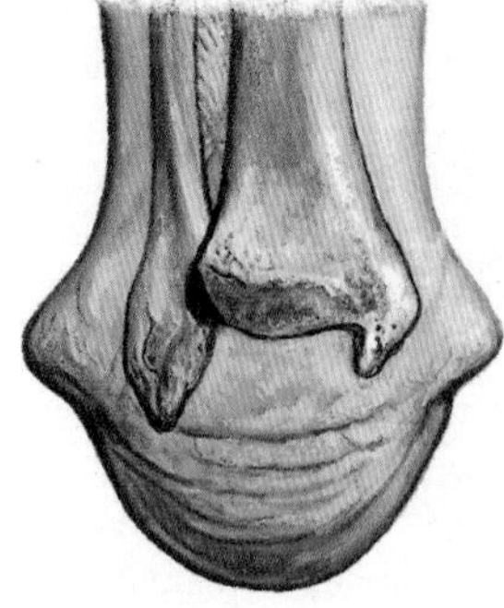

1. "Dog ears" elliptically excised, exposing malleoli.

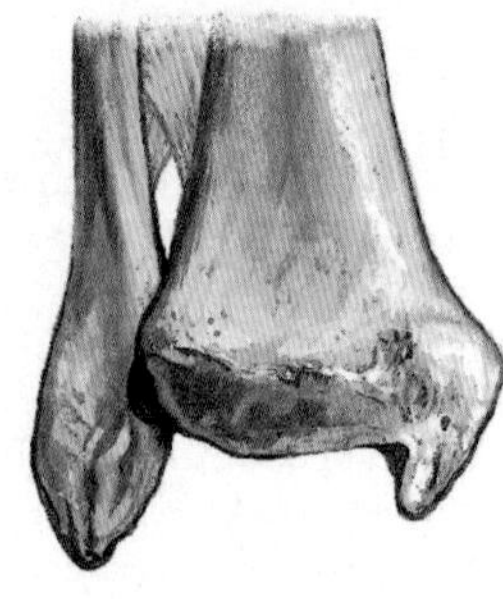

2. Medial and lateral malleoli and flares (shaded area) resected flush with joint.

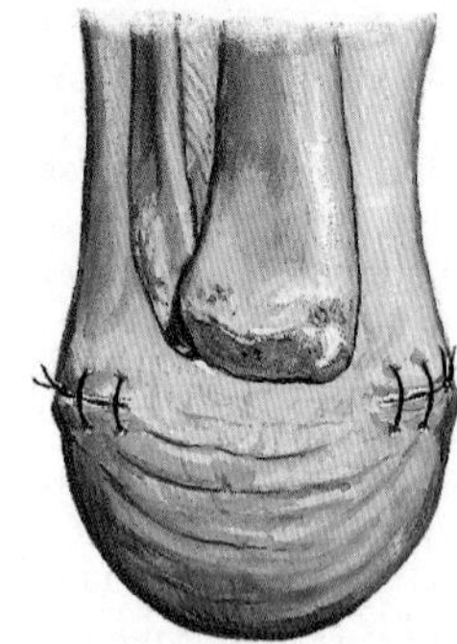

3. Malleoli smoothed and wounds closed.

Amputations in the Foot (Continued)

TRANSMETATARSAL AMPUTATION

One of the most common amputations for forefoot infections in patients with diabetes and for severe forefoot trauma involves removal of the forefoot by transecting the metatarsals to achieve a transmetatarsal amputation. The line of skin incision is positioned more distally on the plantar than on the dorsal aspect of the foot. This approach allows the wound closure to be placed on the dorsum of the foot so that it will not break down with weight-bearing. It also preserves more plantar skin, which is generally better perfused and more durable. The level of metatarsal transaction is determined by the amount of skin available for tension-free closure. The metatarsals are transected in a smooth parabola, with the shaft of the second metatarsal remaining the longest by a few millimeters. In addition, the bones are beveled in a dorsal to plantar direction so that no bone is prominent in the plantar aspect of the foot. The major advantage of this level of amputation is that it preserves enough length to allow the patient to wear a standard shoe using a foam filler in the toe box. Most patients with transmetatarsal amputation are able to walk without a special prosthesis.

CHOPART AMPUTATION

A Chopart amputation is performed at the transverse tarsal articulation through the talonavicular and calcaneocuboid joint. It is not a commonly performed amputation procedure largely because the soft tissues are frequently not adequate for tension-free closure, and a more proximal amputation is required. It is also characterized by a marked tendency for late equinus contracture owing to loss of the ankle dorsiflexors. If this level of amputation is chosen, an Achilles tenotomy and transfer of the anterior compartment tendons to maintain dorsiflexion must be performed as well. Patients with a Chopart amputation require use of an ankle-foot orthosis for ambulation.

SYME AMPUTATION

Syme described a technique for disarticulation of the ankle that preserves the heel pad. This level of amputation preserves most of the leg's length and allows direct weight-bearing on the durable skin of the plantar heel. Wagner popularized performing the Syme amputation in two stages. The first stage disarticulated the ankle but preserved the malleoli. In the second stage, the malleoli were resected to produce a lower profile residual limb that would fit easier in a prosthesis. Today, Syme amputations are usually performed in a single stage. Whether performed in one or two stages, the Syme amputation involves shelling out the talus and calcaneus from the surrounding soft tissues while preserving the heel pad. The pad is then sutured to the tibia to prevent instability. Syme amputation can be successful for the treatment of diabetic complications, gangrene, and trauma. But the heel pad must be healthy and intact for the Syme amputation to be considered. Ulceration or ischemia of the heel pad is an absolute contraindication to Syme amputation.

Section 1 Spine

Bozkus H, Karakas A, Hanci M, Uzan M, Bozdag E, Sarioglu A. Finite element model of the Jefferson fracture: comparison with a cadaver model. Eur Spine J 2001;10(3):257–263.

Broekema AEH et al. Surgical interventions for cervical radiculopathy without myelopathy: a systematic review and meta-analysis. J Bone Joint Surg Am 2020;102:2182–2196.

Bucholz RW, Burkhead WZ. The pathological anatomy of fatal atlanto-occipital dislocations. J Bone Joint Surg Am 1979;61(2):248–250.

Denis F. Spinal instability as defined by the three-column spine concept in acute spinal trauma. Clin Orthop Relat Res 1984;189:65–76.

Goz V, Spiker W, et al. Odontoid fractures: a critical analysis review. J Bone Joint Surg Rev 2019;7(8).

Hsu WK, Anderson PA. Odontoid fractures: update on management. J Am Acad Orthop Surg 2010;18(7):383–394.

Martirosyan NL, Patel AA, Carotenuto A, et al. Genetic alterations in intervertebral disc disease. Front Surg 2016;3:59.

McGrath K, Schmidt E, Rabah N, Abubakr M, Steinmetz M. Clinical assessment and management of Bertolotti syndrome: a review of the literature. Spine J 2021;21(8):1286–1296.

Pryputniewicz DM, Hadley MN. Axis fractures. Neurosurgery 2010;66(3 Suppl):68–82.

Rayes M, Mittal M, Rengachary SS, Mittal S. Hangman's fracture: a historical and biomechanical perspective. J Neurosurg Spine 2011;14(2):198–208.

Sasso RC. C2 dens fractures: treatment options. J Spinal Disord 2001;14(5):455–463.

Section 2 Pelvis, Hip, and Thigh

Edmonds EW, Hughes JL, Bomar JD, Brooks JT, Upasani VV. Ultrasonography in the diagnosis and management of developmental dysplasia of the hip. J Bone Joint Surg Rev 2019; 7(12):1–10.

Foulk DM, Mullis BH. Hip dislocation: evaluation and management. J Am Acad Orthop Surg 2010;18(4):199–209.

Hoaglund FT, Steinbach LS. Primary osteoarthritis of the hip: etiology and epidemiology. J Am Acad Orthop Surg 2001;9(5):320–327.

Kaplan K, Miyamoto R, Levine BR, Egol KA, Zuckerman JD. Surgical management of hip fractures: an evidence-based review of the literature. II: Intertrochanteric fractures. J Am Acad Orthop Surg 2008;16(11):665–673.

Kim HKW. Pathophysiology and new strategies for the treatment of Legg-Calvé-Perthes disease. J Bone Joint Surg Am 2012;94:659–669.

Kuhlman GS, Domb BG. Hip impingement: identifying and treating a common cause of hip pain. Am Fam Physician 2009;80(12): 1429–1434.

Ladenhauf HN, Seitlinger G, Green DW. Osgood-Schlatter disease: a 2020 update of a common knee condition in children. Curr Opin Pediatr (2020); 32:107–112.

Leroux J, Amara SA, Lechevallier J. Legg-Calvé-Perthes disease. Orthop Traumatol Surg Res. 2018;104:S107–S112.

Lindskog DM, Baumgaertner MR. Unstable intertrochanteric hip fractures in the elderly. J Am Acad Orthop Surg 2004;12(3): 179–190.

Lundy D. Subtrochanteric femoral fractures. J Am Acad Orthop Surg 2007;15(11):663–671.

Mathew SE, Larson AN. Natural history of slipped capital femoral epiphysis. J Pediatr Orthop 2019;39:S23–S27.

Miyamoto RG, Kaplan KM, Levine BR, Egol KA, Zuckerman JD. Surgical management of hip fractures: an evidence-based review of the literature. I: femoral neck fractures. J Am Acad Orthop Surg 2008;16(10):596–607.

Murphy RF, Kim YJ. Surgical management of pediatric development dysplasia of the hip. J Am Acad Orthop Surg 2016;24:615–624.

Sierra RJ, Trousdale RT, Ganz R, Leunig M. Hip disease in the young, active patient: evaluation and nonarthroplasty surgical options. J Am Acad Orthop Surg 2008;16(12):689–703.

Sinusas K. Osteoarthritis: diagnosis and treatment. Am Fam Physician 2012;85(1):9–56.

Wylie JD, Novais EN. Evolving understanding of and treatment approaches to slipped capital femoral epiphysis. Curr Rev Musculoskelet Med 2019;12:213–219.

Yang S, Zusman N, Lieberman E, Goldstein RY. Development dysplasia of the hip. Pediatrics 2019;143(1):e20181147.

Section 3 Knee

Fu FH, editor. Master Techniques in Orthopaedic Surgery: Sports Medicine. Lippincott Williams & Wilkins; 2010.

Greene W. Netter's Orthopaedics. Elsevier; 2006.

Hoppenfeld S, deBoer P, Buckley R. Surgical Exposures in Orthopaedics: The Anatomic Approach. Lippincott Williams & Wilkins; 2009.

Hunter RE, Sgaglione NA. AANA Advanced Arthroscopy: The Knee. Elsevier; 2010.

Madden C, Putukian M, McCarty E, Young C. Netter's Sports Medicine. Elsevier; 2009.

Micheli LJ, Kocher M. Micheli & Kocher: The Pediatric and Adolescent Knee. Elsevier; 2006.

Miller MD, Cole BJ, Cosgarea A, Sekiya JK. Operative Techniques: Sports Knee Surgery. Elsevier; 2008.

Noyes FR. Noyes' Knee Disorders: Surgery, Rehabilitation, Clinical Outcomes. 2nd ed. Elsevier; 2016.

Parvizi J, Klatt B. Essentials in Total Knee Arthroplasty. Slack; 2011.

Scott N. Insall & Scott Surgery of the Knee. 6th ed. Elsevier; 2017.

Section 4 Lower Leg

Beaty JH, Kasser JR. Rockwood and Wilkins' Fractures in Children. 6th ed. Lippincott Williams & Wilkins; 2005.

Drake RL, Vogl AW, Mitchell AWM. Gray's Anatomy for Students. Churchill Livingstone; 2009.

Herring JA. Tachdjian's Pediatric Orthopaedics. 4th ed. Elsevier; 2007.

Koval KJ, Zuckerman JD. Handbook of Fractures. 3rd ed. Lippincott Williams & Wilkins; 2006.

Mashru RP, Herman MJ, Pizzutillo PD. Tibial shaft fractures in children and adolescents. J Am Acad Orthop Surg 2005;13:345–352.

Rickert KD, Hosseinzadeh P, Edmonds EW. What's new in pediatric orthopaedic trauma: the lower extremity. J Pediatr Orthop 2018;38:e434–e439.

Section 5 Ankle and Foot

Anderson RB, Hunt KJ, McCormick JJ. Management of common sports-related injuries about the foot and ankle. J Am Acad Orthop Surg 2010;18:546–556.

Coughlin MJ, Mann RA, Saltzman CL. Surgery of the Foot and Ankle. 8th ed. Elsevier; 2007.

Deland JT. Adult acquired flatfoot deformity. J Am Acad Orthop Surg 2008;16:399–406.

Maffulli N, Ferran NA. Management of acute and chronic ankle instability. J Am Acad Orthop Surg 2008;16:608–615.

Manoli A. Posterior tibial tendon insufficiency: diagnosis and treatment. J Am Acad Orthop Surg 1999;12:112–118.

McCormick JJ, Anderson RB. The great toe: failed turf toe, chronic turf toe, and complicated sesamoid injuries. Foot Ankle Clin North Am 2009;14:135–150.

Michaelson JD. Ankle fractures resulting from rotational injuries. J Am Acad Orthop Surg 2003;11:403–412.

Nunley JA, Pfeffer GB, Sanders RW, Trepman E. Advanced Reconstruction: Foot and Ankle. American Academy of Orthopaedic Surgeons; 2004.

INDEX

E

F

M

N

T

U

V

W

Y

Z